Medical Terminology
for Health Professions

4TH EDITION

Ann Ehrlich • Carol L. Schroeder

Delmar
Thomson Learning™

Africa • Australia • Canada • Denmark • Japan • Mexico • New Zealand • Philippines
Puerto Rico • Singapore • Spain • United Kingdom • United States

NOTICE TO THE READER

Delmar Staff:

Health Care Publishing Director: William Brottmiller
Executive Editor: Cathy L. Esperti
Acquisitions Editor: Doris Smith
Development Editor: Deb Flis
Editorial Assistant: Jill Korznat
Executive Marketing Manager: Dawn F. Gerrain
Channel Manager: Tara Carter
Technology Project Manager: Laurie Davis
Executive Production Manager: Karen Leet
Project Editor: Patricia Gillivan
Production Coordinator: Barbara A. Bullock
Art/Design Coordinator: Rich Killar
Cover & Text Design: Charles Cummings Advertising/Art Inc.

COPYRIGHT © 2001
Delmar is a division of Thomson Learning.
The Thomson Learning logo is a registered trademark used herein under license.

Printed in the United States of America
8 9 10 XXX 05 04 03

For more information, contact Delmar, 3 Columbia Circle, PO Box 15015, Albany, NY 12212-0515; or find us on the World Wide Web at http://www.delmar.com

INTERNATIONAL DIVISION LIST

Asia:
Thomson Learning
60 Albert Street, #15-01
Albert Complex
Singapore 189969
Tel: 65 336 6411
Fax: 65 336 7411

Japan:
Thomson Learning
Palaceside Building 5F
1-1-1 Hitotsubashi, Chiyoda-ku
Tokyo 100 0003 Japan
Tel: 813 5218 6544
Fax: 813 5218 6551

Australia/New Zealand:
Nelson/Thomson Learning
102 Dodds Street
South Melbourne, Victoria 3205
Australia
Tel: 61 39 685 4111
Fax: 61 39 685 4199

UK/Europe/Middle East:
Thomson Learning
Berkshire House
168-173 High Holborn
London
WC1V 7AA United Kingdom
Tel: 44 171 497 1422
Fax: 44 171 497 1426

Thomas Nelson & Sons LTD
Nelson House
Mayfield Road
Walton-on-Thames

KT 12 5PL United Kingdom
Tel: 44 1932 2522111
Fax: 44 1932 246574

Latin America:
Thomson Learning
Seneca, 53
Colonia Polanco
11560 Mexico D.F. Mexico
Tel: 525-281-2906
Fax: 525-281-2656

Canada:
Nelson/Thomson Learning
1120 Birchmount Road
Scarborough, Ontario
Canada M1K 5G4
Tel: 416-752-9100
Fax: 416-752-8102

Spain:
Thomson Learning
Calle Magallanes, 25
28015-MADRID
ESPANA
Tel: 34 91 446 33 50
Fax: 34 91 445 62 18

International Headquarters:
Thomson Learning
International Division
290 Harbor Drive, 2nd Floor
Stamford, CT 06902-7477
Tel: 203-969-8700
Fax: 203-969-8751

Library of Congress Cataloging-in-Publication Data
Ehrlich, Ann B. (Ann Beard)
    Medical terminology for health professions / Ann Ehrlich, Carol L. Schroeder.
        p. ; cm
    Includes bibliographical references and index.
    ISBN 0-7668-1297-9 (alk. paper)
    1. Medicine—Terminology--Programmed instruction. I. Schroeder, Carol L. II. Title.
    [DNLM: 1. Terminology--Programmed Instruction. W 18.2 E33m 2000]
R123 .E475 2000
610'.1'4--dc21   00-029757

Contents

Cells

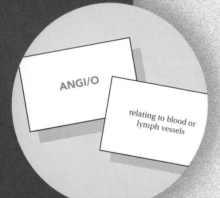

ANGI/O

relating to blood or lymph vessels

Preface

TO THE STUDENT

This is an exciting time to be entering a health care profession. On every level there are almost limitless opportunities to be part of a caring profession, helping people and fully expressing your own special talents and abilities. However, entering a health care field is somewhat like going to live in a foreign country. You can't figure out what's happening until you learn the language.

Here's the good news: learning medical terms is much easier than starting from scratch with a whole new language. In fact, you already know quite a few of the words, such as *appendicitis* and *tonsillectomy*. Even new terms become a lot easier with the discovery that many of them are made up of interchangeable word parts that are used over and over again in different combinations. Once you understand this, you'll be well on your way to "translating" even the toughest medical terms – including terms you have never seen before. You'll be amazed to see how quickly your vocabulary grows!

This text and the accompanying teaching materials make the process as simple as possible. Review the introductory sections – including "How to Use This Book," "How to Use the Student Activity CD-ROM," and the rest of this section – so you can find your way around easily. Once you get comfortable with the materials, you'll find yourself learning faster than you ever imagined possible.

CHAPTER ORGANIZATION

Introductory Chapters

Start your study of medical terminology with **Chapters 1 and 2**. These chapters provide the basics that will help you to master the rest of the book. Chapter 1 introduces key word parts – the building blocks of most medical terms. Chapter 2 introduces more word parts and provides an overview of basic terms used throughout the health field.

After these chapters, complete the **Word Part Review** section that follows Chapter 2. The exercises and test will tell you whether you've mastered the concept of these all-important building blocks.

Body System Chapters

Chapters 3 through 14 are organized according to body systems – one chapter per system. Because each body system stands alone, you can study these chapters in any sequence. Each chapter begins with structures and functions of that system so you can relate these to the specialists, pathology, and diagnostic and treatment procedures that follow.

Chapter 15, **Diagnostic Procedures and Pharmacology** introduces basic diagnostic procedures, imaging procedures and positioning, and pharmacology. This chapter can be studied at any point in the course.

Comprehensive Medical Terminology Review

Located after Chapter 15, this new section helps you prepare for your final examination! It includes study tips, practice exercises, and a simulated final test.

Appendices

Appendix A: Prefixes, Word Roots (Combining Forms), and Suffixes is a handy reference for most medical word parts. When you don't recognize a word part, look it up here.

Appendix B: Abbreviations and Meanings is made up of an extensive list of abbreviations and their commonly accepted meanings. Abbreviations are important in medicine and using them *accurately* is even more important!

Appendix C: Glossary of Pathology and Procedures is a ready reference to quickly find any of the more than 1,500 pathology and procedure terms introduced in the text.

LEARNING SUPPLEMENTS

Flash Cards

Improve your knowledge – and test your mastery – by using the flash cards in the last section of the book. These cards will help you remember many of the more commonly used word parts. Review the suggestions for games and activities using these cards, then carefully remove the pages from the book and separate the cards.

Student Activity CD-ROM

This computer component is an exciting way to gain additional practice in working with medical terms. The exercises and games help you remember even the most difficult terms. See *"How to Use the Student Activity CD-ROM"* for details.

TO THE INSTRUCTOR

From the very first edition, *Medical Terminology for Health Professions* has attempted to break new ground in this complex discipline – by making mastery quick and easy. Now, the fourth edition brings your students fully updated information and more pedagogical tools than ever before.

Also in this edition we welcome Carol L. Schroeder as co-author. Carol brings to the text professional writing skills, superior organizational abilities, and a fresh approach to teaching and learning medical terminology.

GENERAL CHANGES SINCE THE LAST EDITION

This edition continues the emphasis on the **up-to-date language** of the real world of medicine today and includes more than 150 new terms such as *stem cells* and *transesophageal echocardiography*. The other new features are described below. Although changes have been made, you can convert to this new edition quickly and easily by using the Correlation Guide in the Instructor's Manual.

Increased Emphasis on Word Parts

Applying the teaching principal of *"present-use-review"* word parts, their use and meanings are presented in Chapter 1. Word parts are then reviewed and reinforced throughout the text. For additional emphasis, there are word building exercises in the text and on the Student Activity CD-ROM. Different reinforcement and practice modes were designed to accommodate the variety of student learning styles and to maintain student interest.

Vocabulary List

Each chapter begins with a 90 item **vocabulary list**. This includes 15 word parts (for more emphasis) and 75 important terms. This list is conveniently placed on a single page so it can be photocopied for easy reference.

The vocabulary list replaces the audiotape list found in the 3rd edition. Instead of having a separate list, the 60 terms that are on the audiotape and in the Audio Activity on the Student Activity CD-ROM are indicated by an asterisk after the term.

The Human Touch: A Critical Thinking Exercise

At the end of each chapter there is a brief scenario with suggested discussion topics; however, there are no right or wrong answers to these topics. The Human Touch exercises have two important purposes:

- to improve critical thinking skills and stimulate classroom discussion using terms from the chapter
- to encourage students to view each patient as a person, not just a disease

The reviewers were very enthusiastic about this new feature and we think your students will like it too!

Change in the Number of Chapters

To enable the text to fit more effectively in your schedule, it now has **15 chapters**. Nothing has been lost – information from former Chapter 16 has been incorporated elsewhere in the text. Again, the Correlation Guide will help you with these changes.

Comprehensive Medical Terminology Review

The new review section, located after Chapter 15, is an excellent resource for your review sessions in preparation for the final examination. It contains exercises and a practice examination based on information from the entire text.

SPECIAL RESOURCES TO ACCOMPANY THIS TEXT

As with previous editions, special resources help you succeed in teaching *Medical Terminology for Health Professions:*

Audiotapes

Audiotapes containing 60 terms for each chapter are available to accompany this text. In class have students follow the tape by watching for the terms on the vocabulary list that are marked with an asterisk. On the tape these terms are pronounced and defined. The audiotapes can either be packaged with the book for student purchase or sold as a stand-alone item for school purchase that would include duplication rights.

Text/audiotape package, ISBN 0-7668-1298-7
Audiotapes with duplication rights, ISBN 0-7668-1299-5

The Instructor's Manual

Created to meet the challenge of teaching, the Instructor's Manual contains valuable resources for both the experienced and novice instructor:

- A Correlation Guide to help you make the transition from the 3rd to the 4th edition of the text
- Course Planning Tips, including a sample 16-week syllabus and a sample course outline
- Tips for New Teachers that include practical ideas to help new teachers and their students have a successful experience
- Teaching Tools by Chapter that outline resources related to each chapter, including animation and video resources, answer keys for text learning exercises, two 25-question chapter quizzes with answer keys, classroom activities, crossword puzzles, labeling exercises, mid-term and final tests, and a case study to accompany each chapter

Instructor's Guide, ISBN 0-7668-1325-8

Electronic Testbank

By offering 1,600 different questions, 100 for each chapter and the review section, this CD-ROM testbank assists you in creating chapter, midterm, and final examinations.

Features include:

- An interview mode or "wizard" to guide you through the steps to create a test in less than five minutes
- The capability to edit questions or to add an unlimited number of questions
- Online (Internet-based) testing capability
- Online (LAN-based) testing capability
- A sophisticated word processor
- Numerous test layout and printing options
- Link groups of questions to common narratives

Electronic Testbank, ISBN 0-7668-1327-4

Distance Learning Course

A fully developed online course, using this text, is available from Delmar Thomson Learning. This is a great, time-saving way to get your medical terminology online course up and running. The students and teachers who are already using this course are very enthusiastic in their response.

Web Tutor on Web CT is a content-rich, web-based teaching and learning aid that reinforces and clarifies complex concepts in *Medical Terminology for Health Professions, 4th edition.* Web Tutor also includes audio clips, enhanced communication features, customizable instructor tools, and learning links.

To learn more about these exciting new teaching materials, please contact your local Delmar Thomson Learning sales representative or visit our website to complete the online form in the Adopt Web Tutor Section at http://webtutor.delmar.com to set up your personal online course.

Web Tutor and Ehrlich/Medical Terminology for Health Professions, 4e text, ISBN 0-7668-2775-5
Web Tutor, Ehrlich/Medical Terminology for Health Professions, 4e text and audiotapes, ISBN 0-7668-2776-3

Delmar's Medical Terminology CD-ROM Institutional Version

This is an exciting interactive reference, practice, and assessment tool designed to compliment any medical terminology program. Features include the extensive use of multimedia – animations, video, graphics, and activities – to present terms and word building features. Difficult functions, processes, and procedures are included, so learners can more effectively learn from a textbook.

CD-ROM Institutional Version, ISBN 0-7668-0979-X

Delmar's Medical Terminology Video Series

This series of fourteen medical terminology videotapes is designed for allied health and nursing students who are enrolled in medical terminology courses. The videos may be used in class to supplement a lecture or in a resource lab by users who want additional reinforcement. The series can also be used in distance learning programs as a telecourse. The videos simulate a typical medical terminology class, and are organized by body system. The on-cam-

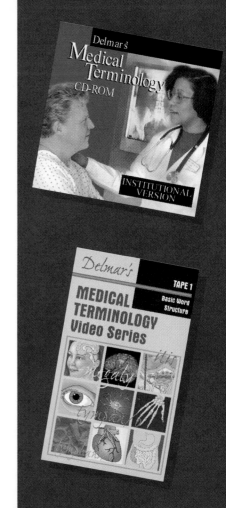

era "instructor" leads students through the various concepts, interspersing lectures with graphics, video clips, and illustrations to emphasize points. This comprehensive series is invaluable to students trying to master the complex world of medical terminology.

Complete Set of Videos, ISBN 0-7668-0976-5
  (Videos can also be purchased individually)

Delmar's Medical Terminology Image Library CD-ROM

This art resource CD-ROM contains 600 graphic files that can be used to enhance your classroom presentations. The CD-ROM is organized by body system and medical specialty areas and includes over 600 word building anatomy, physiology, and pathology illustrations and photographs to enhance learning.

CD-ROM, ISBN 0-7668-0492-5

Delmar's Audiotape Set for Medical Terminology

This audiotape set is an ideal enhancement to any Medical Terminology program or library. These eight, 90-minute audiotapes include the term, word parts, definition of the word parts and term, examples of terms used in context, and then the word pronounced again. Not only will users hear the term to understand correct pronunciation; they will also hear the word parts. The audiotape set is a great reinforcement that can be used in conjunction with any medical terminology book.

Audiotapes Including Duplication Rights, ISBN 0-7668-0491-7

VALUE PACKAGES

You can order the following innovative Delmar products separately – or package them with *Medical Terminology for Health Professions, 4th edition,* in a convenient and affordable value package:

Text & Audiotapes Value Package

With these two 90-minute audiotapes, students learn to pronounce the most difficult medical terms and learn their definitions. The tapes include 60 difficult terms from each chapter; terms marked with an asterisk in the vocabulary list in the text allow students to track their progress. (This value package does not include audiotape duplication rights.)

Text & Audiotapes Value Package, ISBN 0-7668-1298-7

Text & Delmar's Medical Terminology CD-ROM Individual Version Value Package

This is an exciting interactive reference, practice, and assessment tool designed to compliment any medical terminology program. Features include the extensive use of multimedia – animations, video, graphics, and activities – to present terms and word building features. Difficult functions, processes, and procedures are included, so learners can more effectively learn from a textbook.

Text/CD-ROM Individual Version, ISBN 0-7668-7876-7

Acknowledgments

Special thanks to Don Jacobsen for his help in "pronouncing" the terms in this text. Thanks also to the editorial and production staff of Delmar Thomson Learning for their professional, yet personalized, assistance throughout the planning and production processes.

We are particularly grateful to the reviewers who continue to be a valuable resource in guiding this book as it evolves. Their insights, comments, suggestions, and attention to detail were very important in making certain that this book is "on target" for health careers students.

Ann Ehrlich
Carol L. Schroeder

Reviewers

K. Magdalena Andrasevits, AS, BA, Paralegal, NR-CMA
Sanford-Brown College
Kansas City, Missouri

Adrienne L. Carter-Ward, BA, CMA, NRMA
Skadron College, Csi
San Bernardino, California

Kelli Cochran, CAM, EMT-B
Thompson Institute
Philadelphia, Pennsylvania

Patricia Coulson Shivers, PhD, BCLD
Pellissippi State Technical Community College
Knoxville, Tennessee

Marguerite Cummins, MLT, CMA
Thompson Institute
Philadelphia, Pennsylvania

Pamela A. Eugene, LRT
Delgado Community College
New Orleans, Louisiana

Rebecca L. Gibson, MSTE, CMA, ASPT
Community and Technical College
The University of Akron
Akron, Ohio

Susan R. Royce, MS
Maric College
San Diego, California

Lois M. Smith, RN, CMA
Arapahoe Community College
Golden, Colorado

Sylvia Nobles, CRNP, MSN
Trenholm State Technical College
Montgomery, Alabama

Karen Snipe, CPht, AS, BA
Trident Technical College
Charleston, South Carolina

Crystal D. Wilson, CMA
Central Pennsylvania Business School
Summerdale, Pennsylvania

How to Use This Book

Medical Terminology for Health Professions, 4th Edition, helps you learn and remember medical terms with surprising ease. The key lies in the following features.

1 Body System Overview

For handy reference, the first page of each body system chapter includes a chart giving a brief overview of the major structures, related word roots, and primary functions most important to that system.

2 Vocabulary List

New to this edition! The second page of each chapter is a 90-term vocabulary list. Each list includes 15 key word parts and 75 key medical terms for the chapter. This immediately alerts you to the key terms in the chapter and acts as a review guide. Next to each term is a box so you can check off each term as you learn. This list includes the 60 terms pronounced on the Student Activity CD-ROM, which is included with the book, as well as on the optional audiotape.

3 Learning Objectives

The beginning of each chapter lists learning objectives to help you understand what is expected of you as you read the text and complete the exercises. These objectives are set off with a colored bar for easy identification.

4 Illustrations

Complete with detailed labeling, the book's full color illustrations help clarify the text – and contain important information of their own. Review each illustration carefully for easy and effective learning.

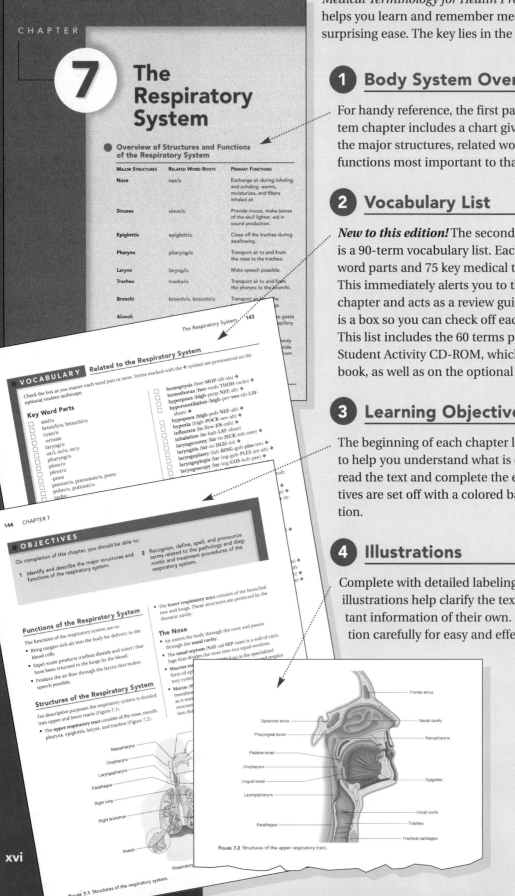

xvi

5 New Terms

Each new term appears in easy-to-spot **bold type**, with the definition following. Even confusing words within a definition are boldfaced and defined.

6 "Sounds Like" Pronunciation System

The "sounds like" pronunciation system makes pronunciation easy by respelling the word with syllables you can understand – and say – at a glance. Simply pronounce the term just as it appears in parentheses, accenting the syllables as follows:

- **Primary** (strongest) **accent**: capital letters and bold type
- **Secondary accent**: lower case letters and bold type

7 Word Parts

Because word parts are such an important part of learning medical terminology, whenever a term made up of word parts is introduced, the definition follows (in parentheses) by the word parts highlighted in red and defined.

8 Learning Exercises

At the end of each chapter are 100 exercises to help you interact with, and review the information in the chapter. The exercises use several formats to provide variety and interest: matching, multiple choice, word building, spellcheck, true/false, labeling, and exercises that require you to write in definitions or missing words. Your instructor has the answers to these exercises in the accompanying Instructor's Guide.

9 The Human Touch: Critical Thinking Exercise

New to this edition! A "real-life" mini story at the end of each chapter that involves patients and pathology helps you practice critical thinking skills, and encourages you to view each patient as a person. These mini stories are a fun classroom activity for discussion of the hot issues in medical care today. There are no right or wrong answers, just questions to get you started using the new terms you have learned.

- **Cilia** (SIL-ee-ah), the thin hairs located just inside the nostrils, filter incoming air to remove debris.
- The **olfactory receptors** (ol-FACK-toh-ree), the receptors for the sense of smell are nerve endings located in the mucous membrane in the upper part of the nasal cavity.

The Tonsils

- The **tonsils**, which have an important function in protecting the body from invading organisms, form a protective circle around the entrance to the respiratory system. Tonsils, which are a type of lymphatic tissue, are discussed in Chapter 6.

The Sinuses

- A **sinus** is an air-filled cavity within a bone that is lined with mucous membrane.
- The functions of sinuses are (1) to make the bones of the skull lighter, (2) to help produce sound by giving resonance to the voice, and (3) to produce mucus that drains into the nasal cavity.
- The **paranasal sinuses** are located in the bones of the skull (para means near, nas means nose, and al means

pertaining to). Shor nasal cavity.

- The sinuses are nam located. The parana Table 7.1.

Table 7.1

PARANASAL SIN

Maxillary sinuses (MACK-sih-ler-ee), located in the maxil bones, are the large the paranasal sinuse

The **ethmoid sinuse** (ETH-moid), locatec the ethmoid bones, irregularly shaped a cells, separated from orbital (eye) cavity c by a thin layer of bo

---

Learning Exercises   CHAPTER **7**

Matching Word Parts—1
Write the letter of the correct answer on the line provided in the left column.

7.1. _____ atel/o

7.2. _____ bronch/o, bronchi/o

7.3. _____ cyan/o

7.4. _____ -ectasis

7.5. _____ laryng/o

A. stretching, dilation, enlargement
B. voice box
C. bronchial tube
D. blue
E. incomplete

7.8. _____ phon/o

7.9. _____ pleur/o

7.10. _____ pneum/o, pneu-

C. multilayered membrane
D. throat
E. voice

Matching Word Parts—3
Write the letter of the correct answer on the line provided in the left column.

7.11. _____ -pnea

7.12. _____ pulmon/o

7.13. _____ tachy-

7.14. _____ thorac/o, -thorax

A. windpipe
B. rapid
C. lung
D. chest or thorax

Matching Word Parts—2
Write the letter of the correct answer on the line provided in the left column.

7.6. _____ ox/i, ox/o, ox/y   A. lung, air

7.7. _____ p

The Human Touch: Critical Thinking Exercise

The following story and questions are designed to stimulate critical thinking through class discussion or as a brief essay response. There are no easy or right-wrong answers to these questions.

Sylvia Gaylord works as a legal aid on the 12th floor of an 18-story glass and steel monument to modern architectural technology in the center of the city. On clear days the views are spectacular. From her cubicle, Sylvia's eye catches the edge of a beautiful blue and white skyscape as she reaches for her medi-haler. This is the third attack since she returned from lunch 4 hours ago — her asthma is really bad today. But if she leaves work early again her boss will write her up. Sylvia concentrates on breathing normally.

Her roommate Kelly is a respiratory therapist at the city's county hospital. Kelly says Sylvia's asthma attacks are probably triggered by the city's high level of air pollution. That can't be true. They both run in the park every morning before work, and Sylvia rarely needs to use her inhaler. The problems start when she gets to work. The wheezing and coughing were so bad today that by the time she got up the elevator and into her cubicle she could hardly breathe.

Last night the cable news ran a story on the unhealthy air found in some buildings. They called it "sick building syndrome" and reported that certain employees developed allergic reactions just by breathing the air. "Hmmm," she thought. "It seems like more and more people are getting sick in our office. John has had the flu twice. Sid's bronchitis turned into bronchopneumonia and Nging complains of sinusitis. Could this building have an air quality problem?"

Suggested Discussion Topics:

1. Discuss which environmental factors might cause an asthma attack.
2. Discuss what Sylvia might do to find out if her building has an air quality problem.
3. Use proper medical terminology to describe what happens to Sylvia's airways during an asthma attack and how medications affect the symptoms.
4. Asthmatic medications, similar to Sylvia's inhaler, are easily available in drugstores without a prescription. Discuss the pros and cons of this practice.
5. If Sylvia's inhaler does not control her attack and her condition worsens, what steps should be taken promptly? Why?

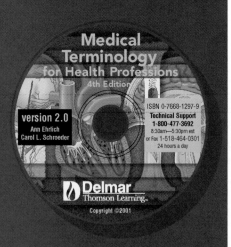

How to Use The Student Activity CD-ROM

The Student Activity CD-ROM was designed as an exciting enhancement to *Medical Terminology for Health Professions, 4th edition* to help you learn difficult medical terms. As you study each chapter in the text, be sure to explore the corresponding unit on the CD-ROM.

Each chapter is divided into two major sections: exercises and fun and games. Exercises can be used for additional practice, review, or self-testing. Fun and games provide an opportunity to play and practice through a variety of activities.

Getting started is easy. Follow the simple directions on the CD label to install the program on your computer. Then take advantage of the following features:

❶ Main Menu

The main menu follows the chapter organization of the text exactly—which makes it easy for you to find your way around. Just click on the button for the chapter you want, and you'll come to the chapter opening screen.

Toolbar

The Back button at the top left of every screen allows you to retrace your steps, while the Exit button gets you out of the program quickly and easily. As you navigate through the software, check the toolbar for other features that help you use individual exercises or games.

Online Help

If you get stuck, just press F1 to get help. The online help includes instructions for all parts of the Student Activity CD-ROM.

❷ The Chapter Screen

Here you have the opportunity to choose how you want to learn. Select one of the exercises for additional practice, review, or self-testing. Or click on a game to practice the terms for that chapter in a fun format.

③ Exercises

The Student Activity CD-ROM acts as your own private tutor. For each exercise, it chooses from a bank of over 800 questions covering all 15 chapters and the Medical Terminology Review. Putting these exercises to work for you is simple:

- Choose a multiple choice, fill-in-the-blank, or labeling exercise, whichever one appeals to you.

- You'll encounter a series of 10 questions for each exercise format; each question gives you two chances to answer correctly.

- Instant feedback tells you whether you're right or wrong —and helps you learn more quickly by explaining why an answer was correct or incorrect.

- The Student Activity CD-ROM displays the percentage of correct answers on the chapter screen. An on-screen score sheet (which you can print) lets you track correct and incorrect answers.

- Review your previous questions and answers in an exercise for more in-depth understanding. Or start an exercise over with a new, random set of questions that gives you a realistic study environment.

- When you're ready for an additional challenge, try the timed Speed Test. Once you've finished, it displays your score and the time you took to complete the test, so you can see how much you've learned.

④ Fun & Games

To have fun while reinforcing your knowledge, enjoy each of the six simple games on this disk. You can play alone, with a partner, or on teams.

- **Concentration:** match terms to their corresponding definitions under the cards as the seconds tick by.

- **Hangman:** review your spelling and vocabulary by choosing the correct letters to spell medical terms before you're "hanged."

- **Crossword Puzzles:** using the definition clues provided, fill in the medical terms to complete each puzzle. A click of the Check button highlights incorrect answers in blue.

- **Medical Terminology Championship Game:** challenge your classmates and increase your knowledge by playing this Jeopardy style question-and-answer game.

- **Listening Activity:** Select medical terms and listen to them to master the pronunciation.

- **Drag & Drop:** Both word building and art labeling exercises are included to help you learn in an interactive environment.

Introduction to Medical Terminology

● Overview of Introduction to Medical Terminology

Word Parts Are the Key!	Introduction to word parts and how they create complex medical terms.
Word Roots (combining forms)	The word parts that usually indicate the part of the body involved.
Suffixes	The word parts that usually indicate the procedure, condition, disorder, or disease.
Prefixes	The word parts that usually indicate location, time, number, or status.
Determining Meanings Based on Word Parts	Use knowledge of word parts to decipher medical terms.
Medical Dictionary Use	Guidelines to make the use of a medical dictionary easier.
Pronunciation	Learn the easy-to-use "Sounds Like" pronunciation system.
Spelling Is Always Important	Discover how one wrong letter can change the entire meaning of a term!
Using Abbreviations	Caution is important when using abbreviations.
Singular and Plural Endings	Unusual singular and plural endings used in medical terms.
Basic Medical Terms	The terms used to describe disease conditions.
Look-Alike Sound-Alike Terms and Word Parts	Clarify confusing terms that look or sound alike.

VOCABULARY   Related to Medical Terminology

Check the box as you master each word part or term. Terms marked with the ❖ symbol are pronounced on the optional student audiotape.

Key Word Parts

- ☐ -algia
- ☐ dys-
- ☐ -ectomy
- ☐ hyper-
- ☐ hypo-
- ☐ -itis
- ☐ -osis
- ☐ -ostomy
- ☐ -otomy
- ☐ -plasty
- ☐ -rrhage
- ☐ -rrhaphy
- ☐ -rrhea
- ☐ -rrhexis
- ☐ -sclerosis

Key Medical Terms

- ☐ abdominocentesis (ab-**dom**-ih-noh-sen-**TEE**-sis) ❖
- ☐ acronym (**ACK**-roh-nim) ❖
- ☐ appendectomy (**ap**-en-**DECK**-toh-mee) ❖
- ☐ appendicitis (ah-**pen**-dih-**SIGH**-tis)
- ☐ arteriogram (ar-**TEER**-ee-oh-gram)
- ☐ arteriography (**ar**-tee-ree-**OG**-rah-fee) ❖
- ☐ arterionecrosis (ar-**tee**-ree-oh-neh-**KROH**-sis)
- ☐ arteriosclerosis (ar-**tee**-ree-oh-skleh-**ROH**-sis)
- ☐ arthralgia (ar-**THRAL**-jee-ah) ❖
- ☐ atheroma (**ath**-er-**OH**-mah)
- ☐ cardiac (**KAR**-dee-ack)
- ☐ colostomy (koh-**LAHS**-toh-mee) ❖
- ☐ colotomy (koh-**LOT**-oh-mee) ❖
- ☐ diagnosis (**dye**-ag-**NOH**-sis) ❖
- ☐ diarrhea (**dye**-ah-**REE**-ah) ❖
- ☐ edema (eh-**DEE**-mah) ❖
- ☐ endarterial (**end**-ar-**TEE**-ree-al) ❖
- ☐ endoscopy (en-**DOS**-koh-pee) ❖
- ☐ eponym (**EP**-oh-nim) ❖
- ☐ erythrocytes (eh-**RITH**-roh-sights)
- ☐ gastralgia (gas-**TRAL**-jee-ah)
- ☐ gastroenteritis (**gas**-troh-en-ter-**EYE**-tis) ❖
- ☐ gastrosis (gas-**TROH**-sis)
- ☐ gerontologist (**jer**-on-**TOL**-oh-jist) ❖
- ☐ hemorrhage (**HEM**-or-idj) ❖
- ☐ hepatomegaly (**hep**-ah-toh-**MEG**-ah-lee) ❖
- ☐ hypertension (**high**-per-**TEN**-shun)
- ☐ hypotension (**high**-poh-**TEN**-shun)

- ☐ ileum (**ILL**-ee-um) ❖
- ☐ ilium (**ILL**-ee-um) ❖
- ☐ infection (in-**FECK**-shun) ❖
- ☐ inflammation (in-flah-**MAY**-shun) ❖
- ☐ interstitial (**in**-ter-**STISH**-al) ❖
- ☐ intramuscular (**in**-trah-**MUS**-kyou-lar) ❖
- ☐ laceration (**lass**-er-**AY**-shun) ❖
- ☐ lesion (**LEE**-zhun) ❖
- ☐ leukocytes (**LOO**-koh-sights)
- ☐ ligation (lye-**GAY**-shun) ❖
- ☐ lithotomy (lih-**THOT**-oh-mee) ❖
- ☐ melanosis (**mel**-ah-**NOH**-sis) ❖
- ☐ mycosis (my-**KOH**-sis) ❖
- ☐ myelopathy (my-eh-**LOP**-ah-thee) ❖
- ☐ myopathy (my-**OP**-ah-thee) ❖
- ☐ myorrhaphy (my-**OR**-ah-fee)
- ☐ myorrhexis (**my**-oh-**RECK**-sis)
- ☐ neonatology (**nee**-oh-nay-**TOL**-oh-jee) ❖
- ☐ neuritis (new-**RYE**-tis) ❖
- ☐ neuroplasty (**NEW**-roh-**plas**-tee) ❖
- ☐ otolaryngology (**oh**-toh-**lar**-in-**GOL**-oh-jee) ❖
- ☐ otorhinolaryngology (oh-toh-**rye**-noh-**lar**-in-**GOL**-oh-jee) ❖
- ☐ palpation (pal-**PAY**-shun) ❖
- ☐ palpitation (**pal**-pih-**TAY**-shun) ❖
- ☐ perinatal (**pehr**-ih-**NAY**-tal) ❖
- ☐ poliomyelitis (**poh**-lee-oh-**my**-eh-**LYE**-tis) ❖
- ☐ postnatal (pohst-**NAY**-tal) ❖
- ☐ prenatal (pre-**NAY**-tal) ❖
- ☐ prognosis (prog-**NOH**-sis) ❖
- ☐ prostate (**PROS**-tayt) ❖
- ☐ prostrate (**PROS**-trayt) ❖
- ☐ pyelitis (**pye**-eh-**LYE**-tis) ❖
- ☐ pyoderma (**pye**-oh-**DER**-mah) ❖
- ☐ pyrosis (pye-**ROH**-sis) ❖
- ☐ subcostal (sub-**KOS**-tal) ❖
- ☐ supination (**soo**-pih-**NAY**-shun) ❖
- ☐ suppuration (**sup**-you-**RAY**-shun) ❖
- ☐ supracostal (**sue**-prah-**KOS**-tal) ❖
- ☐ suturing (**SOO**-chur-ing) ❖
- ☐ symptom (**SIMP**-tum) ❖
- ☐ syndrome (**SIN**-drohm) ❖
- ☐ tonsillectomy (**ton**-sih-**LECK**-toh-mee) ❖
- ☐ tonsillitis (**ton**-sih-**LYE**-tis)
- ☐ trauma (**TRAW**-mah) ❖
- ☐ triage (tree-**AHZH**) ❖
- ☐ viral (**VYE**-ral) ❖
- ☐ virile (**VIR**-ill) ❖

Word Parts Are the Key!

Learning medical terminology is much easier once you understand how word parts work together to form medical terms. This book includes many aids to help you master this skill.

- The types of word parts and the rules for their use are explained in this chapter. Learn these rules and follow them!

- To continue reinforcing your word building skills, each time a term made up of word parts is introduced the definition is followed, in parentheses, by the word parts in red with their meanings.

- After Chapter 2 there is a Word Part Review section. This provides additional word part practice and allows you to evaluate your progress toward mastering the meanings of these word parts.

- The Learning Exercises for each chapter include a "Challenge Word Building" section. These will help you develop your skills in working with word parts.

The Three Types of Word Parts

Three types of word parts may be used to create medical terms. Guidelines for their use are shown in Table 1.1.

- **Word roots**, also known as **combining forms**, contain the basic meaning of the term. They usually, *but not always*, indicate the involved body part.

- **Suffixes** usually, *but not always*, indicate the procedure, condition, disorder, or disease. A suffix always comes at the end of a word.

- **Prefixes** usually, *but not always*, indicate location, time, number, or status. A prefix always comes at the beginning of a word.

Table 1.1

WORD PART GUIDELINES

1. A single word root (combining form) part cannot stand alone. A suffix must be added to complete the term.

2. The rules for the use of combining vowels apply when adding a suffix. These rules are explained in Table 1.3.

3. When a prefix is necessary, it is always placed at the beginning of the word.

Word Roots (Combining Forms)

Word roots, also known as **combining forms**, act as the foundation of most medical terms. They usually, but not always, describe the part of the body that is involved (Figure 1.1). Some word roots indicate color and these are shown in Table 1.2.

Combining Vowels

To make the medical term easier to pronounce, a combining vowel may be needed between the word root and suffix. The rules for using combining vowels are explained in Table 1.3.

- The letter *O* is the most commonly used combining vowel.

- When a word root is shown with a back slash and a combining vowel, such as **cardi/o**, this is referred to as a **combining form** (**cardi/o** means heart).

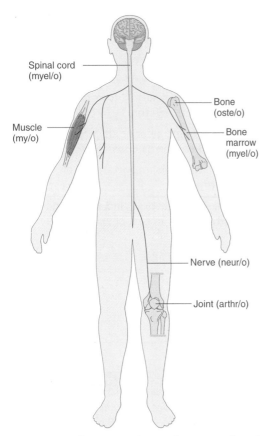

Spinal cord
(myel/o)

Muscle
(my/o)

Bone
(oste/o)

Bone
marrow
(myel/o)

Nerve (neur/o)

Joint (arthr/o)

FIGURE 1.1 A word root (combining form) usually indicates the involved body part.

Table 1.2

WORD ROOTS INDICATING COLOR

cyan/o means blue	**Cyanosis** (**sigh**-ah-**NOH**-sis) is a a blue discoloration of the skin caused by a lack of adequate oxygen (**cyan** means blue and **osis** means condition).
erythr/o means red	**Erythrocytes** (eh-**RITH**-roh-sights) are mature red blood cells (**erythro** means red and **cytes** means cells).
leuk/o means white	**Leukocytes** (**LOO**-koh-sights) are white blood cells (**leuko** means white and **cytes** means cells).
melan/o means black	**Melanosis** (**mel**-ah-**NOH**-sis) is any condition of unusual deposits of black pigment in different parts of the body (**melan** means black and **osis** means condition).
poli/o means gray	**Poliomyelitis** (**poh**-lee-oh-**my**-eh-**LYE**-tis) is a viral infection of the gray matter of the spinal cord that may result in paralysis (**polio** means gray, **myel** means spinal cord, and **itis** means inflammation).

Table 1.3

RULES FOR USING COMBINING VOWELS

1. A combining vowel *is not used* when the suffix begins with a vowel (a-e-i-o-u).

   For example, when **neur/o** (nerve) is joined with the suffix **-itis** (inflammation), the combining vowel is *not used* because **-itis** begins with a vowel.

   Neuritis (new-**RYE**-tis) is an inflammation of a nerve or nerves (**neur** means nerve and **itis** means inflammation).

2. A combining vowel *is used* when the suffix begins with a consonant.

   For example, when **neur/o** (nerve) is joined with the suffix **-plasty** (surgical repair) the combining vowel O *is used* because **-plasty** begins with a consonant.

   Neuroplasty (**NEW**-roh-**plas**-tee) is the surgical repair of a nerve (**neuro** means nerve and **plasty** means surgical repair).

3. A combining vowel *is always used* when two or more root words are joined.

   As an example, when **gastr/o** (stomach) is joined with **enter/o** (small intestine) the combining vowel *is used* with **gastr/o**; however, when the suffix **-itis** (inflammation) is added, the combining vowel is *not used* with **enter/o** because **-itis** begins with a vowel.

   Gastroenteritis (gas-troh-en-ter-**EYE**-tis) is an inflammation of the stomach and small intestine (**gastro** means stomach, **enter** means small intestine, and **itis** means inflammation).

4. A prefix does not require a combining vowel. Do not place a combining vowel between a prefix and the word root.

Commonly Used Word Roots (Combining Forms)

Because word roots (combining forms) describe body parts, most of them are specific to body systems.

- Many of these combining forms are introduced in this chapter and in Chapter 2.
- Learning these word roots *now* will make your study of the other chapters much easier!

Suffixes

A suffix is added to the end of a word root to complete the term. Suffixes usually, but not always, indicate the procedure, condition, disorder, or disease (Figure 1.2).

- For example, **tonsill/o** means tonsils. A suffix is added to complete the term and tell what is happening to the tonsils.
- **Tonsillitis** (**ton**-sih-**LYE**-tis) is an inflammation of the tonsils (**tonsill** means tonsils and **itis** means inflammation).
- A **tonsillectomy** (**ton**-sih-**LECK**-toh-mee) is the surgical removal of the tonsils (**tonsill** means tonsils and **ectomy** means surgical removal).

Suffixes Meaning "Pertaining To"

- Some suffixes complete the term by changing the word root into an **adjective** (a word that describes a noun).
- As an example, **cardiac** (**KAR**-dee-ack) means pertaining to the heart (**cardi** means heart and **ac** means pertaining to).
- Many of these suffixes are defined as "pertaining to." To make such suffixes easy to find, they are listed together in a table at the beginning of Appendix A.

Suffixes as Noun Endings

- Some suffixes complete the term by changing the word root into a **noun** (a word that is the name of a person, place, or thing).
- As an example, the **cranium** (**KRAY**-nee-um) is the portion of the skull that encloses the brain (**crani** means skull and **um** is a noun ending).

- Other suffixes in this group are defined as *noun endings*. These suffixes also are listed in a table at the beginning of Appendix A.

Suffixes Meaning "Abnormal Condition"

- Some suffixes have a general meaning of "abnormal condition or disease."
- As an example, **-osis** means an abnormal condition or disease. **Gastrosis** (gas-**TROH**-sis) means any disease of the stomach (**gastr** means stomach and **osis** means abnormal condition).
- These suffixes are also listed in a table at the beginning of Appendix A.

Suffixes Related to Pathology

Pathology means the study of disease and these suffixes describe specific disease conditions.

- **-algia** means pain and suffering. **Gastralgia** (gas-**TRAL**-jee-ah) means pain in the stomach (**gastr** means stomach and **algia** means pain).
- **-dynia** also means pain. **Gastrodynia** (**gas**-troh-**DIN**-ee-ah) also means pain in the stomach (**gastro** means stomach and **dynia** means pain).
- **-itis** means inflammation. **Gastritis** (gas-**TRY**-tis) is an inflammation of the stomach (**gastr** means stomach and **itis** means inflammation).
- **-malacia** means abnormal softening. **Arteriomalacia** (ar-**tee**-ree-oh-mah-**LAY**-shee-ah) is the abnormal softening of the walls of an artery or arteries (**arterio** means artery and **malacia** means abnormal softening. Notice that **-malacia** is the opposite of **-sclerosis**).
- **-megaly** means enlargement. **Hepatomegaly** (**hep**-ah-toh-**MEG**-ah-lee) is abnormal enlargement of the liver (**hepato** means liver and **megaly** means enlargement).
- **-necrosis** means tissue death. **Arterionecrosis** (ar-**tee**-ree-oh-neh-**KROH**-sis) means the tissue death of an artery or arteries (**arterio** means artery and **necrosis** means tissue death).
- **-sclerosis** means abnormal hardening. **Arteriosclerosis** (ar-**tee**-ree-oh-skleh-**ROH**-sis) is the abnormal hardening of the walls of an artery or arteries (**arterio** means

TONSILL/O (tonsil, tonsils) + -ITIS (inflammation) = TONSILLITIS (inflammation of the tonsils)

FIGURE 1.2 A word root (combining form) plus a suffix creates a new term.

artery and **sclerosis** means abnormal hardening. Notice that **-sclerosis** is the opposite of **-malacia**).

- **-stenosis** means abnormal narrowing. **Arteriostenosis** (ar-**tee**-ree-oh-steh-**NOH**-sis) is the abnormal narrowing of an artery or arteries (**arterio** means artery and **stenosis** means abnormal narrowing.)

Suffixes Related to Procedures

These suffixes identify a procedure that is performed on the body part identified by the word root.

- **-centesis** is a surgical puncture to remove fluid for diagnostic purposes or to remove excess fluid. **Abdominocentesis** (ab-**dom**-ih-noh-sen-**TEE**-sis) is the surgical puncture of the abdominal cavity to remove fluid (**abdomino** means abdomen and **centesis** means a surgical puncture to removal fluid).

- **-ectomy** means surgical removal. An **appendectomy** (**ap**-en-**DECK**-toh-mee) is the surgical removal of the appendix (**append** mean appendix and **ectomy** means surgical removal).

- **-graphy** means the process of recording a picture or record. **Arteriography** (**ar**-tee-ree-**OG**-rah-fee) is the process of recording a picture of an artery or arteries (**arterio** means artery and **graphy** means to record).

- **-gram** means record or picture. An **arteriogram** (ar-**TEER**-ee-oh-gram) is the record produced by arteriography (**arterio** means artery and **gram** means record).

- **-plasty** means surgical repair. **Myoplasty** (**MY**-oh-**plas**-tee) is the surgical repair of a muscle (**myo** means muscle and **plasty** means surgical repair).

- **-scopy** means visual examination. **Endoscopy** (en-**DOS**-koh-pee) is the visual examination of the interior of a body cavity or organ by means of an endoscope (**endo** means within and **scopy** means visual examination).

The Double RRs

These suffixes, which are often referred to as the "double RRs," are particularly confusing. They are grouped together here to help you understand the word parts and to remember the differences.

- **-rrhage** and **–rrhagia** mean bursting forth, an abnormal excessive fluid discharge or bleeding. **Hemorrhage** (**HEM**-or-idj) means the loss of a large amount of blood in a short time (**hemo** means blood and **rrhage** means bursting forth). *Note:* **-rrhage** and **-rrhagia** refer to the flow of blood.

- **-rrhaphy** means to suture or stitch. **Myorrhaphy** (my-**OR**-ah-fee) means to suture a muscle wound (**myo** means muscle and **rrhaphy** means to suture). As an aid to remembering this suffix, think of r-r-wrap as if you were going to wrap the injury in sutures.

- **-rrhea** means an abnormal flow or discharge and refers to the abnormal flow of most body fluids. **Diarrhea** (**dye**-ah-**REE**-ah) is abnormally frequent loose or watery stools (**dia** means through and **rrhea** means abnormal flow). *Note:* Although **-rrhea** and **-rrhage** both describe an abnormal flow, they are *not* used interchangeably.

- **-rrhexis** means rupture. **Myorrhexis** (**my**-oh-**RECK**-sis) means the rupture of a muscle (**myo** means muscle and **rrhexis** means rupture). As an aid to remembering this suffix, think of the *X* being ready to rupture and fly apart.

Prefixes

A prefix is added to the beginning of a word to change the meaning of that term (Figure 1.3). Prefixes usually, but not always, indicate location, time, or number. The term **natal** (**NAY**-tal) means pertaining to birth (**nat** means birth, and **al** means pertaining to). The following examples show how a prefix changes the meaning of this term.

- **Prenatal** (pre-**NAY**-tal) means the time and events before birth (**pre** means before, **nat** means birth, and **al** means pertaining to) (Figure 1.4).

- **Perinatal** (**pehr**-ih-**NAY**-tal) refers to the time and events surrounding birth (**peri** means surrounding, **nat** means birth, and **al** means pertaining to). This is the time just before, during, and just after birth (Figure 1.5).

- **Postnatal** (pohst-**NAY**-tal) means the time and events after birth (**post** means after, **nat** means birth, and **al** means pertaining to) (Figure 1.6).

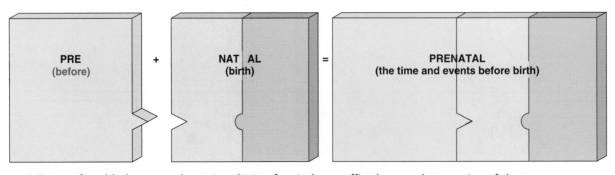

| PRE (before) | + | NAT AL (birth) | = | PRENATAL (the time and events before birth) |

FIGURE 1.3 A prefix added to a word root (combining form) plus a suffix changes the meaning of the term.

FIGURE 1.4 The term *prenatal* refers to the events that occur before birth. Shown here is a diagram of the developing child in the uterus before birth.

Uterus
Umbilical cord
Fetus

FIGURE 1.5 The term *perinatal* refers to the time and events around birth. Shown here is a fetal monitor in use during labor (*Photo courtesy of Memorial Medical Center of Long Beach, CA*)

FIGURE 1.6 The term *postnatal* refers to the time and events after birth. Shown here is a newborn in a neonatal intensive care unit. (*Photo courtesy of Memorial Medical Center of Long Beach, CA*)

Contrasting and Confusing Prefixes

Some prefixes are confusing because they are similar in spelling but opposite in meaning. The more common prefixes of this type are summarized in Table 1.4.

Determining Meanings Based on Word Parts

When you know the meaning of the word parts, it is often possible to figure out the definition of an unfamiliar medical term.

Taking Terms Apart

To determine a word's meaning by looking at the component pieces, you must first separate it into word parts.

- Most people like to start at the end of the word and work toward the beginning.
- Others like to start at the beginning of a word and work toward the end.
- Try it both ways. Then use the system that works best for you.

As an Example

Look at the term **otorhinolaryngology.** It is made up of three combining forms plus a suffix (Figure 1.7).

- The word root **ot/o** means ear. The combining vowel *is used* because **ot/o** is joining another word root.
- The word root **rhin/o** means nose. The combining vowel *is used* because **rhin/o** is joining another word root.
- The word root **laryng/o** means larynx and throat. The combining vowel *is not used* because **laryng/o** is joining a suffix that begins with a vowel.
- The suffix **-ology** means the study of.
- Together they form **otorhinolaryngology** (**oh**-toh-**rye**-noh-**lar**-in-**GOL**-oh-jee), which is the study of the ears, nose, and throat (**oto** means ear, **rhino** means nose, **laryng** means throat, and **ology** means study of).
- Because this is such a long name, this specialty is frequently referred to as **ENT** (ears, nose, throat) or shortened to **otolaryngology** (**oh**-toh-**lar**-in-**GOL**-oh-jee).

Medical Dictionary Use

Learning to use a medical dictionary is an important part of mastering the correct use of medical terms. The following tips for dictionary use apply whether you are working with a traditional book form dictionary or an electronic dictionary on your computer.

Guessing at Meanings

When you are able to "guess" at the meaning of a term based on the word parts that make it up you must always double check for accuracy — because some terms have

Table 1.4

CONTRASTING AND CONFUSING PREFIXES

ab- means away from.	**ad-** means toward or in the direction of.
Abnormal means not normal or away from normal.	**Addiction** means drawn toward or a strong dependence on a drug or substance.
dys- means bad, difficult, painful.	**eu-** means good, normal, well, or easy.
Dysfunctional means an organ or body part that is not working properly.	**Euthyroid** (you-**THIGH**-roid) means a normally functioning thyroid gland.
hyper- means excessive or increased.	**hypo-** means deficient or decreased.
Hypertension (high-per-**TEN**-shun) is higher than normal blood pressure.	**Hypotension** (**high**-poh-**TEN**-shun) is lower than normal blood pressure.
inter- means between or among.	**intra-** means within or inside.
Interstitial (**in**-ter-**STISH**-al) means between, but not within, the parts of a tissue.	**Intramuscular** (**in**-trah-**MUS**-kyou-lar) means within the muscle.
sub- means under, less, or below.	**supra-** means above or excessive.
Subcostal (sub-**KOS**-tal) means below a rib or ribs.	**Supracostal** (**sue**-prah-**KOS**-tal) means above or outside the ribs.

more than one meaning. For example, look at the term *lithotomy* (lih-**THOT**-oh-mee).

- Based on word parts, **lithotomy** means a surgical incision for the removal of a stone (**lith** means stone and **otomy** means a surgical incision). This meaning is discussed in Chapter 9.

- However, lithotomy is also the name of an examination position in which the patient is lying on the back with the feet and legs raised and supported in stirrups. This term is discussed in Chapter 15.

- This possible confusion is only one of the many reasons why a medical dictionary is an important medical terminology tool.

If You Know How to Spell the Word

When starting to work with an unfamiliar dictionary, spend a few minutes reviewing its use guide, table of con-

tents, and appendices. The time you spend here will be saved later when you are looking up unfamiliar terms.

- Based on the first letter of the word, start in the appropriate section of the dictionary. Look at the top of the page for clues. The top left word is the first term on the page. The top right word is the last term on the page.

- Next, alphabetically look for words that start with the first and second letters of the word you are researching. Continue looking through each letter until you find the term you are looking for.

- When you think you have found it, check the spelling very carefully letter-by-letter working from left to right. Terms with similar spellings have very different meanings.

- When you find the term, carefully check *all* of the definitions.

FIGURE 1.7 A medical term may be taken apart to determine its meaning.

If You Do Not Know How to Spell the Word

- Listen carefully to the term and write it down. If you cannot find the word based on your spelling, start looking for alternative spellings based on the beginning sound as shown in Table 1.5. *Note:* All of these examples are in this text; however, you could practice looking them up in the dictionary!

Table 1.5

GUIDELINES TO LOOKING UP UNFAMILIAR TERMS		
If It Sounds Like	**It May Begin With**	**Example**
F	F	flatus (**FLAY**-tus)
	PH	phlegm (**FLEM**)
J	G	gingivitis (jin-jih-**VYE**-tis)
	J	jaundice (**JAWN**-dis)
K	C	crepitus (**KREP**-ih-tus)
	CH	cholera (**KOL**-er-ah)
	K	kyphosis (kye-**FOH**-sis)
	QU	quadriplegia (kwad-rih-**PLEE**-jee-ah)
S	C	cytology (sigh-**TOL**-oh-jee)
	PS	psychologist (sigh-**KOL**-oh-jist)
	S	serology (seh-**ROL**-oh-jee)
Z	X	xeroderma (zee-roh-**DER**-mah)
	Z	zygote (**ZYE**-goht)

Look Under Categories

Most dictionaries use categories such as *Diseases* and *Syndromes* to group disorders with these terms in their titles. As examples:

- **Venereal disease** would be found under **Disease, venereal**. These are sexually transmitted diseases and are discussed in Chapter 14.
- **Fetal alcohol syndrome** would be found under **Syndrome, fetal alcohol**. This is discussed in Chapter 2.
- When you come across such a term and cannot find it listed by the first word, the next step is to look under the appropriate category.

Pronunciation

A medical term is easier to understand and remember when you know how to pronounce it properly. To help you do this, each new term in the text is identified in **bold**, followed (in parentheses) by a commonly accepted pronunciation, and then the definition.

- In this *sounds like* pronunciation system, the word is respelled using normal English letters to create sounds that are familiar. To pronounce a new word, just say it as it is spelled in the parentheses.
- The part of the word that receives the primary (most) emphasis when you say it is in capital letters and bold. For example, **edema** (eh-**DEE**-mah) means excess fluid in body tissues, causing swelling.
- If a part of the word receives secondary emphasis when you say it, this is in lower case letters and bold. For example, **appendicitis** (ah-**pen**-dih-**SIGH**-tis) means an inflammation of the appendix (appendic means appendix and itis means inflammation).

A Word of Caution

Frequently there is more than one correct way to pronounce a medical term!

- The pronunciation of many medical terms is based on their Greek, Latin, or other foreign origins; however, there is a trend toward pronouncing terms as they would sound in English.
- The result is having more than one "correct" pronunciation for a term. In the text sometimes an alternative pronunciation is included to reflect these changes.
- Both are correct and the difference is a matter of preference; however, your instructor will tell you which pronunciation to use in your course.

Spelling Is Always Important

Accuracy in spelling medical terms is extremely important!

- Changing just one or two letters can completely change the meaning of a word — and this difference literally could be a matter of life or death for the patient.
- The section *Look-Alike Sound-Alike Terms and Word Parts* later in this chapter will help you become aware of some terms and word parts that are frequently confused.

Using Abbreviations

Abbreviations are frequently used as a shorthand way to record long and complex medical terms and Appendix B contains an alphabetized list of many of the more commonly used medical abbreviations.

- Abbreviations can also lead to confusion and errors! Therefore, it is important that you be very careful when using or translating an abbreviation.

- For example the abbreviation **BE** means both *below elbow* and *barium enema*. Just imagine what a difference a mix-up here would make for the patient!

- Because the same abbreviation may have more than one meaning, it is important that you be very careful when using or translating an abbreviation. To be safe, always follow the rule: *When in doubt, spell it out.*

Singular and Plural Endings

Many medical terms have Greek or Latin origins. As a result of these different origins, there are unusual rules for changing a singular word into a plural form. Additionally, English endings have been adopted for some commonly used terms.

- Table 1.6 provides guidelines to help you better understand how these plurals are formed.

- Also, throughout the text when a term with an unusual singular or plural form is introduced both forms are included. For example, a **phalanx** (FAY-lanks) is one bone of the fingers or toes (Figure 1.8). (Plural, **phalanges**.)

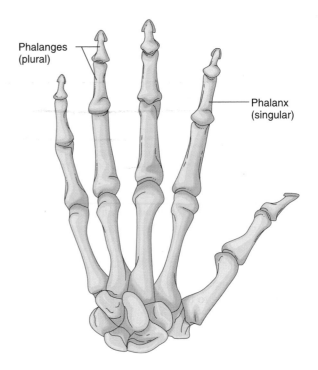

FIGURE 1.8 A phalanx is one finger or toe bone. Two or more of these bones are called phalanges.

Table 1.6

GUIDELINES TO UNUSUAL PLURAL FORMS

Guideline	Singular	Plural
1. If the term ends in **a**, the plural is usually formed by adding an **e**.	bursa vertebra	bursae vertebrae
2. If the term ends in **ex** or **ix**, the plural is usually formed by changing the **ex** or **ix** to **ices**.	appendix index	appendices indices
3. If the term ends in **is**, the plural is usually formed by changing the **is** to **es**.	diagnosis metastasis	diagnoses metastases
4. If the term ends in **itis**, the plural is usually formed by changing the **is** to **ides**.	arthritis meningitis	arthritides meningitides
5. If the term ends in **nx**, the plural is usually formed by changing the **x** to **ges**.	phalanx meninx	phalanges meninges
6. If the term ends in **on**, the plural is usually formed by changing the **on** to **a**.	criterion ganglion	criteria ganglia
7. If the term ends in **um**, the plural usually is formed by changing the **um** to **a**.	diverticulum ovum	diverticula ova
8. If the term ends in **us**, the plural is usually formed by changing the **us** to **i**.	alveolus malleolus	alveoli malleoli

*If you are in doubt as to how a plural is formed, **look it up** in a medical dictionary!*

Basic Medical Terms

The basic medical terms used to describe diseases and disease conditions are shown in Table 1.7.

Look-Alike Sound-Alike Terms and Word Parts

One confusing part of learning medical terminology is dealing with words and word parts that look and sound so much alike. This section highlights some frequently used terms and word parts that you may find most confusing. Pay particular attention to these terms and word parts as you encounter them in the text.

arteri/o, ather/o, and arthr/o

- **arteri/o** means artery. **Endarterial** (end-ar-TEE-ree-al) means pertaining to the interior or lining of an artery (**end** means within, **arteri** means artery, and **al** means pertaining to).
- **ather/o** means plaque or fatty substance. An **atheroma** (ath-er-OH-mah) is a fatty deposit within the wall of an artery (**ather** means fatty substance and **oma** means tumor).

- **arthr/o** means joint. **Arthralgia** (ar-THRAL-jee-ah) means pain in a joint or joints (**arthr** means joint and **algia** means pain).

Ileum and Ilium

- The **ileum** (ILL-ee-um) is part of the small intestine. (Remember, ileum with an e as in intestine.)
- The **ilium** (ILL-ee-um) is part of the hip bone. (Remember, ilium with an i as in hip.)

Infection and Inflammation

- An **infection** (in-FECK-shun) is the invasion of the body by a pathogenic (disease-producing) organism. The infection may remain localized or be systemic (affecting the entire body).
- **Inflammation** (in-flah-MAY-shun) is a localized response to injury or destruction of tissues. The cardinal signs (indications) of inflammation are (1) *redness* (erythema), (2) *heat*, (3) *swelling* (edema), and (4) *pain*. These are caused by extra blood flowing into the area as part of the healing process.
- The suffix **-itis** means inflammation; however, it also is often used to indicate infection.

Table 1.7

BASIC MEDICAL TERMS

A **sign** is evidence of disease, such as fever, that can be observed by the patient and by others. A sign is **objective** because it can be evaluated or measured by others.	A **symptom** (SIMP-tum), such as pain or a headache, can only be observed by the patient. A symptom is **subjective** because it can be evaluated or measured only by the patient.	A **syndrome** (SIN-drohm) is a set of the signs and symptoms that occur together as part of a specific disease process.
Diagnosis (dye-ag-NOH-sis) is the identification of the disease. To **diagnose** is the process of reaching a diagnosis. (Plural, **diagnoses**.)	A **differential diagnosis** attempts to determine which one of several diseases may be producing the symptoms.	**Prognosis** (prog-NOH-sis) is a forecast, or prediction, of the probable course and outcome of a disorder. (Plural, **prognoses**.)
An **acute** disease or symptom has a rapid onset, a severe course, and a relatively short duration.	A **chronic** disease or symptom has a long duration. Although they may be controlled, such diseases are rarely cured.	A **remission** is the partial or complete disappearance of the symptoms of a disease without having achieved a cure. A remission is usually temporary.
Some diseases are named for the **condition described**. For example, **chronic fatigue syndrome** (CFS) is a persistent overwhelming fatigue that does not resolve with bed rest.	An **eponym** (EP-oh-nim) is a disease, structure, operation, or procedure, named for the person who discovered or described it first. For example, **Alzheimer's disease** is named for Alois Alzheimer, a German neurologist who lived from 1864 to 1915 (see Chapter 10).	An **acronym** (ACK-roh-nim) is a word formed from the initial letter or letters of the major parts of a compound term. For example, the acronym **laser** stands for **l**ight **a**mplification by **s**timulated **e**mission of **r**adiation.

Laceration and Lesion

- A **laceration** (**lass**-er-**AY**-shun) is a torn, ragged wound.
- A **lesion** (**LEE**-zhun) is a pathologic change of the tissues due to disease or injury.

Mucous and Mucus

- **Mucous** (**MYOU**-kus) is an adjective that describes the specialized mucous membranes that line the body cavities.
- **Mucus** (**MYOU**-kus) is a noun and is the name of the substance secreted by the mucous membranes.

myc/o, myel/o, and my/o

- **myc/o** means fungus. **Mycosis** (my-**KOH**-sis) means any disease caused by a fungus (**myc** means fungus and **osis** means abnormal condition).
- **myel/o** means bone marrow or spinal cord. **Myelopathy** (my-eh-**LOP**-ah-thee) is any pathologic change or disease in the spinal cord (**myelo** means spinal cord and **pathy** means disease).
- **my/o** means muscle. **Myopathy** (my-**OP**-ah-thee) is any pathologic change or disease of muscle tissue (**myo** means muscle and **pathy** means disease).

-ologist and -ology

- **-ologist** means specialist. A **gerontologist** (jer-on-**TOL**-oh-jist) is a specialist in diagnosing and treating diseases, disorders, and problems associated with aging (**geront** means old age and **ologist** means specialist).
- **-ology** means the study of. **Neonatology** (nee-oh-nay-**TOL**-oh-jee) is the study of disorders of the newborn (**neo** means new, **nat** means birth, and **ology** means study of).

-ostomy and -otomy

- **-ostomy**, which is also used alone as a noun, means to surgically create an artificial opening. A **colostomy** (koh-**LAHS**-toh-mee) is the surgical creation of an opening between the colon and the body surface (**col** means colon and **ostomy** means an artificial opening).
- **-otomy** means cutting into or a surgical incision. A **colotomy** (koh-**LOT**-oh-mee) is a surgical incision into the colon (**col** means colon and **-otomy** means a surgical incision).

Palpation and Palpitation

- **Palpation** (pal-**PAY**-shun) is an examination technique in which the examiner's hands are used to feel the texture, size, consistency, and location of certain body parts. This is discussed in Chapter 16.
- **Palpitation** (**pal**-pih-**TAY**-shun) is a pounding or racing heart. This is discussed in Chapter 5.

Prostate and Prostrate

- **Prostate** (**PROS**-tayt) refers to a male gland that lies under the urinary bladder and surrounds the urethra.
- **Prostrate** (**PROS**-trayt) means to collapse and be lying flat or to be overcome with exhaustion.

pyel/o, py/o, and pyr/o

- **pyel/o** means renal pelvis (which is part of the kidney). **Pyelitis** (pye-eh-**LYE**-tis) is an inflammation of the renal pelvis (**pyel** means renal pelvis and **itis** means inflammation).
- **py/o** means pus. **Pyoderma** (pye-oh-**DER**-mah) is any pus-producing disease of the skin (**pyo** means pus and **derma** means skin).
- **pyr/o** means fever or fire. **Pyrosis** (pye-**ROH**-sis), also known as **heartburn**, is discomfort due to the regurgitation of stomach acid upward into the esophagus (**pyr** means fever or fire and **osis** means abnormal condition).

Supination and Suppuration

- **Supination** (soo-pih-**NAY**-shun) is the act of rotating the arm so that the palm of the hand is forward or upward. It also means the act of assuming the supine (lying down) position.
- **Suppuration** (**sup**-you-**RAY**-shun) is the formation or discharge of pus.

Suturing and Ligation

- **Suturing** (**SOO**-chur-ing) is the act of closing a wound or incision by stitching or a similar means.
- **Ligation** (lye-**GAY**-shun) is the act of binding or tying off blood vessels or ducts.

Triage and Trauma

- **Triage** (tree-**AHZH**) is the medical screening of patients to determine their relative priority of need and the proper place of treatment. For example, emergency personnel arriving on an accident scene must identify which of the injured require care first and determine where they can be treated most effectively.
- **Trauma** (**TRAW**-mah) means wound or injury. These are the types of injuries that might occur in an accident, shooting, natural disaster, or fire.

Viral and Virile

- **Viral** (**VYE**-ral) means pertaining to a virus (**vir** means virus or poison and **al** means pertaining to).
- **Virile** (**VIR**-ill) means possessing masculine traits.

Learning Exercises

● Matching Word Parts—1

Write the letter of the correct answer on the line provided in the left column.

1.1. _____ -algia   A. bad, difficult, painful

1.2. _____ dys-   B. excessive, increased

1.3. _____ -ectomy   C. liver

1.4. _____ hepat/o   D. pain, suffering

1.5. _____ hyper-   E. surgical removal

● Matching Word Parts—2

Write the letter of the correct answer on the line provided in the left column.

1.6. _____ hypo-   A. abnormal condition

1.7. _____ -itis   B. abnormal softening

1.8. _____ -malacia   C. deficient, decreased

1.9. _____ -necrosis   D. inflammation

1.10. ____ -osis   E. tissue death

● Matching Word Parts—3

Write the letter of the correct answer on the line provided in the left column.

1.11. _____ -ostomy   A. bleeding

1.12. _____ -otomy   B. surgical creation of an opening

1.13. _____ -plasty   C. surgical incision

1.14. _____ -rrhage   D. surgical repair

1.15. ____ -rrhaphy   E. to suture

● Matching Word Parts—4

Write the letter of the correct answer on the line provided in the left column.

1.16. _____ -rrhea   A. visual examination

1.17. _____ -rrhexis   B. rupture

1.18. _____ -sclerosis   C. abnormal narrowing

1.19. _____ -scopy   D. abnormal hardening

1.20. ____ -stenosis   E. abnormal flow

● Definitions

Circle the letter next to the correct answer.

1.21. Which word part means plaque or fatty substance?

a. -algia

b. arteri/o

c. ather/o

d. arthr/o

1.22. Which prefix means surrounding?

a. inter-

b. intra-

c. peri-

d. pre-

1.23. Which type of word part is always placed at the end of the term?

a. combining form

b. prefix

c. suffix

d. word root

1.24. Which word part means white?

   a. cyan/o

   b. erythr/o

   c. leuk/o

   d. poli/o

1.25. Which suffix means abnormal softening?

   a. -malacia

   b. -necrosis

   c. -sclerosis

   d. -stenosis

1.26. Pain, which can be observed only by the patient, is a _____ .

   a. prognosis

   b. remission

   c. sign

   d. symptom

1.27. Which prefix means deficient or decreased?

   a. hyper-

   b. hypo-

   c. peri-

   d. supra-

1.28. Which term means a prediction of the probable course and outcome of a disease?

   a. diagnose

   b. diagnosis

   c. prognosis

   d. syndrome

1.29. Which suffix means to rupture?

   a. -rrhage

   b. -rrhaphy

   c. -rrhea

   d. -rrhexis

1.30. Which term is the plural of appendix?

   a. appendexes

   b. appendices

   c. appendixes

   d. appendizes

● Matching Terms and Definitions

Write the letter of the correct answer on the line provided in the left column.

1.31. _____ laceration   A. examination procedure

1.32. _____ lesion   B. male gland

1.33. _____ palpitation   C. pathologic tissue change

1.34. _____ palpation   D. pounding heart

1.35. _____ prostate   E. torn, ragged wound

● Which Word?

Circle the correct term in each sentence.

1.36. The body cavities are lined with specialized *mucous / mucus* membrane.

1.37. The formation of pus is called *supination / suppuration.*

1.38. The term meaning wound or injury is *trauma / triage.*

1.39. The medical term meaning possessing masculine traits is *viral / virile.*

1.40. The medical term for part of the small intestine is *ileum / ilium.*

● Spelling Counts

Find the misspelled word in each sentence. Then write that word, spelled correctly, on the line provided.

1.41. A disease named for the person who discovered it is known as enaponym. _____

1.42. A localized response to injury or tissue destruction is called inflimmation. _____ .

1.43. The act of closing a wound by stitching is sutering. _____

1.44. The medical term meaning the surgical repair of a nerve is neuriplasty. _____

1.45. The medical term meaning inflammation of the tonsils is tonsilitis. _____

● Matching Terms

Write the letter of the correct answer on the line provided in the left column.

1.46. _____ cardiac   A. abnormal stomach condition

1.47. _____ gastralgia   B. pertaining to the heart

1.48. _____ gastrosis   C. rupture of a muscle

1.49. _____ myoplasty   D. stomach pain

1.50. _____ myorrhexis   E. surgical muscle repair

● Term Selection

Circle the letter next to the correct answer.

1.51. Which term means the abnormal narrowing of an artery or arteries?

a. arteriosclerosis

b. arteriostenosis

c. arthrostenosis

d. atherosclerosis

1.52. Based on the word part that indicates color, which term means blue skin coloration due to the lack of oxygen?

a. cyanosis

b. erythrocytes

c. leukocytes

d. melanosis

1.53. Which term contains a combining vowel between two word roots?

a. abdominocentesis

b. endoscopy

c. gastroenteritis

d. hemorrhage

1.54. Which prefix means bad, difficult, or painful?

a. -algia

b. -dynia

c. dys-

d. eu-

1.55. Which term means a specialist in diagnosing and treating diseases, disorders, and problems associated with aging?

a. gerontologist

b. gerontology

c. neurologist

d. neurology

● Sentence Completion

Write the correct term on the line.

1.56. Lower than normal blood pressure is called _____ .

1.57. The process of recording a picture of an artery or arteries is called _____ .

1.58. The term meaning above or outside the ribs is _____ .

1.59. A strong dependence on a drug or substance is known as a/an _____.

1.60. The act of binding or tying off blood vessels or ducts is called _____ .

● True/False

If the statement is true, write T on the line. If the statement is false, write F on the line.

1.61. _____ Arterionecrosis is the abnormal narrowing of an artery or arteries.

1.62. _____ Mucus is the substance secreted by the mucous membranes.

1.63. _____ Supination is the formation or discharging of pus.

1.64. _____ A suffix usually, but not always, indicates location, time, or number.

1.65. _____ A combining vowel is used when the suffix begins with a consonant.

1.66. _____ Ova is the plural of ovum.

1.67. _____ A disease that is in remission has been cured.

1.68. _____ The term phlegm begins with an *F* sound.

1.69. _____ To diagnose is the process of reaching a diagnosis.

1.70. _____ It is not necessary to use a combining vowel when joining two root words.

● Clinical Conditions

Write the correct answer on the line.

1.71. Beverly Gaston suffers from higher than normal blood pressure. This is recorded on her chart as _____ .

1.72. Mrs. Tillson was treated for pulmonary _____ . This condition is an excessive build up of fluid in the lungs.

1.73. Dr. Gusterson is trained in the treatment of the diseases and disorders associated with aging. His specialty is known as _____ .

1.74. In the accident Felipe Valladares suffered a broken toe. The medical term for this is a fractured _____ .

1.75. Hal Jamison received emergency treatment for _____ , which is an inflammation of the appendix.

1.76. Gina Manley told her friends that she has an enlarged liver. The medical term for this condition is _____ .

1.77. As she used her hands to examine the patient, Dr. Liu was using an examination technique called _____ .

1.78. Joan Randolph's medication was administered by an injection into the muscle. This is called an _____ or IM injection.

1.79. Andy Lewis describes that uncomfortable feeling as heartburn. The medical term for this condition is _____ .

1.80. Max Greene's muscle wound required suturing. This procedure is called _____ .

● Which is the correct medical term?

Circle the letter next to the correct answer.

1.81. Which term means an inflammation of a nerve or nerves?

   a. neuralgia

   b. neuritis

   c. neurology

   d. neuroplasty

1.82. Which term means the loss of a large amount of blood in a short time?

   a. diarrhea

   b. hemorrhage

   c. hepatorrhagia

   d. otorrhagia

1.83. Which term means the tissue death of an artery or arteries?

   a. arteriomalacia

   b. arterionecrosis

   c. arteriosclerosis

   d. arteriostenosis

1.84. Which term describes the time and events before birth?

   a. neonatal

   b. perinatal

   c. postnatal

   d. prenatal

1.85. Which term means enlargement of the liver?

   a. hepatitis

   b. hepatomegaly

   c. nephromegaly

   d. nephritis

● Challenge Word Building

These terms are *not* found in this chapter; however, they are made up of the following word parts. You may want to look in the glossary or use a medical dictionary to check your answers.

neo- = new	arteri/o = artery	-algia = pain and suffering
	arthr/o = joint	-itis = inflammation
	cardi/o = heart	-ologist = specialist
	nat/o = birth	-otomy = cutting into, a surgical incision
	neur/o = nerve	-rrhea = abnormal flow
	rhin/o = nose	-scopy = visual examination

1.86.   The medical specialist concerned with the diagnosis and treatment of heart disease is a/an _____ .

1.87.   The medical term meaning a runny nose is _____ .

1.88.   The medical term meaning the inflammation of a joint is _____.

1.89.   A specialist in disorders of the newborn is called a/an _____ .

1.90.   The medical term meaning a surgical incision into a nerve is a/an _____.

1.91.   The medical term meaning the visual examination of the internal structure of a joint is _____ .

1.92.   The medical term meaning an inflammation of an artery is _____.

1.93.   The medical term meaning pain in a nerve or nerves is _____ .

1.94.   The medical term meaning a surgical incision into the heart is a/an _____ .

1.95.   The medical term meaning an inflammation of the nose is _____ .

● **Labeling Exercises**

1.96.   The word part (combining form) meaning spinal cord is _____/_ .

1.97.   The word part (combining form) meaning muscle is _____/_ .

1.98.   The word part (combining form) meaning bone marrow is _____/_ .

1.99.   The word part (combining form) meaning nerve is _____/_ .

1.100. The word part (combining form) meaning joint is _____/_ .

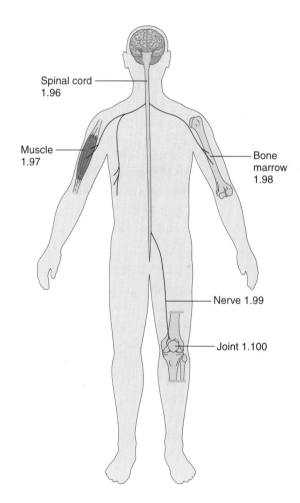

Spinal cord
1.96

Muscle
1.97

Bone
marrow
1.98

Nerve 1.99

Joint 1.100

The Human Touch: Critical Thinking Exercise

The following story and questions are designed to stimulate critical thinking through class discussion or as a brief essay response. There are no easy or right-wrong answers to these questions.

Baylie Hutchins sits at her kitchen table with her medical terminology book opened to the first chapter, highlighter in hand. Her 2-year-old son, Mathias, plays with a box of animal crackers in his highchair, some even finding his mouth. "Arteri/o, ather/o, and arthr/o," she mutters, lips moving to shape unfamiliar sounds. "They're too much alike and they mean totally different things." Mathias sneezes loudly, and spots of animal cracker rain on the page, punctuating her frustration.

"Great job 'Thias," she says wiping the text with her finger. "I planned on using the highlighter to mark with, not your lunch." Mathias giggles and peaks through the tunnel made by one small hand.

"Mucous and mucus," she reads aloud, each sounding the same. Then she remembers her teacher's tip for remembering the difference, "The long word's the membrane and the short one's the secretion."

Matthias picks up an animal cracker and excitedly shouts "Tiger, Mommy! Tiger!" "That's right, 'Thias. Good job!"

Turning back to the page she stares at the red words -rrhagia, -rrhaphy, -rrhea, and -rrhexis. Stumbling over the pronunciation Baylie closes her eyes and tries to silence the voices in her head. "You can't do anything right," her ex-husband says. "Couldn't finish if your life depended on it," her mother's voice snaps.

Baylie keeps at it. "Rhin/o means nose," highlighting those three words, "and a rhinoceros has a big horn on his nose."

"Rhino!" Matthias shouts, holding up an animal cracker. Baylie laughs. We both have new things to learn, she realizes. And we can do it!

Suggested Discussion Topics:

1. Baylie needs to learn medical terminology if she wants a career in the medical field. What study habits would help Baylie accomplish this task?

2. A support group could help empower Baylie to accomplish her goals. What people would you suggest for this group and why?

3. How can this textbook and other resource materials help her (and you) learn medical terminology?

4. Discuss strategies the instructor could, and has already, used to help Baylie improve her terminology skills.

5. Discuss how previous educational or learning experiences influence a student's approach to learning a new skill or subject.

The Human Body in Health and Disease

● Overview of the Human Body in Health and Disease

Anatomic Reference Systems	Descriptive terms used to describe the location of body planes, directions, and cavities.
Cytology	The structures of cells, chromosomes, DNA, and genetics.
Histology	The study of the tissues, which are composed of cells that join together to perform specific functions.
Glands	Specialized cells that secrete material used elsewhere in the body.
Organs and Body Systems	Body parts organized into systems according to function.
Pathology	Study of structural and functional changes caused by disease.

● VOCABULARY   Related to the Human Body in Health and Disease

Check the box as you master each word part or term. Terms marked with the ❖ symbol are pronounced on the optional student audiotape.

Key Word Parts

- ☐ aden/o
- ☐ adip/o
- ☐ caud/o
- ☐ cephal/o
- ☐ col/o
- ☐ coron/o
- ☐ cyt/o
- ☐ hepat/o
- ☐ hist/o
- ☐ hyster/o
- ☐ lapar/o
- ☐ nephr/o
- ☐ oste/o
- ☐ path/o
- ☐ retr/o

Key Medical Terms

- ☐ **abdomen** (ab-DOH-men *or* AB-doh-men) ❖
- ☐ **abdominal** (ab-DOM-ih-nal)
- ☐ **abdominopelvic** (ab-**dom**-ih-noh-PEL-vick) ❖
- ☐ **adenectomy** (ad-eh-NECK-toh-mee) ❖
- ☐ **adenitis** (ad-eh-NIGH-tis) ❖
- ☐ **adenoma** (ad-eh-NOH-mah) ❖
- ☐ **adenomalacia** (ad-eh-noh-mah-LAY-shee-ah) ❖
- ☐ **adenosclerosis** (ad-eh-noh-skleh-ROH-sis) ❖
- ☐ **adenosis** (ad-eh-NOH-sis) ❖
- ☐ **adipose** (AD-ih-pohs) ❖
- ☐ **anaplasia** (an-ah-PLAY-zee-ah) ❖
- ☐ **anatomy** (ah-NAT-oh-mee) ❖
- ☐ **anomaly** (ah-NOM-ah-lee) ❖
- ☐ **anterior** (an-TEER-ee-or) ❖
- ☐ **aplasia** (ah-PLAY-zee-ah) ❖
- ☐ **ascites** (ah-SIGH-teez) ❖
- ☐ **caudal** (KAW-dal) ❖
- ☐ **cephalic** (seh-FAL-ick) ❖
- ☐ **chromosomes** (KROH-moh-sohmes) ❖
- ☐ **communicable** (kuh-MEW-nih-kuh-bul) ❖
- ☐ **congenital** (kon-JEN-ih-tahl) ❖
- ☐ **coronal** (koh-ROH-nal)
- ☐ **cytology** (sigh-TOL-oh-jee) ❖
- ☐ **cytoplasm** (SIGH-toh-plazm)
- ☐ **deoxyribonucleic** (dee-**ock**-see-**rye**-boh-new-KLEE-ick) ❖
- ☐ **distal** (DIS-tal)
- ☐ **dorsal** (DOR-sal)
- ☐ **dysplasia** (dis-PLAY-see-ah) ❖

- ☐ **endemic** (en-DEM-ick) ❖
- ☐ **endocrine** (EN-doh-krin) ❖
- ☐ **epidemic** (ep-ih-DEM-ick) ❖
- ☐ **epidemiologist** (ep-ih-**dee**-mee-OL-oh-jist) ❖
- ☐ **epigastric** (ep-ih-GAS-trick)
- ☐ **epithelial** (ep-ih-THEE-lee-al) ❖
- ☐ **etiology** (ee-tee-OL-oh-jee) ❖
- ☐ **exocrine** (ECK-soh-krin) ❖
- ☐ **geneticist** (jeh-NET-ih-sist) ❖
- ☐ **hemophilia** (hee-moh-FILL-ee-ah) ❖
- ☐ **histologist** (hiss-TOL-oh-jist)
- ☐ **histology** (hiss-TOL-oh-jee) ❖
- ☐ **homeostasis** (hoh-mee-oh-STAY-sis) ❖
- ☐ **hyperplasia** (high-per-PLAY-zee-ah) ❖
- ☐ **hypochondriac** (high-poh-KON-dree-ack)
- ☐ **hypogastric** (high-poh-GAS-trick)
- ☐ **hypoplasia** (high-poh-PLAY-zee-ah) ❖
- ☐ **iatrogenic** (eye-at-roh-JEN-ick) ❖
- ☐ **idiopathic** (id-ee-oh-PATH-ick) ❖
- ☐ **iliac** (ILL-ee-ack)
- ☐ **infectious** (in-FECK-shus) ❖
- ☐ **inguinal** (ING-gwih-nal) ❖
- ☐ **laparoscopy** (lap-ah-ROS-koh-pee) ❖
- ☐ **lumbar** (LUM-bar)
- ☐ **membrane** (MEM-brain)
- ☐ **mesentery** (MESS-en-terr-ee) ❖
- ☐ **midsagittal** (mid-SADJ-ih-tal) ❖
- ☐ **nosocomial** (nos-oh-KOH-mee-al) ❖
- ☐ **nucleus** (NEW-klee-us)
- ☐ **pandemic** (pan-DEM-ick) ❖
- ☐ **parietal peritoneum** (pah-RYE-eh-tal **pehr**-ih-toh-NEE-um) ❖
- ☐ **pathologist** (pah-THOL-oh-jist)
- ☐ **pathology** (pah-THOL-oh-jee) ❖
- ☐ **pelvic** (PEL-vick) ❖
- ☐ **peritoneum** (pehr-ih-toh-NEE-um) ❖
- ☐ **peritonitis** (pehr-ih-toh-NIGH-tis) ❖
- ☐ **phenylketonuria** (fen-il-**kee**-toh-NEW-ree-ah) ❖
- ☐ **physiology** (fiz-ee-OL-oh-jee) ❖
- ☐ **posterior** (pos-TEER-ee-or) ❖
- ☐ **proximal** (PROCK-sih-mal) ❖
- ☐ **retroperitoneal** (ret-roh-**pehr**-ih-toh-NEE-al) ❖
- ☐ **sagittal** (SADJ-ih-tal)
- ☐ **thoracic** (thoh-RAS-ick) ❖
- ☐ **transverse** (trans-VERSE) ❖
- ☐ **umbilical** (um-BILL-ih-kal) ❖
- ☐ **ventral** (VEN-tral) ❖
- ☐ **visceral** (VIS-er-al) ❖

Anatomic Reference Systems

Anatomic reference systems are used to describe the location and functions of body parts. These reference systems include body planes, body directions, body cavities, and structural units.

Anatomy and Physiology Defined

- **Anatomy** (ah-**NAT**-oh-mee) is the study of the structures of the body.

- **Physiology** (**fiz**-ee-**OL**-oh-jee) is the study of the functions of these structures.

The Anatomic Position

Descriptions of the body are based on the **anatomic position**. In this position the individual is

- Standing up so that the body is erect.

- Facing forward.

- Holding the arms at the sides.

- Turning the hands with the palms toward the front.

Body Planes

Planes are imaginary horizontal and vertical lines used to divide the body into sections for descriptive purposes.

Vertical Planes

- A **vertical plane** is an up-and-down line at a right angle to the horizon.

- The **midsagittal plane** (mid-**SADJ**-ih-tal), also known as the **midline**, is the vertical plane that divides the body, from top to bottom, into equal left and right halves (Figure 2.1).

- A **sagittal plane** (**SADJ**-ih-tal) is any vertical plane parallel to the midline that divides the body into unequal left and right portions.

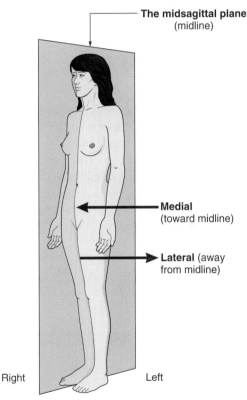

FIGURE 2.1 The midsagittal plane divides the body from top to bottom into equal left and right halves.

- The **coronal plane** (koh-**ROH**-nal) is also known as the **frontal plane** (**coron** means head or crown and **al** means pertaining to). This is any vertical plane, at right angles to the sagittal plane that divides the body into anterior (front) and posterior (back) portions (Figure 2.2).

Horizontal Planes

- A **horizontal plane** is a flat crosswise line like the horizon.

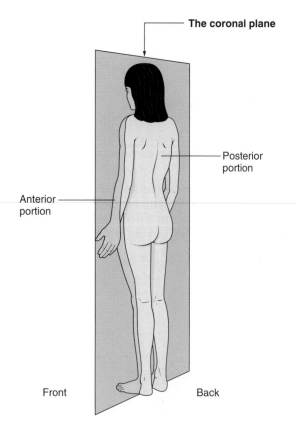

FIGURE 2.2 The coronal plane is located at right angles to the sagittal plane. It divides the body into anterior (front) and posterior (back) portions.

- The **transverse plane** (trans-**VERSE**), also known as the **horizontal plane**, divides the body into superior (upper) and inferior (lower) portions (Figure 2.3).
- A transverse plane can be at the waist or any other level of the body.

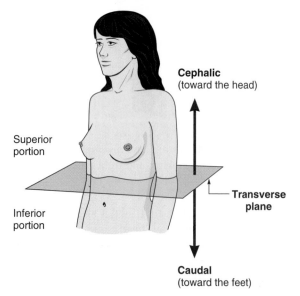

FIGURE 2.3 The transverse plane divides the body into superior (upper) and inferior (lower) portions. This division can be at the waist or any other level across the body.

Body Directions

Relative location of the whole body or an organ is described through the use of pairs of contrasting body direction terms. These are summarized in Table 2.1 and are illustrated in Figures 2.1, 2.2, 2.3, 2.4, and 2.5.

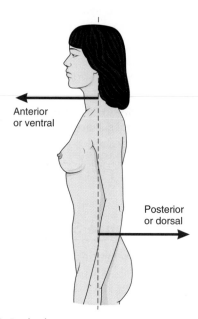

FIGURE 2.4 Body directions. Anterior means toward the front. The ventral surface is the front or belly side. Posterior means toward the back. The dorsal surface is the back side.

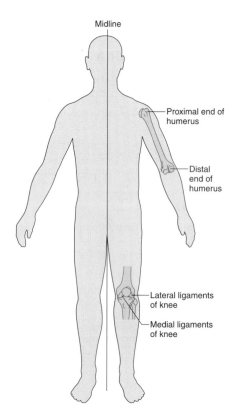

FIGURE 2.5 Body directions.

Table 2.1

TERMS USED TO DESCRIBE BODY DIRECTION

Ventral (**VEN**-tral) refers to the front or belly side of the body or organ (**ventr** means belly side of body and **al** means pertaining to).

Dorsal (**DOR**-sal) refers to the back of the body or organ (**dors** means back of body and **al** means pertaining to).

Anterior (an-**TEER**-ee-or) means situated in the front. It also means on the forward part of an organ (**anter** means front or before and **ior** means pertaining to).

For example, the stomach is located anterior to (in front of) the pancreas. Anterior is also used in reference to the ventral surface of the body.

Posterior (pos-**TEER**-ee-or) means situated in the back. It also means on the back part of an organ (**poster** means back or after and **ior** means pertaining to).

For example, the pancreas is located posterior to (behind) the stomach. Posterior is also used in reference to the dorsal surface of the body.

Superior means uppermost, above, or toward the head.

For example, the lungs are located superior to (above) the diaphragm.

Inferior means lowermost, below, or toward the feet.

For example, the stomach is located inferior to (below) the diaphragm.

Cephalic (seh-**FAL**-ick) means toward the head (**cephal** means head and **ic** means pertaining to).

Caudal (**KAW**-dal) means toward the lower part of the body (**caud** means tail or lower part of the body and **al** means pertaining to).

Proximal (**PROCK**-sih-mal) means situated nearest the midline or beginning of a body structure.

For example, the proximal end of the humerus (the bone of the upper arm) forms part of the shoulder.

Distal (**DIS**-tal) means situated farthest from the midline or beginning of a body structure.

For example, the distal end of the humerus forms part of the elbow.

Medial means the direction toward or nearer the midline.

For example, the medial ligament of the knee is near the inner surface of the leg.

Lateral means the direction toward or nearer the side and away from the midline.

For example, the lateral ligament of the knee is near the side of the leg.

Bilateral means relating to, or having, two sides.

Major Body Cavities

A **body cavity** is a space within the body that contains and protects the internal organs (Figure 2.6).

The Dorsal Cavity

The dorsal cavity, which is divided into two parts, protects the structures of the nervous system that coordinate the bodily functions.

- The **cranial cavity**, located within the skull, protects the brain.
- The **spinal cavity**, located within the spinal column, protects the spinal cord.

The Ventral Cavity

The ventral cavity, which is divided into three parts, contains many of the body organs that maintain homeosta-

sis. **Homeostasis** (**hoh**-mee-oh-**STAY**-sis) means maintaining a constant internal environment (**homeo** means constant and **stasis** means control).

- The **thoracic cavity** (thoh-**RAS**-ick), also known as the **chest cavity**, protects the heart and the lungs. The **diaphragm** is a muscle that separates the thoracic and abdominal cavities.
- The **abdominal cavity** (ab-**DOM**-ih-nal) contains primarily the major organs of digestion. Most frequently referred to simply as the **abdomen**, this term is pronounced as either (ab-**DOH**-men *or* AB-doh-men).
- The **pelvic cavity** (**PEL**-vick) is the space formed by the pelvic (hip) bones. It contains primarily the organs of the reproductive and excretory systems.
- There is no division between the abdominal and pelvic cavities. Together they may be referred to as the **abdominopelvic cavity** (ab-**dom**-ih-noh-**PEL**-vick).

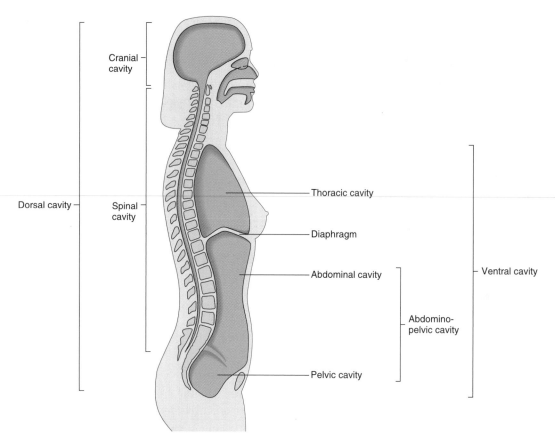

FIGURE 2.6 Major body cavities.

Divisions of the Abdomen

To make it easier to describe where an organ or a pain is located, the abdomen is divided into four imaginary quadrants (Figure 2.7). (**Quadrant** means divided into four.) These are the:

1. Right upper quadrant (RUQ)
2. Left upper quadrant (LUQ)
3. Right lower quadrant (RLQ)
4. Left lower quadrant (LLQ)

Regions of the Thorax and Abdomen

Another descriptive system divides the abdomen and lower portion of the thorax into nine regions (Figure 2.8). These are the:

- **Right and left hypochondriac regions. Hypochondriac** (**high**-poh-**KON**-dree-ack) means below the ribs. This term also means an individual with an abnormal and excessive concern about his or her health.

- **Epigastric region. Epigastric** (ep-ih-**GAS**-trick) means above the stomach.

- **Right and left lumbar regions. Lumbar** (**LUM**-bar) refers to the inward curve of the spine.

- **Umbilical region.** The term **umbilical** (um-**BILL**-ih-kal) means referring to the **umbilicus** (um-**BILL**-ih-kus).

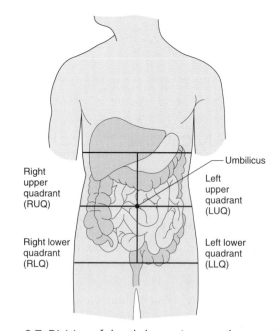

FIGURE 2.7 Division of the abdomen into quadrants.

Also known as the **belly button** or **navel** this is the pit in the center of the abdominal wall marking the point where the umbilical cord was attached to the fetus (**umbilic** means naval and **al** means pertaining to).

Figure 2.8 Regions of the thorax and abdomen.

- **Right and left iliac regions. Iliac** (**ILL**-ee-ack) refers to the hipbone.
- **Hypogastric region. Hypogastric** (**high**-poh-**GAS**-trick) means below the stomach. The entire lower region of the abdomen is also referred to as the **groin** or **inguinal** (**ING**-gwih-nal) area.

Peritoneum

- The **peritoneum** (**pehr**-ih-toh-**NEE**-um) is the membrane that protects and supports (suspends in place) the organs located in the abdominal cavity.
- The **parietal peritoneum** (pah-**RYE**-eh-tal **pehr**-ih-toh-**NEE**-um) is the outer layer of this membrane that lines the abdominal cavity.
- The **visceral peritoneum** (**VIS**-er-al **pehr**-ih-toh-**NEE**-um) is the inner layer of this membrane that surrounds the organs of the abdominal cavity. **Visceral** (**VIS**-er-al) means relating to the internal organs (those enclosed within a cavity) especially the abdominal organs.
- The **mesentery** (**MESS**-en-**terr**-ee) is a layer of the peritoneum that suspends parts of the intestine within the abdominal cavity.
- The term **retroperitoneal** (ret-roh-**pehr**-ih-toh-**NEE**-al) means located behind the peritoneum of the abdominal cavity (**retro** means behind, **periton** means peritoneum, and **eal** means pertaining to).
- **Peritonitis** (**pehr**-ih-toh-**NIGH**-tis) is an inflammation of the peritoneum (**periton** means peritoneum and **itis** means inflammation).

- **Ascites** (ah-**SIGH**-teez) is an abnormal accumulation of clear or milky serous (watery) fluid in the peritoneal cavity.

Laparoscopic Procedures

Laparoscopy (**lap**-ah-**ROS**-koh-pee) is the visual examination of the interior of the abdomen with the use of a laparoscope (**laparo** means abdomen and **scopy** means visual examination).

Laparoscopic surgery involves the use of a laparoscope plus instruments inserted into the abdomen through small incisions (Figure 2.9). These are used to

- Explore and examine the interior of the abdomen.
- Take specimens to be biopsied.
- Perform surgical procedures.

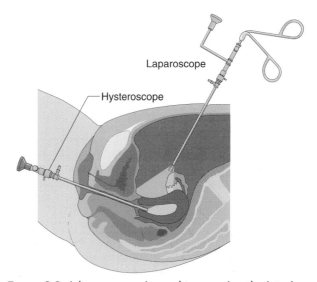

Figure 2.9 A laparoscope is used to examine the interior of the abdomen. A hysteroscope is used to examine the interior of the uterus.

Cytology

Cells are the basic structural units of the body that are specialized and grouped together to form the tissues and organs (Figure 2.10).

- **Cytology** (sigh-**TOL**-oh-jee) is the study of the formation, structure, and function of cells (**cyt** means cell and **ology** means study of).
- The **cell membrane** is the structure that surrounds and protects the cell. A **membrane** (**MEM**-brain) is a thin layer of tissue that covers a surface, lines a cavity, or divides a space or organ.
- **Cytoplasm** (**SIGH**-toh-plazm) is the material within the cell membrane that is *not* part of the nucleus (**cyto** means cell and **plasm** means formative material of cells).

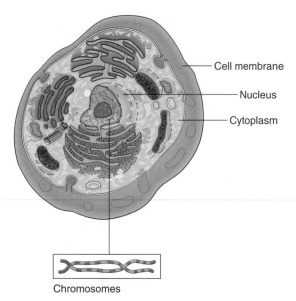

Cell membrane

Nucleus

Cytoplasm

Chromosomes

FIGURE 2.10 Diagrammatic representation of basic cell structure.

- The **nucleus** (**NEW**-klee-us), which is surrounded by the nuclear membrane, is a structure within the cell that has two important functions. (1) It controls the activities of the cell, and (2) it helps the cell divide. (Plural, **nuclei**.)

Chromosomes

- The nucleus of each cell contains 46 **chromosomes** (**KROH**-moh-sohmes) arranged into 23 pairs. There are 22 identical pairs plus the single pair (XX or XY) that determines the sex of the child.
- **Sex cells** (sperm and ovum), also known as **gametes** (**GAM**-eets), are the only cells that do not have 46 chromosomes. Instead, each mature sex cell has 23 single chromosomes. When a sperm and ovum join to form a new life, the embryo receives half of his or her chromosomes from each parent.

DNA

- Chromosomes are organized as long coiled molecules of **deoxyribonucleic acid** (dee-**ock**-see-**rye**-boh-new-**KLEE**-ick) and are commonly referred to as **DNA**.
- **Genes** are the functional units of heredity. Each gene is a segment of DNA that is located in a specific site on a chromosome. Each chromosome contains about 100,000 genes.
- The genes in DNA create a unique pattern for each individual. This pattern can be used to identify the source of tissue specimens and this characteristic makes DNA testing useful in situations such as evidence in some court cases.

Terms Related to Genetics

- **Genetics** is the study of how genes are transferred from the parents to their children and the role of genes in health and disease (**gene** means producing and **tics** means pertaining to).
- A specialist in the field of genetics is known as a **geneticist** (jeh-**NET**-ih-sist).
- **Genetic engineering** is research to identify defective genes and to develop gene therapy to treat or replace these faulty genes.
- The term **genetic mutation** describes changes that occur within genes.
- **Somatic cell mutation** is change within the cells of the body. These changes affect the individual but cannot be transmitted to the next generation.
- **Gametic cell mutation** is change within the genes found in the gametes (sperm or ovum) that can be transmitted by parents to their children.

Genetic Disorders

Genetic disorders, also known as a **hereditary disorders**, are diseases or conditions caused by a defective gene. These genes were transmitted from the parents; however, a genetic disorder may be manifested at any time in life.

There are more than 2,000 known genetic disorders affecting all body systems. The following are examples. Additional genetic disorders are described throughout the text.

- **Cystic fibrosis**, which is discussed in Chapter 7, is a genetic disorder of the exocrine glands. (Exocrine glands are explained later in this chapter in the section titled *Glands*.)
- **Down syndrome**, also known as **trisomy 21**, is a genetic syndrome characterized by varying degrees of mental retardation and multiple physical abnormalities. (*Note:* Down's syndrome is an alternate spelling; however, the preferred spelling is Down syndrome — without the apostrophe and s.)
- **Hemophilia** (**hee**-moh-**FILL**-ee-ah) is a group of hereditary bleeding disorders in which one of the factors needed to clot the blood is missing. Genetic transmission is from a mother to her son(s).
- **Huntington's disease** (HD), also known as **Huntington's chorea** (HC), is a hereditary disorder with symptoms that first appear in midlife and cause the irreversible and progressive loss of muscle control and mental ability. The HD gene, which can be detected through genetic testing, is a dominant gene. This means that 50% of those inheriting it will develop the disease.
- **Muscular dystrophy** (**DIS**-troh-fee), also known as **MD**, is a group of genetic diseases characterized by progressive weakness of muscle fibers (see Chapter 4).

- **Phenylketonuria** (**fen**-il-**kee**-toh-NEW-ree-ah), also known as **PKU**, is a genetic disorder in which an essential digestive enzyme is missing. PKU can be detected by a blood test at birth. If it is not detected and treated early, PKU causes severe mental retardation.

- **Sickle cell anemia**, which is discussed in Chapter 5, is a serious genetic disorder caused by genes that produce abnormal hemoglobin in the red blood cells (Figure 2.11).

- **Tay-Sachs disease**, also known as **TSD**, is a hereditary disease marked by progressive physical degeneration, mental retardation, and early death.

Genetic Counseling

The transmission of genetic disorders is a complex "game of chance" and genetic counseling is a valuable tool for those concerned about genetic disorders. As examples:

- An individual with **sickle cell trait** does *not* have the disease sickle cell anemia. However, he has one gene for sickle cell anemia and one gene for normal hemoglobin. As shown in Figure 2.12, although the potential parents with sickle cell trait are healthy they are *carriers* and can transmit the disease to their children.

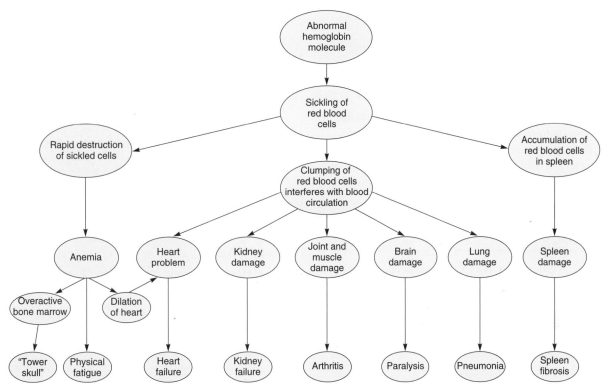

FIGURE 2.11 Sickle cell anemia damages and affects many body systems.

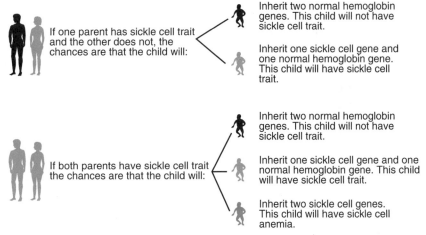

FIGURE 2.12 The genetic probabilities of transmitting sickle cell anemia.

Congenital Disorders

A **congenital disorder** (kon-JEN-ih-tahl) is an abnormal condition that exists at the time of birth and may be caused by a developmental disorder before birth, prenatal influences, premature birth, or injuries during birth.

- A **developmental disorder** may result in an anomaly or malformation such as the absence of a limb or the presence of an extra toe at birth. An **anomaly** (ah-NOM-ah-lee) is a deviation from what is regarded as normal.

- **Prenatal influences** are the mother's health and the prenatal care she receives. As an example, maternal alcohol consumption during pregnancy can cause the congenital disorder **fetal alcohol syndrome**, which is also known as **FAS**. FAS is characterized by prenatal and postnatal physical and behavior traits including growth deficiencies and abnormalities, mental retardation, brain damage, and socialization difficulties.

- **Birth injuries** are congenital disorders that were not present before the events surrounding the time of birth. As an example, **cerebral palsy** (CP), which is discussed in Chapter 10, may be caused by premature birth or be due to inadequate oxygen to the brain during birth.

Histology

A tissue is a group or layer of similarly specialized cells that join together to perform certain specific functions. **Histology** (hiss-TOL-oh-jee) is the study of the structure, composition, and function of tissues (**hist** means tissue and **ology** means a study of). A **histologist** (hiss-TOL-oh-jist) is a specialist in the study of cells and microscopic tissues.

Stem Cells

- **Stem cells**, also known as **precursor cells**, are cells with the ability to divide without limit and to give rise to specialized cells. Stem cells are abundant in a fetus and in the cord blood of a newborn. These cells are present in limited quantities in adults.

- Each type of tissue has its own stem cells and when implanted into the appropriate type of tissue the stem cells can regenerate the full range of cell types normally found there. The research goal is to discover how to use stem cells as a source for organ and tissue regeneration. Some applications, such as bone marrow transplants, are already in use (see Chapter 3).

Types of Tissue

The four main types of tissue are epithelial, connective, muscle, and nerve.

Epithelial Tissues

Epithelial tissues (ep-ih-THEE-lee-al) form a protective covering for all of the internal and external surfaces of the body.

- **Epithelium** (ep-ih-THEE-lee-um) is the specialized epithelial tissue that forms the epidermis of the skin and the surface layer of mucous membranes. The skin is discussed in Chapter 12.

- **Endothelium** (en-doh-THEE-lee-um) is the specialized epithelial tissue that lines the blood and lymph vessels, body cavities, glands, and organs.

- Glands are made up of specialized epithelial tissues that are capable of producing secretions.

Connective Tissues

Connective tissues support and connect organs and other body tissues.

- Bone, cartilage, and other **dense connective tissues** are discussed in Chapter 3.

- **Adipose tissue** (AD-ih-pohs), also known as **fat**, provides protective padding, insulation, support, and acts as a nutrient reserve (**adip** means fat and **ose** means pertaining to).

- **Loose connective tissue** surrounds various organs and supports both nerve cells and blood vessels.

- Blood and lymph, which are discussed in Chapters 5 and 6, are **liquid connective tissues**.

Muscle Tissue

Muscle tissue, which is discussed in Chapter 4, contains cell material with the specialized ability to contract and relax.

Nerve Tissue

Nerve tissue, which is discussed in Chapter 10, contains cells with the specialized ability to react to stimuli and conduct electrical impulses.

Pathology of Tissue Formation

- **Aplasia** (ah-PLAY-zee-ah) means the lack of development of an organ or tissue (**a** means without and **plasia** means formation).

- **Hypoplasia** (high-poh-PLAY-zee-ah) is the incomplete development of an organ or tissue, but less severe in degree than aplasia (**hypo** means deficient and **plasia** means formation).

- **Hyperplasia** (high-per-PLAY-zee-ah) is an abnormal increase in the number of normal cells in normal arrangement in a tissue (**hyper** means excessive and **plasia** means formation).

- **Dysplasia** (dis-PLAY-see-ah) means abnormal development or growth, especially of cells (**dys-** means bad and **plasia** means formation).

- **Anaplasia** (an-ah-PLAY-zee-ah) is a change in the structure of cells and in their orientation to each other (**ana** means excessive and **plasia** means formation). These abnormal cells are characteristic of malignancy and are discussed in Chapter 6. (A **malignancy** is a life-threatening tumor that tends to spread to distant body sites.)

Glands

A gland is a group of specialized epithelial cells that form secretions. A **secretion** is the substance produced by a gland. The two types of glands are exocrine and endocrine glands (Figure 2.13).

- **Exocrine glands** (**ECK**-soh-krin), such as sweat glands, secrete their chemical substances into ducts that lead either to other organs or out of the body (**exo** means out of and **crine** means to secrete).

- **Endocrine glands** (**EN**-doh-krin), which secrete hormones, do *not* have ducts (**endo** means within and **crine** means to secrete). These secretions flow directly into the bloodstream for transportation to organs and other structures throughout the body. (The endocrine system is discussed in Chapter 13.)

Pathology and Procedures of Glands

- **Adenectomy** (**ad**-eh-**NECK**-toh-mee) is the surgical removal of a gland (**aden** means gland and **ectomy** means surgical removal).

- **Adenitis** (**ad**-eh-**NIGH**-tis) is inflammation of a gland (**aden** means gland and **itis** means inflammation).

- An **adenoma** (**ad**-eh-**NOH**-mah) is a benign tumor in which the cells form recognizable glandular structures (**aden** means gland and **oma** means tumor). (Benign means not life-threatening).

- **Adenomalacia** (**ad**-eh-noh-mah-**LAY**-shee-ah) is the abnormal softening of a gland (**adeno** means gland and **malacia** means abnormal softening).

- **Adenosclerosis** (**ad**-eh-noh-skleh-**ROH**-sis) is the abnormal hardening of a gland (**adeno** means gland and **sclerosis** means abnormal hardening).

- **Adenosis** (**ad**-eh-**NOH**-sis) is any disease condition of a gland (**aden** means gland and **osis** means an abnormal condition.)

Organs and Body Systems

An **organ** is a somewhat independent part of the body that performs a special function or functions.

The tissues and organs of the body are organized into systems that perform specialized functions (Figure 2.14). These systems are outlined in Table 2.2.

Pathology

- **Pathology** (pah-**THOL**-oh-jee) is the study of structural and functional changes caused by disease (**path/o** and **pathy** mean disease; however, they also mean suffering, feeling, and emotion). Pathology also means a condition caused by disease.

- A **pathologist** (pah-**THOL**-oh-jist) specializes in the laboratory analysis of tissue samples removed at operations and postmortem (after death) examinations to confirm or establish a diagnosis (**path** means disease and **ologist** means specialist). A postmortem examination is also known as an **autopsy** (**AW**-top-see).

- **Etiology** (ee-tee-**OL**-oh-jee) is the study of the causes of diseases (**eti** means cause and **ology** means study of). The organisms that cause diseases are discussed in Chapter 6.

- Terms used to describe different types of diseases are summarized in Table 2.3.

Disease Transmission

- A **communicable disease** (kuh-**MEW**-nih-kuh-bul), also known as a **contagious disease**, is any disease transmitted from one person to another either by direct contact or indirectly by contact with contaminated objects.

- **Contaminated** means the possible presence of an infectious agent. Contamination may occur through a lack of proper hygiene standards such as handwashing or taking proper precautions.

- **Bloodborne transmission** is through contact with blood or body fluids that are contaminated with blood. Examples include acquired immunodeficiency syn-

(continues on page 32)

FIGURE 2.13 Exocrine glands secrete their chemical substances into ducts that lead either to other organs or out of the body. Endocrine glands pour their secretions directly into the bloodstream.

LEVEL   EXAMPLES

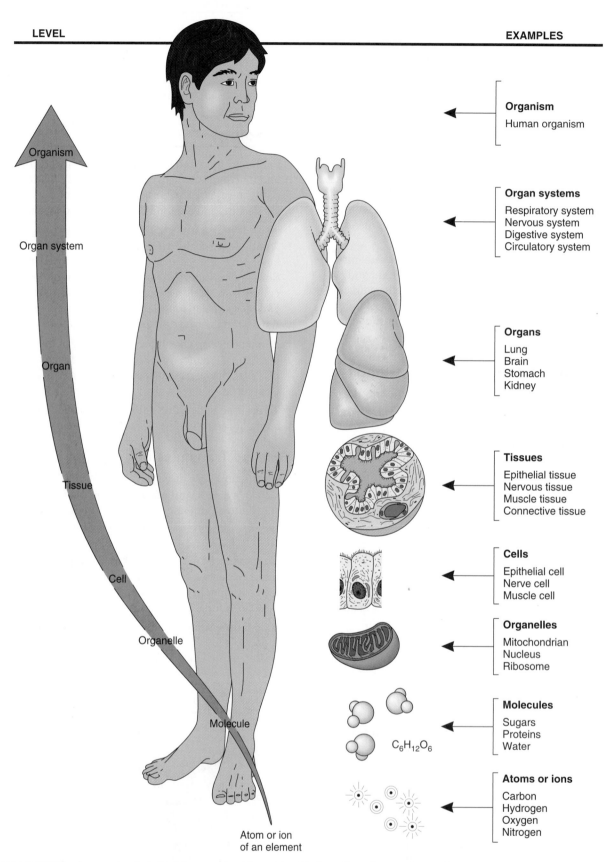

Organism
Human organism

Organ systems
Respiratory system
Nervous system
Digestive system
Circulatory system

Organs
Lung
Brain
Stomach
Kidney

Tissues
Epithelial tissue
Nervous tissue
Muscle tissue
Connective tissue

Cells
Epithelial cell
Nerve cell
Muscle cell

Organelles
Mitochondrian
Nucleus
Ribosome

Molecules
Sugars
Proteins
Water

$C_6H_{12}O_6$

Atoms or ions
Carbon
Hydrogen
Oxygen
Nitrogen

Organism

Organ system

Organ

Tissue

Cell

Organelle

Molecule

Atom or ion
of an element

FIGURE 2.14 The human body is highly organized from the single cell to the total organism.

Table 2.2

MAJOR BODY SYSTEMS

Body System	Major Structures and Related Word Parts	Major Functions
Skeletal System	bones (oste/o) joints (arthr/o) cartilage (chondr/o)	Supports and shapes the body. Protects the internal organs. Forms some blood cells and stores minerals.
Muscular System	muscles (my/o) fascia (fasci/o) tendons (ten/o, tend/o, tendin/o)	Holds the body erect. Makes movement possible. Moves body fluids and generates body heat.
Cardiovascular System	heart (card/o, cardi/o) arteries (arteri/o) veins (phleb/o, ven/o) blood (hem/o, hemat/o)	Pumps blood that carries oxygen and nutrients throughout the body. Carries liquid waste to the lungs and kidneys.
Lymphatic and Immune Systems	lymph, lymph vessels, and lymph nodes (lymph/o) tonsils (tonsill/o) spleen (splen/o) thymus (thym/o) specialized blood cells	Protects the body from harmful substances. Brings oxygen and nutrients to cells. Removes waste from the cells.
Respiratory System	nose (nas/o) pharynx (pharyng/o) trachea (trache/o) larynx (laryng/o) lungs (pneum/o, pneumon/o)	Brings oxygen into the body for transportation to the cells. Removes carbon dioxide and some water waste from the body.
Digestive System	mouth (or/o) esophagus (esophag/o) stomach (gastr/o) small intestines (enter/o) large intestines (col/o) liver (hepat/o) pancreas (pancreat/o)	Digests ingested food so it can be absorbed into the bloodstream. Eliminates solid wastes.
Urinary System	kidneys (nephr/o, ren/o) ureters (ureter/o) urinary bladder (cyst/o, vesic/o) urethra (urethr/o)	Filters blood to remove waste. Maintains the electrolyte and fluid balance within the body.
Nervous System	nerves (neur/o) brain (encephal/o) spinal cord (myel/o) eyes (ocul/o, ophthalm/o) ears (acoust/o, ot/o)	Coordinates the reception of stimuli. Transmits messages throughout the body.
Integumentary System	skin (cutane/o, dermat/o, derm/o) sebaceous glands (seb/o) sweat glands (hidr/o)	Protects the body against invasion by bacteria. Regulates the body temperature and water content.

(continues)

Table 2.2 (continued)

MAJOR BODY SYSTEMS

Body System	Major Structures and Related Word Parts	Major Functions
Endocrine System	adrenals (**adren/o**) gonads (**gonad/o**) pancreas (**pancreat/o**) pineal (**pineal/o**) pituitary (**pituit/o**) thyroid (**thyroid/o**) parathyroids (**parathyroid/o**) thymus (**thym/o**)	Integrates all body functions.
Reproductive System	**Male:** testicles (**orch/o, orchid/o**) **Female:** ovaries (**oophor/o, ovari/o**) uterus (**hyster/o, metr/o, metri/o, uter/o**)	Produces new life.

Table 2.3

TYPES OF DISEASES

An **infectious disease** (in-**FECK**-shus) is an illness caused by a pathogenic organism.

An **idiopathic disorder** (id-ee-oh-**PATH**-ick) is an illness without known cause.

In an **organic disorder** (or-**GAN**-ick) there are pathologic physical changes that explain the symptoms being experienced by the patient. As an example, a gastric ulcer is an organic disorder (see Chapter 8).

In a **functional disorder** there are no detectable physical changes to explain the symptoms being experienced by the patient. As an example, a panic attack is a functional disorder (see Chapter 10).

An **iatrogenic illness** (eye-**at**-roh-**JEN**-ick) is an unfavorable response to medical treatment for a different disorder.

A **nosocomial infection** (nos-oh-**KOH**-mee-al) is a hospital-acquired infection that was not present on admission but appears 72 hours or more after hospitalization.

drome (AIDS) and hepatitis. Bloodborne diseases are also transmitted through sexual contact. These disorders are discussed in Chapters 5 and 6.

- **Sexually transmitted diseases**, also known as **STDs** and **venereal diseases**, require direct person-to-person contact or contact with lesions. These disorders are discussed in Chapter 14.
- **Airborne transmission** is through respiratory droplets such as contact with material from the cough or sneeze. Examples include tuberculosis, influenza, colds, and measles. These disorders are discussed in Chapter 7.
- **Food and waterborne transmission**, also known as **fecal/oral transmission**, is by eating or drinking contaminated food or water that has not been prepared properly to kill the contamination. These disorders are discussed in Chapter 8.

Outbreaks of Diseases

- An **epidemiologist** (ep-ih-dee-mee-**OL**-oh-jist) specializes in the study of outbreaks of disease within a population group (epidemi means epidemic and ologist means specialist).
- **Endemic** (en-**DEM**-ick) means the ongoing presence of a disease within a population, group, or area. For example, the common cold is endemic because it is always present within the population.
- An **epidemic** (ep-ih-**DEM**-ick) is a sudden and widespread outbreak of a disease within a population group or area. For example, a sudden widespread outbreak of measles is an epidemic.
- **Pandemic** (pan-**DEM**-ick) means occurring over a large geographic area, possibly worldwide. For example, the spread of AIDS is pandemic.

Learning Exercises

● Word Part Matching—1

Write the letter of the correct answer on the line provided in the left column.

2.1. _____ adip/o

2.2. _____ aden/o

2.3. _____ caud/o

2.4. _____ cephal/o

2.5. _____ coron/o

A. crown, coronary

B. fat

C. gland

D. lower part of body

E. relating to the head

● Word Part Matching—2

Write the letter of the correct answer on the line provided in the left column.

2.6. _____ cyt/o

2.7. _____ epi-

2.8. _____ hist/o

2.9. _____ home/o

2.10. _____ lapar/o

A. abdomen

B. above

C. cell

D. constant

E. tissue

● Word Part Matching—3

Write the letter of the correct answer on the line provided in the left column.

2.11. _____ path/o

2.12. _____ retr/o

2.13. _____ -plasm

2.14. _____ co/o

2.15. _____ -stasis

A. colon

B. control

C. disease, suffering, feeling, and emotion

D. formation

E. behind

● Definitions

Circle the letter next to the correct answer.

2.16. Which term describes a hospital-acquired infection?

   a. iatrogenic

   b. idiopathic

   c. nosocomial

   d. organic

2.17. Which genetic change can be transmitted from parents to their children?

   a. cytoplasm mutation

   b. gametic cell mutation

   c. genetically engineered alterations

   d. somatic cell mutation

2.18. The dorsal cavity contains the _____ .

   a. heart and lungs

   b. major organs of digestion

   c. organs that maintain a constant internal environment

   d. structures of the central nervous system

2.19. Lateral means _____ .

   a. near the beginning of the structure

   b. near the front of the body

   c. toward the midline

   d. toward the side

2.20. Which type of tissue covers the internal and external surfaces of the body?

   a. adipose

   b. connective

   c. cytoplasm

   d. epithelial

2.21. Which genetic disorder is characterized by a missing digestive enzyme?

    a. Huntington's disease

    b. phenylketonuria

    c. Tay-Sachs

    d. trisomy 21

2.22. Which term means the surgical removal of a gland?

    a. adenectomy

    b. adenitis

    c. adenoma

    d. adenosis

2.23. Which type of peritoneum surrounds the organs located in the abdominal cavity?

    a. abdominal

    b. mesentery

    c. parietal

    d. visceral

2.24. Which structures are the biologic units of heredity?

    a. cells

    b. cytoplasm

    c. genes

    d. protoplasm

2.25. Which term describes the study of the structure, composition, and function of tissues?

    a. anatomy

    b. cytology

    c. histology

    d. pathology

● Matching Structures and Word Parts

Write the letter of the correct answer on the line provided in the left column.

2.26. _____ chondr/o   A. vein

2.27. _____ derm/o   B. uterus

2.28. _____ hyster/o   C. cartilage

2.29. _____ orchid/o   D. skin

2.30. _____ phleb/o   E. testicles

● Which Word?

Circle the correct term in each sentence.

2.31. The lower area of the abdomen is referred to as the *inguinal / umbilical* region.

2.32. The study of how traits are transferred from the parents to their children is called *genetics / histology.*

2.33. A specialist in the study of the outbreaks of disease is a/an *epidemiologist / pathologist.*

2.34. Glands that excrete their secretions through ducts are known as *endocrine / exocrine* glands.

2.35. The location of the stomach is *inferior / superior* to the diaphragm.

● Spelling Counts

Find the misspelled word in each sentence. Then write that word, spelled correctly, on the line provided.

2.36. The term hemiostasis means to maintain a constant internal environment. _____

2.37. The abdominel cavity contains primarily the major organs of digestion. _____

2.38. A bloodborn disease is transmitted through contact with blood or with body fluids that are contaminated with blood. _____

2.39. An infectous disease is an illness caused by a pathogenic organism. _____

2.40. An anamoly is any deviation from what is regarded as normal. _____

● Matching Pathology of Tissue Formation

Write the letter of the correct answer on the line provided in the left column.

2.41. _____ anaplasia

2.42. _____ aplasia

2.43. _____ dysplasia

2.44. _____ hyperplasia

2.45. _____ hypoplasia

A. Abnormal development or growth, especially of cells.

B. A change in the structure of cells and in their orientation to each other.

C. An abnormal increase in the number of normal cells in normal arrangement in a tissue.

D. Incomplete development of an organ or tissue.

E. Lack of development of an organ or tissue.

● Term Selection

Circle the letter next to the correct answer.

2.46. Which term describes the surface of a structure that is nearest the midline?

a. distal

b. lateral

c. medial

d. proximal

2.47. Which term means situated in the back?

a. anterior

b. cephalic

c. posterior

d. ventral

2.48. Which plane divides the body into front and back portions?

a. coronal

b. horizontal

c. sagittal

d. transverse

2.49. The midsagittal plane divides the body into _____ .

a. anterior and posterior portions

b. cephalic and caudal halves

c. left and right halves

d. upper and lower sections

2.50. Which end of the humerus (upper arm bone) forms part of the elbow?

a. distal

b. lateral

c. medial

d. proximal

● Sentence Completion

2.51. The inherited disorder that begins in midlife and causes the progressive loss of muscle control and mental ability is _____ disease (HD).

2.52. The study of the functions of the structures of the body is known as _____ .

2.53. Also known as the chest, the _____ cavity protects the heart and lungs.

2.54. The term meaning located behind the peritoneum is _____ .

2.55. The visual examination of the interior of the abdomen using a laparoscope is known as _____ .

● True/False

If the statement is true, write T on the line.
If the statement is false, write F on the line.

2.56. _____ Somatic cell mutation cannot be transmitted to the offspring.

2.57. _____ Deoxyribonucleic acid (DNA) is found only in sperm and ovum.

2.58. _____ Hypogastric means above the stomach.

2.59. _____ Ascites is an abnormal accumulation of watery fluid in the peritoneal cavity.

2.60. _____ The lumbar region refers to the inward curvature of the spine.

2.61. _____ An organ is a group of specialized cells that secrete fluids used elsewhere in the body.

2.62. _____ A congenital disorder is present at birth.

2.63. _____ Sickle cell anemia and sickle cell trait are two names for the same disease.

2.64. _____ Cerebral palsy is a hereditary disorder.

2.65. _____ Exocrine glands do not have ducts.

● Clinical Conditions

Write the correct answer on the line.

2.66. Mr. Lui died of cholera during a sudden and widespread outbreak of this disease in his country. Such an outbreak is described as being a/an _____ .

2.67. Brenda Farmer's doctor could not find any physical changes to explain her symptoms. The doctor refers to this as a/an _____ disorder.

2.68. Gerald Carlson inherited a bleeding disorder in which one of the clotting factors is missing. This disease, which he inherited from his mother, is known as _____ .

2.69. Wally Foster has a kidney disease. His doctor is performing tests to determine the cause or _____ of this illness.

2.70. Mrs. Reynolds has an inflammation of the peritoneum. The medical term for this condition is _____ .

2.71. On a camping trip Ralph Jenkins drank contaminated water. Now he is very sick and his doctor says he contracted the illness through _____ transmission.

2.72. Jose Ortega complained of pain in the lower right area of his abdomen. Using the system that divides the abdomen into four sections his doctor recorded this as being in the lower right _____ .

2.73. Tracy Ames has an inflammation within the area formed by the hipbones. Her doctor describes this area as the _____ cavity.

2.74. In college Gerald McClelland wants to learn more about the structure and functions of cells. To accomplish this he has signed up for a course in _____ .

2.75. Ashley Goldberg is fascinated by how traits and characteristics are transmitted. She wants to specialize in the this field and is studying to become a/an _____ .

● Which is the Correct Term?

2.76. Scott Asbury has pain in the lower left quadrant. Which term is also used to describe this area?

   a. groin or inguinal area

   b. hypochondriac region

   c. lumbar region

   d. umbilical region

2.77. Which genetic disorder is also known as trisomy 21?

   a. Down syndrome

   b. fetal alcohol syndrome

   c. hemophilia

   d. phenylketonuria

2.78. Roger and Beth are expecting! Roger has sickle cell trait and Beth does not. Which statement is true about their baby?

   a. It is possible that the child will not inherit sickle cell trait.

   b. Because Beth does not have sickle cell trait, the child cannot have it.

   c. Because Roger has sickle cell trait, the child will definitely have it.

   d. The child will have sickle cell anemia.

2.79. Which one the following is liquid connective tissue?

   a. blood

   b. epithelial tissue

   c. muscle

   d. nerve

2.80. The word part **esophag/o** means esophagus. This structure is part of the _____ system?

   a. cardiovascular

   b. digestive

   c. respiratory

   d. urinary

● Challenge Word Building

This group of exercises provides an opportunity to work with the word parts you have learned in Chapters 1 and 2. To answer the question, combine the appropriate parts. While doing this, pay attention to the use of combining vowels! You may want to look in the glossary or use a medical dictionary to check your answers.

gastr/o = stomach   **-algia** = pain
laryng/o = larynx   **-ectomy** = surgical removal
my/o = muscle   **-itis** = inflammation
nephr/o = kidney   **-osis** = abnormal condition
neur/o = nerve   **-plasty** = surgical repair

2.81. The medical term meaning the surgical repair of a muscle is _____ .

2.82. The medical term meaning pain in a nerve is _____ .

2.83. The medical term meaning an abnormal condition of the stomach is _____ .

2.84. The medical term meaning inflammation of the larynx is _____ .

2.85. The medical term meaning the surgical removal of part of a muscle is a/an _____ .

2.86. The medical term meaning pain in the stomach is _____ .

2.87. The medical term meaning surgical removal the larynx is _____ .

2.88. The medical term meaning an abnormal condition of the kidney is _____ .

2.89. The medical term meaning surgical repair of a nerve is _____ .

2.90. The medical term meaning inflammation of the kidney is _____ .

● Labeling Exercises

Identify the numbered items on these diagrams.

2.91. This is the _____ _____ region.

2.92. This is the _____ region.

2.93. This is the _____ region.

2.94. This is the _____ _____ region.

2.95. This is the _____ _____ region.

2.96. This is the midline or _____ plane.

2.97. This is known as the ventral or _____ surface.

2.98. This arrow is pointing in a/an _____ direction.

2.99. This is known as the dorsal or _____ surface.

2.100. This is the frontal or _____ plane.

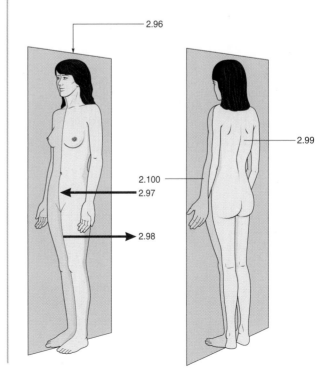

The Human Touch: Critical Thinking Exercise

The following story and questions are designed to stimulate critical thinking through class discussion or as a brief essay response. There are no easy or right-wrong answers to these questions.

Tahriah and Justise Brown have three wonderful children. The oldest is in her second year at the community college. The middle one plays third base for his high school varsity team, and the youngest is a freshman with an eye on the tennis team. The Browns are looking forward to planning weddings and spoiling "grand-babies." But then, at age 44, Tahriah discovers she is pregnant.

Her obstetrician, Dr. Makay, suggests performing genetic testing using amniotic fluid gathered by a procedure called amniocentesis. He tells her, "Technical advances allow a glimpse into the womb to discover genetic anomalies. Because of your age, Tahriah, I am concerned about Down syndrome." He waits, gauging her reaction, then continues.

"This genetic disorder causes various degrees of mental retardation and physical defects. Severe cases produce a child unable to feed or care for itself. Life-threatening physical defects may require expensive, painful surgical procedures. Although they do exhibit the typical Down's facial appearance, some of these children display only marginal symptoms and function within societal norms."

Dr. Makay discusses choices the Browns would need to make if genetic testing indicates Down syndrome. Finally he says, "We can detect its presence, but not the degree or severity. Don't decide now. Go home, talk with your family, and call me soon with your decision."

Tahriah, Justise, and their children discuss the possibilities that amniocentesis presents. They talk late into the night. The decision is difficult, but in the morning Tahriah calls Dr. Makay to . . .

Suggested Discussion Topics:

1. Discuss the challenges a Down syndrome child would present to the Brown family.

2. Genetic testing can determine gender, negative and positive genetic characteristics, and whether or not a fetus will grow up to have a high risk of certain diseases (such as breast cancer). Discuss how this type of information could be used by parents, health care providers, and insurance companies.

3. Discuss the options available to Tahriah if the genetic test is positive for Down syndrome.

4. If you knew that your genes could cause your child to be born with a severe handicap, would you want to know? Why or why not?

5. Children with severe handicaps require expensive care whether they live at home or in an institution. Who should pay for this burden and why?

Word Part Review

In the first two chapters you were introduced to many prefixes, word roots (combining forms), and suffixes. As you study the body system chapters, you will learn even more word parts as they relate to each system. Your study of the body systems will be much easier if you have mastered *at least* the word parts in this section.

These questions give you additional word part practice plus opportunities to work with the correct use of combining vowels and building unfamiliar terms based on familiar word parts.

The 50-question post-test at the end of this section enables you to evaluate your mastery of these word parts.

WORD PART PRACTICE SESSION

● **Matching Word Parts**

Write the letter of the correct answer on the line provided in the left column.

WP.1. _____ dys-   A. within, inside

WP.2. _____ hyper-   B. between, among

WP.3. _____ hypo-   C. excessive, increased

WP.4. _____ inter-   D. deficient, decreased

WP.5. _____ intra-   E. bad, difficult, painful

● **Matching Word Parts**

Write the letter of the correct answer on the line provided in the left column.

WP.6. _____ pre-   A. above, excessive

WP.7. _____ peri-   B. before

WP.8. _____ poly-   C. many

WP.9. _____ sub-   D. surrounding

WP.10. _____ supra-   E. under, less, below

● **Matching Word Parts**

Write the letter of the correct answer on the line provided in the left column.

WP.11. _____ -algia   A. inflammation

WP.12. _____ -centesis B. pain, suffering

WP.13. _____ -ectomy   C. recording a picture or record

WP.14. _____ -itis   D. surgical puncture to remove fluid

WP.15. _____ -graphy   E. surgical removal

● **Matching Word Parts**

Write the letter of the correct answer on the line provided in the left column.

WP.16. _____ -dynia   A. surgical repair

WP.17. _____ -malacia   B. abnormal softening.

WP.18. _____ -necrosis C. pain

WP.19. _____ -oma   D. tissue death

WP.20. _____ -plasty   E. tumor or neoplasm

● **Matching Word Parts**

Write the letter of the correct answer on the line provided in the left column.

WP.21. _____ -ac   A. abnormal condition, disease

WP.22. _____ -ostomy   B. abnormal hardening

WP.23. _____ -osis   C. cutting, surgical incision

WP.24. _____ -otomy   D. pertaining to

WP.25. _____ -sclerosis E. surgical creation of an opening

● **Matching Word Parts**

Write the letter of the correct answer on the line provided in the left column.

WP.26. _____ -rrhagia, -rrhage   A. abnormal flow, discharge

WP.27. _____ -rrhaphy   B. abnormal tightening or narrowing

WP.28. _____ -rrhea   C. bleeding

WP.29. _____ -rrhexis   D. rupture

WP.30. _____ -stenosis E. to suture

● **True/False**

If the statement is true, write T on the line. If the statement is false, write F on the line.

WP.31. _____ myc/o means mucous.

WP.32. _____ peri- means surrounding.

WP.33. _____ hyper- means below, under, decreased.

WP.34. _____ ather/o means plaque or fatty substance.

WP.35. _____ -gram means an instrument for recording.

WP.36. _____ arthr/o means joint.

WP.37. _____ **cardi/o** means heart.

WP.38. _____ **gastr/o** means kidney.

WP.39. _____ **-centesis** means to see or a visual examination.

● Word Building

WP.40. **rhin/o** means nose. The medical term for an abnormal flow commonly known as a runny nose is _____ .

WP.41. **nephr/o** means kidney. The term meaning the surgical removal of a kidney is a/an _____ .

WP.42. **ot/o** means ear. The term meaning inflammation of the ear is _____ .

WP.43. **cardi/o** means heart. The term meaning an enlarged heart is _____ .

WP.44. **hepat/o** means liver. The term meaning inflammation of the liver is _____ .

WP.45. **arthr/o** means joint. The term meaning the visual examination of the interior of a joint is _____ .

WP.46. **ur/o** means urine. The study of the urinary system is known as _____ .

WP.47. **hemat/o** means blood. A specialist in disorders of the blood is known as a/an _____ .

WP.48. **col/o** means colon. A surgical incision into the colon is a/an _____ .

WP.49. **phleb/o** means vein. The medical term meaning inflammation of a vein is _____ .

WP.50. **electr/o** means electric and **cardi/o** means heart. A record of the electrical activity of the heart is called an ECG or a/an _____ .

WORD PART POST-TEST

Write the word part in the space below.

PT.1. The suffix meaning surgical removal is _____ .

PT.2. The prefix meaning excessive, increased is _____ .

PT.3. The suffix meaning surgical repair is _____ .

PT.4. The suffix meaning enlargement is _____ .

PT.5. The word root (combining form) meaning bone marrow or spinal cord is _____ .

PT.6. The word root (combining form) meaning muscle is _____ .

PT.7. The prefix meaning between, among is _____ .

PT.8. The word root (combining form) meaning nerve is _____ .

PT.9. The suffix meaning to see or a visual examination is _____ .

PT.10. The suffix meaning the study of is _____ .

● Matching Word Parts

Write the letter of the correct answer on the line provided in the left column.

PT.11. _____ **arteri/o**   A. tumor

PT.12. _____ **-oma**   B. to suture

PT.13. _____ **peri-**   C. surrounding

PT.14. _____ **-rrhaphy**   D. rupture

PT.15. _____ **-rrhexis**   E. artery

● Matching Word Parts

Write the letter of the correct answer on the line provided in the left column.

PT.16. _____ **-itis**   A. abnormal hardening

PT.17. _____ **neo-**   B. ear

PT.18. _____ **-ologist**   C. inflammation

PT.19. _____ **ot/o**   D. new

PT.20. _____ **-sclerosis**   E. specialist

● True/False

If the statement is true, write T on the line. If the statement is false, write F on the line.

PT.21. _____ **hem/o** means blood.

PT.22. _____ **-algia** means pain.

PT.23. _____ **oste/o** means bone.

PT.24. _____ **dys-** means abnormal.

PT.25. _____ **hepat/o** means liver.

PT.26. _____ **Tonsillitis** is an inflammation of the tonsils.

PT.27. _____ A **myectomy** is a surgical incision into a muscle.

PT.28. _____ **Gastralgia** means a pain in the stomach.

PT.29. _____ A **gerontologist** specializes in the diseases of women.

PT.30. _____ **Gastritis** is an enlargement of the stomach.

● Word Building

Regarding Nerves (**neur/o** means nerve)

PT.31. A surgical incision into a nerve is a
_____ .

PT.32. A benign tumor made up of nerve tissue is a
_____ .

PT.33. The surgical repair of a nerve or nerves is
_____ .

PT.34. The term meaning to suture the ends of a severed nerve is _____ .

PT.35. Abnormal softening of the nerves is called
_____ .

PT.36. A specialist in diagnosing and treating disorders of the nervous system is a/an
_____ .

PT.37. The term meaning inflammation of a nerve or nerves is _____ .

Relating to Blood Vessels (**angi/o** means relating to the blood vessels)

PT.38. The death of the walls of blood vessels is
_____ .

PT.39. The abnormal hardening of the walls of blood vessels is _____ .

PT.40. The abnormal narrowing of a blood vessel is
_____ .

PT.41. The surgical removal of a blood vessel is a/an
_____ .

PT.42. The process of recording a picture of an artery is called _____ .

● Missing Words

Write the missing word on the line.

PT.43. **arteri/o** means artery. The surgical repair of an artery is a/an_____ .

PT.44. **laryng/o** means larynx. The medical term meaning inflammation of the larynx is
_____ .

PT.45. **col/o** means colon. The surgical removal of all or part of the colon is a/an
_____ .

PT.46. **my/o** means muscle. The abnormal softening of muscle tissue is _____ .

PT.47. **gastr/o** means stomach. The term meaning any abnormal condition of the stomach is
_____ .

PT.48. **cardi/o** means heart. The term meaning the study of the heart is _____ .

PT.49. **col/o** means colon. The term meaning inflammation of the colon is _____ .

PT.50. **phleb/o** means vein. A surgical incision into a vein is _____ .

The Skeletal System

3

● **Overview of Structures, Word Parts, and Functions of the Skeletal System**

MAJOR STRUCTURES	RELATED WORD ROOTS	PRIMARY FUNCTIONS
Bones	oss/e, oss/i, oste/o, ost/o	Act as the framework for the body, protect the internal organs, and store the mineral calcium.
Bone marrow	myel/o *(also means spinal cord)*	Forms some blood cells.
Cartilage	chondr/o	Creates a smooth surface for motion within the joints and protect the ends of bones.
Ligaments	ligament/o	Connects one bone to another.
Joints	arthr/o	Work with the muscles to make a variety of motions possible.
Synovial membrane	synovi/o, synov/o	Forms the lining of synovial joints and secretes synovial fluid.
Synovial fluid	synovi/o, synov/o	Lubricant to make smooth joint movements possible.
Bursa	burs/o	Cushions areas subject to friction during movement.

● VOCABULARY   Related to the Skeletal System

Check the box as you master each word part or term. Terms marked with the ❖ symbol are pronounced on the optional student audiotape.

Word Parts

- [ ] ankyl/o
- [ ] arthr/o
- [ ] chondr/o
- [ ] cost/o
- [ ] crani/o
- [ ] -desis
- [ ] kyph/o
- [ ] lord/o
- [ ] -lysis
- [ ] myel/o
- [ ] oss/e, oss/i, ost/o, oste/o
- [ ] -poietic
- [ ] spondyl/o
- [ ] -um

Key Medical Terms

- [ ] **allogenic** (**al**-oh-**JEN**-ick) ❖
- [ ] **ankylosing spondylitis** (**ang**-kih-**LOH**-sing spon-dih-**LYE**-tis) ❖
- [ ] **ankylosis** (**ang**-kih-**LOH**-sis) ❖
- [ ] **arthrocentesis** (**ar**-throh-sen-**TEE**-sis) ❖
- [ ] **arthrodesis** (ar-throh-**DEE**-sis) ❖
- [ ] **arthrolysis** (ar-**THROL**-ih-sis) ❖
- [ ] **arthroplasty** (**AR**-throh-**plas**-tee) ❖
- [ ] **arthrosclerosis** (ar-throh-skleh-**ROH**-sis) ❖
- [ ] **arthroscopic** (ar-throh-**SKOP**-ick)
- [ ] **arthroscopy** (ar-**THROS**-koh-pee) ❖
- [ ] **autologous** (aw-**TOL**-uh-guss) ❖
- [ ] **bursectomy** (ber-**SECK**-toh-mee) ❖
- [ ] **bursitis** (ber-**SIGH**-tis) ❖
- [ ] **callus** (**KAL**-us) ❖
- [ ] **chondroma** (kon-**DROH**-mah) ❖
- [ ] **chondromalacia** (**kon**-droh-mah-**LAY**-shee-ah) ❖
- [ ] **chondroplasty** (**KON**-droh-**plas**-tee) ❖
- [ ] **comminuted** (**KOM**-ih-**newt**-ed) ❖
- [ ] **craniectomy** (kray-nee-**EK**-toh-mee) ❖
- [ ] **cranioplasty** (**KRAY**-nee-oh-**plas**-tee) ❖
- [ ] **crepitation** (**krep**-ih-**TAY**-shun)
- [ ] **crepitus** (**KREP**-ih-tus) ❖
- [ ] **cruciate** (**KROO**-shee-ayt)
- [ ] **Ewing's sarcoma** (**YOU**-ingz sar-**KOH**-mah) ❖
- [ ] **exostosis** (**eck**-sos-**TOH**-sis) ❖
- [ ] **fontanel** (**fon**-tah-**NELL**)
- [ ] **gouty arthritis** (**GOW**-tee ar-**THRIGH**-tis) ❖
- [ ] **hallux valgus** (**HAL**-ucks **VAL**-guss) ❖
- [ ] **hematopoietic** (**hee**-mah-toh-poi-**ET**-ick *or* **hem**-ah-toh-poi-**ET**-ick)
- [ ] **kyphosis** (kye-**FOH**-sis) ❖

- [ ] **laminectomy** (**lam**-ih-**NECK**-toh-mee) ❖
- [ ] **lordosis** (lor-**DOH**-sis) ❖
- [ ] **lumbago** (lum-**BAY**-goh) ❖
- [ ] **luxation** (luck-**SAY**-shun) ❖
- [ ] **manubrium** (mah-**NEW**-bree-um)
- [ ] **maxillary** (**MACK**-sih-**ler**-ee)
- [ ] **myeloma** (**my**-eh-**LOH**-mah) ❖
- [ ] **orthopedist** (**or**-thoh-**PEE**-dist) ❖
- [ ] **orthotics** (or-**THOT**-icks) ❖
- [ ] **ostectomy** (oss-**TECK**-toh-mee)
- [ ] **osteitis** (oss-tee-**EYE**-tis) ❖
- [ ] **osteitis deformans** (oss-tee-**EYE**-tis dee-**FOR**-manz)
- [ ] **osteoarthritis** (oss-tee-oh-ar-**THRIGH**-tis) ❖
- [ ] **osteochondroma** (oss-tee-oh-kon-**DROH**-mah) ❖
- [ ] **osteoclasis** (oss-tee-**OCK**-lah-sis) ❖
- [ ] **osteomalacia** (oss-tee-oh-mah-**LAY**-shee-ah) ❖
- [ ] **osteomyelitis** (oss-tee-oh-**my**-eh-**LYE**-tis) ❖
- [ ] **osteonecrosis** (oss-tee-oh-neh-**KROH**-sis) ❖
- [ ] **osteoplasty** (**OSS**-tee-oh-**plas**-tee) ❖
- [ ] **osteoporosis** (oss-tee-oh-poh-**ROH**-sis) ❖
- [ ] **osteorrhaphy** (oss-tee-**OR**-ah-fee) ❖
- [ ] **osteotomy** (oss-tee-**OT**-oh-mee) ❖
- [ ] **Paget's** (**PAJ**-its) ❖
- [ ] **patella** (pah-**TEL**-ah)
- [ ] **percutaneous diskectomy** (**per**-kyou-**TAY**-nee-us dis-**KECK**-toh-mee) ❖
- [ ] **periosteotomy** (**pehr**-ee-oss-tee-**OT**-oh-mee) ❖
- [ ] **periosteum** (**pehr**-ee-**OSS**-tee-um)
- [ ] **periostitis** (**pehr**-ee-oss-**TYE**-tis) ❖
- [ ] **podiatrist** (poh-**DYE**-ah-trist) ❖
- [ ] **popliteal** (pop-**LIT**-ee-al)
- [ ] **rheumatoid arthritis** (**ROO**-mah-toyd ar-**THRIGH**-tis) ❖
- [ ] **rheumatologist** (roo-mah-**TOL**-oh-jist) ❖
- [ ] **rickets** (**RICK**-ets) ❖
- [ ] **sacroiliac** (**say**-kroh-**ILL**-ee-ack)
- [ ] **scoliosis** (skoh-lee-**OH**-sis) ❖
- [ ] **spina bifida** (**SPY**-nah **BIF**-ih-dah) ❖
- [ ] **spondylitis** (spon-dih-**LYE**-tis) ❖
- [ ] **spondylolisthesis** (spon-dih-loh-liss-**THEE**-sis) ❖
- [ ] **spondylosis** (spon-dih-**LOH**-sis) ❖
- [ ] **subluxation** (sub-luck-**SAY**-shun)
- [ ] **synovectomy** (sin-oh-**VECK**-toh-mee) ❖
- [ ] **synovitis** (sin-oh-**VYE**-tiss) ❖
- [ ] **talipes** (**TAL**-ih-peez) ❖
- [ ] **vertebrae** (**VER**-teh-bray *or* **VER**-teh-bree) ❖
- [ ] **vertebral** (**VER**-tee-bral *or* **VER**-teh-bral)

● OBJECTIVES

On completion of this chapter, you should be able to:

1 Identify and describe the major functions and structures of the skeletal system.

2 Describe three types of joints.

3 Differentiate between the axial and appendicular skeletons.

4 Identify the medical specialists who treat disorders of the skeletal system.

5 Recognize, define, spell, and pronounce terms related to the pathology and diagnostic and treatment procedures of the skeletal system.

Functions of the Skeletal System

The skeletal system has many important functions.

- Bones act as the framework of the body.
- Bones support and protect the internal organs.
- Joints, in conjunction with muscles, ligaments, and tendons make possible the wide variety of body movements.
- Calcium required for normal nerve and muscle function is stored in bones.
- Red bone marrow, which is located in spongy bone, has an important function in the formation of blood.

Structures of the Skeletal System

The structures of the skeletal system include bones, cartilage, ligaments, joints, and bursa.

The Structure of Bones

Bone is a form of connective tissue and is almost the hardest tissue in the human body (only dental enamel is harder).

The Tissues of Bone

Although it is very hard and dense, bone is a living structure that changes and is capable of healing itself. The tissues that make up a bone are summarized in Table 3.1.

Bone Marrow

- **Red bone marrow**, located within the spongy bone, is hematopoietic and manufactures red blood cells, hemoglobin, white blood cells, and megakaryocytes that produce thrombocytes. These types of blood cells are discussed in Chapter 5. ■ **Caution:** The word part **myel/o** means either bone marrow *or* spinal cord.

  Hematopoietic (**hee**-mah-toh-poi-**ET**-ick *or* hem-ah-toh-poi-**ET**-ick) means pertaining to the formation of blood cells (**hemato** means blood and **poietic** means

Table 3.1

TISSUES OF A BONE	
Periosteum (**pehr**-ee-**OSS**-tee-um)	The tough, fibrous tissue that forms the outermost covering of bone (**peri** means surrounding, **oste** means bone, and **um** is a noun ending).
Compact Bone	The hard, dense, and very strong bone that forms the outer layer of the bones.
Spongy Bone	Lighter and not as strong as compact bone, it is commonly found in ends and inner portions of long bones such as the femur. Red bone marrow is located within this spongy bone.
Medullary Cavity (**MED**-you-**lehr**-ee)	Located in the shaft of a long bone, the medullary cavity is surrounded by compact bone, lined with **endosteum** (en-**DOS**-tee-um), and contains yellow bone marrow.

pertaining to formation). The term **hemopoietic** (hee-moh-poy-**ET**-ick) also means pertaining to the formation of blood cells (**hemo** means blood and **poietic** means pertaining to formation).

- **Yellow bone marrow**, found in medullary cavity, is composed chiefly of fat cells and functions as a fat storage area.

Cartilage

- **Cartilage** (**KAR**-tih-lidj) is the smooth, rubbery blue-white connective tissue that acts as a shock absorber between bones. Cartilage, which is more elastic than bone, makes up the flexible parts of the skeleton such as the outer ear and the tip of the nose.

- **Articular cartilage** (ar-**TICK**-you-lar **KAR**-tih-lidj) covers the surfaces of bones that form joints to make smooth joint movement possible and to protect the bones from rubbing against each other (see Figure 3.1 on the proximal epiphysis and in Figure 3.5).

- The **meniscus** (meh-**NIS**-kus) is the curved fibrous cartilage found in some joints, such as the knee and the temporomandibular joint of the jaw (see Figure 3.4).

Anatomic Landmarks of a Bone

- The **diaphysis** (dye-**AF**-ih-sis) is the shaft of a long bone (see Figure 3.1).

- The **epiphysis** (eh-**PIF**-ih-sis), which is covered with articular cartilage, is the wide end of a long bone.

- The **proximal epiphysis** is the end of the bone that is located nearest to the midline of the body.

- The **distal epiphysis** is the end of the bone that is located farthest away from the midline.

- A **foramen** (foh-**RAY**-men) is an opening in a bone through which blood vessels, nerves, and ligaments pass. (Plural, **foramina**.) For example, the spinal cord runs through the vertebral foramen shown in Figure 3.13.

- A **process** is a normal projection on the surface of a bone that serves as attachments for muscles and tendons. For example, the mastoid process is a bony projection located on each temporal bone just behind the ear (see Figure 3.9).

Joints

Joints, also known as **articulations**, are connections between bones.

- As used here, the term **articulate** (ar-**TICK**-you-late) means to join or to come together in a manner that allows motion between the parts.

- Articulate also means to speak clearly.

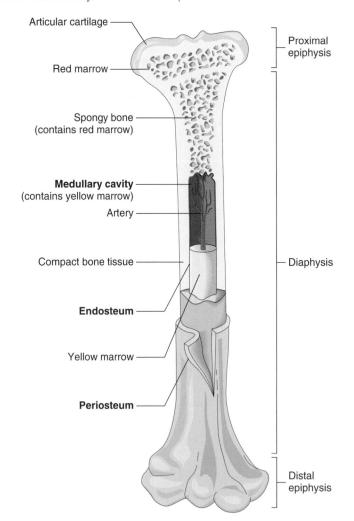

Articular cartilage

Red marrow

Spongy bone (contains red marrow)

Medullary cavity (contains yellow marrow)

Artery

Compact bone tissue

Endosteum

Yellow marrow

Periosteum

Proximal epiphysis

Diaphysis

Distal epiphysis

FIGURE 3.1 Anatomic features of a typical long bone.

Types of Joints

Different types of joints make a wide range of motions possible. These include sutures, symphyses, and synovial joints.

Sutures

- A **suture** is the jagged line where bones join and form a joint that does not move. (Suture also means to stitch.) Figure 3.2 shows the coronal and sagittal sutures across the top of the skull in an adult.
- On a baby's head the **fontanel** (**fon**-tah-**NELL**), also known as the **soft spot**, is where the sutures between the frontal and parietal bones have not yet closed. This disappears as the child grows and the sutures close. (This is also spelled **fontanelle**.)

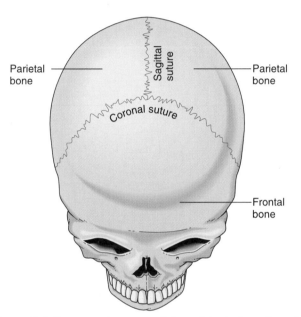

FIGURE 3.2 Bones and sutures of the adult skull as viewed from above.

Symphyses

- A **symphysis** (**SIM**-fih-sis), also known as a **cartilaginous joint** (**kar**-tih-**LADJ**-ih-nus), is where two bones join and are held firmly together so that they function as one bone. For example the pubic symphysis as shown in Figure 3.15.

Synovial Joints

- **Synovial joints** (sih-**NOH**-vee-al) are the movable joints of the body. Although these joints are described in simple terms, they are actually very complex structures (Figure 3.3).
- **Ball and socket joints**, such as the hips and shoulders, are synovial joints that allow a wide range of movement in many directions (Figure 3.3A).
- **Hinge joints**, such as the knees and elbows, are synovial joints that allow movement primarily in one direction or plane (Figure 3.3B and C).

Structures of Synovial Joints

Ligaments

- A **ligament** (**LIG**-ah-ment) is a band of fibrous connective tissue that connects one bone to another bone (Figure 3.4)
- Be careful not to confuse ligaments and tendons. A **tendon** attaches a muscle to bone. Tendons are discussed in Chapter 4.

Synovial Membrane and Fluid

- Synovial joints are surrounded by a fibrous capsule and are lined with synovial membrane. The synovial membrane secretes synovial fluid that acts as a lubricant to make the smooth movement of the joint possible (Figure 3.5).

Bursa

- A **bursa** (**BER**-sah) is a fibrous sac that is lined with a synovial membrane and contains synovial fluid. A

FIGURE 3.3 Examples of synovial joints. (A) Ball and socket joint of the hip. (B) Hinge joint of the elbow. (C) Hinge joint of the knee.

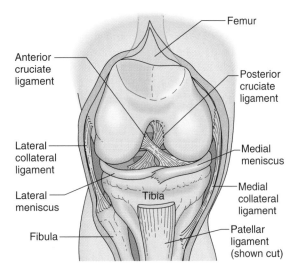

FIGURE 3.4 Major ligaments of the knee. This schematic representation, with the patella removed, shows the complex system of ligaments that make movement of the knee possible.

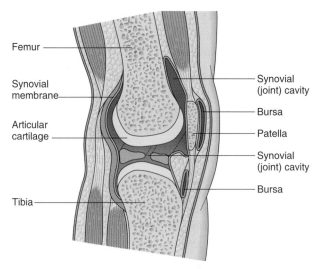

FIGURE 3.5 Structures of a synovial joint and bursa. (This is a lateral view of the knee.)

bursa acts as a cushion to ease movement in areas that are subject to friction such as in shoulder, elbow, and knee joints where a tendon passes over a bone (see Figures 3.5 and 4.16). (The plural of bursa is **bursae**.)

The Skeleton

The 206 bones in the adult human body are shown in Figures 3.6, 3.7, and 3.8. For descriptive purposes, the skeleton is divided into the axial and appendicular skeletal systems.

Axial Skeleton

- The **axial skeleton** (80 bones) protects the major organs of the nervous, respiratory, and circulatory systems. The term axial refers to an imaginary line or axis that runs through the center of the body.
- The axial skeleton consists of the skull, spinal column, ribs, and sternum.

Appendicular Skeleton

- The **appendicular skeleton** (126 bones) makes body movement possible and also protects the organs of digestion, excretion, and reproduction. The term appendicular means referring to an appendage, which is anything that is attached to a major part of the body.
- The appendicular skeleton is organized into the **upper extremities** (shoulders, arms, forearms, wrists, and hands) and the **lower extremities** (hips, thighs, legs, ankles, and feet.)

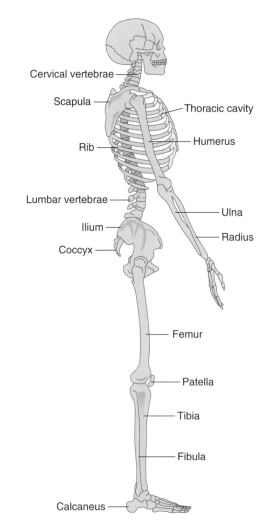

FIGURE 3.6 Lateral view of the adult human skeleton.

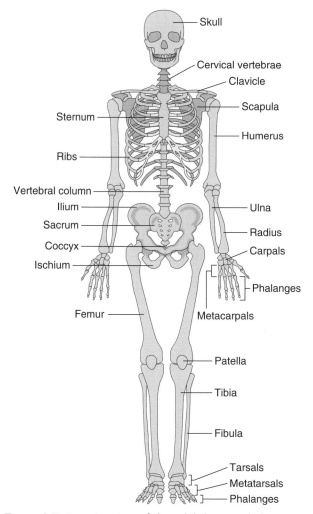

FIGURE 3.7 Anterior view of the adult human skeleton.

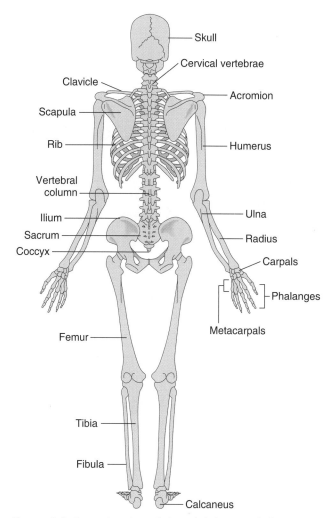

FIGURE 3.8 Posterior view of the adult human skeleton.

Bones of the Skull

As you study the following bones of the skull, refer to Figures 3.9, and 3.10.

Bones of the Cranium

- The **cranium** (**KRAY**-nee-um) is the portion of the skull that encloses the brain (**crani** means skull and **um** is a noun ending). The cranium is made up of the following bones.
- The **frontal bone** forms the forehead.
- The **parietal bones** (pah-**RYE**-eh-tal) form most of the roof and upper sides of the cranium.
- The **occipital bone** (ock-**SIP**-ih-tal) forms the posterior floor and walls of the cranium. The spinal cord passes through the **foramen magnum** of the occipital bone.
- The **temporal bones** form the sides and base of the cranium.

- The **sphenoid bone** (**SFEE**-noid) forms part of the base of the skull and parts of the floor and sides of the bony socket surrounding and protecting the eyeball.
- The **ethmoid bone** (**ETH**-moid) forms part of the nose, the orbit, and the floor of the cranium.

Auditory Ossicles

- The **auditory ossicles** (**OSS**-ih-kulz), which are the bones of the middle ear, are discussed in Chapter 11.
- The **external auditory meatus** (mee-**AY**-tus), which is the external opening of the ear, is located in the temporal bone.

Bones of the Face

- The **zygomatic bones** (zye-goh-**MAT**-ick), also known as the **cheekbones**, articulate with the frontal bones.
- The **maxillary bones** (**MACK**-sih-**ler**-ee) form most of the upper jaw.

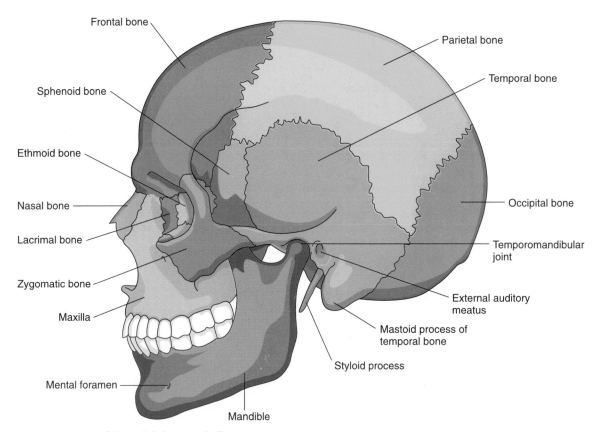

FIGURE 3.9 Lateral view of the adult human skull.

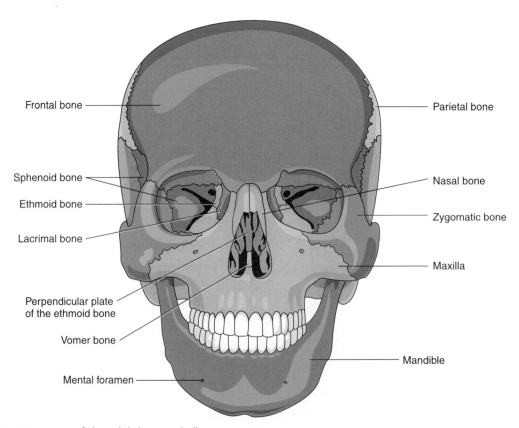

FIGURE 3.10 Anterior view of the adult human skull.

- The **palatine bones** (**PAL**-ah-tine) form part of the hard palate of the mouth and the floor of the nose.
- The **lacrimal bones** (**LACK**-rih-mal) make up part of the orbit at the inner angle of the eye.
- The **inferior conchae** (**KONG**-kee *or* **KONG**-kay) are the thin, scroll-like bones that form part of the interior of the nose (singular, **concha**).
- The **vomer bone** (**VOH**-mer) forms the base for the nasal septum. The **nasal septum** is the cartilage structure that divides the two nasal cavities and forms the base of the nose.
- The **mandible** (**MAN**-dih-bul), also known as the **lower jawbone**, is the only movable bone of the skull. The mandible is attached to the skull at the **temporomandibular joint** (**tem**-poh-roh-man-**DIB**-you-lar), which is also known as the **TMJ**.
- The **hyoid bone** (**HIGH**-oid) is unique in that it does not articulate with any other bone. Instead it is suspended between the mandible and the laryngopharynx (see Figure 7.5).

Thoracic Cavity, Ribs, and Sternum

Thoracic Cavity
- The **thoracic cavity** (thoh-**RAS**-ick) is made up of the ribs, sternum, and thoracic vertebrae (see Figure 3.6). Also known as the **rib cage**, this structure protects the heart and lungs.

Ribs
- There are 12 pairs of ribs, called **costals** (**KOSS**-tulz), that attach posteriorly to the thoracic vertebrae (**cost** means rib and **al** means pertaining to).
- The first 7 pairs of ribs, called **true ribs**, are attached anteriorly to the sternum (Figure 3.11).
- The next 3 pairs of ribs, called **false ribs**, are attached anteriorly to cartilage that joins with the sternum.
- The last 2 pairs of ribs, called **floating ribs**, are not attached anteriorly.

Sternum
- The **sternum** (**STER**-num), also known as the **breastbone**, forms the middle of the front of the rib cage. It is divided into three parts. (see Figure 3.11).
- The **manubrium** (mah-**NEW**-bree-um), which is bone, is the upper portion of the sternum.
- The **body** of the sternum, which is bone, is the middle portion of the sternum.
- The **xiphoid process** (**ZIF**-oid), which is cartilage, is the lower portion of the sternum.

Shoulders

As you study the bones of the shoulder, refer to Figures 3.8 and 3.11.

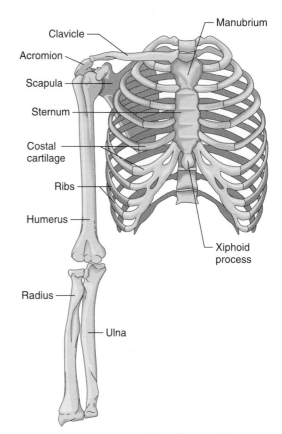

FIGURE 3.11 Anterior view of the ribs, shoulder, and arm. (Cartilage structures are shown in blue.)

- The shoulders form the **pectoral girdle** (**PECK**-toh-rahl), also known as the **shoulder girdle**, that supports the arms and hands. (As used here, the term **girdle** means a structure that encircles the body.)
- The **clavicle** (**KLAV**-ih-kul), also known as the **collar bone**, is a slender bone that connects the sternum to the scapula.
- The **scapula** (**SKAP**-you-lah) is also known as the **shoulder blade** (plural, **scapulae**).
- The **acromion** (ah-**KROH**-mee-on) is an extension of the scapula that forms the high point of the shoulder.

Arms

As you study the following bones of the arms, refer to Figures 3.11 and 3.12.
- The **humerus** (**HEW**-mer-us) is the bone of the upper arm (plural, **humeri**).
- The **radius** (**RAY**-dee-us) is the smaller bone in the forearm. The radius runs up the thumb side of the forearm.
- The **ulna** (**ULL**-nah) is the larger bone of the forearm. It articulates with the humerus to form the elbow joint.
- The **olecranon process** (oh-**LEK**-rah-non), commonly known as the **funny bone**, is a large projection on the upper end of the ulna that forms the point of the elbow that tingles when struck.

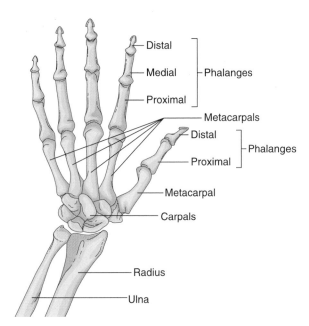

FIGURE 3.12 Dorsal view of the bones of the lower left arm, wrist, and hand.

Wrists and Hands

As you study the following bones of the wrists and hands, refer to Figure 3.12.

- The **carpals** (**KAR**-palz) are the bones of the wrist.
- The **metacarpals** (met-ah-**KAR**-palz) are the bones that form the palm of the hand.
- The **phalanges** (fah-**LAN**-jeez) are the bones of the fingers (and of the toes) (singular, **phalanx**).
- Each finger has three bones. These are the **distal** (outermost), **medial** (middle), and **proximal** (nearest the hand) phalanges.
- The thumb has only **distal** and **proximal** phalanges.

Spinal Column

- The **spinal column** is also known as the **vertebral column** (VER-teh-bral *or* VER-tee-bral).
- This vertebral column consists of 26 **vertebrae** (VER-teh-bray *or* VER-teh-bree) (singular, **vertebra**).
- The functions of the spinal column are to support the head and body and to protect the spinal cord.

Structures of Vertebrae

- The **body** is the solid anterior portion of a vertebra (Figure 3.13).
- A **lamina** (**LAM**-ih-nah) is the posterior portion of a vertebra (plural, **laminae**). Several **processes** extend from this area.
- The **vertebral foramen** is the opening in the middle of the vertebra. The spinal cord passes through this opening.

FIGURE 3.13 Structures of a thoracic vertebra.

Types of Vertebrae

- The **cervical vertebrae** (**SER**-vih-kal) are the first set of seven vertebrae that form the neck. They are also known as **C1** through **C7** (Figure 3.14). (**Cervical** means pertaining to the neck.)
- The **thoracic vertebrae** (thoh-**RASS**-ick) make up the second set of 12 vertebrae. They form the outward curve of the spine and are known as **T1** through **T12**.
- The **lumbar vertebrae** (**LUM**-bar) make up the third set of five vertebrae. They are known as **L1** through **L5**. The lumbar vertebrae are the largest and strongest of the vertebrae and form the inward curve of the spine.

Intervertebral Disks

- The **intervertebral disks** (**in**-ter-**VER**-teh-bral), which are made of cartilage, separate and cushion the vertebrae from each other. These disks act as the shock absorbers and allow for movement of the spinal column (see Figure 3.21A).

Sacrum

- The **sacrum** (**SAY**-krum) is a slightly curved, triangular-shaped bone near the base of the spine (Figure 3.15). At birth it is composed of five separate sacral bones; however, in the young child they fuse together to form a single bone.

Coccyx

- The **coccyx** (**KOCK**-sicks), also known as the **tailbone**, forms the end of the spine and is made up of four small vertebrae fused together (see Figure 3.15).

Pelvic Girdle

- The **pelvic girdle**, also known as the **hips** or **pelvic bone**, protects internal organs and supports the lower extremities. This structure is made up of several bones fused together (see Figure 3.15).
- The **ilium** (**ILL**-ee-um) is the upper, blade-shaped part of the hip on each side of the pelvic girdle.
- The **sacroiliac** (**say**-kroh-**ILL**-ee-ack) is the slightly movable articulation between the sacrum and the ilium.

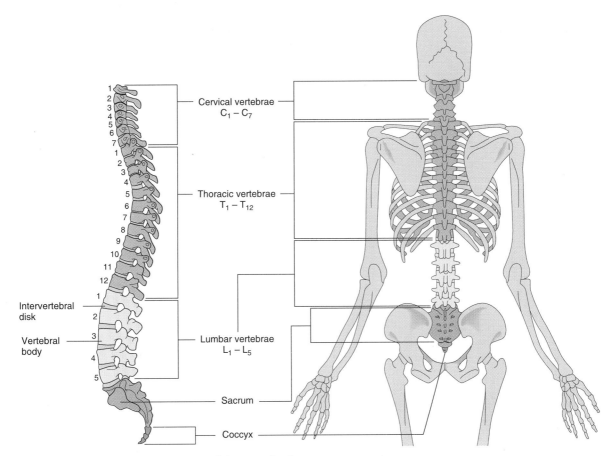

Figure 3.14 Lateral and posterior views of the spinal column.

- The **ischium** (**ISS**-kee-um) is the lower and posterior portion of the pelvic girdle.
- These three bones, which are also known as the **pubic bones**, fuse together and in the posterior they fuse with the sacrum.
- The **pubis** (**PEW**-bis) is the anterior portion of the pelvic girdle.
- The two pubic bones join at the anterior midline to form the **pubic symphysis** (**PEW**-bick **SIM**-fih-sis). This is a cartilaginous joint that holds the bones firmly together.

- The **acetabulum** (**ass**-eh-**TAB**-you-lum), the large socket in the pelvic bones, forms the hip socket for the head of the femur.

Legs and Knees

As you study the following bones, refer to Figures 3.16 and 3.17.

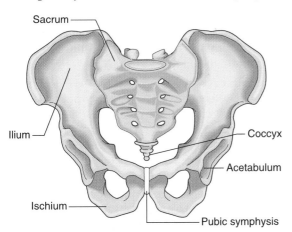

Figure 3.15 Anterior view of the pelvis.

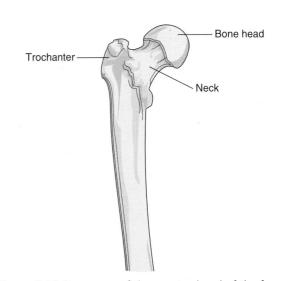

Figure 3.16 Structures of the proximal end of the femur.

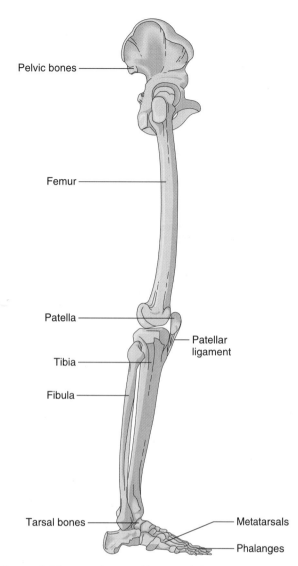

Pelvic bones

Femur

Patella

Tibia

Patellar ligament

Fibula

Tarsal bones

Metatarsals

Phalanges

FIGURE 3.17 Lateral view of bones of the lower extremity.

Femur

- The **femur** (**FEE**-mur) is the upper leg bone (see Figure 3.16). Also known as the **thigh bone**, it is the largest bone in the body.
- The **head** of the femur articulates with the acetabulum (hip socket).
- The **femoral neck** (**FEM**-or-al) is the narrow area just below the head of the femur.
- The **trochanter** (tro-**KAN**-ter) is one of the two large bony projections on the upper end of the femur just below the femoral neck.

Knees

- The **patella** (pah-**TEL**-ah) is the bony anterior portion of the kneecap.
- The term **popliteal** (pop-**LIT**-ee-al) refers to the posterior surface of the knee and is used to describe the space, ligaments, vessels, and muscles in this area.

- The **anterior cruciate ligament** (ACL) and **posterior cruciate ligament** (PCL), which are shown in Figure 3.4, make possible the movements of the knee. These are known as **cruciate ligaments** (**KROO**-shee-ayt) because they are shaped like a cross.

Lower Leg

- The **tibia** (**TIB**-ee-ah), also known as the **shinbone**, is the larger weight-bearing bone in the anterior of the lower leg.
- The **fibula** (**FIB**-you-lah) is the smaller of the two bones of the lower leg.

Ankles and Feet

- The **tarsals** (**TAHR**-salz) are the bones that make up the ankles (Figure 3.18).
- The **malleolus** (mal-**LEE**-oh-lus) is the rounded bony protuberance on each side of the ankle (plural, **malleoli**).
- The **talus** (**TAY**-luss) is the anklebone that articulates with the tibia and fibula (see Figure 3.17).
- The **calcaneus** (kal-**KAY**-nee-uss), or **heel bone**, is the largest of the tarsal bones (see Figure 3.18).
- The **metatarsals** (**met**-ah-**TAHR**-salz) are the bones of the foot.
- The **phalanges** (fah-**LAN**-jeez) are the bones of the toes (and of the fingers) (singular, **phalanx**).

Medical Specialties Related to the Skeletal System

- A **chiropractor** (**KYE**-roh-**prack**-tor) holds a Doctor of Chiropractic (DC) degree and specializes in manipulative treatment of disorders originating from misalignment of the spine.
- An **orthopedic surgeon**, also known as an **orthopedist** (or-thoh-**PEE**-dist), specializes in diagnosing and treating diseases and disorders involving the bones, joints, and muscles.
- **Orthotics** (or-**THOT**-icks) is the field of knowledge relating to making and fitting of orthopedic appliances, such as a brace or splint to support, align, prevent, or correct deformities or to improve the function of movable parts of the body.
- **Osteopathic physicians** (**oss**-tee-oh-**PATH**-ick) hold a Doctor of Osteopathy (DO) degree and specialize in treating health problems by manipulation (changing the positions of the bones). They may also use traditional forms of medical treatment. The term **osteopathy** (**oss**-tee-**OP**-ah-thee) also refers to any bone disease.
- A **podiatrist** (poh-**DYE**-ah-trist) holds a Doctor of Podiatry (DP) or Doctor of Podiatric Medicine (DPM) degree and specializes in diagnosing and treating disorders of the foot (**pod** mean foot and **iatrist** means specialist).

FIGURE 3.18 Superior and medial views of the bones of the right ankle and foot.

- A **rheumatologist** (roo-mah-**TOL**-oh-jist) is a physician who specializes in the diagnosis and treatment of rheumatic diseases that are characterized by inflammation in the connective tissues.

- **Rheumatism** (**ROO**-mah-tizm) is a general term for a variety of acute and chronic conditions characterized by inflammation and deterioration of connective tissues. This group of disorders includes joint diseases, such as arthritis, and muscle disorders such as fibromyalgia (see Chapter 4).

Pathology of the Skeletal System

Joints

- **Ankylosis** (ang-kih-**LOH**-sis) is the loss or absence of mobility in a joint due to disease, an injury, or a surgical procedure (**ankyl** means crooked, bent, or stiff and **osis** means abnormal condition).

- **Arthralgia** (ar-**THRAL**-jee-ah) is pain in a joint (**arthr** means joint and **algia** means pain).

- **Arthrosclerosis** (ar-throh-skleh-**ROH**-sis) is stiffness of the joints, especially in the elderly (**arthro** means joint and **sclerosis** means abnormal hardening).

- **Bursitis** (ber-**SIGH**-tis) is an inflammation of a bursa that is typically caused by repetitive movements (**burs** means bursa and **itis** means inflammation). Repetitive stress disorders are discussed in Chapter 4.

- A **chondroma** (kon-**DROH**-mah) is a slow-growing benign tumor derived from cartilage cells (**chondr** means cartilage and **oma** means tumor).

- **Chondromalacia** (**kon**-droh-mah-**LAY**-shee-ah) is abnormal softening of the cartilage (**chondro** means cartilage and **malacia** means abnormal softening).

- **Hallux valgus** (**HAL**-ucks **VAL**-guss), commonly known as a **bunion**, is an abnormal enlargement of the joint at the base of the great toe (hallux means big toe and val-

FIGURE 3.19 Superior view of a hallux valgus (bunion).

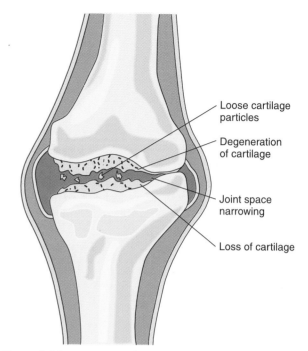

FIGURE 3.20 Damage to the knee caused by osteoarthritis.

gus means bent). This shift in the joint creates pressure on the other toes as the great toe is forced laterally (Figure 3.19).

- **Luxation** (luck-SAY-shun), also known as **dislocation**, is the dislocation or displacement of a bone from its joint. **Subluxation** (sub-luck-SAY-shun) is the partial displacement of a bone from its joint.

- **Synovitis** (sin-oh-VYE-tiss) is inflammation of the synovial membrane that results in swelling and pain (**synov** means synovial membrane and **itis** means inflammation). It may be caused by an injury, infection, or irritation produced by damaged cartilage.

Arthritis

- **Arthritis** (ar-THRIGH-tis) is an inflammatory condition of one or more joints (**arthr** means joint and **itis** means inflammation). There are many different forms and causes of arthritis (plural, **arthritides**).

- **Osteoarthritis** (oss-tee-oh-ar-THRIGH-tis), known as **wear-and-tear arthritis** or **OA** (**osteo** means bone, **arthr** means joint, and **itis** means inflammation). This **degenerative joint disease** (DJD) is most commonly associated with aging (Figure 3.20).

- **Gouty arthritis** (GOW-tee ar-THRIGH-tis), also known as **gout**, is a type of arthritis associated with the formation of uric acid crystals in the joint as the result of

hyperuricemia (excess uric acid concentrates in the blood).

Rheumatoid Arthritis

- **Rheumatoid arthritis** (ROO-mah-toyd ar-THRIGH-tis), also known as **RA**, is an autoimmune disorder. In contrast to osteoarthritis, the symptoms are generalized and usually more severe. In RA, the synovial membranes are inflamed and thicken. Other tissues are also attacked causing the joints to become swollen, painful, and immobile.

- **Ankylosing spondylitis** (ang-kih-LOH-sing spon-dih-LYE-tis) is a form of rheumatoid arthritis characterized by progressive stiffening of the spine caused by fusion of the vertebral bodies.

- **Juvenile rheumatoid arthritis** affects children. Symptoms include pain and swelling in the joints, skin rash, fever, slowed growth, and fatigue.

Spinal Column

- A **herniated disk** (HER-nee-ayt-ed), also known as a **ruptured disk**, is a rupture of the intervertebral disk that results in pressure on spinal nerve roots (Figure 3.21B).

- **Lumbago** (lum-BAY-goh), also known as **low back pain**, is pain of the lumbar region (**lumb** means lumbar and **ago** means diseased condition).

- **Spondylitis** (spon-dih-LYE-tis) is an inflammation of the vertebrae (**spondyl** means vertebrae and **itis** means inflammation).

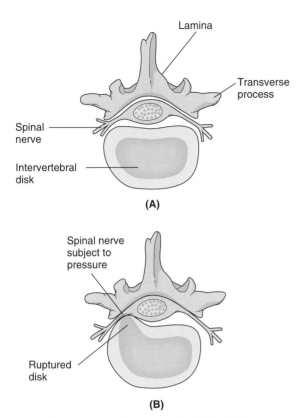

FIGURE 3.21 (A) Normal intervertebral disk. (B) Ruptured disk causing pressure on a spinal nerve.

- **Spondylolisthesis** (**spon**-dih-loh-liss-**THEE**-sis) is the forward movement of the body of one of the lower lumbar vertebra on the vertebra below it or on the sacrum (**spondyl** means vertebrae and **listhesis** means slipping).

- **Spondylosis** (**spon**-dih-**LOH**-sis) is any degenerative condition of the vertebrae (**spondyl** means vertebrae and **osis** means abnormal condition).

Spina Bifida

- **Spina bifida** (**SPY**-nah **BIF**-ih-dah) is the congenital defect that occurs during early pregnancy in which the spinal canal fails to close around the spinal cord (**spina** means pertaining to the spine and **bifida** means split.). Many cases of spina bifida are caused by a lack of folic acid (a vitamin) during the early stages of pregnancy.

Curvatures of the Spine

- **Kyphosis** (kye-**FOH**-sis) is an abnormal increase in the outward curvature of the thoracic spine as viewed from the side (**kyph** means hump and **osis** means abnormal condition). This condition is also known as **humpback** or **dowager's hump** (see Figure 3.22A).

- **Lordosis** (lor-**DOH**-sis) is an abnormal increase in the forward curvature of the lower or lumbar spine (**lord** means bent backward and **osis** means abnormal condition). This condition is also known as **swayback** (see Figure 3.22B).

- **Scoliosis** (skoh-lee-**OH**-sis) is an abnormal lateral (sideways) curvature of the spine (**scoli** means curved and **osis** means abnormal condition). See Figure 3.22C.

Bone

- An **exostosis** (**eck**-sos-**TOH**-sis) is a benign growth on the surface of a bone (**ex** means outside, **ost** means bone, and **osis** means abnormal condition).

- **Ostealgia** (**oss**-tee-**AL**-jee-ah) is any pain linked to an abnormal condition within a bone (**oste** means bone and **algia** means pain).

- **Osteitis** (**oss**-tee-**EYE**-tis) is an inflammation of bone (**oste** means bone and **itis** means inflammation).

FIGURE 3.22 Abnormal curvatures of the spine. (A) Kyphosis. (B) Lordosis. (C) Scoliosis. (Normal curvatures are shown in shadow.)

- **Osteomalacia** (oss-tee-oh-mah-**LAY**-shee-ah) is the abnormal softening of bones due to disease (**osteo** means bone and **malacia** means abnormal softening).

- **Osteomyelitis** (oss-tee-oh-**my**-eh-**LYE**-tis) is an inflammation of the bone and bone marrow (**osteo** means bone, **myel** means bone marrow, and **itis** means inflammation).

- **Osteonecrosis** (oss-tee-oh-neh-**KROH**-sis) is the destruction and death of bone tissue caused by an insufficient blood supply, infection, malignancy, or trauma (**osteo** means bone and **necrosis** means tissue death).

- **Paget's disease** (**PAJ**-its), also known as **osteitis deformans** (oss-tee-**EYE**-tis dee-**FOR**-manz), is a disease of unknown cause that is characterized by extensive bone destruction followed by abnormal bone repair. As the disease progresses, the bones become deformed and weakened and may bend or break easily.

- **Periostitis** (pehr-ee-oss-**TYE**-tis) is an inflammation of the periosteum (**peri** means surrounding, **ost** means bone, and **itis** means inflammation).

- **Rickets** (**RICK**-ets), which is caused by calcium and vitamin D deficiencies in early childhood, results in demineralized bones and related deformities.

- **Talipes** (**TAL**-ih-peez), also known as **clubfoot**, is a congenital deformity in which the foot may be turned outward or inward as shown in Figure 3-23.

Figure 3.23 Talipes, also known as clubfoot, with the feet turned inward.

Tumors of Bones

- **Ewing's sarcoma** (**YOU**-ingz sar-**KOH**-mah), also known as **Ewing's family of tumors**, is a group of cancers that most frequently affects children or adolescents. A sarcoma is a malignant tumor of connective tissue and in Ewing's sarcoma they usually occur in the diaphyses (shaft) of long bones in the arms and legs and then may spread rapidly to other body sites.

- A **myeloma** (my-eh-**LOH**-mah) is a malignant tumor composed of cells derived from hemopoietic (blood-forming) tissues of the bone marrow. Myeloma is usually progressive, may cause pathologic fractures, and is often fatal (**myel** means bone marrow and **oma** means tumor).

- An **osteochondroma** (oss-tee-oh-kon-**DROH**-mah) is the most common benign bone tumor (**osteo** means bone, **chondr** means cartilage, and **oma** means tumor). These tumors are growths on the surface of a bone that protrude as hard lumps covered with a cap of cartilage.

Osteoporosis

Osteoporosis (oss-tee-oh-poh-**ROH**-sis) is a marked loss of bone density and an increase in bone porosity frequently associated with aging (**osteo** means bone and **porosis** means porous condition). Osteoporosis is primarily responsible for three types of fractures.

- **Vertebral crush fractures**, also known as **compression fractures** of the spine, occur when one or more of the vertebrae become so weak that they collapse spontaneously or under minimal stress. This results in pain, loss of height, and development of the spinal curvature known as **dowager's hump**. These changes in the spine cause the loss of height, crowding of the internal organs, and reduced lung capacity (Figure 3.24).

- **Colles' fracture**, also know as a **fractured wrist**, is a fracture of the lower end of the radius. This occurs when a person tries to break a fall by landing on his hands and the trauma causes the weakened bone to break (Figure 3.25).

- An **osteoporotic hip fracture** (oss-tee-oh-pah-**ROT**-ick), also known as a **broken hip**, can occur spontaneously or as the result of a fall. Complications from these fractures may result in death or the loss of function, mobility, and independence.

Fractures

- A **fracture**, which is abbreviated as **Fx**, is a broken bone. Fractures are described in terms of their complexity (Figure 3.26).

- A **greenstick fracture**, or **incomplete fracture**, is one in which the bone is partially bent and only partially broken. This type of fracture is usually longitudinal and occurs primarily in children.

- A **closed fracture**, also known as a **simple** or **complete fracture**, is one in which the bone is broken but there is no open wound in the skin (see Figure 3.26). A **transverse fracture** is straight across the bone. An **oblique fracture** is at an angle.

- An **open fracture**, also known as a **compound fracture**, is one in which the bone is broken and there is an open wound in the skin.

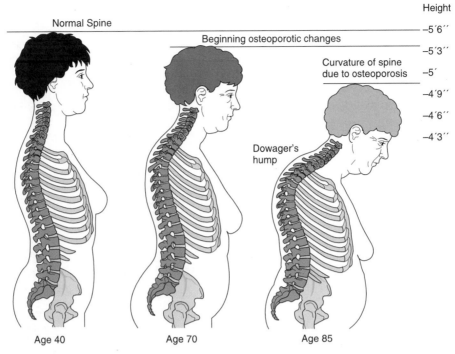

FIGURE 3.24 Curvature of the spine due to osteoporosis.

FIGURE 3.25 A Colles' fracture of the left wrist.

- A **comminuted fracture** is one in which the bone is splintered or crushed. **Comminuted** (**KOM**-ih-**newt**-ed) means crushed into small pieces.

- A **compression fracture** occurs when the bone is pressed together (compressed) on itself (see Osteoporosis).

- A **spiral fracture** is a fracture in which the bone has been twisted apart. This occurs as the result of a severe twisting motion as in a sports injury.

- A **stress fracture** is a small crack in bones that often develop from chronic, excessive impact. These fractures are usually due to a sports injury.

- A **fat embolus** (**EM**-boh-lus) may form when a long bone is fractured and fat cells from yellow bone mar-

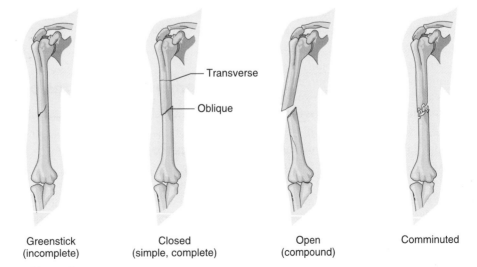

FIGURE 3.26 Types of bone fractures.

row are released into the blood. (An **embolus** is any foreign matter circulating in the blood that may become lodged and block the blood vessel. Emboli are discussed in Chapter 5.)

- **Crepitation** (**krep**-ih-**TAY**-shun), also know as **crepitus** (**KREP**-ih-tus), is the crackling sensation that is felt and heard when the ends of a broken bone move together.

- As the bone heals a **callus** (**KAL**-us) forms a bulging deposit around the area of the break. This tissue eventually becomes bone.

Diagnostic Procedures of the Skeletal System

- **Arthrocentesis** (ar-throh-sen-**TEE**-sis) is a surgical puncture of the joint space to remove synovial fluid for analysis (**arthro** means joint and **centesis** means a surgical puncture to remove fluid).

- **Arthroscopy** (ar-**THROS**-koh-pee) is the visual examination of the internal structure of a joint (**arthro** means joint and **scopy** means visual examination) using an **arthroscope** (see Figure 15.18).

- **Bone density testing** (BDT), also known as **bone mass measurement** or **densitometry**, is the use of several types of radiation tests to determine bone density. These tests are indicated for conditions such as osteoporosis, osteomalacia, and Paget's disease.

- A **bone marrow biopsy**, also known as a **BMB**, is performed by inserting a sharp needle into the hipbone or sternum and removing bone marrow cells. This is performed as a diagnostic test to determine why blood cells are abnormal. This is also performed to find a donor match for a bone marrow transplant.

- A **bone scan** is the use of nuclear medicine to detect bone cancer and osteomyelitis before these pathologies become visible on traditional radiographs (see Chapter 15 and Figure 15.29).

- **Dual x-ray absorptiometry** (ab-**sorp**-shee-**OM**-eh-tree), also known as **DXA**, is a low-exposure radiographic measurement that is most often used to detect early signs of osteoposoris.

  Ultrasonic bone density testing, called a **bone sonometer**, uses sound waves to take measurements of the heel bone. This is a screening test for osteoposoris or other conditions causing a loss of bone mass. If the test indicates risks, more definitive testing is indicated.

- **Magnetic resonance imaging** (MRI) is used to image soft tissue structures such as the interior of complex joints and spinal disorders. It is not the most effective method of imaging hard tissues such as bone.

- **Radiographs**, also known as **x-rays**, are used to visualize fractured bones (Figure 3.27).

FIGURE 3.27 Radiographs of a simple fracture of the femur. The top picture is an anterior-posterior (AP) view. The bottom picture is a lateral view that more exactly locates the fractured ends of the bone.

Treatment Procedures of the Skeletal System

Medications

- **Nonsteroidal anti-inflammatory drugs**, also known as **NSAIDs**, are administered to control pain and to reduce inflammation and swelling. Aspirin is an example of a NSAID; however, medications in this group may thin the blood and attack the stomach lining.

- **Acetaminophen** also controls pain without the same side effects as NSAIDs; however, it does not have the ability to reduce inflammation and swelling.
- Aspirin and acetaminophen are also used as antipyretics. An **antipyretic** (an-tih-pye-RET-ick) reduces or relieves fever.
- **COX-2 inhibitors**, a newer class of medications, control the pain and inflammation of osteoarthritis and rheumatoid arthritis while greatly reducing the side effects of NSAIDs. These medications are named for the two *cyclooxygenase* (COX) enzymes that are associated with arthritic pain and inflammation.

Bone Marrow Transplants

A **bone marrow transplant**, also known as **BMT** or a **stem cell transplant**, is used to treat certain types of cancers such as leukemia and lymphomas that affect bone marrow. These cancers are discussed in Chapters 5 and 6.

- In this treatment both the cancer and the patient's bone marrow are destroyed with high-intensity radiation and chemotherapy.
- Next, healthy bone marrow cells are transfused into the recipient's blood. These cells migrate to the spongy bone where they grow into cancer-free red bone marrow.

Autologous Transplants

- Most frequently, the BMT is an **autologous transplant** (aw-TOL-uh-guss) using some of the patient's own bone marrow that was harvested before treatment began. (Autologous means originating within an individual.)

Allogenic Transplants

- If the patient's own marrow cannot be used, an **allogenic transplant** (al-oh-JEN-ick), using bone marrow from a donor, may be a possibility. However unless this is a perfect match there is the danger that the recipient's body will reject the transplant. (Allogenic means originating within another.)

Cord Blood

- **Cord blood**, collected immediately after birth, is a rich source of stem cells and has the potential of being an alternative to bone marrow transplants.

Joints

- **Arthroscopic surgery** (ar-throh-SKOP-ick) is the treatment of the interior of a joint, such as the removal of torn cartilage, with the use of an arthroscope and instruments inserted through small incisions (see Figure 15.18).
- A **bursectomy** (ber-SECK-toh-mee) is the surgical removal of a bursa (**burs** means the bursa and **ectomy** means surgical removal).

- **Chondroplasty** (KON-droh-plas-tee) is the surgical repair of cartilage (**chondro** means cartilage and **plasty** means surgical repair).
- A **synovectomy** (sin-oh-VECK-toh-mee) is the surgical removal of a synovial membrane from a joint (**synov** means synovial membrane and **ectomy** means surgical removal). This procedure is performed to repair a joint damaged by rheumatoid arthritis.
- **Arthrodesis** (ar-throh-DEE-sis), also known as **fusion** or **surgical ankylosis**, is a surgical procedure to stiffen a joint or join spinal vertebrae (**arthro** means joint and **desis** means surgical fixation of bone or joint).
- **Arthrolysis** (ar-THROL-ih-sis) is the surgical loosening of an ankylosed joint (**arthro** means joint and **lysis** means loosening or setting free). *Note:* The suffix -lysis also means breaking down or destruction and may indicate either a pathologic state or a therapeutic procedure.
- A **periosteotomy** (peer-ee-oss-tee-OT-oh-mee) is an incision through the periosteum (**peri** means surrounding, **oste** means bone, and **otomy** means surgical incision).

Joint Replacement

- **Arthroplasty** (AR-throh-plas-tee) is any surgical repair of a damaged joint (**arthro** means joint and **plasty** means surgical repair); however, this term has come to mean the surgical replacement of a joint. These procedures are named for the involved joint and the amount of the joint that is replaced.
- The replacement part is called a **prosthesis** (pros-THEE-sis) or an **implant** (Figure 3.28). The broader definition of prosthesis is a substitute for a diseased or missing part of the body (plural, **prostheses**).
- A **total knee replacement**, also known as a **TKR**, means that all of the parts of the knee were replaced (see Figures 3.28 and 3.29).
- A **partial knee replacement**, also known as a **PKR**, means that only part of the knee was replaced.
- A **total hip replacement**, also known as a **THR**, consists of two components. The thigh component is a metal shaft fitted into the femur with a metal ball at the top end. The ball fits into a plastic lined cup-shaped socket that replaces the acetabulum within the hipbone.
- **Revision surgery** is the replacement of a worn or failed implant.

Spinal Column

- **Diskectomy** (dis-KECK-toh-mee) is the surgical removal of an intervertebral disk.
- In a **percutaneous diskectomy** (per-kyou-TAY-nee-us dis-KECK-toh-mee) a thin tube is inserted through the skin of the back to suction out the ruptured disk or to

FIGURE 3.28 Components of a total hip replacement and a total knee replacement. Polyethylene, a smooth tough plastic, makes smooth movement possible.

FIGURE 3.29 Radiograph of a total knee replacement. The metallic components are lighter than the bone.

vaporize it with a laser. (**Percutaneous** means through the skin.)

- A **laminectomy** (**lam**-ih-**NECK**-toh-mee) is the surgical removal of a lamina from a vertebra.

- **Spinal fusion** is a technique to immobilize part of the spine by joining together (fusing) two or more vertebrae. This may be performed with a diskectomy or laminectomy. See also **arthrodesis**.

Bones

- A **craniectomy** (**kray**-nee-**EK**-toh-mee) is the surgical removal of a portion of the skull (**crani** means skull and **ectomy** means surgical removal).

- A **craniotomy** (**kray**-nee-**OT**-oh-mee) is also known as a **bone flap** (**crani** means skull and **otomy** means a surgical incision). This procedure is a surgical incision or opening into the skull that is performed to gain access to part of the brain (Figure 3.30).

- A **cranioplasty** (**KRAY**-nee-oh-**plas**-tee) is the surgical repair of the skull (**cranio** means skull and **plasty** means surgical repair).

- **Osteoclasis** (**oss**-tee-**OCK**-lah-sis) is the surgical fracture of a bone to correct a deformity (**osteo** means bone and **clasis** means to break).

- An **ostectomy** (oss-**TECK**-toh-mee) is the surgical removal of bone (**ost** means bone and **ectomy** means the surgical removal. Notice that the root word **ost** is

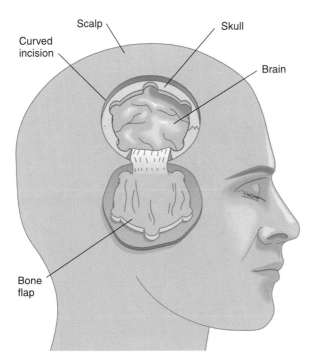

FIGURE 3.30 A craniotomy is performed to gain access to a portion of the brain.

used to avoid having two e's together when it joins the suffix **ectomy**).

- **Osteoplasty** (**OSS**-tee-oh-**plas**-tee) is the surgical repair of bones (**osteo** means bone and **plasty** means surgical repair).
- **Osteorrhaphy** (**oss**-tee-**OR**-ah-fee) is the suturing or wiring together of bones (**osteo** means bone and **rrhaphy** means to suture).
- **Osteotomy** (**oss**-tee-**OT**-oh-mee) is a surgical incision or sectioning of a bone (**oste** means bone and **otomy**

means a surgical incision). This procedure may be performed to realign a joint damaged by arthritis.

Treatment of Fractures

- **Manipulation**, in relation to fractures and dislocations, is the attempted realignment of the bone involved in a fracture or joint dislocation. Also known as **closed reduction**, the affected bone is returned to its normal anatomic alignment by application of manually applied forces and then is usually immobilized to maintain the realigned position (Figure 3.31).
- **Traction** is a pulling force exerted on a limb in a distal direction in an effort to return the bone or joint to normal alignment.
- **Immobilization**, also known as **stabilization**, is the act of holding, suturing, or fastening the bone in a fixed position with strapping or a cast.

FIGURE 3.31 Closed reduction of a fractured left humerus.

External Fixation

- **External fixation** is a fracture treatment procedure in which pins are placed through the soft tissues and bone so that an external appliance can be used to hold the pieces of bone firmly in place during healing. When healing is complete the appliance is removed (Figure 3.32).

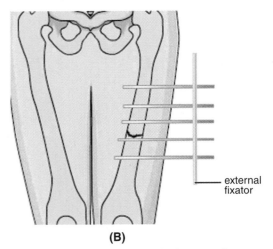

(A)   **(B)**

FIGURE 3.32 External fixation. (A) Fracture of the epiphysis of a femur. (B) External fixation stabilizes the bone and is removed after the bone has healed.

Internal Fixation

- **Internal fixation**, which is also known as open reduction internal fixation (ORIF), is a fracture treatment procedure in which pins or a plate are placed directly into the bone to hold the broken pieces in place. This form of fixation is not usually removed after the fracture has healed (Figure 3.33).

(A) **(B)**

FIGURE **3.33** Internal fixation. (A) Fracture of the femoral neck. (B) Internal fixation pins are placed to stabilize the bone. These are not removed.

Learning Exercises

Matching Word Parts—1

Write the letter of the correct answer on the line provided in the left column.

3.1. _____ ankly/o   A. hump

3.2. _____ arthr/o   B. cartilage

3.3. _____ -um   C. crooked, bent, or stiff

3.4. _____ kyph/o   D. joint

3.5. _____ chondr/o   E. noun ending

Matching Word Parts—2

Write the letter of the correct answer on the line provided in the left column.

3.6. _____ cost/o   A. cranium, skull

3.7. _____ crani/o   B. rib

3.8. _____ -desis   C. setting free, loosening

3.9. _____ -lysis   D. spinal cord, bone marrow

3.10. _____ myel/o   E. surgical fixation of bone or joint

Matching Word Parts—3

Write the letter of the correct answer on the line provided in the left column.

3.11. _____ oss/e, oss/i, ost/o, oste/o   A. vertebra, vertebral column

3.12. _____ spondyl/o   B. curved

3.13. _____ lord/o   C. bent backward

3.14. _____ -poietic   D. pertaining to formation

3.15. _____ scolio   E. bone

Definitions

Circle the letter next to the correct answer.

3.16. Which term describes the shaft of a long bone?

     a. diaphysis

     b. distal epiphysis

     c. endosteum

     d. proximal epiphysis

3.17. The tarsals are the bones that make up the _____ .

     a. ankles

     b. fingers

     c. toes

     d. wrist

3.18. The manubrium is the _____ .

     a. lower jaw

     b. lower portion of the sternum

     c. thin, scroll-like bone of the nose

     d. upper portion of the sternum

3.19. Which term describes the movable joints of the body?

     a. cartilaginous

     b. fibrous

     c. suture

     d. synovial

3.20. The sacrum is _____ .

     a. also known as the tailbone

     b. the lower portion of the sternum

     c. the anterior portion of the pelvis

     d. triangular in shape

3.21.   The opening in a bone through which blood vessels, nerves, and ligaments pass is a _____ .

   a. fontanel

   b. foramen

   c. meatus

   d. suture

3.22.   Which term describes the band of fibrous tissue that connects one bone to another?

   a. articular cartilage

   b. ligament

   c. synovial membrane

   d. tendon

3.23.   The acetabulum is also known as the _____ .

   a. collar bone

   b. hip socket

   c. kneecap

   d. shinbone

3.24.   The bones of the fingers and toes are called _____ .

   a. carpals

   b. metatarsals

   c. tarsals

   d. phalanges

3.25.   Which term describes a normal projection on the surface of a bone?

   a. cruciate

   b. exostosis

   c. popliteal

   d. process

● **Matching Structures**

Write the letter of the correct definition on the line next to each term.

3.26. _____ clavicle   A. breastbone

3.27. _____ olecranon   B. cheek bone

3.28. _____ sternum   C. collar bone

3.29. _____ patella   D. kneecap

3.30. _____ zygomatic   E. point of the elbow

● **Which Word?**

Circle the correct term in each sentence.

3.31.   The surgical loosening of an ankylosed joint is called *arthrodesis* / *arthrolysis*.

3.32.   A physician who specializes in the diagnosis and treatment of diseases characterized by inflammation in the connective tissues is a/an *orthopedist* / *rheumatologist*.

3.33.   A bone marrow transplant using marrow from a donor is an *allogenic* / *autologous* transplant.

3.34.   The medical term meaning the surgical repair of the skull is a *craniectomy* / *cranioplasty*.

3.35.   The medical term for the type of arthritis commonly known as wear-and-tear arthritis is *osteoarthritis* / *rheumatoid arthritis*.

● **Spelling Counts**

Find the misspelled word in each sentence. Then write that word, spelled correctly, on the line provided.

3.36.   The medical term for the condition commonly known as low back pain is lumbaego. _____

3.37.   Ostealgea means any pain that is linked to an abnormal condition with a bone. _____ .

3.38.   Ankylosing spondilitis is an inflammatory joint disease characterized by progressive stiffening of the spine caused by fusion of the vertebral bodies. _____

3.39.   The medical term meaning suturing or wiring together of bones is osterrhaphy. _____

3.40.   The sound heard when the ends of a broken bone move together is called crepetation. _____

● Matching Abbreviations

Write the letter of the correct answer on the line provided in the left column.

3.41. _____ THR   A. bone marrow biopsy

3.42. _____ Fx   B. total knee replacement

3.43. _____ OA   C. osteoarthritis

3.44. _____ TKR   D. fracture

3.45. _____ BMB   E. total hip replacement

● Term Selection

Circle the letter next to the correct answer.

3.46. Which term means the death of bone tissue?

a. osteitis deformans

b. osteomyelitis

c. osteonecrosis

d. osteoporosis

3.47. Which medical term means an abnormal increase in the forward curvature of the lower or lumbar spine?

a. kyphosis

b. lordosis

c. Paget's disease

d. scoliosis

3.48. Which of these diseases is an autoimmune disorder?

a. osteoarthritis

b. rheumatoid arthritis

c. spina bifida

d. spondylosis

3.49. Which of these conditions is a group of cancers that most frequently affects children or adolescents?

a. Ewing's sarcoma

b. myeloma

c. osteochondroma

d. talipes

3.50. Which term describes the bulging deposit that forms around the area of the break during the healing of a fractured bone?

a. callus

b. comminuted

c. crepitation

d. crepitus

● Sentence Completion

Write the correct term on the line provided.

3.51. The general term used to describe a variety of acute and chronic conditions characterized by inflammation and deterioration of connective tissues is _____ .

3.52. The partial displacement of a bone from its joint is known as _____ .

3.53. The medical term for the procedure also known as fusion, that stiffens a joint or joining of several vertebrae is

_____ .

3.54. The medical term for the surgical removal of a spinal lamina is a/an _____ .

3.55. A hallux valgus is commonly known as a/an

_____ .

● True/False

If the statement is true, write T on the line. If the statement is false, write F on the line.

3.56. _____ A percutaneous diskectomy is performed through the skin of the back.

3.57. _____ A craniotomy is a surgical incision into the collar bone.

3.58. _____ Spondylolisthesis is a subluxation of one vertebra over the one below it.

3.59. _____ Osteoclasis is a pathologic condition that involves abnormal hardening of the bones.

3.60. _____ Arthrocentesis is the surgical removal of fluid from a joint.

3.61. _____ When a bone is broken at an angle it is said to be an oblique fracture.

3.62. _____ Paget's disease is caused by a deficiency of calcium and vitamin D in early childhood.

3.63. _____ Stiffness of the joints, especially in the aged, is known as atherosclerosis.

3.64. _____ The loss or absence of mobility in a joint because the bones have abnormally fused together is known as ankylosis.

3.65. _____ The surgical removal of a bursa is a bursitis.

● **Clinical Conditions**

Write the correct answer on the line.

3.66. Bobby Kuhn fell out of a tree and broke his arm. Dr. Parker described this as a closed or _____ fracture because, although the bone was broken, there was no open wound of the skin.

3.67. Eduardo Sanchez has an inflammation of the bone and bone marrow. The medical term for this condition is _____ .

3.68. Ashley Hargraves was diagnosed as having a/an _____ . This is a tumor composed of cells derived from hemopoietic tissues of the bone marrow.

3.69. Mrs. Morton suffers from dowager's hump. This medical term for this abnormal curvature of the spine is _____ .

3.70. Henry Turner specializes in creating _____ . These are orthopedic appliances to align, prevent or correct deformities or to improve the function of movable parts of the body.

3.71. Howard Jamison was born with a congenital failure of the spinal canal to close over the spinal cord. The medical term for this condition is spina _____ .

3.72. Mrs. Gilmer, who is 84 years old, fell and broke her hip. Her doctor repaired this fracture by placing pins to hold the bone together as it heals. These pins, which will not be removed, are known as _____ fixation.

3.73. Betty Greene has been running for several years; however, now her knees hurt. Dr. Baskin diagnosed that she has _____ . This is an abnormal softening of the cartilage in these joints.

3.74. Patty Turner (age 7) has symptoms that include a skin rash, fever, slowed growth, fatigue and swelling in the joints. She was diagnosed as having juvenile _____ arthritis.

3.75. Robert Young has a very sore shoulder. Dr. Wilson diagnosed it as an inflammation of the bursa and called it _____ .

● **Which is the correct medical term?**

Circle the letter next to the correct answer.

3.76. Rodney Horner is being treated for a fracture in which the ends of the bones were crushed together. Which type of fracture is this?

a. Colles'

b. comminuted

c. compound

d. simple

3.77. Alex Jordon's doctor surgically repaired her damaged cartilage. Which term describes the surgical repair of cartilage?

a. arthroplasty

b. chondritis

c. chondroplasty

d. osteoplasty

3.78. Jane Parker was concerned about bone loss after menopause. To evaluate the condition of her bones, which test did Jane's doctor order?

a. a bone scan

b. an MRI

c. a blood calcium test

d. dual x-ray absorptiometry

3.79. Which procedure did Dr. Wong order for his injured patient in an effort to return the joint to normal alignment?

a. external fixation

b. immobilization

c. manipulation

d. traction

3.80. Juanita was treated for an inflammation of the tissue that surrounds a bone. Which is the medical term for this condition?

    a. ostealgia

    b. osteitis

    c. osteomyelitis

    d. periostitis

● Challenge Word Building

These terms are *not* found in this chapter; however, they are made up of these familiar word parts. You may want to look in the glossary or use a medical dictionary to check your answers!

poly-	arthr/o	-ectomy
	chondr/o	-itis
	cost/o	-malacia
	crani/o	-otomy
	oste/o	-pathy
		-sclerosis

3.81. Abnormal hardening of bone is called
_____ .

3.82. The surgical removal of a rib is a/an
_____ .

3.83. The medical term for a disease of the cartilage is _____ .

3.84. A surgical incision into a joint is a/an
_____ .

3.85. The medical term meaning inflammation of cartilage is _____ .

3.86. The surgical removal of a joint is a/an
_____ .

3.87. The medical term meaning inflammation of more than one joint is _____ .

3.88. The medical term meaning any disease involving the bones and joints is
_____ .

3.89. A surgical incision or division of a rib is a/an
_____ .

3.90. The medical term meaning abnormal softening of the skull is _____ .

● Labeling Exercises

Identify the numbered items on these diagrams.

3.91._____ vertebrae

3.92._____

3.93._____

3.94._____

3.95._____

3.96._____

3.97._____

3.98._____

3.99._____

3.100._____

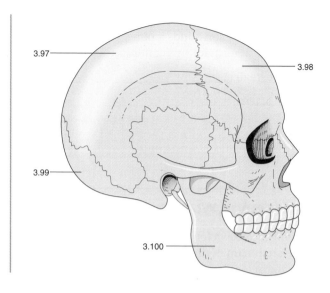

3.97

3.98

3.99

3.100

The Human Touch: Critical Thinking Exercise

The following story and questions are designed to stimulate critical thinking through class discussion or as a brief essay response. There are no easy or right-wrong answers to these questions.

Dr. Johnstone didn't like what he saw. The x-rays of Gladys Gwynn's hip showed a fracture of the femoral neck and severe osteoporosis of the hip. Mrs. Gwynn had been admitted to the orthopedic ward of Hamilton Hospital following a fall that morning at Sunny Meadows, an assisted living facility. The accident had occurred when Sheri Smith, a new aide, lost her grip while helping Mrs. Gwynn in the shower.

A frail but alert and cheerful woman of 85, Gladys Gwynn has osteoarthritis and osteoporosis that forced her to rely on a walker. She had been living at Sunny Meadows since her husband's death 4 years ago. Dr. Johnstone knew that she did not have any relatives in the area, and he did not think that she had signed a health care power-of-attorney designating someone to help with medical decisions like this.

A total hip replacement (THP) would be the logical treatment for a younger patient because it could restore some of her lost mobility. However, for a frail patient like Mrs. Gwynn internal fixation of the fracture might be the treatment of choice. This would repair the break, but not improve her mobility.

Dr. Johnstone needed to make a decision soon, but Mrs. Gwynn was still groggy from the pain medication. With one more look at the x-ray, Dr. Johnstone sighed and walked toward Mrs. Gwynn's room . . .

Suggested Discussion Topics:

1. Gladys Gwynn has no children or other relatives in the area and is unable to speak for herself. Who should decide which surgery should be performed?

2. Do you think Sheri Smith or Sunny Meadows should be held responsible for Mrs. Gwynn's accident? If so, who should be held responsible?

3. A total hip replacement is more expensive than the internal fixation procedure and has a longer more strenuous recovery period. Given the patient's condition, and the limited dollars available for health care, which procedure should be performed?

4. How would you have answered question 3 differently if Mrs. Gwynn were your mother?

5. If Mrs. Gwynn's recovery does not go well and she is no longer able to get around by herself will she be allowed to continue living at Sunny Meadows?

The Muscular System

CHAPTER

● **Overview of Structures, Word Parts, and Functions of the Muscular System**

MAJOR STRUCTURES	RELATED WORD ROOTS	PRIMARY FUNCTIONS
Muscles	my/o, myos/o	Make body movement possible, hold body erect, move body fluids, and produce body heat.
Fascia	fasci/o	Cover, support, and separate muscles.
Tendons	ten/o, tend/o, tendin/o	Attach muscle to bone.

VOCABULARY   Related to the Muscular System

Check the box as you master each word part or term. Terms marked with the ❖ symbol are pronounced on the optional student audiotape.

Key Word Parts

- [ ] bi-
- [ ] -cele
- [ ] -desis
- [ ] fasci/o
- [ ] -ia
- [ ] -ic
- [ ] kinesi/o
- [ ] -lysis
- [ ] my/o
- [ ] -plegia
- [ ] –rrhexis
- [ ] tax/o
- [ ] ten/o, tend/o, tendin/o
- [ ] ton/o
- [ ] tri-

Key Medical Terms

- [ ] **abduction** (ab-**DUCK**-shun)
- [ ] **Achilles tendinitis** (**ten**-dih-**NIGH**-tis) ❖
- [ ] **adduction** (ah-**DUCK**-shun)
- [ ] **adhesion** (ad-**HEE**-zhun) ❖
- [ ] **anticholinergic drug** (**an**-tih-**koh**-lin-**ER**-jik)
- [ ] **ataxia** (ah-**TACK**-see-ah) ❖
- [ ] **atonic** (ah-**TON**-ick) ❖
- [ ] **atrophy** (**AT**-roh-fee) ❖
- [ ] **atropine** (**AT**-roh-peen)
- [ ] **Becker's muscular dystrophy** (**BECK**-urz) ❖
- [ ] **bradykinesia** (**brad**-ee-kih-**NEE**-zee-ah *or* **brad**-ee-kih-**NEE**-zhuh) ❖
- [ ] **cardioplegia** (**kar**-dee-oh-**PLEE**-jee-ah)
- [ ] **carpal tunnel syndrome** (**KAR**-pul) ❖
- [ ] **cervical radiculopathy** (rah-**dick**-you-**LOP**-ah-thee) ❖
- [ ] **circumduction** (**ser**-kum-**DUCK**-shun)
- [ ] **claudication** (**klaw**-dih-**KAY**-shun) ❖
- [ ] **contracture** (kon-**TRACK**-chur) ❖
- [ ] **dorsiflexion** (**dor**-sih-**FLECK**-shun)
- [ ] **Duchenne's muscular dystrophy** (doo-**SHENZ**) ❖
- [ ] **dyskinesia** (**dis**-kih-**NEE**-zee-ah) ❖
- [ ] **dystaxia** (dis-**TACK**-see-ah) ❖
- [ ] **dystonia** (dis-**TOH**-nee-ah) ❖
- [ ] **electromyography** (ee-**leck**-troh-my-**OG**-rah-fee) ❖
- [ ] **electroneuromyography** (ee-**leck**-troh-**new**-roh-my-**OG**-rah-fee) ❖
- [ ] **epicondylitis** (**ep**-ih-**kon**-dih-**LYE**-tis) ❖
- [ ] **ergonomics** (**er**-goh-**NOM**-icks) ❖
- [ ] **fasciitis** (**fas**-ee-**EYE**-tis) ❖
- [ ] **fascioplasty** (**FASH**-ee-oh-**plas**-tee) ❖

- [ ] **fasciotomy** (**fash**-ee-**OT**-oh-mee) ❖
- [ ] **fibromyalgia syndrome** (**figh**-broh-my-**AL**-jee-ah) ❖
- [ ] **hemiparesis** (**hem**-ee-pah-**REE**-sis)
- [ ] **hemiplegia** (**hem**-ee-**PLEE**-jee-ah) ❖
- [ ] **hyperkinesia** (**high**-per-kye-**NEE**-zee-ah) ❖
- [ ] **hypertonia** (**high**-per-**TOH**-nee-ah) ❖
- [ ] **hypokinesia** (**high**-poh-kye-**NEE**-zee-ah) ❖
- [ ] **hypotonia** (**high**-poh-**TOH**-nee-ah) ❖
- [ ] **impingement syndrome** (im-**PINJ**-ment) ❖
- [ ] **kinesiology** (kih-**nee**-see-**OL**-oh-jee) ❖
- [ ] **muscular dystrophy** (**DIS**-troh-fee) ❖
- [ ] **myalgia** (my-**AL**-jee-ah) ❖
- [ ] **myasthenia** (**my**-as-**THEE**-nee-ah) ❖
- [ ] **myasthenia gravis** (**my**-as-**THEE**-nee-ah **GRAH**-vis) ❖
- [ ] **myectomy** (my-**ECK**-toh-mee)
- [ ] **myocele** (**MY**-oh-seel) ❖
- [ ] **myoclonus** (my-oh-**KLOH**-nus *or* my-**OCK**-loh-nus) ❖
- [ ] **myofascial** (my-oh-**FASH**-ee-ahl) ❖
- [ ] **myolysis** (my-**OL**-ih-sis) ❖
- [ ] **myomalacia** (**my**-oh-mah-**LAY**-shee-ah) ❖
- [ ] **myoparesis** (**my**-oh-**PAR**-eh-sis)
- [ ] **myoplasty** (**MY**-oh-**plas**-tee) ❖
- [ ] **myorrhaphy** (my-**OR**-ah-fee) ❖
- [ ] **myorrhexis** (**my**-oh-**RECK**-sis) ❖
- [ ] **myositis** (**my**-oh-**SIGH**-tis) ❖
- [ ] **myotonia** (**my**-oh-**TOH**-nee-ah) ❖
- [ ] **oblique** (oh-**BLEEK**)
- [ ] **paraplegia** (**par**-ah-**PLEE**-jee-ah) ❖
- [ ] **polymyositis** (**pol**-ee-**my**-oh-**SIGH**-tis) ❖
- [ ] **pronation** (proh-**NAY**-shun)
- [ ] **quadriplegia** (**kwad**-rih-**PLEE**-jee-ah) ❖
- [ ] **rectus** (**RECK**-tus)
- [ ] **singultus** (sing-**GUL**-tus) ❖
- [ ] **spasmodic torticollis** (spaz-**MOD**-ick **tor**-tih-**KOL**-is) ❖
- [ ] **sphincter** (**SFINK**-ter)
- [ ] **supination** (**soo**-pih-**NAY**-shun)
- [ ] **tardive dyskinesia** (**TAHR**-div **dis**-kih-**NEE**-zee-ah) ❖
- [ ] **tenalgia** (ten-**AL**-jee-ah) ❖
- [ ] **tendinitis** (**ten**-dih-**NIGH**-tis) ❖
- [ ] **tendonitis** (**ten**-doh-**NIGH**-tis) ❖
- [ ] **tenectomy** (teh-**NECK**-toh-mee) ❖
- [ ] **tenodesis** (ten-**ODD**-eh-sis) ❖
- [ ] **tenolysis** (ten-**OL**-ih-sis) ❖
- [ ] **tenonectomy** (**ten**-oh-**NECK**-toh-mee) ❖
- [ ] **tenoplasty** (**TEN**-oh-**plas**-tee) ❖
- [ ] **tenorrhaphy** (ten-**OR**-ah-fee) ❖
- [ ] **tenotomy** (teh-**NOT**-oh-mee) ❖

Functions of the Muscular System

- Muscles hold the body erect and make movements possible.
- Muscle movement generates nearly 85% of the heat that keeps the body warm.
- Muscles move food through the digestive system (see Chapter 8).
- Muscle movements, such as walking, aids the flow of blood through veins as it returns to the heart (see Chapter 5).
- Muscle action moves fluids through ducts and tubes associated with other body systems.

Structures of the Muscular System

The body has more than 600 muscles that make up about 40% to 45% of the body's weight. These muscles are made up of fibers, covered with fascia, and attached to bones by tendons.

Muscle Fibers

- The muscles are composed of long, slender cells known as **muscle fibers**. (A fiber is a thread-like structure.) Each muscle consists of a group of fibers held together by connective tissue and enclosed in a fibrous sheath.

Fascia

- **Fascia** (**FASH**-ee-ah) is the sheet or band of fibrous connective tissue that covers, supports, and separates muscles.

Tendons

- A **tendon** is a narrow band of nonelastic, dense, fibrous connective tissue that attaches a muscle to a bone (Figure 4.1).
- For example, the **Achilles tendon** attaches the gastrocnemius muscle (the major muscle of the calf of the leg) to the heel bone (see Figure 4.10).

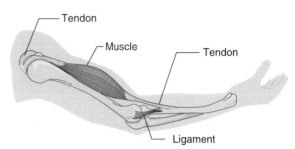

FIGURE 4.1 Tendons attach muscle to bone. Ligaments join bone to bone.

- Be careful not to confuse tendons with ligaments. As shown in Figure 4.1, ligaments connect one bone to another bone. Ligaments are discussed in Chapter 3.

Aponeurosis

- An **aponeurosis** (**ap**-oh-new-**ROH**-sis) is a flat fibrous sheet of connective tissue that is very similar to a tendon; however, an aponeurosis attaches a muscle to bone *or* to other tissues (plural, **aponeuroses**). As an example, the abdominal aponeurosis can be seen in Figure 4.9.

Types of Muscle Tissue

The three types of muscle tissue are skeletal, smooth, and cardiac (Figure 4.2). These types are described according to their appearance and function.

Skeletal Muscles

- **Skeletal muscles** attach to the bones of the skeleton and are the muscles that make possible body motions such as walking and smiling (see Figure 4.2A).
- Skeletal muscles are also known as **striated** (**STRYE**-ayt-ed) muscles because dark and light bands in the muscle fibers create a striped (striated) appearance.
- Skeletal muscles are also known as **voluntary muscles** because we have conscious (voluntary) control over these muscles.

(A) Skeletal muscle

A fiber

Many nuclei per fiber

Striations (cross-stripes)

(B) Smooth muscle

Spindle-shaped fiber

Nucleus

Cell (fiber) membrane

(C) Cardiac muscle

A fiber

Centrally located nucleus

Striations (cross-stripes)

Branching of fiber

Figure 4.2 Types of muscle tissue. (A) Skeletal muscle. (B) Smooth muscle. (C) Cardiac muscle.

Smooth Muscles

- **Smooth muscles** are located in the walls of internal organs such as the digestive tract, blood vessels, and ducts leading from glands (see Figure 4.2B). Their function is to move and control the flow of fluids through these structures.

- Smooth muscles are also known as **unstriated muscles** because they do *not* have the dark and light bands that produce the striped (striated) appearance seen in striated muscles.

- Smooth muscles are also known as **involuntary muscles** because they are under the control of the autonomic nervous system and are not under voluntary control.

- Smooth muscles are also known as **visceral muscles** (VIS-er-al) because they are found in the large internal organs (except the heart) and in hollow structures such as the digestive and urinary systems.

Cardiac Muscle

- **Cardiac muscle**, also known as **myocardial muscle** (my-oh-KAR-dee-al), forms the muscular wall of the heart (**myo** means muscle, **cardi** means heart, and **al** means pertaining to). The heart is discussed in Chapter 5.

- This muscle is also known as the **myocardium** (my-oh-KAR-dee-um) (**myo** means muscle, **card** means heart, and **ium** means tissue).

- **Cardiac muscle** is specialized tissue that is like striated muscle in its appearance, but like smooth muscle in its action (see Figure 4.2C). It is the contraction and relaxation of this muscle that causes the heartbeat.

Characteristics of Muscles

Kinesiology (kih-**nee**-see-**OL**-oh-jee) is the study of muscular activity and the resulting movement of body parts (**kinesi** means movement and **ology** means the study of).

Antagonistic Muscle Pairs

- The muscles of the body are arranged in antagonistic pairs. **Antagonistic** means to work in opposition to each other.
- In an antagonistic pair, one muscle produces movement in one direction and the other muscle produces movement in the opposite direction.

Contraction and Relaxation

- Muscles are made up of specialized cells that can change length or shape by contracting and relaxing. It is these contrasting actions that make motion possible.
- **Contraction** is the tightening of a muscle. As the muscle contracts it becomes shorter and thicker causing the belly (center) of the muscle to enlarge.
- **Relaxation** occurs when a muscle returns to its original form. As the muscle relaxes it becomes longer and thinner and the belly is no longer enlarged.
- When one muscle of a pair contracts, the other usually relaxes (Figure 4.3).
- **Muscle tone**, also known as **tonus** (**TOH**-nus), is the normal state of balanced muscle tension (contraction and relaxation) that is required to hold the body in an awake position.

Muscle Innervation

- **Muscle innervation** (in-err-**VAY**-shun) is the stimulation of the muscle by an impulse transmitted by a motor nerve. This stimulation causes the muscle to contract. When the stimulation stops, the muscle relaxes.
- **Neuromuscular** (**new**-roh-**MUS**-kyou-lar) means pertaining to the relationship between nerve and muscle. If the nerve impulse is interrupted due to injury or pathology of the nervous system, the muscle is paralyzed and cannot contract.

Range of Motion

Range of motion (ROM) is the change in joint position that is produced by muscle movements. These muscle motions, which occur as pairs of opposites, are described below, contrasted in Table 4.1, and illustrated in Figures 4.4 through 4.8.

Abduction and Adduction

- **Abduction** (ab-**DUCK**-shun) is movement away from the midline of the body (see Figure 4.4). For example, during abduction the arm moves outward, away from the side of the body.
- An **abductor** is a muscle that moves a part away from the midline.
- **Adduction** (ah-**DUCK**-shun) is movement toward the midline of the body (see Figure 4.4). For example, during adduction the arm moves inward, toward the side of the body.
- An **adductor** is a muscle that moves a part toward the midline.

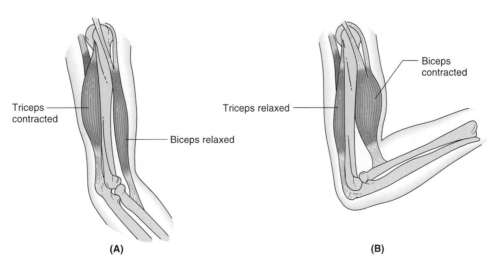

(A)   **(B)**

FIGURE 4.3 Antagonistic muscle pair of the upper arm in action. (A) During extension of the elbow, the triceps is contracted and the biceps is relaxed. (B) During flexion of the elbow, the triceps is relaxed and the biceps is contracted.

Table 4.1

CONTRASTING MUSCLE MOTIONS

Abduction moves away from the midline.	**Adduction** moves toward the midline.
Flexion (bending) decreases an angle as in bending a joint.	**Extension** (straightening) increases an angle as in straightening a joint.
Elevation raises a body part.	**Depression** lowers a body part.
Rotation turns a bone on its own axis.	**Circumduction** turns at the far end.
Supination turns the palm upward or forward.	**Pronation** turns the palm downward or backward.
Dorsiflexion bends the foot upward at the ankle.	**Plantar flexion** bends the foot downward at the ankle.

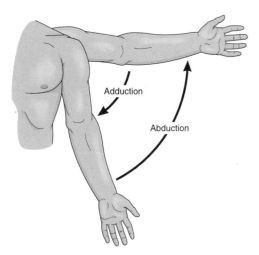

FIGURE 4.4 Abduction moves the arm away from the body. Adduction moves the arm toward the body.

Flexion and Extension

- **Flexion** (FLECK-shun) means decreasing the angle between two bones or bending a limb at a joint (see Figure 4.5). During flexion of the arm, the elbow is bent and the lower arm is brought upward. During flexion of the leg, the knee is bent and the lower leg is brought backward.
- A **flexor** is a muscle that bends a limb at a joint.
- **Extension** means increasing the angle between two bones or straightening out a limb (see Figure 4.5). During extension of the arm, the elbow is straightened and the lower arm is brought downward. During extension of the leg, the knee is straightened and the lower leg brought forward.

- An **extensor** is a muscle that straightens a limb at a joint.
- **Hyperextension** is the extreme or overextension of a limb or body part beyond its normal limit. For example, movement of the head far backward or far forward beyond the normal range of motion causes hyperextension of the muscles of the neck.

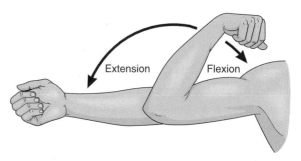

FIGURE 4.5 Extension increases the angle of the elbow. Flexion decreases the angle of the elbow.

Elevation and Depression

- **Elevation** is the act of raising or lifting a body part, such as raising the ribs when breathing in.
- A **levator** (lee-VAY-tor) is a muscle that raises a body part. For example, the *levator anguli oris* raises the corner of the mouth. (**Anguli** means angle and **oris** means mouth.)
- **Depression** is the act of lowering a body part such as lowering the ribs when breathing out.
- A **depressor** is a muscle that lowers a body part. For example, the *depressor anguli oris* lowers the corner of the mouth.

Rotation and Circumduction

- **Rotation** is a circular movement around an axis. Turning the head as when saying no is an example of rotation.
- A **rotator muscle** turns a body part on its axis. (An **axis** is the central line of the body or any of its parts.) For example, the head of the humerus (upper arm bone) rotates within the shoulder joint (see Figure 4.6).

FIGURE 4.6 Circumduction is movement at the far end of the arm. Rotation is the movement of the humerus in the shoulder joint.

- The **rotator cuff** is the group of muscles that hold the head of the humerus securely in place as it rotates within the shoulder joint (see Figure 4.15).
- **Circumduction** (**ser**-kum-**DUCK**-shun) is the circular movement of a limb at the far end. An example of circumduction is the swinging motion of the far end of the arm when throwing (see Figure 4.6).

Supination and Pronation

- **Supination** (**soo**-pih-**NAY**-shun) is the act of rotating the arm or the leg so the palm of the hand or sole of the foot is turned forward or upward (see Figure 4.7).
- **Pronation** (proh-**NAY**-shun) is the act of rotating the arm or leg so the palm of the hand or sole of the foot is turned downward or backward (see Figure 4.7).

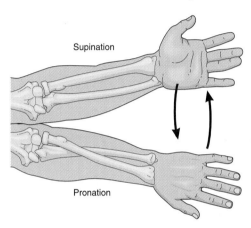

Supination

Pronation

FIGURE 4.7 Supination is turning the arm so the palm of the hand is turned upward. Pronation is turning the arm so the palm of the hand is downward.

Dorsiflexion and Plantar Flexion

- **Dorsiflexion** (**dor**-sih-**FLECK**-shun) bends the foot upward at the ankle. This action narrows the angle between the top of the foot and the front of the leg (see Figure 4.8).

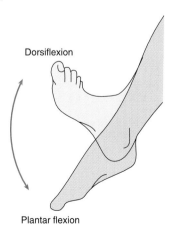

Dorsiflexion

Plantar flexion

FIGURE 4.8 Dorsiflexion bends the foot upward at the ankle. Plantarflexion bends the foot downward at the ankle.

- **Plantar flexion** (**PLAN**-tar **FLECK**-shun) bends the foot downward at the ankle. This action increases the angle between the top of the foot and the front of the leg. The term **plantar** means pertaining to the sole of the foot.

How Muscles are Named

As you study this section please refer to Figures 4.9 through 4.13.

Origin and Insertion

Some muscles are named by joining the name of the place of origin to the name of the place of insertion.

- **Muscle origin** is the place where the muscle begins (originates). This is the more fixed attachment and/or the end of the muscle nearest the midline of the body.
- **Muscle insertion** is the place where the muscle ends (inserts). It is the more moveable end and/or the portion of the muscle farthest from the midline of the body.
- For example, the **sternocleidomastoid** (**ster**-noh-**kly**-doh-**MASS**-toid) muscle that helps flex the neck and rotate the head is named for its origin and insertion (see Figure 4.11). This muscle originates near the midline from the sternum (breastbone) and clavicle (collar bone). It inserts away from the midline into the mastoid process of the temporal bone (located just behind the ear).

Muscles Named for Their Action

Some muscles are named for their action such as flexing or extending.

- For example, the **flexor carpi muscles** work with the **extensor carpi muscles** to make possible the flexion and extension motions of the wrist (see Figure 4.9).

Muscles Named for Their Location

Some muscles are named for their location on the body or the organ they are near.

- For example, the **pectoralis major** is an important muscle of the chest and **pectoral** (**PECK**-toh-rahl) means relating to the chest (see Figure 4.9).
- Other muscles, such as **vastus lateralis** and **vastus medialis**, indicate their location by including lateral (toward the side) and medial (toward the midline) in their names (see Figures 4.9 and 4.10).
- Some muscles show location by including external (near the surface) and internal (deeper location) in their names. For example the **external oblique** and **internal oblique** muscles (see Figures 4.9 and 4.12).

FIGURE 4.9 Major muscles of body (anterior view).

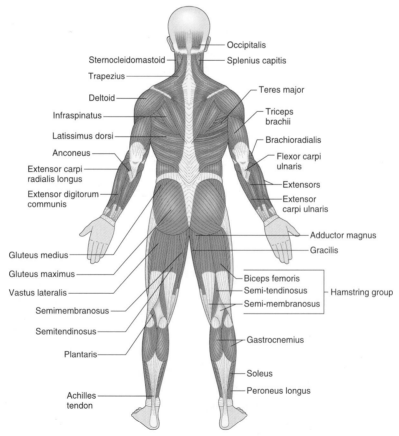

FIGURE 4.10 Major muscles of body (posterior view).

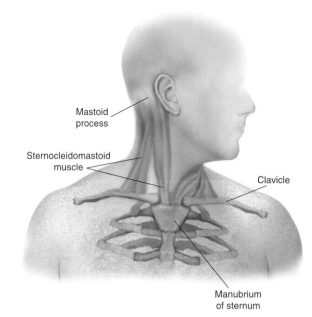

Mastoid process

Sternocleidomastoid muscle

Clavicle

Manubrium of sternum

Figure 4.11 The sternocleidomastoid muscle is named for its origins and insertion.

Muscles Named for Fiber Direction

Some muscles are named for the direction in which their fibers run.

- **Rectus** (**RECK**-tus) means straight. For example, **rectus abdominis** is an abdominal muscle in straight alignment with the vertical axis of the body (see Figures 4.9 and 4.12).
- **Oblique** (oh-**BLEEK**) means slanted or at an angle. For example, the **external abdominal oblique** is an abdom-

inal muscle that slants outward, at an oblique angle, away from the midline.

- **Transverse** means in a crosswise direction. For example, the **transverse abdominis** is an abdominal muscle with a crosswise alignment.
- A **sphincter** (**SFINK**-ter) is a ringlike muscle that tightly constricts the opening of a passageway. A sphincter is named for the passage involved. For example, the **anal sphincter** closes the anus.

Muscles Named for Number of Divisions

Muscles may be named according to the number of divisions forming them (Figure 4.13).

- For example, the **biceps brachii** (**BRAY**-kee-eye), also known as the **biceps** muscle, is formed from two divisions (**bi** means two and **ceps** means head). This is the muscle of the anterior upper arm that flexes the elbow.
- For example, the **triceps brachii** (**BRAY**-kee-eye), also known as the **triceps** muscle, is formed from three divisions (**tri** means three and **ceps** means head). This is the muscle of the posterior upper arm that extends the elbow.
- For example, the **quadriceps femoris** (**FEM**-or-iss) is formed from four muscle divisions (**quadri** means four and **ceps** means head). This large muscle, which is located on the anterior thigh, assists in extending the femur (bone of the upper leg).

Muscles Named for Their Size

Some muscles are named because they are broad or narrow, large or small.

- For example, **gluteus maximus** (**GLOO**-tee-us) is the largest muscle of the buttock (see Figure 4.10).

Rectus abdominis

External oblique

Internal oblique

Transversus abdominis

Figure 4.12 Examples of muscles named for their direction.

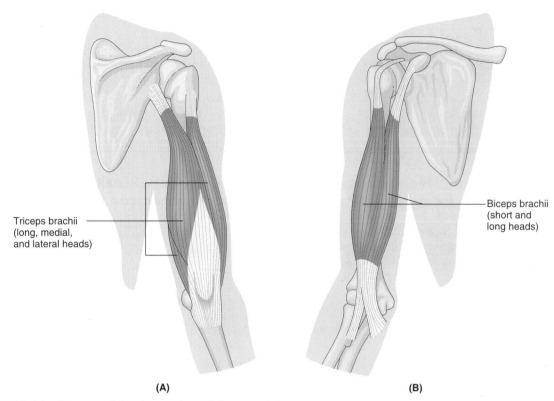

Triceps brachii
(long, medial,
and lateral heads)

Biceps brachii
(short and
long heads)

(A)   **(B)**

FIGURE 4.13 Muscles named for the number of divisions. (A) Posterior view. (B) Anterior view.

Muscles Named for Their Shape

Other muscles are named because they are shaped like a familiar object.

- For example, the **deltoid muscle**, which forms the muscular shoulder cap, is shaped like an inverted triangle or the Greek letter delta (see Figures 4.9 and 4.10).

Medical Specialties Related to the Muscular System

Skeletal Muscle Disorders

- An **orthopedic surgeon** treats injuries and disorders involving bones, joints, muscles, and tendons.
- A **rheumatologist** (roo-mah-**TOL**-oh-jist) treats disorders that involve the inflammation of connective tissues including muscles.
- A **neurologist** (new-**ROL**-oh-jist) treats the cause of paralysis and similar muscular disorders in which there is a loss of function.
- A specialist in **sports medicine** treats sports-related injuries of the bones, joints, and muscles.

Smooth Muscle Disorders

- Smooth muscles are a key component in most body systems. The specialist who treats the involved body system also cares for any involved muscles.

Cardiac Muscle Disorders

- A **cardiologist** treats disorders of the cardiac muscles.

Pathology of the Muscular System

Fibers, Fascia, and Tendons

- **Fasciitis** (fas-ee-**EYE**-tis) is inflammation of a fascia (**fasci** means fascia and **itis** means inflammation and this term is spelled correctly with two letter *i*s next to each other; however a secondary spelling that is also acceptable is fascitis).
- **Tenalgia** (ten-**AL**-jee-ah) is pain in a tendon (**ten** means tendon and **algia** means pain). It is also known as **tenodynia** (ten-oh-**DIN**-ee-ah).
- **Tendinitis** (ten-dih-**NIGH**-tis) is an inflammation of the tendons caused by excessive or unusual use of the joint (**tendin** means tendon and **itis** means inflammation). This is also known as **tendonitis** (ten-doh-**NIGH**-tis).

  Overuse tendinitis is an inflammation of tendons caused by excessive or unusual use of a joint.

Muscles

- An **adhesion** (ad-**HEE**-zhun) is a band of fibrous tissue that holds structures together abnormally. Adhesions may form in muscles and internal organs as the result of an injury or surgery.

- **Muscle atrophy** (AT-roh-fee) is weakness and wasting away of muscle tissue. It may be caused by pathology or by disuse of the muscle over a long period of time.

- **Myalgia** (my-AL-jee-ah) means muscle tenderness or pain (**my** means muscle and **algia** means pain).

- **Myolysis** (my-OL-ih-sis) is the degeneration (breaking down) of muscle tissue (**myo** means muscle and **lysis** means destruction or breaking down in disease).

- **Myositis** (my-oh-SIGH-tis) is inflammation of a muscle tissue, especially skeletal muscles (**myos** means muscle and **itis** means inflammation).

- **Polymyositis** (pol-ee-my-oh-SIGH-tis) is a chronic, progressive disease affecting the skeletal muscles that is characterized by muscle weakness and atrophy (**poly** means many, **myos** means muscle, and **itis** means inflammation).

- **Myomalacia** (my-oh-mah-LAY-shee-ah) is abnormal softening of muscle tissue (**myo** means muscle and **malacia** means abnormal softening).

- **Myorrhexis** (my-oh-RECK-sis) is the rupture of a muscle (**myo** means muscle and **rrhexis** means rupture).

- **Myosclerosis** (my-oh-skleh-ROH-sis) is abnormal hardening of muscle tissue (**myo** means muscle and **sclerosis** means abnormal hardening).

Hernias

- A **hernia** (HER-nee-ah) is the protrusion of a part or structure through the tissues normally containing it.

- A **myocele** (MY-oh-seel) is the protrusion of a muscle through its ruptured sheath or fascia (**myo** means muscle and **cele** means hernia).

Muscle Tone

- **Atonic** (ah-TON-ick) means the lack of normal muscle tone (**a** means without, **ton** means tone, and **ic** means pertaining to).

- **Dystonia** (dis-TOH-nee-ah) is a condition of abnormal muscle tone (**dys** means bad, **ton** means tone, and **ia** means condition).

- **Hypertonia** (high-per-TOH-nee-ah) is a condition of excessive tone of the skeletal muscles with increased resistance of muscle to passive stretching (**hyper** means excessive, **ton** means tone, and **ia** means condition).

- **Hypotonia** (high-poh-TOH-nee-ah) is a condition of diminished tone of the skeletal muscles with decreased resistance of muscle to passive stretching (**hypo** means deficient, **ton** means tone, and **ia** means condition).

- **Myotonia** (my-oh-TOH-nee-ah) is the delayed relaxation of a muscle after a strong contraction (**myo** means muscle, **ton** means tone, and **ia** means condition).

Voluntary Muscle Movement

- **Ataxia** (ah-TACK-see-ah) is an inability to coordinate the muscles in the execution of voluntary movement (**a** means without, **tax** means coordination, and **ia** means condition).

- **Dystaxia** (dis-TACK-see-ah), also known as **partial ataxia**, is difficulty in controlling voluntary movement (**dys** means bad, **tax** means coordination and **ia** means condition).

- A **contracture** (kon-TRACK-chur) is an abnormal shortening of muscle tissues making the muscle resistant to stretching.

- **Intermittent claudication** (klaw-dih-KAY-shun) is a complex of symptoms including cramplike pain of the leg muscles caused by poor circulation and may be an indication of a larger cardiovascular problem.

- A **spasm**, also known as a **cramp**, is a sudden, violent, involuntary contraction of a muscle or a group of muscles.

- **Spasmodic torticollis** (spaz-MOD-ick tor-tih-KOL-is), also known as **wryneck**, is a stiff neck due to spasmodic contraction of the neck muscles that pull the head toward the affected side.

Muscle Function

- **Bradykinesia** (brad-ee-kih-NEE-zee-ah *or* brad-ee-kih-NEE-zhuh) means extreme slowness in movement (**brady** means slow, **kines** means movement, and **ia** means condition).

- **Dyskinesia** (dis-kih-NEE-zee-ah) means distortion or impairment of voluntary movement as in a tic or spasm (**dys** means bad, **kines** means movement, and **ia** means condition).

- **Hyperkinesia** (high-per-kye-NEE-zee-ah), also known as **hyperactivity**, means abnormally increased motor function or activity (**hyper** means excessive, **kines** means movement, and **ia** means condition).

- **Hypokinesia** (high-poh-kye-NEE-zee-ah) is abnormally decreased motor function or activity (**hypo** means deficient, **kines** means movement, and **ia** means condition).

- **Tardive dyskinesia** (TAHR-div dis-kih-NEE-zee-ah) is the late appearance of dyskinesia as a side effect of long-term treatment with certain antipsychotic drugs. (**Tardive** means lateness in appearance.)

Myoclonus

- **Myoclonus** (my-oh-KLOH-nus *or* my-OCK-loh-nus) is a spasm or twitching of a muscle or group of muscles (**myo** means muscle and **clonus** mean violent action).

- **Nocturnal myoclonus** (nock-TER-nal my-oh-KLOH-nus *or* my-OCK-loh-nus) is jerking of the limbs that may occur normally as a person is falling asleep. (**Nocturnal** means pertaining to night.)

- **Singultus** (sing-GUL-tus), also known as **hiccups**, is myoclonus of the diaphragm that causes the characteristic hiccup sound with each spasm. (The diaphragm is the muscle separating the chest and abdomen.)

Myasthenia Gravis

- **Myasthenia** (my-as-THEE-nee-ah) is muscle weakness from any cause (**my** means muscle and **asthenia** means weakness or lack of strength).

- **Myasthenia gravis** (my-as-THEE-nee-ah GRAH-vis), also known as **MG**, is a chronic autoimmune disease in which there is an abnormality in the neuromuscular function causing episodes of muscle weakness. MG most frequently affects the muscles that control eye movements, eyelids, chewing, swallowing, coughing, and facial expression.

Muscular Dystrophy

- **Muscular dystrophy** (DIS-troh-fee) is a group of inherited muscle disorders that cause muscle weakness without affecting the nervous system. The most common forms, which affect only males, are Duchenne's muscular dystrophy (DMD) and Becker's muscular dystrophy (BMD).

- **Duchenne's muscular dystrophy** (doo-SHENZ) appears between 2 to 6 years of age, and progresses slowly; however, survival is rare beyond the late twenties.

- **Becker's muscular dystrophy** (BECK-urz) is a less severe illness and does not appear until early adolescence or adulthood. The progression is slower with survival well into mid to late adulthood.

Fibromyalgia Syndrome

- **Fibromyalgia syndrome** (figh-broh-my-AL-jee-ah) is a chronic disorder of unknown cause characterized by widespread aching pain, tender points, and fatigue (**fibro** means fibrous connective tissue, **my** means muscle, and **algia** means pain). Also known as **FMS**, this syndrome does not cause joint deformity, is not progressive, and is not crippling.

- **Tender points**, which are abnormal localized areas of soreness, are important diagnostic indicators of FMS. As shown in Figure 4.14, these points occur at predictable locations at the base of the neck, along the backbone, in front of the hip and elbow, and at the rear of the knee and shoulder.

Repetitive Stress Disorders

- **Repetitive stress disorders** have symptoms caused by repetitive motions that involve muscles, tendons, nerves, and joints. These conditions most commonly occur as workplace or sports injuries.

- **Ergonomics** (er-goh-NOM-icks) is the study of human factors that affect the design and operation of tools and the work environment (**ergo** means work, **nom** means control, and **ics** means pertaining to). This term is also applied to the design of sports equipment.

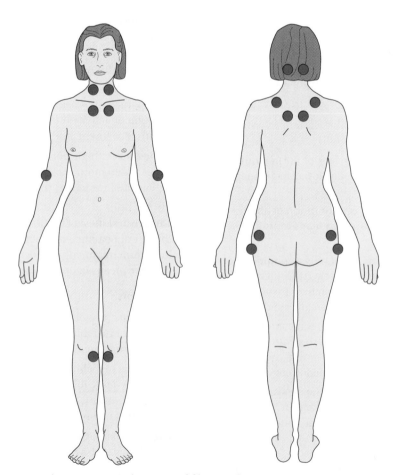

FIGURE **4.14** Tender points are characteristic indications of fibromyalgia.

ROTATOR CUFF

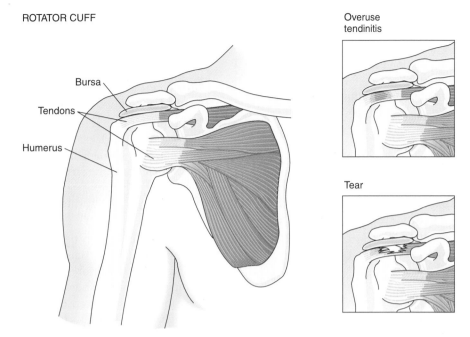

FIGURE 4.15 The rotator cuff in health (left) and with injuries (right).

- **Overuse injuries** occur when minor tissue injuries due to overuse are not given time to heal. This type of injury may be caused by factors such as spending hours at the keyboard or by lengthy sports training sessions.

Myofascial Damage

- **Myofascial damage** (**my**-oh-**FASH**-ee-ahl), which can be caused by overworking muscles, results in tenderness and swelling of the muscles and their surrounding tissues (**myo** means muscle, **fasci** means fascia, and **al** means pertaining to).

Rotator Cuff Injuries

- **Rotator cuff tendinitis** (**ten**-dih-**NIGH**-tis) is an inflammation of the tendons of the rotator cuff (Figure 4.15). This condition is often named for the cause such as **tennis shoulder** or **pitcher's shoulder**.

- **Impingement syndrome** (im-**PINJ**-ment) occurs when the tendons become inflamed and get caught in the narrow space between the bones within the shoulder joint.

- **Calcium deposits** may form within the tendons of the rotator cuff. These deposits cause chronic irritation of the tendons.

- **Torn tendon**. If left untreated, or if the overuse continues, the irritated tendon may weaken and tear.

Carpal Tunnel Syndrome

- The **carpal tunnel** (**KAR-pul**) is a narrow bony passage under the carpal ligament located 1/4 inch below the inner surface of the wrist (Figure 4.16). The median nerve and the tendons that bend the fingers pass through this tunnel. (**Carpal** means pertaining to the wrist.)

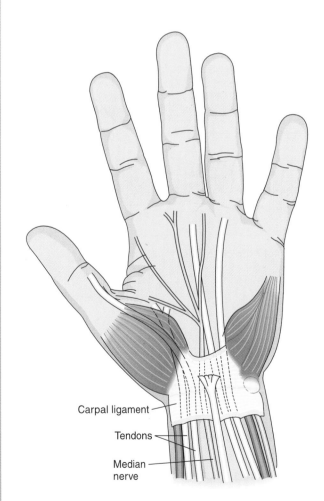

FIGURE 4.16 Carpal tunnel syndrome.

- **Carpal tunnel syndrome** occurs when the tendons passing through the carpal tunnel are chronically overused and become inflamed and swollen. This swelling creates compression (pressure) on the median nerve as it passes through the carpal tunnel. This causes pain, burning, and paresthesia (tingling) in the fingers and hand.

Cervical Radiculopathy

- **Cervical radiculopathy** (rah-**dick**-you-**LOP**-ah-thee) is nerve pain caused by pressure on the spinal nerve roots in the neck region (**radiculo** means nerve root, and **pathy** means disease). This pressure may be due to muscle spasms due to repetitive motions or can be caused by compression of cervical vertebral disks.

Epicondylitis

- **Epicondylitis** (ep-ih-**kon**-dih-**LYE**-tis) is inflammation of the tissues surrounding the elbow.
- **Lateral epicondylitis**, with pain on the outer side of the arm of the forearm, is also known as **tennis elbow** (Figure 4.17).
- **Medial epicondylitis**, with pain on the palm-side of the forearm, is also known as **golfer's elbow**.

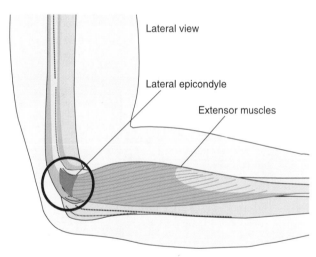

Lateral view

Lateral epicondyle

Extensor muscles

FIGURE 4.17 Epicondylitis.

Heel Spurs

- **Heel spurs**, which are associated with **plantar fasciitis**, are benign bony growths on the dorsal surface of the calcaneus (heel bone). The pain associated with this condition is due to inflammation of the plantar fascia as it rubs against these bony growths.

Sports Injuries

- A **sprain** is an injury to a joint such as ankle, knee, or wrist. Frequently caused by overuse, a sprain frequently involves a stretched or torn ligament.

- A **strain** is an injury to the body of the muscle or attachment of the tendon. Strains usually are associated with overuse injuries that involve a stretched or torn muscle or tendon attachment.
- Although these terms have slightly different meanings, they are frequently used interchangeably.
- A **shin splint** is pain caused by the muscle tearing away from the tibia, which is also known as the **shinbone**. Shin splints can develop in the anterolateral (front and side) muscles or in the posteromedial (back and side) muscles of the lower leg (see Figures 4.9 and 4.10). This type of injury is usually caused by repeated stress to the lower leg.
- A **hamstring injury** may be a strain or tear of the posterior femoral muscles. (Hamstring refers to the three muscles on the posterior of the thigh that straighten the hip and bend the knee as shown in Figure 4.10.) These injuries usually cause sudden pain in the back of the thigh as these muscles contract suddenly.
- **Achilles tendinitis** (ten-dih-**NIGH**-tis) is a painful inflammation of the Achilles tendon caused by excessive stress being placed on the tendon.

Paralysis

- **Myoparesis** (**my**-oh-**PAR**-eh-sis) is a weakness or slight paralysis of a muscle (**myo** means muscle and **paresis** means partial or incomplete paralysis).
- **Hemiparesis** (**hem**-ee-pah-**REE**-sis) means slight paralysis of one side of the body (**hemi** means half and **paresis** means partial or incomplete paralysis).
- **Paralysis** (pah-**RAL**-ih-sis) is the loss of sensation and voluntary muscle movements through disease or injury to its nerve supply. Damage may be either temporary or permanent (plural, **paralyses**).
- Paralysis is frequently caused by a **spinal cord injury**, also known as an **SCI**, that prevents nerve impulses from being carried below the level of the injury (see Figure 3.14).
- **Paraplegia** (par-ah-**PLEE**-jee-ah) is the paralysis of both legs and the lower part of the body. An individual affected with paraplegia is known as a **paraplegic**. An SCI below the cervical vertebrae results in paraplegia.
- **Quadriplegia** (kwad-rih-**PLEE**-jee-ah) is the paralysis of all four extremities (**quadri** means four and **plegia** means paralysis). An SCI involving the cervical vertebrae causes quadriplegia. If the injury is above C5, it also affects respiration.
- **Hemiplegia** (hem-ee-**PLEE**-jee-ah) is the total paralysis of one side of the body (**hemi** means half and **plegia** means paralysis). This form of paralysis is usually associated with a stroke or brain damage. Damage to one side of the brain causes paralysis on the opposite side of the body.

- **Cardioplegia** (**kar**-dee-oh-**PLEE**-jee-ah) is paralysis of the muscles of the heart (**cardio** means heart and **plegia** means paralysis).

Diagnostic Procedures of the Muscular System

- **Deep tendon reflexes**, also known as **DTR**, are tested with a reflex hammer used to strike the tendon. Figure 4.18 shows reflex testing on the kneecap (patellar reflex) and Achilles tendon (calcaneous reflex). An abnormal response, or the absence of a response, is an indication of pathology that may be caused by disrupted innervation of the involved muscles. Reflexes also are lost in deep coma or due to medication such as heavy sedation.
- **Electromyography** (ee-**leck**-troh-my-**OG**-rah-fee), also known as an EMG, records the strength of muscle contractions as the result of electrical stimulation. The resulting record is called an **electromyogram** (**electro** means electricity, **myo** means muscle, and **gram** means record).
- **Electroneuromyography** (ee-**leck**-troh-**new**-roh-my-**OG**-rah-fee), also known as **nerve conduction studies**, is a procedure for testing and recording neuromuscular activity by the electric stimulation of nerve trunk carrying fibers to and from the muscle.
- **Range of motion testing** (ROM) is a diagnostic procedure to evaluate joint mobility and muscle strength (see Figure 4.19).

Treatment Procedures of the Muscular System

Medications

- An **anti-inflammatory**, such as ibuprofen (Motrin), acts as an analgesic (relieves pain) and as an anti-inflammatory (relieves inflammation).
- An **antispasmodic**, also known as an **anticholinergic drug** (**an**-tih-**koh**-lin-**ER**-jik), acts to control spasmodic activity of the smooth muscles such as those of the intestine.
- **Atropine** (**AT**-roh-peen) is an antispasmodic that may be administered preoperatively to relax smooth muscles.
- A **muscle relaxant**, such as diazepam (Valium), acts on the central nervous system to relax muscle tone and relieve spasms. Many of these medications also relieve anxiety and tension.

Physical Therapy

- **Physical therapy**, also known as **PT**, is treatment to prevent disability or to restore functioning through the use of exercise, heat, massage, and other methods to improve circulation, flexibility, and muscle strength.
- **Range of motion exercises**, also known as **ROM**, are one form of PT. The goal of these therapeutic measures is to increase strength, flexibility, and mobility (Figure 4.19).

(A)

(B)

FIGURE 4.18 Assessment of deep tendon reflexes. (A) Testing the patellar reflex. (B) Testing the Achilles tendon reflex.

FIGURE 4.19 Range of motion exercises aid in restoring joint mobility and muscle strength.

Activities of Daily Living

The minimum goal of therapy is to restore the individual to the level of self help known as **activities of daily living**. Also known as **ADL**, these activities include

- Personal hygiene
- Dressing
- Grooming
- Eating
- Toileting

Fascia

- A **fasciotomy** (fash-ee-OT-oh-mee) is a surgical incision of fascia (**fasci** means fascia and **otomy** means a surgical incision).
- **Fascioplasty** (FASH-ee-oh-plas-tee) is the surgical repair of a fascia (**fasci** means fascia and **plasty** means surgical repair).

Tendons

- **Carpal tunnel release** is surgical enlargement of the carpal tunnel or cutting of the carpal ligament to relieve nerve pressure. This treatment is used to relieve the pressure on tendons and nerves in severe cases of carpal tunnel syndrome.
- A **tenectomy** (teh-NECK-toh-mee) is the surgical removal of a lesion from a tendon or tendon sheath (**ten** means tendon and **ectomy** means surgical removal).
- **Tenodesis** (ten-ODD-eh-sis) means to suture the end of a tendon to bone (**teno** means tendon and **desis** means to bind or tie together).
- **Tenolysis** (ten-OL-ih-sis) means to free a tendon from adhesions (**teno** means tendon and **lysis** means to set free).
- A **tenonectomy** (ten-oh-NECK-toh-mee) is the surgical removal of part of a tendon for the purpose of shortening it (**tenon** means tendon and **ectomy** means surgical removal). Notice that tenectomy and tenonectomy are similar in spelling but different in meaning.)
- A **tenotomy** (teh-NOT-oh-mee), also known as **tendotomy**, is the surgical division of a tendon for relief of a deformity caused by abnormal shortening of a muscle such as strabismus (crossed eyes).
- **Tenoplasty** (TEN-oh-plas-tee), also known as **tendoplasty**, is the surgical repair of a tendon (**teno** means tendon and **plasty** means surgical repair).
- **Tenorrhaphy** (ten-OR-ah-fee) is the suturing of a divided tendon (**teno** means tendon and **rrhaphy** means to suture).

Muscles

- A **myectomy** (my-ECK-toh-mee) is the surgical removal of a portion of a muscle (**my** means muscle and **ectomy** means surgical removal).
- **Myoplasty** (MY-oh-plas-tee) is the surgical repair of a muscle (**myo** means muscle and **plasty** means surgical repair).
- **Myorrhaphy** (my-OR-ah-fee) means to suture a muscle wound (**myo** means muscle and **rrhaphy** means to suture).

Learning Exercises

● Matching Word Parts—1

Write the letter of the correct answer on the line provided in the left column.

4.1. _____ -cele   A. movement, motion

4.2. _____ fasci/o   B. hernia

4.3. _____ fibr/o fibros/o   C. fibrous connective tissue

4.4. _____ -ia   D. fascia

4.5. _____ kinesi/o   E. condition

● Matching Word Parts—2

Write the letter of the correct answer on the line provided in the left column.

4.6. _____ my/o   A. tone, tension, stretching

4.7. _____ –rrhexis   B. tendon

4.8. _____ tax/o   C. rupture

4.9. _____ ten/o, tend/o, tendin/o   D. muscle

4.10. _____ ton/o   E. coordination

● Matching Muscle Directions and Positions—3

Write the letter of the correct answer on the line provided in the left column.

4.11. _____ lateralis   A. cross-wise

4.12. _____ oblique   B. ring-like

4.13. _____ rectus   C. slanted at an angle

4.14. _____ sphincter   D. straight

4.15. _____ transverse   E. toward the side

Definitions

Circle the letter next to the correct answer.

4.16. Muscles under voluntary control are known as _____ .

a. involuntary

b. nonstriated

c. skeletal

d. visceral

4.17. The origin of a muscle is _____ .

a. away from the midline

b. the more flexible end

c. the place where the muscle begins

d. the point of contraction

4.18. Which term means turning the hand so the palm is upward?

a. circumduction

b. pronation

c. rotating

d. supination

4.19. Which term means extreme slowness of movement?

a. bradykinesia

b. dyskinesia

c. hypotonia

d. myotonia

4.20. Where is the point of insertion for the sternocleidomastoid muscle?

a. breastbone

b. clavicle

c. mastoid process

d. sternum

4.21. The quadriceps femoris _____ .

a. forms the rotator cuff

b. is formed from four divisions

c. is the large muscle of the buttocks

d. is the major muscle of the lower leg

4.22. A narrow band of fibrous tissue that attaches a muscle to bone is called a/an _____ .

a. aponeurosis

b. fascia

c. ligament

d. tendon

4.23. Which term means a band of fibers that hold structures together abnormally?

a. adhesion

b. aponeurosis

c. atrophy

d. contracture

4.24. Which muscle makes possible the bending motion of the wrist?

a. extensor carpi

b. flexor carpi

c. vastus lateralis

d. vastus medialis

4.25. Which term means pain in a tendon?

a. tenalgia

b. tendenalgia

c. tendinitis

d. tendonalgia

Matching Pathology

Write the letter of the correct answer on the line provided in the left column.

4.26. _____ contracture

A. sudden involuntary contraction of a muscle

4.27. _____ epicondylitis

B. inflammation of tissues surrounding the elbow

4.28. _____ myolysis

C. inflammation of a voluntary muscle

4.29. _____ myositis

D. breaking down of muscle tissue

4.30. _____ spasm

E. abnormal shortening of muscle tissue

Which Word?

Circle the correct term.

4.31. The muscles found in hollow structures are known as *striated / involuntary* muscles.

4.32. Pectoralis major is a major muscle of the *chest / thigh.*

4.33. The term meaning a condition of abnormal muscle tone is *dystaxia / dystonia.*

4.34. The form of muscular dystrophy in which survival is rarely beyond the late twenties is *Becker's / Duchenne's.*

4.35. The term meaning the study of human factors that affect the work environment is *ergonomics / impingement syndrome.*

Spelling Counts

Find the misspelled term and spell it correctly on the line at the end of the sentence.

4.36. The tricips brachii is the muscle of the posterior upper arm. _____

4.37. The medical term for hiccups is singulutas. _____

4.38. Muscle tone, also known as tonis, is the normal state of balanced tension that is present in the body when one is awake. _____

4.39. Jamie Vaughn suffers from a lack of muscle coordination that is known as ataxis. _____

4.40. The gleoteus maximus is the largest muscle of the buttock. _____

Term Selection

4.41. Which term means the rupture of a muscle?

a. myocele

b. myorrhaphy

c. myorrhexis

d. myotomy

4.42. Which term describes a fibrous sheet that attaches a muscle to bone *or* to other tissues?

a. aponeurosis

b. fascia

c. fibrous sheath

d. ligament

4.43. Which statement describes nocturnal myoclonus?

a. It is a normal occurrence.

b. It is also known as hiccups.

c. It is an inherited condition.

d. It is due to a lack of muscle tone.

4.44. Which term describes the study of muscular activity and the resulting movement of body parts?

a. ergonomics

b. kinesiology

c. pathophysiology

d. physiology

4.45. Which term means distortion or impairment of voluntary movement?

a. bradykinesia

b. dyskinesia

c. hyperkinesia

d. hypokinesia

● Sentence Completion

Write the missing word on the line.

4.46. The diagnostic procedure for testing and recording neuromuscular activity by the electric stimulation of nerve trunk carrying fibers to and from the muscle is called _____ .

4.47. A muscle that raises a body part is called a/an _____ .

4.48. The group of muscles that hold the head of the humerus securely in place as it rotates within the shoulder joint form the _____ cuff.

4.49. When tendons become inflamed and get caught in the narrow space between the bones within the shoulder joint this is known as the _____ syndrome.

4.50. The sheet or band of fibrous connective tissue that covers, supports, and separates muscles is called _____ .

4.51. The term meaning difficulty in controlling voluntary movement is _____ .

4.52. The medical term meaning to suture the end of a tendon to bone is _____ .

4.53. The opposite of extension is _____ .

4.54. Inflammation of a tendon is called _____ .

4.55. A surgical incision into fascia is known as a/an _____ .

● True/False

If the statement is true, write T on the line. If the statement is false, write F on the line.

4.56. _____ Electromyography records the strength of muscle contractions as the result of electrical stimulation.

4.57. _____ Hypertonia is a condition of diminished tone of the skeletal muscles.

4.58. _____ Tender points are symptomatic of myasthenia gravis.

4.59. _____ When the nerve impulse to a muscle is interrupted, that muscle is paralyzed.

4.60. _____ Plantar flexion is turning the hand downward.

4.61. _____ Carpal tunnel syndrome pain is due to bone spurs in the wrist.

4.62. _____ Pain on movement of the shoulder joint may be due to calcium deposits in tissues.

4.63. _____ A hamstring injury is also known as tennis elbow.

4.64. _____ Shin splints are stress fractures of the tibia.

4.65. _____ Cardiac muscle is a specialized type of muscle found only in the heart.

● Clinical Conditions

Write the correct answer on the line.

4.66. George Quinton suffered from spasmodic _____ . This is also known as wryneck.

4.67. Nina Burleson suffers from a chronic autoimmune disease in which there is an abnormality in the neuromuscular function causing episodes of muscle weakness. This condition is known as _____ gravis.

4.68. Due to the lack of exercise while he was confined to bed, Gerald Hastings experienced muscle _____ .

4.69. Jill Franklin has abnormal hardening of muscle tissue. This condition is called _____ .

4.70. Based on the presence of tender points, Allison Cox's doctor diagnosed her condition as _____ syndrome.

4.71. Chuan Lee was injured in an accident and suffered the rupture of a muscle through its sheath or fascia. This is called a/an _____ .

4.72. After her abdominal surgery, Beth Hill suffered from intestinal _____ , which abnormally held the structures together.

4.73. Several months after the accident, Jackson Brooks underwent _____ to free the tendons in his arm from the adhesions caused by his injury.

4.74. Steve Reeves suffered paralysis of all four limbs caused by a spinal injury. This condition is called _____ .

4.75. After suffering a stroke, Juan Hernandez has slight paralysis on one side of his body. His doctor describes this as _____ .

● Which is the Correct Medical Term?

Circle the letter next to the correct answer.

4.76. Which term means delayed relaxation of a muscle after a strong contraction?

   a. atonic

   b. dystaxia

   c. dystonia

   d. myotonia

4.77. Which term means the surgical repair of a tendon?

   a. tenectomy

   b. tenodesis

   c. tenolysis

   d. tenoplasty

4.78. Which type of muscle tissue makes walking possible?

   a. smooth

   b. striated

   c. involuntary

   d. visceral

4.79. Which term means abnormal softening of a muscle?

   a. myasthenia

   b. myomalacia

   c. myorrhexis

   d. myosclerosis

4.80. Which is the common name for spasmodic torticollis?

   a. cramp

   b. hiccup

   c. limping

   d. wryneck

● Challenge Word Building

These terms are not found in this chapter; however, they are made up of these familiar word parts: You may want to look in the glossary or use a medical dictionary to check your answers!

poly-	card/o	-algia
	fasci/o	-desis
	herni/o	-ectomy
	my/o	-itis
	sphincter/o	-necrosis
		-otomy
		-pathy
		-rrhaphy

4.81. The medical term meaning any abnormal condition of skeletal muscles is

   _____ .

4.82. The medical term meaning pain in several muscle groups is _____ .

4.83. The medical term meaning the necrosis, or death, of individual muscle fibers is

   _____ .

4.84. The medical term meaning the suturing of torn fascia is _____ .

4.85. The medical term meaning a surgical incision into, or division of, a muscle is a/an

   _____ .

4.86. The medical term meaning suturing (binding) fascia to a skeletal attachment is

   _____ .

4.87. The medical term meaning inflammation of the muscle of the heart is

   _____ .

4.88. The medical term meaning the surgical removal of fascia is a/an

   _____ .

4.89. The medical term meaning the surgical suturing of a defect in a muscular wall such as the repair of a hernia is
   a/an_____ .

4.90. The medical term meaning an incision into or division of a sphincter muscle is
   a/an_____ .

● Labeling Exercises

- abduction
- adduction
- circumduction
- dorsiflexion
- extension
- flexion
- plantar flexion
- pronation
- rotation
- supination

Identify the movements in the pictures below by writing the correct term on the line provided. As a hint the terms are listed above.

4.91. _____
4.92. _____
4.93. _____
4.94. _____
4.95. _____
4.96. _____
4.97. _____
4.98. _____
4.99. _____
4.100. _____

4.91
4.92

4.93
4.94

4.95

4.96
4.97

4.98
4.99

4.100

The Human Touch: Critical Thinking Exercise

The following story and questions are designed to stimulate critical thinking through class discussion or as a brief essay response. There are no easy or right-wrong answers to these questions.

"Leg muscles save back muscles . . . Mandatory OSHA meeting Tuesday at noon. Bring lunch," states the company memo. Sandor Padilla, a 28-year-old cargo loader, sighs. "Third meeting this year and its not even June yet!" He only has two minutes to reach the tarmac. "Oh well, cargo waits for no man," he thinks as he jogs off to work.

Sandor enjoys his job. It keeps him fit, but lets his mind follow more creative avenues. Today his thoughts stray to his daughter Reina's 5th birthday party, just two weeks away. "A pony, or a clown? Hot dogs or tacos?" he muses. Single parenting has its moments. As he is busy thinking of other things the heavy crate slips, driving him into a squatting position that injures his thigh muscles. His cry of pain brings Janet Wilson, his supervisor, running to help.

The first aid station ices his leg to reduce swelling and pain. After the supervisor completes the incident report, she drives Sandor to the emergency room. Dr. Basra, the orthopedic specialist on call, diagnoses myorrhexis of the left rectus femoris with myoparesis. A myotomy with myorrhaphy is performed. After 4 days in the hospital Sandor is sent home with a Vicodin prescription for pain and orders for physical therapy sessions three times a week. He is not expected to return to work for at least 90 days.

AirFreight Systems receives the first report of injury and compares it with the supervisor's incident report. Ruling: Safety Violation. No Liability. Return to work in 30 days or dismissal.

Suggested Discussion Topics:

1. On what basis do you think AirFreight determined that this was a safety violation?
2. Who do you think should be liable for Sandor's accident and the cost of his medical care? Why?
3. Do you think the air freight company can take away Sandor's job if he does not return in 30 calendar days?
4. What do you think are Sandor's options if he cannot return to work at the airport within 30 calendar days?
5. Use your knowledge of medical terminology to describe the extent of Sandor's injury, diagnosis, and treatment to someone with no medical background.

The Cardiovascular System

● **Overview of Structures, Word Parts, and Functions of the Cardiovascular System**

MAJOR STRUCTURES	RELATED WORD ROOTS	PRIMARY FUNCTIONS
Heart	card/o, cardi/o	Pumps blood into the arteries.
Arteries	arteri/o	Transport blood to all body parts.
Capillaries	capill/o	Exchange nutrients and waste products with cells.
Veins	phleb/o, ven/o	Return blood to the heart.
Blood	hem/o, hemat/o	Brings oxygen and nutrients to all cells and carries away waste.
		Plays several important roles in the immune and endocrine systems.

VOCABULARY Related to the Cardiovascular System

Check the box as you master each word part or term. Terms marked with the ❖ symbol are pronounced on the optional student audiotape.

Word Parts

- [ ] angi/o
- [ ] aort/o
- [ ] arteri/o
- [ ] ather/o
- [ ] brady-
- [ ] cardi/o
- [ ] coron/o
- [ ] -emia
- [ ] erythr/o
- [ ] hem/o, hemat/o
- [ ] leuk/o
- [ ] phleb/o
- [ ] tachy-
- [ ] thromb/o
- [ ] ven/o

Key Medical Terms

- [ ] **aneurysm** (AN-you-rizm) ❖
- [ ] **aneurysmectomy** (**an**-you-riz-**MECK**-toh-mee) ❖
- [ ] **aneurysmorrhaphy** (**an**-you-riz-**MOR**-ah-fee) ❖
- [ ] **angiitis** (an-je-**EYE**-tis) ❖
- [ ] **angina** (an-**JIGH**-nah *or* AN-jih-nuh) ❖
- [ ] **angiocardiography** (an-jee-oh-**kar**-dee-**OG**-rah-fee) ❖
- [ ] **angiography** (an-jee-**OG**-rah-fee)
- [ ] **angionecrosis** (**an**-jee-oh-neh-**KROH**-sis)
- [ ] **angiostenosis** (AN-jee-oh-steh-**NOH**-sis)
- [ ] **antiarrhythmic** (an-tih-ah-**RITH**-mick) ❖
- [ ] **anticoagulant** (an-tih-koh-**AG**-you-lant) ❖
- [ ] **antihypertensive** (an-tih-**high**-per-**TEN**-siv) ❖
- [ ] **aplastic anemia** (ay-**PLAS**-tick ah-**NEE**-mee-ah) ❖
- [ ] **arrhythmia** (ah-**RITH**-mee-ah) ❖
- [ ] **arteriectomy** (ar-teh-ree-**ECK**-toh-mee) ❖
- [ ] **arteriosclerosis** (ar-**tee**-ree-oh-skleh-**ROH**-sis) ❖
- [ ] **arteritis** (ar-teh-**RYE**-tis) ❖
- [ ] **atherectomy** (ath-er-**ECK**-toh-mee) ❖
- [ ] **atheroma** (ath-er-**OH**-mah) ❖
- [ ] **atherosclerosis** (ath-er-oh-skleh-**ROH**-sis) ❖
- [ ] **basophils** (**BAY**-soh-fills) ❖
- [ ] **bradycardia** (brad-ee-**KAR**-dee-ah) ❖
- [ ] **cardiac catheterization** (**KAR**-dee-ack **kath**-eh-ter-eye-**ZAY**-shun) ❖
- [ ] **cholesterol** (koh-**LES**-ter-ol) ❖
- [ ] **defibrillation** (dee-**fib**-rih-**LAY**-shun) ❖
- [ ] **diastolic** (dye-ah-**STOL**-ick) ❖
- [ ] **dyscrasia** (dis-**KRAY**-zee-ah) ❖
- [ ] **echocardiography** (eck-oh-**kar**-dee-**OG**-rah-fee) ❖
- [ ] **electrocardiogram** (ee-**leck**-troh-**KAR**-dee-oh-gram) ❖

- [ ] **embolism** (**EM**-boh-lizm) ❖
- [ ] **embolus** (**EM**-boh-lus) ❖
- [ ] **endarterectomy** (**end**-ar-ter-**ECK**-toh-mee) ❖
- [ ] **endocarditis** (**en**-doh-kar-**DYE**-tis) ❖
- [ ] **eosinophils** (ee-oh-**SIN**-oh-fills) ❖
- [ ] **erythrocytes** (eh-**RITH**-roh-sights)
- [ ] **fibrillation** (fih-brih-**LAY**-shun) ❖
- [ ] **hemangioma** (hee-**man**-jee-**OH**-mah) ❖
- [ ] **hemochromatosis** (hee-moh-**kroh**-mah-**TOH**-sis) ❖
- [ ] **hemoglobin** (hee-moh-**GLOH**-bin)
- [ ] **hemolytic anemia** (hee-moh-**LIT**-ick ah-**NEE**-mee-ah) ❖
- [ ] **hemostasis** (hee-moh-**STAY**-sis) ❖
- [ ] **homocysteine** (hoh-moh-**SIS**-teen) ❖
- [ ] **hypoperfusion** (**high**-poh-per-**FYOU**-zhun) ❖
- [ ] **ischemia** (iss-**KEE**-me-ah) ❖
- [ ] **leukemia** (loo-**KEE**-me-ah) ❖
- [ ] **leukocytes** (**LOO**-koh-sites)
- [ ] **leukopenia** (loo-koh-**PEE**-nee-ah) ❖
- [ ] **lymphocytes** (**LIM**-foh-sights)
- [ ] **megaloblastic anemia** (**MEG**-ah-loh-**blas**-tick ah-**NEE**-mee-ah) ❖
- [ ] **monocytes** (**MON**-oh-sights)
- [ ] **myocardial infarction** (**my**-oh-**KAR**-dee-al in-**FARK**-shun) ❖
- [ ] **myocarditis** (my-oh-kar-**DYE**-tis) ❖
- [ ] **neutrophils** (**NEW**-troh-fills)
- [ ] **palpitation** (**pal**-pih-**TAY**-shun) ❖
- [ ] **pericarditis** (**pehr**-ih-kar-**DYE**-tis) ❖
- [ ] **pernicious anemia** (per-**NISH**-us ah-**NEE**-mee-ah) ❖
- [ ] **phlebitis** (fleh-**BYE**-tis) ❖
- [ ] **phlebography** (fleh-**BOG**-rah-fee) ❖
- [ ] **plaque** (**PLACK**)
- [ ] **polyarteritis** (**pol**-ee-**ar**-teh-**RYE**-tis) ❖
- [ ] **Raynaud's** (ray-**NOHZ**) ❖
- [ ] **septicemia** (sep-tih-**SEE**-mee-ah) ❖
- [ ] **systolic** (sis-**TOL**-ick) ❖
- [ ] **tachycardia** (tack-ee-**KAR**-dee-ah) ❖
- [ ] **thrombocytes** (**THROM**-boh-sights)
- [ ] **thrombocytopenia** (**throm**-boh-**sigh**-toh-**PEE**-nee-ah) ❖
- [ ] **thrombolytic** (**throm**-boh-**LIT**-ick) ❖
- [ ] **thrombosis** (throm-**BOH**-sis) ❖
- [ ] **thrombus** (**THROM**-bus) ❖
- [ ] **triglycerides** (try-**GLIS**-er-eyeds) ❖
- [ ] **valvoplasty** (**VAL**-voh-**plas**-tee) ❖
- [ ] **valvulitis** (val-view-**LYE**-tis) ❖
- [ ] **valvuloplasty** (**VAL**-view-loh-**plas**-tee) ❖
- [ ] **varicose veins** (**VAR**-ih-kohs **VAYNS**) ❖
- [ ] **vasculitis** (vas-kyou-**LYE**-tis) ❖

● OBJECTIVES

On completion of this chapter, you should be able to:

1 Describe the heart in terms of chambers, valves, blood flow, heartbeat, blood supply, and heart sounds.

2 Differentiate among the three different types of blood vessels and describe the major function of each.

3 Identify the major components of blood and the major functions of each.

4 State the difference between pulmonary and systemic circulation.

5 Recognize, define, spell, and pronounce the terms related to the pathology, diagnostic and treatment procedures of the cardiovascular system.

Functions of the Cardiovascular System

The term **cardiovascular** means pertaining to the heart and the blood vessels. These structures work together as an efficient pumping system to supply all body tissues with oxygen and nutrients and to transport cellular waste products to the appropriate organs for removal from the body.

▪ In addition, the blood cells play important roles in the immune system (see Chapter 6) and endocrine system (see Chapter 13).

Structures of the Cardiovascular System

The major structures of the cardiovascular system are the heart, blood vessels, and blood.

The Heart

The heart, which is a hollow muscular organ located between the lungs and above the diaphragm, is a very effective pump that furnishes the power to maintain blood flow throughout both the pulmonary and systemic circulatory systems (Figures 5.1 and 5.2).

Superior vena cava

Right pulmonary artery

Right pulmonary veins

Right atrium

Right ventricle

Aorta

Left pulmonary artery

Left pulmonary veins

Left atrium

Left ventricle

Apex

FIGURE 5.1 External view of the heart.

FIGURE 5.2 Cross section of the heart.

The Pericardium

- The **pericardium** (pehr-ih-**KAR**-dee-um) is the double-walled membranous sac that encloses the heart.
- **Pericardial fluid** between the layers prevents friction when the heart beats.

The Walls of the Heart

The walls of the heart are made up of three layers: the epicardium, myocardium, and endocardium (Figure 5.3).

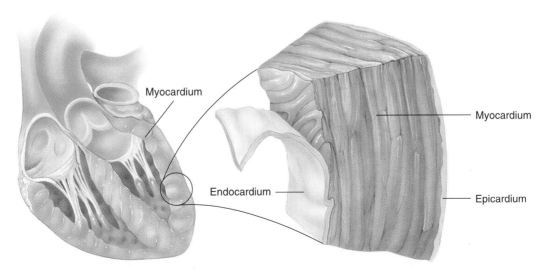

FIGURE 5.3 Schematic of the tissues of the walls of the heart.

- The **epicardium** (ep-ih-**KAR**-dee-um) is the external layer of the heart and also is part of the inner layer of the pericardial sac.
- The **myocardium** (my-oh-**KAR**-dee-um), which is the middle and thickest of the three layers, consists of cardiac muscle (See Cardiac Muscle in Chapter 4.)
- The **endocardium** (en-doh-**KAR**-dee-um), which is the lining of the heart, forms the inner surface that comes in direct contact with blood being pumped through the heart.

The Blood Supply to the Myocardium

- The myocardium is specialized muscle that beats constantly and *must* have a continuous supply of oxygen and nutrients and the prompt removal of waste.
- The **coronary arteries and veins** supply the blood needs of the myocardium. If this blood supply is disrupted, the myocardium in the affected area dies (Figure 5.4).

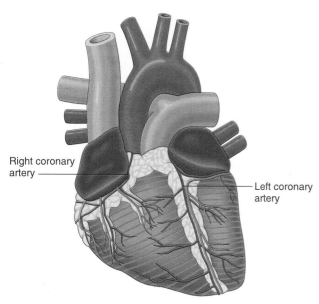

Right coronary artery

Left coronary artery

FIGURE 5.4 The coronary arteries supply blood to the myocardium.

The Heart Chambers

The heart is divided into left and right sides. Each side is subdivided, thus forming four chambers (see Figure 5.2).

- The **atria** (**AY**-tree-ah), the two upper chambers of the heart, are the receiving chambers. All blood vessels coming into the heart enter here (singular, **atrium**).
- The atria are separated by the **interatrial septum**. A **septum** (**SEP**-tum) is a separating wall or partition.
- The two **ventricles** (**VEN**-trih-kuhls) are the lower chambers of the heart. All vessels leaving the heart emerge from the ventricles. (The term ventricle refers to both the ventricles of the heart and of the brain.)

- The ventricles, separated by the **interventricular septum**, are the pumping chambers. The ventricular walls are thicker than the atrial walls because the ventricles pump blood longer distances.
- The narrow tip of the heart is called the **cardiac apex**.

The Heart Valves

The flow of blood through the heart is controlled by the tricuspid, pulmonary semilunar, mitral, and aortic semilunar valves. If any of these valves is not working correctly, blood does not flow properly through the heart and cannot be pumped effectively to all parts of the body (see Figures 5.2 and 5.5).

- The **tricuspid valve** (try-**KUS**-pid), also known as the **TV**, controls the opening between the right atrium and the right ventricle. (Tricuspid means having three points or cusps and this valve is shaped with three points.)
- The **pulmonary semilunar valve** (sem-ee-**LOO**-nar) is located between the right ventricle and the pulmonary artery. (Semilunar means half-moon and this valve is shaped like a half-moon.)
- The **mitral valve** (**MY**-tral), also known as the **MV** or **bicuspid valve**, is located between the left atrium and left ventricle. (Bicuspid means having two points and this valve is shaped with two points.)
- The **aortic semilunar valve** (ay-**OR**-tick sem-ee-**LOO**-nar) is located between the left ventricle and the aorta. Semilunar also means half-moon and this valve is shaped like a half-moon.

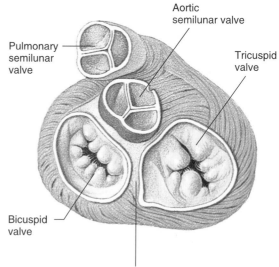

Aortic semilunar valve

Pulmonary semilunar valve

Tricuspid valve

Bicuspid valve

Fibrous connective tissue

FIGURE 5.5 The valves of the heart. This is a superior view with the atria removed.

Systemic and Pulmonary Circulation

The flow of blood through the heart is summarized in Table 5.1. The red arrows indicate oxygenated (oxygen-

Table 5.1

BLOOD FLOW THROUGH THE HEART

↓ The **right atrium** (**RA**) receives oxygen-poor blood from all tissues, except the lungs, through the **superior** and **inferior venae cavae**. Blood flows out of the RA through the **tricuspid valve** into the right ventricle.

↓ The **right ventricle** (**RV**) pumps the oxygen-poor blood through the **pulmonary semilunar valve** and into the **pulmonary artery**, which carries it to the lungs.

↓ The **left atrium** (**LA**) receives oxygen-rich (oxygenated) blood from the lungs through the **four pulmonary veins**. The blood flows out of the LA, through the **mitral valve**, and into the left ventricle.

↓ The **left ventricle** (**LV**) receives oxygen-rich blood from the left atrium. Blood flows out of the LV through the **aortic semilunar valve** and into the **aorta**, which carries it to all parts of the body, except the lungs.

↓ Oxygen-poor blood is returned by the venae cavae to the right atrium and the cycle continues.

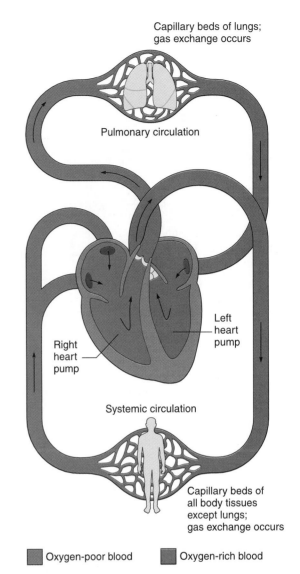

Oxygen-poor blood ▢ Oxygen-rich blood ▢

FIGURE 5.6 Systemic and pulmonary circulation.

rich) blood and blue arrows indicate deoxygenated (oxygen-poor) blood. This flow travels through both systemic and pulmonary circulation, which makes possible the important function of blood that is bringing oxygen to the cells and removing waste products (Figure 5.6).

Systemic Circulation

- Systemic circulation includes blood flow to all parts of the body *except* the lungs.
- Oxygen-rich blood flows out of the heart from the left ventricle into arterial circulation.
- Oxygen-poor blood returns to the heart through the veins and flows into the right atrium.

Pulmonary Circulation

- **Pulmonary circulation** is the flow of blood between the heart and lungs.
- Blood flows out of the heart from the right ventricle and through the pulmonary arteries to the lungs. This is the only place in the body where arteries carry oxygen-poor blood.
- In the lungs, waste material (carbon dioxide) from the body is exchanged for oxygen from the inhaled air.
- The pulmonary veins carry the oxygen-rich blood into the left atrium of the heart. This is the only place in the body where veins carry oxygen-rich blood.

The Heartbeat

- To pump blood effectively throughout the body, the contraction and relaxation (beating) of the heart must occur in exactly the correct sequence.
- The rate and regularity of the heartbeat is determined by **electrical impulses** from nerves that stimulate the myocardium of the chambers of the heart.
- Also known as the **conduction system**, these electrical impulses are controlled by the sinoatrial (S-A) node, atrioventricular (A-V) node, and bundle of His (Figure 5.7).

The Sinoatrial Node

- The **sinoatrial node** (**sigh-noh-AY-tree-ahl**), also known as the **S-A node**, is located in the posterior wall of the right atrium near the entrance of the superior vena cava.

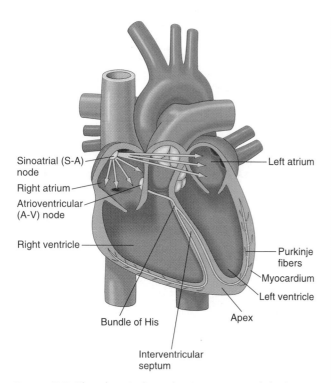

Sinoatrial (S-A) node

Right atrium

Atrioventricular (A-V) node

Right ventricle

Left atrium

Purkinje fibers

Myocardium

Left ventricle

Apex

Bundle of His

Interventricular septum

FIGURE 5.7 The electrical conduction system of the heart.

- Because the S-A node establishes the basic rhythm of the heartbeat, it is called the **natural pacemaker** of the heart.
- Electrical impulses from the S-A node start each wave of muscle contraction in the heart.
- The impulse in the right atrium spreads over the muscles of both atria, causing them to contract simultaneously.
- This contraction forces blood into the ventricles.

The Atrioventricular Node

- The impulses from the S-A node also travel to the **atrioventricular node** (ay-tree-oh-ven-**TRICK**-you-lahr)
- Also known as the **A-V node**, it is located on the floor of the right atrium near the interatrial septum.
- The A-V node transmits the electric impulses on to the bundle of His.

The Bundle of His

- The **bundle of His** (**HISS**), named for Wilhelm His, Jr., a 19th century Swiss physician, is located within the interventricular septum.
- Branches of the bundle of His carry the impulse to the right and left ventricles and the **Purkinje fibers**.
- Stimulation of the **Purkinje fibers**, named for Johannes Purkinje, a 19th century physiologist, causes the ventricles to contract simultaneously forcing blood into the aorta and pulmonary arteries.

Electrical Waves

The activities of the electrical conduction system of the heart can be visualized as wave movements on a monitor or an electrocardiogram (Figure 5.8).

- The **P wave** is due to the contraction (stimulation) of the atria.
- The **QRS complex** shows the contraction (stimulation) of the ventricles. The atria relax as the ventricles contract.
- The **T wave** is the relaxation (recovery) of the ventricles.

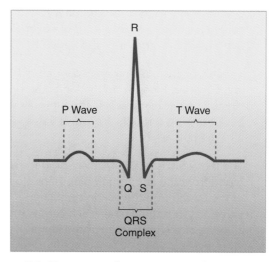

FIGURE 5.8 The waves of contraction and relaxation of the heart can be visualized on a monitor or on an EKG.

Heart Sounds

When a stethoscope is used to listen to the heartbeat, two distinct sounds are heard. They are called the "lubb-dupp" sounds.

- Heard first is the **lubb sound**. This is caused by the tricuspid and mitral valves closing between the atria and the ventricles.
- Heard next is the **dupp sound**, which is shorter and higher pitched. It is caused by the closing of the semilunar valves in the aorta and pulmonary arteries as blood is pumped out of the heart.

The Blood Vessels

There are three major types of blood vessels in the body. These are the arteries, capillaries, and veins.

- The **lumen** (**LOO**-men) is the opening within these vessels through which the blood flows.

The Arteries

The arteries are the large blood vessels that carry blood away from the heart to all regions of the body. It is the high oxygen content that gives arterial blood its bright red color (Figure 5.9).

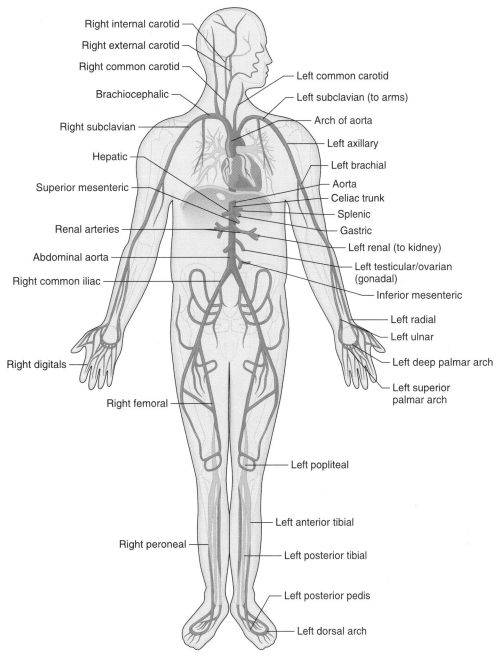

Right internal carotid
Right external carotid
Right common carotid
Brachiocephalic
Right subclavian
Hepatic
Superior mesenteric
Renal arteries
Abdominal aorta
Right common iliac
Right digitals
Right femoral
Right peroneal

Left common carotid
Left subclavian (to arms)
Arch of aorta
Left axillary
Left brachial
Aorta
Celiac trunk
Splenic
Gastric
Left renal (to kidney)
Left testicular/ovarian (gonadal)
Inferior mesenteric
Left radial
Left ulnar
Left deep palmar arch
Left superior palmar arch
Left popliteal
Left anterior tibial
Left posterior tibial
Left posterior pedis
Left dorsal arch

FIGURE 5.9 Arterial circulation.

- The term **endarterial** (**end**-ar-**TEE**-ree-al) means pertaining to the interior or lining of an artery (**end** means within, **arteri** means artery, and **al** means pertaining to).

- The walls of the arteries are composed of three layers. This structure makes them both muscular and elastic so they can expand and contract with the pumping beat of the heart. It is this contraction and expansion that causes blood to spurt out when an artery is cut.

- The **aorta** (ay-**OR**-tah) is the main trunk of the arterial system and begins from the left ventricle of the heart (see Figure 5.1).

- The **coronary artery** (**KOR**-uh-**nerr**-ee) branches from the aorta and supplies blood to the myocardium (see Figure 5.4).

- The **arterioles** (ar-**TEE**-ree-ohlz), which are the smaller thinner branches of arteries, carry blood to the capillaries.

The Capillaries

- **Capillaries** serve as the anatomic units connecting the arterial and venous circulatory systems. The capillaries, which are only one epithelial cell in thickness, are the smallest vessels in the body.

- Blood flows rapidly along the arteries and veins. However, this flow is much slower through the expanded vascular bed provided by the network of capillaries.

- This slower flow allows time for the exchange of oxygen, nutrients, and waste materials between the tissue fluids and the surrounding cells.

The Veins

The veins form a low-pressure collecting system to return the waste-filled blood to the heart (Figures 5.10 and 5.11).

- Veins have thinner walls and are less elastic than the arteries. Contractions of the skeletal muscles cause the blood to flow through the veins toward the heart.

- Veins have valves that allow blood to flow toward the heart but prevent it from flowing away from the heart.

- **Venules** (VEN-youls) are small veins that join to form the larger veins.

The Venae Cavae

- The **venae cavae** (VEE-nee KAY-vee) are the two large veins that enter the heart (singular, **vena cava**).

FIGURE 5.10 Venous circulation.

(A)   (B)   (C)

FIGURE 5.11 Veins contain valves to prevent the backward flow of blood. (A) External view of the vein shows wider area of valve. (B) Internal view with the valve open as blood flows through. (C) Internal view with the valve closed.

- The **superior vena cava** (VEE-nah KAY-vah), also known as the **SVC**, brings blood from the upper portion of the body (see Figure 5.1).
- The **inferior vena cava**, also known as the **IVC**, brings blood from the lower portion of the body (see Figure 5.2).

The Pulse and Blood Pressure

- The **pulse** is the rhythmic expansion and contraction of an artery produced by the pressure of the blood moving through the artery (see Chapter 15).
- **Blood pressure** is a measurement of the amount of pressure exerted against the walls of the vessels.
- **Systolic pressure** (sis-TOL-ick), which occurs when the ventricles contract, is the highest pressure against the walls of the blood vessels.
- **Diastolic pressure** (dye-ah-STOL-ick), which occurs when the ventricles are relaxed, is the lowest pressure against the walls of the blood vessels.
- Blood pressure is recorded as systolic over diastolic. A normal blood pressure reading for a seated adult is about 130/84 mm Hg. (**Hg** is the abbreviation for mercury.)

The Blood

Blood is composed of 55% liquid plasma and 45% formed elements (Figure 5.12). The **formed elements**, also known as **blood corpuscles**, include the red blood cells, white blood cells, and platelets.

Plasma (55% of total volume)

Formed elements (45% of total volume)

Test tube containing whole blood

Erythrocytes

Thrombocytes (platelets)

Neutrophil

Monocyte

Eosinophil

Lymphocyte

Leukocytes

Basophil

FIGURE 5.12 The major components of blood.

Plasma

- **Plasma** (**PLAZ**-mah) is a straw-colored fluid that contains nutrients, hormones, and waste products. Plasma is 91% water. The remaining 9% consists mainly of proteins including the clotting proteins.
- **Serum** (**SEER**-um) is plasma with these clotting proteins removed.
- **Fibrinogen** (figh-**BRIN**-oh-jen) and **prothrombin** (proh-**THROM**-bin) are clotting proteins found in plasma. They have an important role in clot formation to control bleeding.

Erythrocytes

- **Erythrocytes** (eh-**RITH**-roh-sights), which are also known as **red blood cells** or **RBCs**, are mature red blood cells.
- These cells, which are produced by the red bone marrow, are shaped like a doughnut with a thin central portion instead of a hole (see Figure 5.16).
- **Hemoglobin** (**hee**-moh-**GLOH**-bin), which is the iron-containing pigment of the erythrocytes, transports oxygen from the lungs to the tissues of the body.
- A **reticulocyte** (reh-**TICK**-you-loh-**site**) is an immature erythrocyte that is characterized by a meshlike pattern of threads.
- The normal life span of a RBC is about 120 days. After this, **macrophages** in the spleen, liver, and bone marrow destroy erythrocytes that are no longer useful.

Leukocytes

- **Leukocytes** (**LOO**-koh-sites), also known as **white blood cells** or **WBCs**, protect the body against harmful invaders such as bacteria. The following are the major groups of leukocytes.
- **Neutrophils** (**NEW**-troh-fills), which are formed in red bone marrow, are the most prevalent type of WBC. These cells fight infection by phagocytosis. **Phagocytosis** (**fag**-oh-sigh-**TOH**-sis) is the process of engulfing and swallowing germs. An elevated neutrophil count indicates a bacterial infection.
- **Basophils** (**BAY**-soh-fills), which are formed in red bone marrow, promote the inflammatory response. An elevated basophil count may indicate an allergic condition.
- **Eosinophils** (**ee**-oh-**SIN**-oh-fills), which are formed in red bone marrow, increase in response to allergic reactions. An elevated eosinophil count indicates an allergic condition.
- **Lymphocytes** (**LIM**-foh-sights) are formed in red bone marrow, lymph nodes, and the spleen. These cells have an important role in protecting the body against disease (see Chapter 6).
- **Monocytes** (**MON**-oh-sights) are formed in red bone marrow, lymph nodes, and the spleen. They also are important in protecting against disease and an elevated monocyte count usually indicates a chronic infection.

Thrombocytes

- **Thrombocytes** (**THROM**-boh-sights), also known as **platelets**, are the smallest formed elements of the blood. They are not cells, but are fragments of specialized large bone marrow cells known as megakaryocytes.
- Thrombocytes play an important role in the clotting of blood. When the blood vessel is damaged platelets are activated. Once activated the platelets become sticky and clump together to form a clot.

Blood Types

The four major types of blood are A, AB, B, and O. These groups are based on the presence of the A and/or B antigens on red blood cells. In type O, both antigens are absent.

Table 5.2 explains how these types interact in terms of donating and receiving blood.

- The safe administration of blood from donor to recipient requires careful typing and crossmatching to ensure a correct match.
- A patient receiving blood incompatible with his own can experience serious and possibly fatal reactions.

Table 5.2

BLOOD TYPES AS DONORS AND RECIPIENTS		
Blood Type	**Can Donate To**	**Can Receive From**
A	**A** or **AB** only	**A** or **O** only
B	**B** or **AB** only	**B** or **O** only
AB (the universal recipient)	**AB** only	A, B, AB, O
O (the universal donor)	A, B, AB, O	**O** only

The Rh Factor

In addition to having antigens A and/or B, red blood cells also contain the Rh antigen. Since this was first found in Rhesus monkeys, this factor was named for them. Each individual is either positive or negative for the **Rh factor**.

- About 85% of Americans are **Rh positive (Rh+)**. This means that they *have* the Rh antigen.
- The remaining 15% are **Rh negative (Rh–)**. This means that they *do not have* the Rh antigen.

- The Rh factor is an important consideration in cross-matching blood for transfusions.
- The Rh factor also causes difficulties when an Rh+ infant is born to an Rh– mother (see Chapter 14).

Blood Gases

- A **blood gas** is a gas that is dissolved in the liquid part of the blood. The major blood gases are **oxygen** (O_2), **carbon dioxide** (CO_2), and **nitrogen** (N_2).

Medical Specialties Related to the Cardiovascular System

- A **cardiologist** (**kar**-dee-**OL**-oh-jist) specializes in diagnosing and treating abnormalities, diseases, and disorders of the heart (**cardi** means heart and **ologist** means specialist).

- A **hematologist** (**hee**-mah-**TOL**-oh-jist *or* **hem**-ah-**TOL**-oh-jist) specializes in diagnosing and treating diseases and disorders of the blood and blood-forming tissues (**hemat** means blood and **ologist** means specialist).

Pathology of the Cardiovascular System

Coronary Artery Disease

- **Coronary artery disease**, also known as **CAD**, is atherosclerosis of the coronary arteries that may cause angina pectoris, myocardial infarction, and sudden death (Figure 5.13).

- **End-stage coronary artery disease** is the final phase of CAD characterized by unrelenting angina pain and a

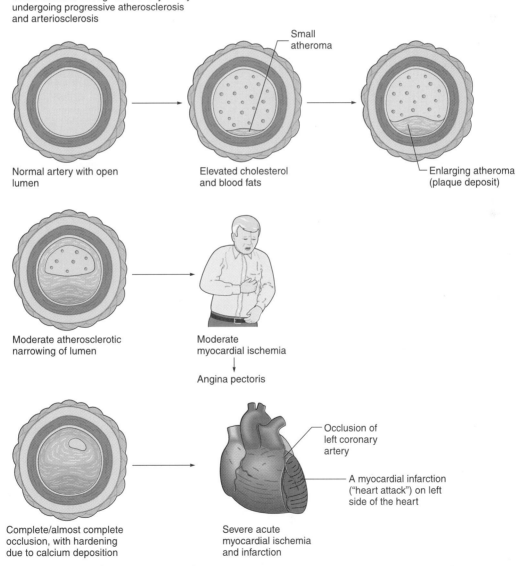

Cross sections through a coronary artery undergoing progressive atherosclerosis and arteriosclerosis

Small atheroma

Normal artery with open lumen

Elevated cholesterol and blood fats

Enlarging atheroma (plaque deposit)

Moderate atherosclerotic narrowing of lumen

Moderate myocardial ischemia

Angina pectoris

Complete/almost complete occlusion, with hardening due to calcium deposition

Severe acute myocardial ischemia and infarction

Occlusion of left coronary artery

A myocardial infarction ("heart attack") on left side of the heart

FIGURE 5.13 The progression of coronary heart disease.

severely limited lifestyle in which medication is the only remaining treatment option.

- **Atherosclerosis** (**ath-er-oh**-skleh-**ROH**-sis) is hardening and narrowing of the arteries due to a buildup of cholesterol plaques (**athero** means plaque or fatty substance and **sclerosis** means abnormal hardening) (Figures 5.13 and 5.14).

- An **atheroma** (**ath-er-OH**-mah), which is characteristic of atherosclerosis, is a plaque (fatty deposit) within the arterial wall (**ather** means plaque and **oma** means tumor).

- This type of **plaque** (**PLACK**) is similar to the buildup of rust inside a pipe and it may protrude outward into the opening of the vessel or move inward into the wall of the vessel. (Compare with dental plaque discussed in Chapter 8.)

- **Ischemia** (iss-**KEE**-mee-ah) is a deficiency in blood supply due to either the constriction or the obstruction of a blood vessel (**isch** means to hold back and **emia** means blood).

- **Ischemic heart disease** (iss-**KEE**-mick), also known as **IHD**, is a group of cardiac disabilities resulting from an insufficient supply of oxygenated blood to the heart that is usually associated with CAD.

- **Angina pectoris** (an-**JIGH**-nah *or* **AN**-jih-nuh **PECK**-toh-riss) is severe episodes of spasmodic choking or suffocating chest pain. This is usually due to interference with, but not complete blockage of, the supply of oxygen to the myocardium.

- A **myocardial infarction** (**my-oh-KAR**-dee-al in-**FARK**-shun), also known as a **heart attack** or **MI**, is the occlusion (closing off) of a coronary artery resulting in an infarct of the affected myocardium. Damage to the myocardium impairs the heart's ability to pump blood through the body.

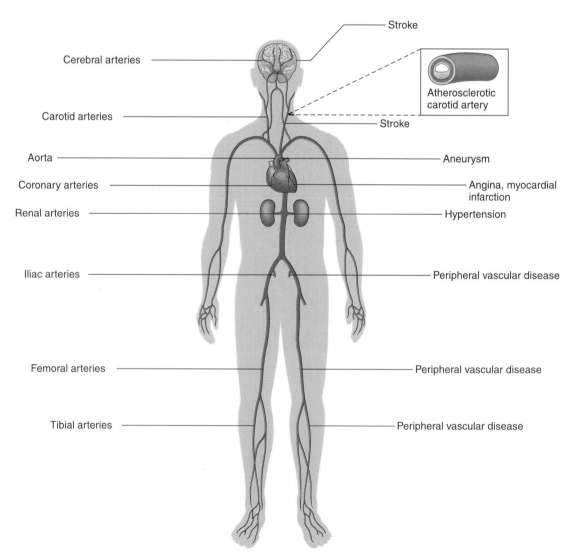

FIGURE 5.14 The risks of atherosclerosis. (Left) Affected sites. (Right) Potential complications.

- An **infarct** (IN-farkt) is a localized area of necrosis (tissue death) caused by an interruption of the blood supply.

Congestive Heart Failure

- **Congestive heart failure**, also known as **CHF**, is a syndrome in which the heart is unable to pump enough blood to meet the body's needs for oxygen and nutrients. In response to the reduced blood flow, the kidneys retain more fluid within the body and this fluid accumulates in the legs, ankles, and lungs. The term congestive refers to this fluid buildup.

Forms of Carditis

- The term **carditis** (kar-DYE-tis) means an inflammation of the heart (**card** means heart and **itis** means inflammation). *Note the spelling of carditis.* The word roots **cardi/o** and **card/o** both mean heart. In this term **card/o** is used to avoid having a double *i* when it is joined with the suffix **-itis**.
- **Endocarditis** (en-doh-kar-DYE-tis) is an inflammation of the inner layer of the heart (**endo** means within, **card** means heart, and **itis** means inflammation).
- **Bacterial endocarditis** is an inflammation of the lining or valves of the heart caused by bacteria.
- **Myocarditis** (my-oh-kar-DYE-tis) is an inflammation of the myocardium (**myo** means muscle, **card** means heart, and **itis** means inflammation).
- **Pericarditis** (pehr-ih-kar-DYE-tis) is an inflammation of the pericardium (**peri** means surrounding, **card** means heart, and **itis** means inflammation).

Heart Valves

- **Valvulitis** (val-view-LYE-tis) is an inflammatory condition of a heart valve (**valvul** means valve and **itis** means inflammation).
- **Mitral valve prolapse** is an abnormal protrusion of the mitral value that results in the incomplete closure of the valve. (**Prolapse** means falling down.)
- **Mitral stenosis** (steh-NOH-sis) is abnormal narrowing of the opening of the mitral valve. **Tricuspid stenosis** is abnormal narrowing of the opening of the tricuspid valve.
- A valve that does not function properly may allow blood to flow back into the heart chamber. The sound of this abnormal flow is called a **heart murmur**.

Arrhythmias

- **Cardiac arrhythmia** (ah-RITH-mee-ah), also called **dysrhythmia** (dis-RITH-me-ah), is an irregularity or the loss of normal rhythm of the heartbeat.
- **Bradycardia** (brad-ee-KAR-dee-ah) is an abnormally slow heartbeat (**brady** means slow, **card** means heart,

and **ia** means abnormal condition). This term is usually applied to rates under 60 beats per minute. (Compare this with tachycardia.)
- A **flutter** is a cardiac arrhythmia in which the atrial contractions are rapid but regular. (Compare this with atrial fibrillation.).
- **Palpitation** (pal-pih-TAY-shun) is a pounding or racing heart with or without irregularity in rhythm. This is associated with certain heart disorders, or it may be a response accompanying a panic attack (see Chapter 10).
- **Tachycardia** (tack-ee-KAR-dee-ah) is an abnormally fast heartbeat (**tachy** means rapid, **card** means heart, and **ia** means abnormal condition). This term is usually applied to rates over 100 beats per minute. (Compare this with bradycardia.)
- **Paroxysmal tachycardia** is a fast heartbeat of sudden onset. **Paroxysm** (PAR-ock-sizm) means a sudden convulsion, seizure, or spasm.

Fibrillation

- **Fibrillation** (fih-brih-LAY-shun) is rapid, random, and ineffective contractions of the heart.
- In **atrial fibrillation**, also known as **A fib**, the atria beat faster than the ventricles. This produces an irregular quivering action of the atria and a very rapid ventricular heartbeat.
- **Ventricular fibrillation**, also known as **V fib**, is the result of irregular contractions of the ventricles and is fatal unless reversed by electric defibrillation.

Blood Vessels

- **Angiitis** (an-je-EYE-tis), also known as **vasculitis** (vas-kyou-LYE-tis), is the inflammation of a blood or lymph vessel (**angi** means vessel and **itis** means inflammation. *Note:* This term is spelled with a double *i*).
- **Angionecrosis** (an-jee-oh-neh-KROH-sis) is the necrosis (death) of the walls of blood vessels (**angio** means vessel and **necrosis** means tissue death).
- An **angiospasm** (AN-jee-oh-spazm) is a spasmodic contraction of the blood vessels (**angio** means vessel and **spasm** means tightening or cramping).
- **Angiostenosis** (AN-jee-oh-steh-NOH-sis) is the narrowing of a blood vessel (**angio** means vessel and **stenosis** means abnormal narrowing).
- A **hemangioma** (hee-man-jee-OH-mah) is a benign tumor made up of newly formed blood vessels (**hemangi** means blood vessel and **oma** means tumor). (See also Chapter 12.)
- **Hypoperfusion** (high-poh-per-FYOU-zhun) is a deficiency of blood passing through an organ or body part. **Perfusion** (per-FYOU-zuhn) means the flow of blood through the vessels of an organ.

Arteries

- An **aneurysm** (AN-you-rizm) is a localized weak spot or balloon-like enlargement of the wall of an artery. Most aneurysms occur in large blood vessels and are named for the involved blood vessels such as an aortic aneurysm. If an aneurysm ruptures it is often fatal because of the rapid loss of blood.

- **Arteritis** (ar-teh-RYE-tis) is inflammation of an artery (**arter** means artery and **itis** mean inflammation).

- **Polyarteritis** (pol-ee-ar-teh-RYE-tis) is an inflammation involving several arteries (**poly** means many, **arter** means artery, and **itis** mean inflammation).

- **Arteriosclerosis** (ar-**tee**-ree-oh-skleh-**ROH**-sis) is hardening of the arteries, which reduces the flow of blood through these vessels (**arterio** means artery and **sclerosis** mean abnormal hardening).

- **Raynaud's phenomenon** (ray-**NOHZ**) consists of intermittent attacks of pallor (paleness), cyanosis (blue color), and redness of the fingers and toes. These symptoms are due to arterial and arteriolar contraction and are usually caused by cold or emotion.

Veins

- **Phlebitis** (fleh-BYE-tis) is the inflammation of a vein (**phleb** means vein and **itis** mean inflammation). (See also thrombophlebitis.)

- **Varicose veins** (VAR-ih-kohs VAYNS) are abnormally swollen veins usually occurring in the legs (Figure 5.15). A **varicosity** (var-ih-KOS-ih-tee) is one area of swelling (plural, **varices**).

Valve closes, pushing the venous blood toward the heart.

Valves remain open, pooling the blood in the veins.

(A) Normal veins   **(B) Varicose veins**

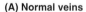

Figure 5.15 Normal veins and varicose veins compared.

Thromboses and Embolisms

- A **thrombosis** (throm-BOH-sis) (plural, **thromboses**) is an abnormal condition in which a thrombus develops within a blood vessel (**thromb** means clot and **osis** means abnormal condition).

- A **thrombus** (THROM-bus) is a blood clot attached to the interior wall of a vein or artery (**thromb** means clot and **us** is a singular noun ending).

- A **thrombotic occlusion** (throm-BOT-ick ah-KLOO-zhun) is the blocking of an artery by a clot (**thrombo**

means clot and **tic** means pertaining to). As used here, **occlusion** means a blockage in a canal, vessel, or passageway in the body.

- A **coronary thrombosis** (KOR-uh-**nerr**-ee throm-BOH-sis) is damage to the heart caused by a thrombus blocking a coronary artery.

- An **embolus** (EM-boh-lus) is a foreign object, such as a blood clot, quantity of air or gas, or a bit of tissue or tumor that is circulating in the blood (**embol** means something inserted and **us** is a singular noun ending). (Plural, **emboli.**)

- An **embolism** (EM-boh-lizm) is the blockage of a vessel by an embolus. An embolism occurs when the embolus is larger than the blood vessel and blocks the flow of blood (**embol** means something inserted and **ism** means condition).

Blood Disorders

- **Dyscrasia** (dis-KRAY-zee-ah) is any abnormal or pathologic condition of the blood (**dys** means bad and **crasia** means a mixture or blending).

- **Hemochromatosis** (hee-moh-**kroh**-mah-TOH-sis) is also known as **iron overload disease** (**hemo** means blood, **chromat** means color, and **osis** means abnormal condition). This is a genetic disorder in which the intestines absorb too much iron. The excess iron enters the bloodstream and accumulates in organs where it causes damage.

- **Septicemia** (sep-tih-SEE-mee-ah), also known as **blood poisoning**, is the presence of pathogenic microorganisms or their toxins in the blood.

Cholesterol

- **Cholesterol** (koh-LES-ter-ol) are lipids (fatty substances) that travel in the blood in packages called **lipoproteins**. The presence of cholesterol at certain levels is normal and essential for good health. A pathologic condition is present when these fats are present in excessive amounts. Table 5.3 shows the desirable levels of each substance for people without heart disease. These are expressed as milligrams per deciliter (mg/dL).

- **Low-density lipoprotein cholesterol** is also known as **LDL** or **bad cholesterol** because excess quantities contribute to plaque buildup in the arteries.

- **High-density lipoprotein cholesterol** is also known as **HDL** or **good cholesterol** because it carries unneeded cholesterol back to the liver for processing and does not contribute to plaque buildup.

- **Triglycerides** (try-GLIS-er-eyeds) are combinations of fatty acids attached to glycerol that are also found normally in the blood in limited quantities.

- **Homocysteine** (hoh-moh-SIS-teen) is an amino acid normally found in the blood and used by the body to build and maintain tissues. However, when present in elevated levels, homocysteine can damage arterial walls and increase the risk of coronary artery disease.

Table 5.3

BLOOD LIPOPROTEIN LEVELS			
Test	Desirable (mg/dL)	Borderline (mg/dL)	Undesirable (mg/dL)
Total cholesterol	Below 200	200–240	Above 240
LDL cholesterol	Below 130	130–160	Above 160
HDL cholesterol	Above 45	35–45	Below 35
Triglycerides	Below 200	200–400	Above 400
Homocysteine	less than 14 micromoles per liter is considered normal; however, firm standards have not yet been established.		

Such increases may be caused by a diet severely lacking in several B vitamins.

- **Hyperlipidemia** (**high**-per-**lip**-ih-**DEE**-mee-ah), also known as **hyperlipemia** (**high**-per-lye-**PEE**-mee-ah), is a general term for elevated plasma concentrations of cholesterol, triglycerides, and lipoproteins. The levels of each of these substances can be measured by a blood test.

Blood Cells

- **Erythrocytosis** (eh-**rith**-roh-sigh-**TOH**-sis) is an abnormal increase in the number of circulating red blood cells (**erythro** means red, **cyt** means cell, and **osis** means abnormal condition).

- **Thrombocytopenia** (**throm**-boh-**sigh**-toh-**PEE**-nee-ah), also known as **thrombopenia**, is an abnormal decrease in the number of platelets (**thrombo** means clot, **cyto** means cell, and **penia** means a deficiency of).

- **Leukopenia** (**loo**-koh-**PEE**-nee-ah) is an abnormal decrease in the number of white blood cells. It may affect one or all kinds of white blood cells (**leuko** means white and **penia** means a deficiency of).

- **Leukemia** (loo-**KEE**-mee-ah) is a malignancy characterized by a progressive increase of abnormal leukocytes (**leuk** means white and **emia** means blood condition).

Anemias

- **Anemia** (ah-**NEE**-mee-ah) is a disorder characterized by lower than normal levels of red blood cells in the blood (**an** means without or less than and suffix **emia** means blood condition).

- **Aplastic anemia** (ay-**PLAS**-tick ah-**NEE**-mee-ah) is marked by an absence of *all* formed blood elements (**a** means without, **plast** means growth, and **ic** means pertaining to). This is caused by the failure of blood cell production in the bone marrow.

- In **hemolytic anemia** (**hee**-moh-**LIT**-ick ah-**NEE**-mee-ah) red blood cells are destroyed faster than the bone marrow can replace them (**hemo** means relating to blood and **lytic** means to destroy).

- **Iron-deficiency anemia** develops if not enough iron is available to bone marrow to make hemoglobin. It may be caused by inadequate iron intake, malabsorption of iron, pregnancy and lactation, or chronic blood loss.

- In **megaloblastic anemia** (**MEG**-ah-loh-**blas**-tick ah-**NEE**-mee-ah) the bone marrow produces megaloblasts. These are large abnormal red blood cells with a reduced capacity to carry oxygen. This type of anemia is almost always caused by a vitamin deficiency.

- In **pernicious anemia** (per-**NISH**-us ah-**NEE**-mee-ah) an autoimmune disorder results in the inability of the body to absorb vitamin B_{12} normally.

- **Sickle cell anemia** is a genetic disorder that causes abnormal hemoglobin that results in the red blood cells assuming an abnormal sickle shape (Figure 5.16). This abnormal shape interferes with normal blood flow resulting in damage to most of the body systems (see Chapter 2).

Normal red blood cell   Sickle-shaped red blood cell

FIGURE 5.16 Blood cells magnified through a scanning electron microscope. *(Courtesy of Philips Electronic Instruments Company.)*

- **Thalassemia** (thal-ah-SEE-mee-ah), also known as **Cooley's anemia**, is a group of genetic disorders characterized by short-lived red blood cells that lack the normal ability to produce hemoglobin.

Hypertension

- **Essential hypertension**, also known as **primary hypertension** or **idiopathic hypertension**, is consistently elevated blood pressure of unknown origin. (**Idiopathic** means of unknown cause.) The classifications of blood pressure for adults are summarized in Table 5.4.

- **Secondary hypertension** is caused by a different medical problem such as a kidney disorder or a tumor on the adrenal glands. When the other problem is cured, the secondary hypertension should be resolved.

- **Malignant hypertension** is characterized by the sudden onset of severely elevated blood pressure. It can be life-threatening and commonly damages small vessels in the brain, retina, heart, and kidneys.

Table 5.4

BLOOD PRESSURE CLASSIFICATIONS FOR ADULTS		
Category	**Systolic (mm Hg)**	**Diastolic (mm Hg)**
Optimal	120 or less	80 or less
Normal	129 or less	84 or less
High-normal	130–139	85–89
Hypertension		
Stage 1 (mild)	140–159	90–99
Stage 2 (moderate)	160–179	100–109
Stage 3 (severe)	180 or higher	110 or higher

Based on information from the Joint National Committee on Detection, Evaluation, and Treatment of High Blood Pressure, 1997.

Diagnostic Procedures of the Cardiovascular System

- **Blood tests** are discussed in Chapter 15.

- An ongoing measurement of **blood oxygen levels** can be obtained through a monitor attached to a finger. The levels of other blood gases are measured with a blood test.

- **Angiography** (an-jee-OG-rah-fee) is a radiographic (x-ray) study of blood vessels after the injection of a contrast medium (Figure 5.17). The resulting film is an **angiogram**. This procedure is frequently performed in conjunction with cardiac catheterization.

- **Angiocardiography** (an-jee-oh-**kar**-dee-**OG**-rah-fee) uses a contrast medium and chest x-rays to visualize the dimensions of the heart and large blood vessels (**angio** means blood vessel, **cardio** means heart and **graphy** means the process of recording). The contrast medium, which appears white on the film, is used to make these soft tissue structures visible on the resulting **angiocardiogram**.

- **Cardiac catheterization** (KAR-dee-ack **kath**-eh-ter-eye-**ZAY**-shun), also known as **CC**, is a procedure in which a catheter is passed into a vein or artery and is guided into the heart. When the catheter is in place, a contrast medium is introduced to produce an angiogram to determine how well the heart is working. This procedure is also used for treatment purposes (see Clearing Blocked Arteries).

FIGURE 5.17 An angiogram showing the femoral arteries. The use of a contrast medium makes the arteries visible.

- **Phlebography** (fleh-**BOG**-rah-fee) is the technique of preparing an x-ray image of veins injected with a contrast medium material. The resulting film is a **phlebogram**.

Electrocardiography

- An **electrocardiogram** (ee-**leck**-troh-**KAR**-dee-oh-gram), also known as **ECG** or **EKG**, is a record of the electrical activity of the myocardium (see Figure 5.8). **Electrocardiography** (ee-**leck**-troh-kar-dee-**OG**-rah-fee) is the process of recording this activity (**electro** means electric, **cardio** means heart, and **graphy** means the process of recording).

- A **Holter monitor** uses electrodes attached similarly to an ECG but is worn by the patient to record heart rates and rhythms over a 24-hour period.

- **Stress tests** are ECGs used to assess cardiovascular health and function during and after the application of stress such as exercise on a treadmill.

   In a **thallium stress test** (**THAL**-ee-um) the flow of blood through the heart during activity is assessed through the use of thallium (a radiopharmaceutical) during a stress test. (Radiopharmaceuticals are discussed in Chapter 15.)

Ultrasonic Diagnostic Procedures

- **Echocardiography** (**eck**-oh-**kar**-dee-**OG**-rah-fee), also known as an **ECHO**, is an ultrasonic diagnostic procedure used to evaluate the structures and motion of the heart (**echo** means sound, **cardio** means heart, and **graphy** means to record). The resulting record is an **echocardiogram**.

- **Transesophageal echocardiography** (**trans**-eh-**sof**-ah-**JEE**-al **eck**-oh-**kar**-dee-**OG**-rah-fee), also known as **TEE**, is an ultrasonic procedure that images the heart from inside the esophagus. Because the esophagus is so close to the heart, this technique produces clearer images than those obtained with echocardiography.

Treatment Procedures of the Cardiovascular System

Antihypertensive Medications

An **antihypertensive** (**an**-tih-**high**-per-**TEN**-siv) is administered to lower blood pressure. The following are medications used for this purpose.

- **ACE inhibitors** (angiotensin-converting enzyme inhibitors), which are used to treat hypertension and CHF, interfere with the action of the kidney hormone renin that causes the heart muscles to squeeze.

- **Beta-blockers** slow the heartbeat.

- **Calcium channel blockers** reduce the contraction of the muscles that squeeze blood vessels tight. These medications are used to treat hypertension, angina, and arrhythmia.

- **Diuretics** (**dye**-you-**RET**-icks), which increase urine secretion to rid the body of excess sodium and water, are administered to treat hypertension and CHF.

Additional Medications

- **Statins**, a type of **cholesterol-lowering drug**, are used to reduce LDL cholesterol or other lipids in the blood.

- **Digoxin** (dih-**JOCK**-sin) also known as **digitalis** (**dij**-ih-**TAL**-is), slows and strengthens the heart muscle contractions and is used in the treatment of atrial fibrillation and CHF.

- **Nitroglycerin**, a vasodilator, is used to relieve the pain of angina. It may be administered sublingually (under the tongue), through the skin (by a patch), or orally as a spray.

- An **anticoagulant** (**an**-tih-koh-**AG**-you-lant), also known as a **thrombolytic** (**throm**-boh-**LIT**-ick) agent, slows blood clotting (coagulation) and prevents new clots from forming.

- An **antiarrhythmic** (**an**-tih-ah-**RITH**-mick) is administered to control irregularities of the heartbeat.

- **Tissue plasminogen activator** (**TISH**-you plaz-**MIN**-oh-jen **ACK**-tih-**vay**-tor), also known as **TPA**, is a clot-dissolving enzyme used for the immediate treatment of heart attack victims.

- A **vasoconstrictor** (**vas**-oh-kon-**STRICK**-tor) constricts (narrows) the blood vessels.

- A **vasodilator** (**vas**-oh-dye-**LAYT**-or) dilates (expands) the blood vessels.

Clearing Blocked Arteries

- **Percutaneous transluminal coronary angioplasty** (**AN**-jee-oh-**plas**-tee) is also called **PTCA** or **balloon angioplasty** (Figure 5.18). In this procedure, a small balloon on the end of a catheter is used to open a partially blocked coronary artery by flattening the plaque deposit and stretching the lumen. After the plaque has been flattened the balloon is deflated and the catheter and balloon are removed.

- **Percutaneous** (**per**-kyou-**TAY**-nee-us) means through the skin and **transluminal** means within the lumen of an artery.

- In a similar technique, a **stent** is implanted in a coronary artery to provide support to the arterial wall to prevent restenosis (Figure 5.19). **Restenosis** describes the condition when an artery that has been opened by angioplasty closes again (**re** means again and **stenosis** means narrowing).

- An **atherectomy** (**ath**-er-**ECK**-toh-mee) is the surgical removal of plaque from the interior lining of an artery (**ather** means plaque and **ectomy** means surgical removal). After the catheter and balloon are in place,

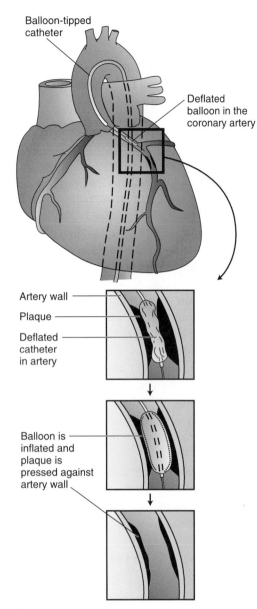

FIGURE 5.18 Balloon angioplasty is used to reopen a blocked coronary artery.

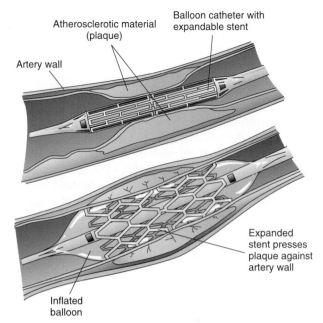

FIGURE 5.19 A stent is placed to prevent restenosis of the treated artery.

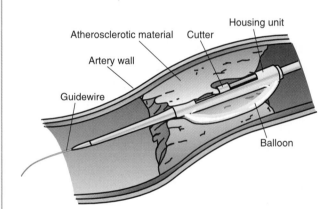

FIGURE 5.20 A cutting instrument is used to remove plaque from the artery wall.

the balloon is inflated and a cutting tool is used to shave off pieces of the plaque buildup (Figure 5.20).

- An **endarterectomy** (**end**-ar-ter-**ECK**-toh-mee) is the surgical removal of the lining of an artery that is clogged with plaque (**end** means within, **arter** means artery, and **ectomy** means surgical removal).

- A **carotid endarterectomy** is the surgical removal of the lining of a portion of a clogged carotid artery leading to the brain. The artery may be reinforced with a piece of vein taken from the leg. This procedure is performed to reduce the risk of stroke by ensuring the blood flow to the brain.

Coronary Artery Bypass Graft

- **Coronary artery bypass graft** (**CABG**) is also known as **bypass surgery** (Figure 5.21). In this surgery, which requires opening the chest, a piece of vein from the leg is implanted on the heart to bypass a blockage in the coronary artery and to improve the flow of blood to the heart.

- A **minimally invasive direct coronary artery bypass** (**MIDCAB**), also known as a **keyhole** or **buttonhole bypass** is an alternative technique for some bypass cases. This procedure is performed with the aid of a fiberoptic camera through small openings between the ribs.

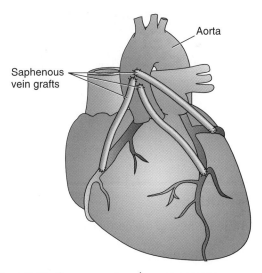

FIGURE 5.21 Coronary artery bypass surgery.

Heart

- **Defibrillation** (dee-**fib**-rih-**LAY**-shun), also known as **cardioversion** (**kar**-dee-oh-**VER**-zhun), is the use of electrical shock to restore the heart's normal rhythm. This can be performed externally as an emergency procedure or a device may be implanted to control severe arrhythmias.

- **Valvoplasty** (**VAL**-voh-**plas**-tee), also known as **valvuloplasty** (**VAL**-view-loh-**plas**-tee), is the surgical repair of a heart valve. This term also describes the surgical replacement of a heart valve.

- A **pacemaker** is an electronic device that may be attached externally or implanted under the skin, with connections leading into the heart to regulate the heartbeat (Figure 5.22). Pacemakers are used primarily as treatment for bradycardia or atrial fibrillation.

- **Cardiopulmonary resuscitation**, commonly known as **CPR**, is an emergency procedure for life support consisting of artificial respiration and manual external cardiac compression.

Blood Vessels, Blood, and Bleeding

- An **aneurysmectomy** (**an**-you-riz-**MECK**-toh-mee) is the surgical removal of an aneurysm (aneurysm means aneurysm and ectomy means surgical removal).

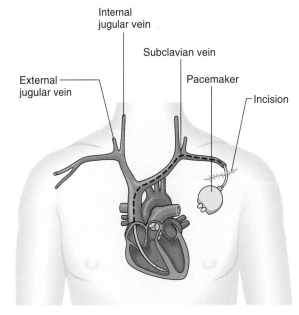

FIGURE 5.22 This type of artificial pacemaker is implanted under the skin.

- **Aneurysmorrhaphy** (**an**-you-riz-**MOR**-ah-fee) means to suture an aneurysm (aneurysm means aneurysm and rrhaphy means to suture).

- An **arteriectomy** (**ar**-teh-ree-**ECK**-toh-mee) is the surgical removal of part of an artery (arteri means artery and ectomy means surgical removal).

- **Hemostasis** (**hee**-moh-**STAY**-sis) means to control bleeding (hemo means blood and stasis means stopping or controlling).

- **Plasmapheresis** (**plaz**-mah-feh-**REE**-sis) is a procedure in which the plasma is removed from donated blood and the remaining components, mostly RBCs, are returned to the donor. This is performed to reduce or eliminate harmful substances present in the plasma.

- A **transfusion** is the introduction of whole blood or blood components into the bloodstream of the recipient. Unless the blood for transfusion has been carefully typed and crossmatched, the patient may suffer a severe transfusion reaction. Donated blood is also tested to prevent the transmission of bloodborne diseases such as the human immunodeficiency virus (HIV) and hepatitis.

5 ● Learning Exercises

● Matching Word Parts—1

Write the letter of the correct answer on the line provided in the left column.

5.1. _____ angi/o   A. aorta

5.2. _____ aort/o   B. artery

5.3. _____ arteri/o   C. plaque, fatty substance

5.4. _____ ather/o   D. relating to blood or lymph vessels

5.5. _____ brady-   E. slow

● Matching Word Parts—2

Write the letter of the correct answer on the line provided in the left column.

5.6. _____ cardi/o   A. blood or blood condition

5.7. _____ coron/o   B. crown, coronary

5.8. _____ ech/o   C. heart

5.9. _____ -emia   D. red

5.10. _____ erythr/o   E. sound

● Matching Word Parts—3

Write the letter of the correct answer on the line provided in the left column.

5.11. _____ hemat/o, hem/o   A. white

5.12. _____ leuk/o   B. vein

5.13. _____ phleb/o   C. fast, rapid

5.14. _____ tachy-   D. clot

5.15. _____ thromb/o   E. blood, relating to blood

● Definitions

Circle the letter next to the correct answer.

5.16. Leukocytes are _____ .

a. hemoglobin carriers

b. destroyed in the spleen

c. important clotting factors

d. important in fighting disease in the body

5.17. Which term means any abnormal or pathologic condition of the blood?

a. anemia

b. dyscrasia

c. hemochromatosis

d. septicemia

5.18. The myocardium receives its blood supply from the _____ .

a. aorta

b. coronary arteries

c. inferior vena cava

d. superior vena cava

5.19. Which term describes a diagnostic procedure using ultrasound to evaluate the structures and motion of the heart?

a. echocardiography

b. echoencephalography

c. electrocardiography

d. electroencephalography

5.20. Which heart valve is also known as the bicuspid valve?

a. aortic semilunar

b. mitral

c. pulmonary semilunar

d. tricuspid

5.21. Which heart chamber pumps blood to the lungs?

    a. left atrium

    b. left ventricle

    c. right atrium

    d. right ventricle

5.22. Which is the smallest formed element in the blood?

    a. erythrocytes

    b. leukocytes

    c. monocytes

    d. thrombocytes

5.23. Which term describes a foreign object circulating in the blood?

    a. embolism

    b. embolus

    c. thrombosis

    d. thrombus

5.24. Hemostasis means to _____ .

    a. control bleeding

    b. destroy worn-out red blood cells

    c. form new red blood cells

    d. maintain a stable body temperature

5.25. Which term means immature red blood cells?

    a. erythrocytes

    b. leukocytes

    c. reticulocytes

    d. thrombocytes

● Matching Structures

Write the letter of the correct answer on the line provided in the left column.

5.26. _____ endocardium   A. a hollow muscular organ

5.27. _____ epicardium   B. cardiac muscle

5.28. _____ heart   C. external layer of the heart

5.29. _____ myocardium   D. inner lining of the heart

5.30. _____ pericardium   E. sac enclosing the heart

● Which Word?

Circle the correct term in each sentence.

5.31. The substance known as good cholesterol is *high-density lipoprotein / low-density lipoprotein.*

5.32. An abnormally slow heartbeat is described as *bradycardia / tachycardia.*

5.33. Rapid, random, and ineffective contractions of the heart are described as *fibrillation / flutter.*

5.34. In recording blood pressure the higher reading is *diastolic / systolic* pressure.

5.35. The medical term for condition in which there is an abnormal decrease in the number of white blood cells is *leukemia / leukopenia.*

● Spelling Counts

Find the misspelled word in each sentence. Then write that word, spelled correctly, on the line provided.

5.36. The autopsy indicated the cause of death was a ruptured aneuryism. _____

5.37. The inflammation of a vein is known as flebitis. _____

5.38. Any abnormal heart rhythm is described as a cardiac arrhythemia. _____

5.39. Thallassemia is a genetic disorder characterized by short-lived red blood cells.

_____

5.40. Cholestarol is a fatty substance that circulates in the blood. _____

● Matching Abbreviations

Write the letter of the correct answer on the line provided in the left column.

5.41. _____ A-V   A. mitral valve

5.42. _____ LV   B. sinoatrial node

5.43. _____ MV   C. right atrium

5.44. _____ RA   D. atrioventricular node

5.45. _____ S-A   E. left ventricle

● Term Selection

Circle the letter next to the correct answer.

5.46. Which term indicates the presence of pathogens in the blood?

    a. dyscrasia

    b. pericarditis

    c. Raynaud's phenomenon

    d. septicemia

5.47. Which term describes chronic hypertension caused by a different medical problem?

    a. essential

    b. primary

    c. malignant

    d. secondary

5.48. Which form of anemia is characterized by large abnormal RBCs with a reduced capacity to carry hemoglobin?

    a. aplastic

    b. hemolytic

    c. megaloblastic

    d. pernicious

5.49. Which type of medication is administered to lower high blood pressure?

    a. antihypertensives

    b. digoxin

    c. TPA (tissue plasminogen activator)

    d. statins

5.50. Which diagnostic procedure involves the use of a radiopharmaceutical?

    a. angiography

    b. phlebography

    c. thallium stress test

    d. transesophageal echocardiography

● Sentence Completion

Write the correct term on the line.

5.51. Plasma with the clotting proteins removed is called _____ .

5.52. A localized balloon-like enlargement of an artery is called a/an _____ .

5.53. The medical term meaning the surgical removal of the lining of an artery is a/an _____ .

5.54. The name of the protein found in red blood cells that plays an essential role in oxygen transport is _____ .

5.55. The name of an amino acid normally found in the blood and used by the body to build and maintain tissues is _____ .

● True/False

If the statement is true, write T on the line. If the statement is false, write F on the line.

5.56. _____ The interatrial septum separates the lower chambers of the heart.

5.57. _____ Angiography is a study of the heart using sound waves.

5.58. _____ Arteries have valves to allow blood to flow away from the heart.

5.59. _____ The Rh factor is an antigen present on the erythrocytes of most people.

5.60. _____ Thrombocytopenia is an abnormal decrease in the number of platelets.

5.61. _____ An embolus is a blood clot attached to the interior wall of a vein or artery.

5.62. _____ Hemochromatosis is also known as iron overload disease.

5.63. _____ Plasmapheresis is a procedure in which the plasma is removed from donated blood and the remaining components are returned to the donor.

5.64. _____ A vasoconstrictor is a drug that enlarges the blood vessels.

5.65. _____ When erythrocytes are no longer useful, they are destroyed by macrophages in the spleen, liver, and bone marrow.

● Clinical Conditions

Write the correct answer on the line.

5.66. Allen Franklin was rushed to the hospital when he suffered a/an _____ _____ , which is commonly known as a heart attack.

5.67. Ramon Martinez has an abnormally slow heartbeat. The medical term for this is _____ .

5.68. During her pregnancy, Polly Olson suffered from _____ veins (abnormally swollen veins) in her legs.

5.69. Thomas Willis suffers from spasmodic, choking, or suffocating pain caused by a lack of oxygen to his heart muscle. The medical term for this condition is _____ pectoris.

5.70. Gary Klein suffers from a malignancy characterized by a progressive increase of abnormal leukocytes. The medical term for this condition is _____ .

5.71. Helen Grovenor had a/an _____ implanted as treatment to control atrial fibrillation.

5.72. Dr. Lawson read the patient's _____ . This is also known as an ECG or EKG.

5.73. Jason Turner suffered from cardiac arrest. The paramedics saved his life by using _____ resuscitation (CPR).

5.74. Darlene Nolan has mitral _____ . This is an obstructive lesion in the mitral valve of the heart.

5.75. Hamilton Edwards Sr. suffers from _____ heart disease. This is a group of cardiac disabilities resulting from an insufficient supply of oxygenated blood to the heart.

● Which is the correct medical term?

Circle the letter next to the correct answer.

3.76. Which term describes a fatty plaque buildup within an artery?
a. angiitis
b. angiostenosis
c. arteriosclerosis
d. atheroma

3.77. Which term describes a syndrome in which the heart is unable to pump enough blood to meet the body's needs?
a. cardiac arrhythmia
b. congestive heart failure
c. coronary artery disease
d. ischemia

3.78. Which term describes the blocking of an artery by a clot?
a. aneurysm
b. phlebitis
c. thrombotic occlusion
d. thrombophlebitis

3.79. Which term describes intermittent attacks of paleness, cyanosis, and redness of the fingers and toes?
a. angina pectoris
b. hemochromatosis
c. plasmapheresis
d. Raynaud's phenomenon

3.80. Which term means to suture an aneurysm?
a. aneurysmectomy
b. aneurysmoplasty
c. aneurysmorrhaphy
d. aneurysmotomy

● Challenge Word Building

These terms are *not* found in this chapter; however, they are made up of these familiar word parts. You may want to look in the glossary or use a medical dictionary to check your answers!

peri-	angi/o	-ectomy
	cardi/o	-megaly
	phleb/o	-rrhaphy
		-rrhexis
		-stenosis

5.81. Abnormal enlargement of the heart is known as _____ .

5.82. The surgical removal of a portion of a blood vessel is a/an _____ .

5.83. The abnormal narrowing of the lumen of a vein is called _____ .

5.84. The surgical removal of a portion of the tissue surrounding the heart is a/an _____ .

5.85. The procedure to suture the heart wall is a/an _____ .

5.86. The term meaning the rupture of a vein is _____ .

5.87. The suture repair of any vessel, especially of a blood vessel is called a/an _____ .

5.88. The term meaning rupture of the heart is _____ .

5.89. The procedure to suture the tissue surrounding the heart is a/an _____ .

5.90. The abnormal enlargement of blood vessels is known as _____ .

● Labeling Exercises

Identify the numbered items on these diagrams.

5.91. Superior _____ _____

5.92. Right _____

5.93. Right _____

5.94. Left pulmonary _____

5.95. Left pulmonary _____

5.96. _____ _____ valve

5.97. _____ valve

5.98. _____

5.99. _____ _____ valve

5.100. _____ valve

The Human Touch: Critical Thinking Exercise

The following story and questions are designed to stimulate critical thinking through class discussion or as a brief essay response. There are no easy or right-wrong answers to these questions.

Randi Marchant, a 42-year-old waitress, was vacuuming the family room when she felt that painful squeezing in her chest again. Third time today, but this one really hurt. She sat down to catch her breath and stubbed out the cigarette smoldering in the half-filled ashtray by the couch. Her husband Jimmy and stepdaughter Melonie had pestered her until she finally had taken time off work to see her doctor. Dr. Harris found that her blood pressure was 168/98 — probably due to the noon rush stress at work she rationalized. At least her cholesterol test was only 30 points above average this time. It had been slowly coming down, even though she cheated on her diet.

As another wave of pain tightened its icy fingers around her heart, and the pain moved up into both sides of her jaw. Randi remembered the doctor's words. "Probably just a little heartburn . . . women have less risk for heart attack than men . . ." This didn't feel like heartburn but the pain didn't radiate down her left arm so it couldn't be her heart, could it?

"Don't think about the pain," she told herself. "Think of something else . . . Melonie's prom dress . . needs altering . ." Randi fell to the floor, clutching her chest, just as Melonie walked in. She saw her stepmother slumped on the floor and screamed "Oh my God! Help, somebody help!"

Suggested Discussion Topics:

1. What information in the story indicates that Randi might be a candidate for heart disease?
2. Discuss why you think Dr. Harris didn't consider Randi as a candidate for heart attack.
3. What can Melonie do immediately to possibly save Randi's life?
4. Discuss why it is important that Randi receive appropriate treatment immediately.
5. What steps should someone at risk for heart disease take to help prevent the problem from becoming more serious?

The Lymphatic and Immune Systems

● Overview of Structures, Word Parts, and Functions of the Lymphatic and Immune Systems

MAJOR STRUCTURES	RELATED WORD ROOTS	PRIMARY FUNCTIONS
Lymph fluid and vessels	lymph/o	Return cellular waste and tissue fluid to the circulatory system.
Lymph nodes	lymphaden/o	Produce lymphocytes and filter harmful substances from lymph.
Tonsils and adenoids	tonsill/o, adenoid/o	Protect the entry into the respiratory system.
Spleen	splen/o	Filters foreign materials from the blood.
		Stores red blood cells, and maintains the appropriate balance between cells and plasma in the blood.
		Destroys old worn out blood cells, acts as a blood reservoir, and stores platelets.
Bone marrow	myel/o	Produces blood cells (see chapters 3 and 5).
Lymphocytes	lymph/o, -cyte	Play an important role in immune reactions.
Thymus	thym/o	Produces T lymphocytes for the immune system.
Immune system	immun/o	Defends the body against harmful substances such as pathogenic microorganisms, allergens, toxins, and malignant cells.

VOCABULARY Related to the Lymphatic and Immune Systems

Check the box as you master each word part or term. Terms marked with the ❖ symbol are pronounced on the optional student audiotape.

Key Word Parts

- [ ] blast/o
- [ ] carcin/o
- [ ] cervic/o
- [ ] -cide
- [ ] -genesis
- [ ] immun/o
- [ ] -lytic
- [ ] neo-
- [ ] -oma
- [ ] onc/o
- [ ] phag/o
- [ ] -plasm
- [ ] sarc/o
- [ ] splen/o
- [ ] -tic

Key Medical Terms

- [ ] acquired immunodeficiency syndrome
- [ ] allergen (AL-er-jen) ❖
- [ ] anaphylaxis (an-ah-fih-LACK-sis) ❖
- [ ] antibody
- [ ] antigen (AN-tih-jen)
- [ ] antiviral (an-tih-VYE-ral) ❖
- [ ] aspergillosis (ass-per-jil-OH-sis) ❖
- [ ] autoimmune disorder (aw-toh-ih-MYOUN) ❖
- [ ] axillary lymph nodes (AK-sih-lar-ee) ❖
- [ ] bacilli (bah-SILL-eye) ❖
- [ ] bacteria (back-TEER-ree-ah) ❖
- [ ] bactericide (back-TEER-ih-sighd)
- [ ] bacteriostatic (bac-tee-ree-oh-STAT-ick)
- [ ] brachytherapy (brack-ee-THER-ah-pee) ❖
- [ ] carcinoma (kar-sih-NOH-mah) ❖
- [ ] cervical lymph nodes (SER-vih-kal) ❖
- [ ] complement (KOM-pleh-ment)
- [ ] cytomegalovirus (sigh-toh-meg-ah-loh-VYE-rus) ❖
- [ ] cytotoxic (sigh-toh-TOK-sick) ❖
- [ ] ductal carcinoma in situ
- [ ] ELISA
- [ ] herpes zoster (HER-peez ZOS-ter) ❖
- [ ] Hodgkin's disease (HODJ-kinz) ❖
- [ ] human immunodeficiency virus
- [ ] immunodeficiency disorder (im-you-noh-deh-FISH-en-see) ❖
- [ ] immunoglobulin (im-you-noh-GLOB-you-lin) ❖
- [ ] immunologist (im-you-NOL-oh-jist) ❖
- [ ] immunosuppressant (im-you-noh-soo-PRES-ant) ❖

- [ ] immunosuppression (im-you-noh-sup-PRESH-un)
- [ ] immunotherapy (ih-myou-noh-THER-ah-pee) ❖
- [ ] infectious mononucleosis (mon-oh-new-klee-OH-sis) ❖
- [ ] infiltrating ductal carcinoma
- [ ] infiltrating lobular carcinoma
- [ ] inguinal lymph nodes (ING-gwih-nal) ❖
- [ ] interferon (in-ter-FEAR-on) ❖
- [ ] Kaposi's sarcoma (KAP-oh-seez sar-KOH-mah) ❖
- [ ] lumpectomy (lum-PECK-toh-mee) ❖
- [ ] lymphadenitis (lim-fad-eh-NIGH-tis) ❖
- [ ] lymphadenopathy (lim-fad-eh-NOP-ah-thee) ❖
- [ ] lymphangiogram (lim-FAN-jee-oh-gram) ❖
- [ ] lymphangioma (lim-fan-jee-OH-mah) ❖
- [ ] lymphedema (lim-feh-DEE-mah) ❖
- [ ] lymphocytes (LIM-foh-sights) ❖
- [ ] lymphokines (LIM-foh-kyeens) ❖
- [ ] lymphoma (lim-FOH-mah) ❖
- [ ] macrophage (MACK-roh-fayj) ❖
- [ ] metastasis (meh-TAS-tah-sis) ❖
- [ ] metastasize (meh-TAS-tah-sighz) ❖
- [ ] moniliasis (mon-ih-LYE-ah-sis) ❖
- [ ] myoma (my-OH-mah) ❖
- [ ] myosarcoma (my-oh-sahr-KOH-mah) ❖
- [ ] neoplasm (NEE-oh-plazm) ❖
- [ ] neuroblastoma (new-roh-blas-TOH-mah) ❖
- [ ] non-Hodgkin's lymphoma (non-HODG-kinz lim-FOH-mah) ❖
- [ ] oncologist (ong-KOL-oh-jist) ❖
- [ ] oncology (ong-KOL-oh-jee) ❖
- [ ] opportunistic infection (op-ur-too-NIHS-tick) ❖
- [ ] osteosarcoma (oss-tee-oh-sar-KOH-mah) ❖
- [ ] parasite (PAR-ah-sight) ❖
- [ ] pathogen (PATH-oh-jen) ❖
- [ ] phagocyte (FAG-oh-sight) ❖
- [ ] phagocytosis (fag-oh-sigh-TOH-sis) ❖
- [ ] rabies (RAY-beez) ❖
- [ ] retinoblastoma (ret-ih-noh-blas-TOH-mah) ❖
- [ ] rickettsia (rih-KET-see-ah) ❖
- [ ] rubella (roo-BELL-ah) ❖
- [ ] sarcoma (sar-KOH-mah) ❖
- [ ] spirochetes (SPY-roh-keets) ❖
- [ ] splenomegaly (splee-noh-MEG-ah-lee) ❖
- [ ] splenorrhagia (splee-noh-RAY-jee-ah) ❖
- [ ] staphylococci (staf-ih-loh-KOCK-sigh) ❖
- [ ] streptococci (strep-toh-KOCK-sigh) ❖
- [ ] teletherapy (tel-eh-THER-ah-pee) ❖
- [ ] thymus (THIGH-mus)
- [ ] Western blot test

● OBJECTIVES

On completion of this chapter, you should be able to:

1. Describe the major functions and structures of the lymphatic and immune systems.

2. Recognize, define, spell, and pronounce the major terms related to pathology and diagnostic and treatment procedures of the lymphatic and immune systems.

3. Recognize, define, spell, and pronounce terms related to oncology.

Medical Specialties Related to the Lymphatic and Immune Systems

- An **allergist** (AL-er-jist) specializes in diagnosing and treating conditions of altered immunologic reactivity such as allergic reactions.

- A **hematologist** (hee-mah-TOL-oh-jist *or* hem-ah-TOL-oh-jist) specializes in diagnosing and treating diseases and disorders of the blood and blood-forming tissues (**hemat** means blood and **ologist** means specialist).

- An **immunologist** (im-you-NOL-oh-jist) is a specialist in the study, diagnosis, and treatment of disorders of the immune system (**immun** means protected and **ologist** means specialist).

- An **oncologist** (ong-KOL-oh-jist) is a specialist in diagnosing and treating malignant disorders such as tumors and cancer (**onc** means tumor and **ologist** means specialist).

Functions and Structures of the Lymphatic System

Functions of the Lymphatic System

The lymphatic system has three primary functions. These are to:

- Return cellular waste products and excess fluid from the tissues to the circulatory system.

- Absorb fats and fat-soluble vitamins from the digestive system and transport them to the cells.

- Serve as an important part of the immune system.

Structures of the Lymphatic System

The major structures of the lymphatic system are **lymph fluid**, **lymph vessels**, **lymph nodes**, **tonsils**, **spleen**, **thymus**, and **lymphocytes** (these specialized white blood cells [WBCs] are discussed with the immune system).

Lymph Fluid

- **Intercellular fluid**, also known as **interstitial fluid** (in-ter-STISH-al) or **tissue fluid**, is plasma that flows out of

the capillaries of the circulatory system into the spaces between the cells. This fluid carries food, oxygen, and hormones to the cells (Figure 6.1).

- **Lymph fluid**, usually referred to as **lymph**, returns intercellular fluid containing waste products from the cells to the venous circulatory system (Figure 6.2). It also returns any blood cells that escaped from the capillaries.

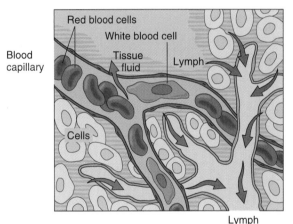

FIGURE 6.1 Lymph circulation showing interaction with blood vessels and cells.

Lymph Vessels

- **Lymph capillaries** are thin-walled tubes that carry lymph fluid from the tissues to the larger **lymphatic vessels** (Figure 6.3).

- Like veins, lymphatic vessels have valves to prevent the backward flow of fluid and lymph always flows *toward* the thoracic cavity.

- The **right lymphatic duct** and the **thoracic duct** empty lymph into veins in the upper thoracic region.

- **Lacteals** (LACK-tee-ahls) are specialized lymph capillaries located in the villi of the small intestine. Here fats and fat-soluble vitamins are absorbed and carried into the bloodstream.

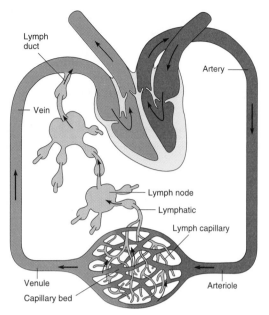

FIGURE 6.2 Fluids that leave circulation through the capillaries are returned to venous circulation by the lymphatic system.

Lymph Nodes

- Lymph nodes are small bean-shaped structures located in lymph vessels that provide a site for lymphocyte production (see Figures 6.2 and 6.3, and Table 6.1).
- These nodes filter lymph to remove harmful substances such as bacteria, viruses, and malignant cells

Table 6.1

MAJOR LYMPH NODE SITES

Cervical lymph nodes (**SER**-vih-kal) are located in the neck (**cervic** means neck and **al** means pertaining to).

Axillary lymph nodes (**AK**-sih-**lar**-ee) are located under the arms (**axill** means arm pit and **ary** means pertaining to).

Inguinal lymph nodes (**ING**-gwih-nal) are located in the inguinal (groin) area of the lower abdomen (**inguin** means groin and **al** means pertaining to).

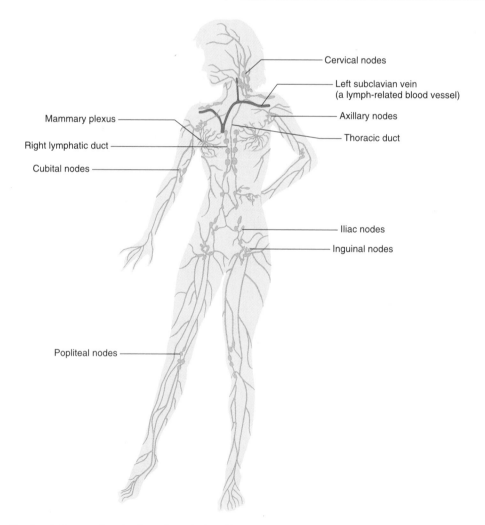

FIGURE 6.3 Lymphatic circulation and major lymph node locations.

as lymph flows through the node. Because of this function, swollen lymph nodes are often an indication of a disease process.

The Tonsils

The **tonsils** (**TON**-sils) are masses of lymphatic tissue that form a protective ring around the nose and upper throat (Figure 6.4 and Table 6.2).

The Vermiform Appendix and Peyer's Patches

These structures protect against the entry of invaders through the digestive system.

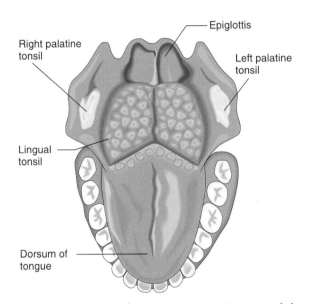

FIGURE 6.4 The tonsils form a protective ring around the entrance to the respiratory system.

Table 6.2

LOCATIONS OF THE TONSILS

The **adenoids** (**AD**-eh-noids), also known as the **nasopharyngeal tonsils** (**nay**-zoh-fah-**RIN**-jee-al), are located in the nasopharynx.

The **palatine tonsils** (**PAL**-ah-tine) are located in the portion of the throat that is visible through the mouth.

The **lingual tonsils** (**LING**-gwal) are located at the base of the tongue.

- The **vermiform appendix** is lymphatic tissue that hangs from the lower portion of the cecum of the large intestine (see Figure 6.6).
- **Peyer's patches** are small areas of lymphatic tissue located on the walls of the large intestine.

The Spleen

The spleen is a saclike mass of lymphatic tissue located in the left upper quadrant of the abdomen, just inferior to (below) the diaphragm and posterior to (behind) the stomach (Figure 6.5).

- The spleen filters microorganisms and other foreign material from the blood.
- The spleen forms lymphocytes and monocytes, which are specialized WBCs with roles in the immune system.
- The spleen is **hemolytic** (**hee**-moh-**LIT**-ick). This means that it removes and destroys worn-out red blood cells (**hemo** means blood and **lytic** means to destroy).

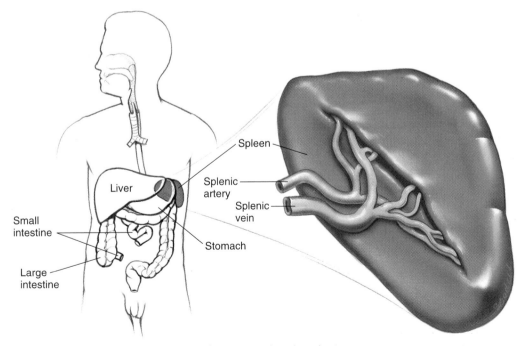

FIGURE 6.5 The spleen performs many important functions related to the immune system.

- The spleen stores extra erythrocytes and maintains the appropriate balance between the red blood cells and plasma in the circulation.

The Thymus

The **thymus** (**THIGH**-mus) is located superior to (above) the heart (see Figure 6.6). Although it is composed largely of lymphatic tissue, the thymus plays important roles in the endocrine (see Chapter 13) and immune systems.

Pathology and Diagnostic Procedures of Lymphatic Structures

- **Lymphadenitis** (lim-**fad**-eh-**NIGH**-tis), also known as **swollen glands**, is an inflammation of the lymph nodes (**lymphaden** means lymph node and **itis** means inflammation).

- **Lymphadenopathy** (lim-**fad**-eh-**NOP**-ah-thee) is any disease process usually involving enlargement of the lymph nodes (**lymphadeno** means lymph node and **pathy** means disease).

- **Persistent generalized lymphadenopathy**, also known as **PGL**, is the continued presence of enlarged lymph nodes. PGL is often an indication of the presence of a malignancy or deficiency in immune system function.

- A **lymphangiogram** (lim-**FAN**-jee-oh-**gram**) is a radiographic study of the lymphatic vessels and nodes with the use of a contrast medium to make these structures visible (**lymphangio** means lymph vessel and **gram** means record).

- A **lymphangioma** (lim-**fan**-jee-**OH**-mah) is a benign abnormal collection of lymphatic vessels forming a mass (**lymphangi** means lymph vessel and **oma** means tumor).

- **Lymphedema** (lim-feh-**DEE**-mah) is an abnormal accumulation of fluid primarily in the legs and ankles that occurs when veins or lymph vessels do not drain properly (**lymph** means lymph and **edema** means swelling). Compare with lipedema in Chapter 12.

- **Splenomegaly** (splee-noh-**MEG**-ah-lee) is an enlargement of the spleen (**spleno** means spleen and **megaly** means abnormal enlargement). Notice that the word root for spleen is always spelled with only one *e*).

- **Splenorrhagia** (splee-noh-**RAY**-jee-ah) is bleeding from the spleen (**spleno** means spleen and **rrhagia** means bleeding).

Functions and Structures of the Immune System

Functions of the Immune System

The functions of the immune system are to protect the body from harmful substances including pathogens (disease-producing microorganisms), allergens (substances producing an allergic reaction), toxins (poisons), and malignant cells.

Structures of the Immune System

Unlike other body systems, the immune system is not contained within a single set of organs or vessels. Instead it depends on structures from several other body systems (Figure 6.6).

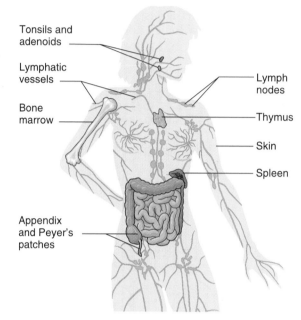

FIGURE 6.6 The immune system involves structures from many body systems.

The First Lines of Defense

The first role of the immune system is to prevent foreign substances from entering the body. However, several other body systems make up this important first line of defense.

- **Intact skin** wraps the body in a physical barrier that prevents invading organisms from entering the body. (**Intact** means there are no cuts, scrapes, or open sores.)

- The **respiratory system** traps breathed in foreign matter with nose hairs and the moist mucous membranes that line the respiratory system. Coughing and sneezing help expel foreign matter from the respiratory system.

- The **digestive system** uses the acids and enzymes produced by the stomach to destroy invaders that are swallowed or consumed with food.

- The **lymphatic system** structures and cells are essential components in fighting invaders once they have entered the body.

The Immune Response

When infectious microorganisms do enter the body one way in which the immune system destroys them is through antigen-antibody reactions.

- An **antigen** (AN-tih-jen), also known as **Ag**, is any substance such as a virus, bacterium, or toxin that the body regards as foreign. As foreign substances, antigens stimulate an immune response.
- An **antibody**, also known as **Ab**, is a disease-fighting protein created by the immune system in response to the presence of that specific antigen.
- The **immune reaction**, also known as the **antigen-antibody** reaction, involves binding these foreign antigens to antibodies to form antigen-antibody complexes. This tags the potentially dangerous antigen so that it can be recognized and destroyed.

Specialized Cells of the Immune Reactions

The immune response requires the actions of many specialized cells.

Lymphocytes

- **Lymphocytes** (LIM-foh-sights) are WBCs that specialize so they can attack specific microorganisms. Lymphocytes are formed in bone marrow and undergo further maturation and differentiation in lymphatic tissue throughout the body including the lymph nodes, spleen, thymus, tonsils, and Peyer's patches.
- The two major classes of lymphocytes are B cells and T cells.

B Cells

- Each **B cell**, also known as a **B lymphocyte**, is designed to make only one specific antibody against a specific antigen. B cells are most effective against viruses and bacteria that are circulating in the blood.
- When confronted with this type of antigen, B cells are transformed into plasma cells. **Plasma cells** produce and secrete antibodies coded to match the antigen. This enables the body to destroy the antigen in the antigen-antibody response.
- **Complement** (KOM-pleh-ment) is a complex series of proteins that circulate in normal serum. They are activated on contact with an antigen and aid the antibodies by puncturing the cell membrane of the antigen.
- **Immunoglobulin** (im-you-noh-GLOB-you-lin), also known as **Ig**, is a synonym for the term antibody. The five classes of immunoglobulins (antibodies) are summarized in Table 6.3.

T Cells

- **T cells**, also known as **T lymphocytes**, are small circulating lymphocytes that have traveled to the thymus. Here they mature as a result of their exposure to thymosin (the hormone secreted by the thymus).
- The primary function of the T cells is to coordinate immune defenses and to kill invading organisms on contact.

Table 6.3

IMMUNOGLOBULINS

Immunoglobulin M	IgM is the first immunoglobulin the body produces when challenged by an antigen and is found in circulating fluids.
Immunoglobulin G	IgG is the most common type of antibody found in the plasma. It is formed after a second exposure to an antigen.
Immunoglobulin A	IgA is the major antibody that protects against invasion through the mucous membranes and is found primarily in tissues other than blood.
Immunoglobulin E	IgE provides defenses against environmental antigens. It also is the antibody that causes acute allergic reactions such as hay fever.
Immunoglobulin D	IgD is found in small amounts in serum and is thought is play a role in B-cell differentiation.

- **Interferon** (in-ter-FEAR-on), which is produced by the T cells, is a family of proteins released by cells when invaded by a virus. Interferon causes noninfected cells to form an antiviral protein that slows or stops viral multiplication.
- **Lymphokines** (LIM-foh-kyeens), which are produced by the T cells, direct the immune response by signaling between the cells of the immune system. Lymphokines attract macrophages to the infected site and prepare them to attack.
- A **macrophage** (MACK-roh-fayj), which is a type of phagocyte, protects the body by ingesting (eating) invading cells and by interacting with the other cells of the immune system (**macro** means large and **phage** means a cell that eats).
- A **phagocyte** (FAG-oh-sight) is a WBC with the ability to ingest (eat) and destroy substances such as cell debris, dust, pollen, and pathogens (**phago** means eat or swallow and **cyte** means cell). This process is known as **phagocytosis** (fag-oh-sigh-TOH-sis).

Immunity

Immunity is the state of being resistant or not susceptible to a specific disease.

- **Natural immunity** is passed from mother to fetus before birth. Immediately after birth additional immunity is passed from mother to child through breast milk.

- **Acquired immunity** is obtained by the development of antibodies during an attack of an infectious disease. As an example, after having chickenpox antibodies are present against it.

- **Artificial immunity**, which is also known as **immunization**, is immunity that was acquired through **vaccination**. Examples of currently available vaccines include chickenpox, diphtheria, hepatitis B, influenza (some types), measles, meningitis, mumps, pertussis (whooping cough), pneumonia (some types), poliomyelitis, smallpox, tetanus, and typhoid.

Immune System Response Factors

Important factors that influence the immune system's ability to respond are health, age, and heredity.

- **Health**. The better the individual's general health, the more likely that the immune system can respond effectively. Diseases strike more easily when general health, and in particular the functioning of the immune system, is compromised.

- **Age**. Older individuals usually have more acquired immunity; however, their immune systems tend to respond less quickly and effectively to new challenges.

- **Heredity**. Genes, and genetic disorders, shape the makeup of antibodies and other immune cells. These factors influence the body's ability to respond (see Chapter 2).

- An **opportunistic infection** (op-ur-too-NIHS-tick) is a pathogen that normally does not cause disease but is able to cause illness in a weakened host whose resistance has been decreased by a different disorder.

Pathology and Diagnostic Procedures of the Immune System

Allergic Reactions

- An **allergy**, also known as **hypersensitivity**, is an overreaction by the body to a particular antigen.

- An allergic reaction occurs when the body's immune system reacts to a harmless allergen such as pollen, food, or animal dander, as if it were a dangerous invader. An **allergen** (AL-er-jen) is an antigen that is capable of inducing an allergic response.

- In a **cellular response**, also known as a **localized** or **delayed allergic response**, the body does not react the first time it is exposed to the allergen. However, sensitivity is established and future contacts cause symptoms that include itching, erythema (redness of the skin), and large hives. As an example, contact dermatitis is a skin reaction caused by a localized allergic response (see Chapter 12).

- A **systemic reaction**, also described as **anaphylaxis** (an-ah-fih-LACK-sis), is a severe response to a foreign substance such as a drug, food, insect venom, or chemical. Symptoms develop very quickly and include swelling, blockage of air passages, and a drop in blood pressure. Without appropriate care, the patient may die within minutes.

- A **scratch test** is a diagnostic test to identify commonly troublesome allergens such as tree pollen and ragweed. Swelling and itching indicate an allergic reaction (Figure 6.7).

- **Antihistamines** are medications administered to block and control allergic reactions.

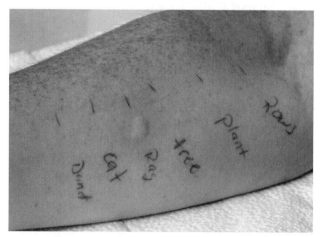

FIGURE 6.7 In scratch tests, allergens are placed on the skin, the skin is scratched, and the allergen is labeled. Reactions usually occur within 20 minutes. Pictured is a reaction to ragweed.

Autoimmune Disorders

An **autoimmune disorder** (aw-toh-ih-MYOUN) is a condition in which the immune system misreads normal antigens and creates antibodies and directs T cells against the body's own tissues. Many of these disorders appear to be genetically transmitted and they affect most body systems (Table 6.4). For reasons that are not understood, 75% of these diseases occur most frequently in women during the childbearing years.

Immunodeficiency

- An **immunodeficiency disorder** (im-you-noh-deh-FISH-en-see) is a condition that occurs when one or more parts of the immune system are deficient or missing.

- When the immune system is weakened it is also described as being **compromised**.

- Some immunodeficiency disorders, such as **congenital immunodeficiency**, are hereditary. Other forms are caused by pathogens.

- The **human immunodeficiency virus**, also known as **HIV** (pronounced H-I-V), is a bloodborne pathogen

Table 6.4

EXAMPLES OF AUTOIMMUNE DISORDERS AND AFFECTED BODY SYSTEMS

Disease	Affected Area
Crohn's disease	Intestines, the ileum, or the colon (see Chapter 8)
Diabetes mellitus, type 1	Insulin-producing pancreatic cells (see Chapter 13)
Graves' disease	Thyroid gland (see Chapter 13)
Hashimoto's thyroiditis	Thyroid gland (see Chapter 13)
Lupus erythematosus	Skin and other body systems (see Chapter 12)
Myasthenia gravis	Nerve/muscle synapses (see Chapter 4)
Multiple sclerosis	Brain and spinal cord (see Chapter 10)
Psoriasis	Skin (see Chapter 12)
Rheumatoid arthritis	Connective tissue (see Chapter 3)
Scleroderma	Skin and other tissues (see Chapter 12)

that invades and then progressively impairs or kills cells of the immune system.

- **Acquired immunodeficiency syndrome**, also known as **AIDS**, describes the advanced stages of HIV infection.

- **ELISA**, which is the abbreviation for **enzyme-linked immunosorbent assay**, is a blood test used to screen for the presence of HIV antibodies; however, this test may produce a false-positive result. (A **false-positive** result is an inaccurate test result indicating the presence of HIV when it is not true.)

- When the results of the ELISA test are positive, a **Western blot test** is performed to confirm the diagnosis. The Western blot test, which detects the presence of specific viral proteins, produces more accurate results.

Treatment Procedures of the Immune System

Immunotherapy

- **Immunotherapy** (ih-**myou**-noh-**THER**-ah-pee) is a treatment of disease either by enhancing or repressing the immune response.

- In the treatment of allergies, immunotherapy is used to repress the immune response.
- In the treatment of cancers, immunotherapy is used to stimulate the immune response.

Antibody Therapy

- **Synthetic immunoglobulins**, also known as **immune serum**, are used as a postexposure preventive measure against certain viruses including rabies and some types of hepatitis.

- **Synthetic interferon** is used in the treatment of hepatitis B and C and in some cancers.

- **Monoclonal antibodies**, also known as **MAbs**, are antibodies produced in the laboratory. Currently MAbs are used in laboratory research, medical tests, and the treatment of some Non-Hodgkin's lymphoma, and melanoma, breast and colon cancers.

Immunosuppression

- **Immunosuppression** (**im**-you-noh-sup-**PRESH**-un) is treatment used to interfere with the ability of the immune system to respond to stimulation by antigens.

- An **immunosuppressant** (**im**-you-noh-soo-**PRES**-ant) is a drug that prevents or reduces the body's normal reactions to invasion by disease or by foreign tissues. Immunosuppressants are used to prevent the rejection of donor tissue or to depress autoimmune disorders.

- A **corticosteroid drug** is a hormone-like preparation used primarily as an anti-inflammatory and as an immunosuppressant.

- A **cytotoxic drug** (**sigh**-toh-**TOK**-sick) kills or damages cells (**cyto** means cell, **tox** means poison, and **ic** means pertaining to). It is used as an immunosuppressant and as an antineoplastic.

- An **antineoplastic** (**an**-tih-nee-oh-**PLAS**-tick) blocks the growth of neoplasms and is used to treat cancer.

Pathogenic Organisms

A **pathogen** (**PATH**-oh-jen) is a microorganism that causes a disease (Figure 6.8). A **microorganism** is a living organism that is so small it can only be seen with the aid of a microscope.

Bacteria

Bacteria (back-**TEER**-ree-ah) are a group of one-celled microscopic organisms. (singular, **bacterium**). The pathogenic types of bacteria include bacilli, rickettsia, spirochetes, staphylococci, and streptococci.

- **Bacilli** (bah-**SILL**-eye) are rod-shaped spore-forming bacteria (singular, **bacillus**). **Tetanus** and **tuberculosis** are caused by bacilli.

- A **rickettsia** (rih-**KET**-see-ah) is a small bacterium that lives in lice, fleas, ticks and mites (plural, **rickettsiae**). They transmit the infection to humans. **Rocky**

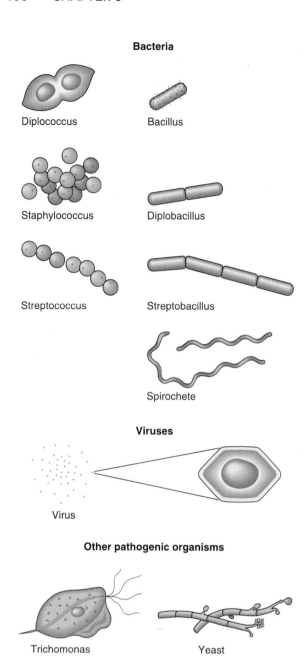

Bacteria

Diplococcus

Bacillus

Staphylococcus

Diplobacillus

Streptococcus

Streptobacillus

Spirochete

Viruses

Virus

Other pathogenic organisms

Trichomonas

Yeast

FIGURE 6.8 Types of pathogens.

Mountain spotted fever is caused by a rickettsia that was transmitted by a tick bite.

- **Spirochetes** (**SPY**-roh-keets) are spiral-shaped bacteria that have flexible walls and are capable of movement. **Lyme disease**, which is transmitted to man by an infected deer tick, is caused by the spirochete *Borrellia burgdorferi*.

- **Staphylococci** (**staf**-ih-loh-**KOCK**-sigh) are bacteria that form irregular groups or clusters (singular, **staphylococcus**). **Endocarditis**, **pneumonia**, and some **skin infections** are caused by staphylococci.

- **Streptococci** (**strep**-toh-**KOCK**-sigh) are bacteria that form a chain (singular, **streptococcus**). Severe **pharyn-**

gitis, also known as a strep throat, is caused by streptococci.

Fungus, Yeast, and Parasites

- A **fungus** (**FUNG**-gus) is a simple parasitic plant. Some of these plants are harmless to humans and others are pathogenic (plural, **fungi**). **Aspergillosis** (**ass**-per-jil-**OH**-sis) is an infection caused by a fungus of the genus *Aspergillus*. It may cause inflammation and lesions on or in any organ.

- **Yeast** is a type of fungus. **Moniliasis** (mon-ih-**LYE**-ah-sis) is an infection of the skin or mucous membranes caused by the pathogenic yeast *Candida albicans*. These infections are usually localized in the mouth or the vagina.

- A **parasite** (**PAR**-ah-sight) is a plant or animal that lives on or within another living organism at the expense of that organism. **Malaria** (mah-**LAY**-ree-ah) is caused by a parasite that lives within certain mosquitoes and is transferred to humans by the bite of the mosquito.

Viruses

- **Viruses** (**VYE**-rus-ez) are very small infectious agents that live only by invading cells. Within the cell they reproduce and then break the cell walls so the newly formed virus can spread to other cells.

Viral Infections

- **Chickenpox**, also known as **varicella** or **VZV**, is an acute highly contagious viral disease characterized by fever and pustules. It is caused by the herpes virus *Varicella zoster* and is transmitted by respiratory droplets or direct contact with sores.

- **Cytomegalovirus** (sigh-toh-**meg**-ah-loh-**VYE**-rus), also known as **CMV**, is an infection caused by a group of large herpes-type viruses with a wide variety of disease effects.

- **Herpes zoster** (**HER**-peez **ZOS**-ter), also known as **shingles** or **HZ**, is an acute viral infection characterized by painful skin eruptions that follow the underlying route of the inflamed nerve. This inflammation, which is caused by the chickenpox virus that remained dormant in a nerve, is reactivated years later when the immune system is compromised.

- **Infectious mononucleosis** (**mon**-oh-**new**-klee-**OH**-sis), which is caused by the Epstein-Barr virus (one of the herpes viruses), is characterized by fever, a sore throat, and enlarged lymph nodes.

- **Measles** is an acute, highly contagious viral disease transmitted by respiratory droplets. It is characterized first by the appearance of Koplik's spots and then followed by a spreading skin rash. **Koplik's spots** are small red spots with blue-white centers that appear on the lining of the mouth. (Compare measles with rubella.)

- **Mumps** is an acute viral disease characterized by swelling of the parotid glands. (The parotid glands are salivary glands located on the face just in front of the ears.)
- **Rabies** (RAY-beez) is an acute viral infection that may be transmitted to humans by the blood, tissue, or saliva of an infected animal.
- **Rubella** (roo-BELL-ah), also known as **German measles** or **3-day measles**, is a viral infection characterized by fever and a diffuse, fine, red rash. If the mother has rubella during the early stages of pregnancy, the disease may cause congenital abnormalities in the infant. (Compare rubella with measles.)

Medications to Control Infections

- An **antibiotic** is a chemical substance that is capable of inhibiting growth or killing pathogenic microorganisms (**anti** means against, **bio** means life, and **tic** means pertaining to). Antibiotics are used to combat bacterial infections.
- A **bactericide** (back-TEER-ih-sighd) is a substance that causes the death of bacteria (**bacteri** means bacteria and **cide** means causing death). Bactericides include primarily the antibiotic groups of **penicillins** and **cephalosporins**.
- A **bacteriostatic** (bac-tee-ree-oh-STAT-ick) is an agent that inhibits, slows, or retards the growth of bacteria.

These include primarily the antibiotic groups of **tetracyclines**, **sulfonamides**, and **erythromycin**.
- An **antiviral drug** (an-tih-VYE-ral), such as acyclovir, is used to treat viral infections or to provide temporary immunity. Antibiotics are not effective against viruses.

Oncology

Oncology (ong-KOL-oh-jee) is the study of the prevention, causes, and treatment of tumors and cancer (**onc** means tumor and **ology** means study of).

The term *cancer* is used to describe over 200 different kinds of malignancies. It attacks all body systems and is the second leading cause of death in the United States (Figure 6.9). Most cancers are named for the part of the body where the cancer first starts.

Terms Related to Tumors

- A **tumor**, also known as a **neoplasm** (NEE-oh-plazm), is a new and abnormal tissue formation (**neo** means new or strange and **plasm** means formation).
- Through a process known as **angiogenesis** (an-jee-oh-JEN-eh-sis) the tumor supports its growth by creating its own blood supply (**angio** means vessel and **genesis** means reproduction). **Antiangiogenesis** is a form of

FIGURE 6.9 Leading sites of cancer incidence and death in 1998. *From the American Cancer Society's Cancer Facts and Figures - 1998, reprinted with permission.*

treatment that is being developed to cut off this blood supply to the tumor.

- Within a tumor the multiplication of cells is uncontrolled, more rapid than normal, and progressive. A **tumor** may be either benign or malignant.

- **Memory aid**: Benign sounds like *be nice* and malignant sounds like *malicious* or *mean*!

Benign

- **Benign** means not recurring, nonmalignant, and with a favorable chance for recovery. As an example, a **myoma** (my-OH-mah) is a benign neoplasm made up of muscle tissue (**my** means muscle and **oma** means tumor). Although not malignant, these tumors can cause problems through pressure on adjacent structures.

Malignant

- **Malignant** means harmful, tending to spread, becoming progressively worse, and life-threatening. Malignant tumors tend to spread to distant body sites.

Class A colorectal cancer

Class B colorectal cancer

Class C colorectal cancer

FIGURE 6.10 Stages of colorectal cancer. *Class A* the polyp has formed but not yet invaded the surrounding tissue. *Class B* the cancer has invaded the underlying tissue. *Class C* the cancer has spread to surrounding lymph nodes.

- The term **carcinoma in situ**, also known as **CIT**, describes a malignant tumor in its original position that has not yet disturbed or invaded the surrounding tissues.

- An **invasive malignancy** grows and spreads into healthy adjacent tissue. Figure 6.10 shows the progression as colorectal cancer invades the surrounding tissues.

- **Metastasize** (meh-TAS-tah-sighz) is the verb that describes the process by which cancer spreads from one place to another. The cancer starts at the primary site and spreads to a secondary site.

- A **metastasis** (meh-TAS-tah-sis) is the new cancer site that results from the spreading process (**meta** means beyond and **stasis** means stopping). The metastasis may be within the same body system or distance from the primary site in another body system (plural, **metastases**).

Staging

- **Staging** is the process of classifying tumors with respect to how far the disease has progressed, the potential for its responding to therapy, and the patient's prognosis. Specific staging systems are used for different types of cancer (see Tables 6.5 and 6.6).

Carcinomas

- A **carcinoma** (kar-sih-NOH-mah), also known as **CA** or **Ca**, is a malignant tumor that occurs in epithelial tissue (**carcin** means cancer and **oma** means tumor). Epithelial tissue covers the internal and external surfaces of the body (Figure 6.11).

- These cancers tend to infiltrate, produce metastases, and affect any organ or part of the body.

- As an example, an **adenocarcinoma** (ad-eh-noh-kar-sih-NOH-mah) is any one of a large group of carcinomas derived from glandular tissue (**adeno** means gland, **carcin** means cancer, and **oma** means tumor).

FIGURE 6.11 Carcinoma of the lip. *(Courtesy of Dr. Joseph Konzelman, School of Dentistry, Medical College of Georgia)*

Sarcomas

- A **sarcoma** (sar-KOH-mah) is a malignant tumor that arises from connective tissue (**sarc** means flesh and **oma** means tumor). (Plural, **sarcomas** or **sarcomata**.)

Tissues affected by sarcomas include bones, the bladder, kidneys, liver, lungs, muscles, and spleen.

- Hard tissue sarcomas arise from bone or cartilage (see also Chapter 3). As an example, **osteosarcoma** (**oss**-tee-oh-sar-**KOH**-mah) is a malignant tumor usually involving the upper shaft of long bones, the pelvis, or knee (**osteo** means bone, **sarc** means flesh, and **oma** means tumor).

- Soft tissue sarcomas arise from tissues such as fat, muscle, and nerves. As an example, a **myosarcoma** (**my**-oh-sahr-**KOH**-mah) is a malignant tumor derived from muscle tissue (**myo** means muscle, **sarc** means flesh, and **oma** means tumor).

- **Kaposi's sarcoma** (**KAP**-oh-seez sar-**KOH**-mah), also known as **KS**, is an opportunistic infection frequently associated with HIV. It may affect the skin, mucous membranes, lymph nodes and internal organs.

Lymphomas

- **Lymphoma** (lim-**FOH**-mah) is a general term applied to malignancies that develop in the lymphatic system (**lymph** means lymph and **oma** means tumor). The two most common types are Hodgkin's disease and non-Hodgkin's lymphoma.

Hodgkin's Disease

- **Hodgkin's disease** (**HODJ**-kinz), also known as **Hodgkin's lymphoma** or **HL**, is distinguished by the presence of *Reed-Sternberg cells*. These are large cancerous lymphocytes that are identified by microscopic examination of a biopsy specimen taken from an enlarged lymph node. The staging system to describe this disease is shown in Table 6.5.

Non-Hodgkin's Lymphomas

- The term **non-Hodgkin's lymphomas** (non-**HODJ**-kinz lim-**FOH**-mah), also known as **NHL**, is used to describe all lymphomas *other than* Hodgkin's lymphoma.

- In NHL, the cells of the lymphatic system divide and grow without any order or control. This causes tumors to develop in different locations on the body and these cancer cells can also spread to other organs.

- The disease is described as low-grade (growing slowly), intermediate-grade (growing moderately), and high-grade (growing rapidly).

- Treatment depends on the type and stage of NHL and usually includes chemotherapy, radiation therapy, and possibly a bone marrow transplant (see Chapter 3).

Blastomas

- A **blastoma** (blas-**TOH**-mah) is a neoplasm composed chiefly or entirely of immature undifferentiated cells (**blast** means immature or embryonic and **oma** means tumor). Blastomas are frequently named for the tissues involved.

- A **neuroblastoma** (**new**-roh-blas-**TOH**-mah) is a sarcoma of nervous system origin (**neuro** means nerve, **blast** means immature or embryonic, and **oma** means tumor).

- A **retinoblastoma** (**ret**-ih-noh-blas-**TOH**-mah) is a malignant tumor of childhood arising from cells of the retina of the eye and usually occurring before the third year of life (**retino** means retina, **blast** means immature or embryonic, and **oma** means tumor).

Breast Cancer

Breast cancer is a malignant tumor that develops from the cells of the breast and may spread to adjacent lymph nodes and other body sites (Figure 6.12).

Types of Breast Cancer

- **Invasive ductal carcinoma**, also known as **infiltrating ductal carcinoma** or **IDC**, starts in the milk duct, breaks through the wall of that duct, and invades fatty breast tissue. IDC accounts for the majority of all breast cancers.

- **Ductal carcinoma in situ**, also known as **DCIS**, is breast cancer at its earliest stage (stage 0) before the cancer has broken through the wall of the duct. At this stage the cure rate is nearly 100%.

- **Invasive lobular carcinoma**, also known as **infiltrating lobular carcinoma** or **ILC**, is cancer that starts in the milk glands (lobules), breaks through the wall of the gland and invades the fatty tissue of the breast. Once the cancer reaches the lymph nodes, it can rapidly spread to distant parts of the body.

Table 6.5

STAGING FOR HODGKIN'S DISEASE

Stage	Has Spread to	15-Year Cure Rate
I	Limited to lymph nodes in one area of the body such as one side of the neck.	95% plus
II	Involves lymph nodes in two or more areas on the same side of the diaphragm (either above or below).	90%
III	Involves lymph nodes above and below the diaphragm.	80%
IV	Involves lymph nodes plus other tissues including bone marrow, lungs, or liver	60 to 70%

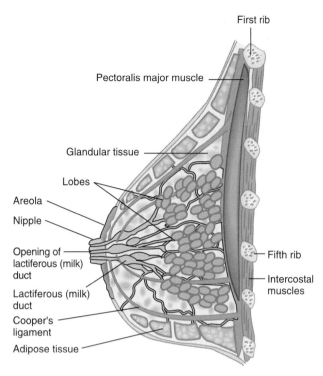

First rib

Pectoralis major muscle

Glandular tissue

Lobes

Areola

Nipple

Opening of
lactiferous (milk)
duct

Lactiferous (milk)
duct

Cooper's
ligament

Adipose tissue

Fifth rib

Intercostal
muscles

Figure 6.12 Invasive ductal carcinoma is the most common form of breast cancer.

- **Male breast cancer** can occur in the small amount of breast tissue that is normally present in men. The types of cancers are similar to those occurring in women.

Detection of Breast Cancer

Early detection is possible through **breast self-examination** (BSE), **mammograms**, and professional palpation. Diagnosis is confirmed by biopsy. These are discussed in Chapter 14.

A **biopsy** is the removal of tissue to confirm a diagnosis. After a diagnosis has been established, treatment is then based on the stage of the cancer (Table 6.6).

Treatment of Breast Cancer

- A **lumpectomy** is the surgical removal of only the cancerous tissue and a margin (rim) of normal tissue (Figure 6.13).
- A **modified radical mastectomy** is the surgical removal of the entire breast and lymph nodes under the arm (Figure 6.14).

Cancer Treatments

The three most common forms of cancer treatments are surgery, chemotherapy, and radiation therapy.

Surgery

- When possible, cancer surgery involves removing the malignancy plus a margin of normal surrounding tissue.

Table 6.6

STAGING BREAST CANCER

Stage	Explanation
I	The cancer is no larger than 2 centimeters (about 1 inch) and has not spread outside the breast.
II	Any of the following may be true: The cancer is no larger than 2 centimeters but has spread to the axillary lymph nodes. The cancer is between 2 and 5 centimeters (from 1 to 2 inches) and may or may not have spread to the axillary lymph nodes. The cancer is larger than 5 centimeters (greater than 2 inches) but has not spread to the axillary lymph nodes.
IIIA	Either of the following is true: The cancer is smaller than 5 centimeters and has spread to the axillary lymph nodes and the lymph nodes are attached to each other or to other structures. The cancer is larger than 5 centimeters and has spread to the axillary lymph nodes
IIIB	Either of the following is true: The cancer has spread to tissues near the breast (skin or chest wall, including the ribs and muscles of the chest). The cancer has spread to lymph nodes inside the chest wall along the breastbone.
IV	The cancer has spread to other organs of the body, most often the bones, lungs, liver, or brain. Or, the cancer has spread locally to the skin and lymph nodes inside the neck, near the collarbone.

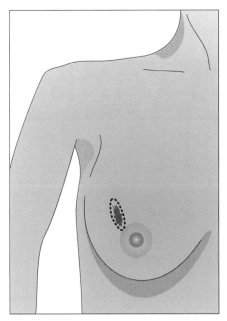

FIGURE 6.13 A lumpectomy is the removal of the cancerous tissue plus a rim of healthy tissue.

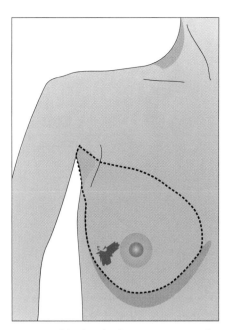

FIGURE 6.14 A modified radical mastectomy is the removal of the entire breast and the adjacent lymph nodes.

Chemotherapy

- **Chemotherapy** is the use of chemical agents and drugs in combinations selected to effectively destroy malignant cells and tissues.

Radiation Therapies

- **Radiation therapy** is the treatment of cancers through the use of x-rays. The goal of these therapies is to destroy the cancer while sparing healthy tissues.

- **Brachytherapy** (**brack**-ee-**THER**-ah-pee) is the use of radioactive materials in contact with, or implanted into, the tissues to be treated (Figure 6.15).

- **Teletherapy** (**tel**-eh-**THER**-ah-pee) is radiation therapy administered at a distance from the body. With 3-dimensional computer imaging it is possible to aim doses more precisely.

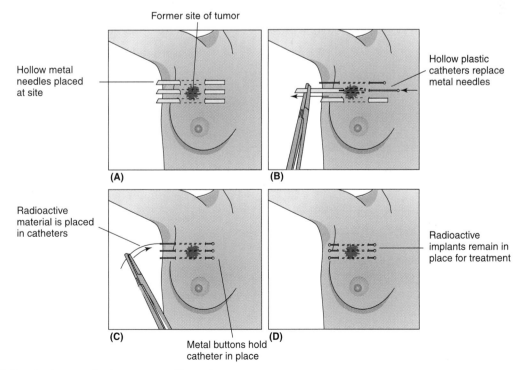

Former site of tumor

Hollow metal needles placed at site

Hollow plastic catheters replace metal needles

Radioactive material is placed in catheters

Radioactive implants remain in place for treatment

Metal buttons hold catheter in place

(A) (B) (C) (D)

FIGURE 6.15 Brachytherapy for treatment of breast cancer.

Learning Exercises

Matching Word Parts—1

Write the letter of the correct answer on the line provided in the left column.

6.1. _____ blast/o   A. to destroy

6.2. _____ carcin/o   B. neck

6.3. _____ cervic/o   C. eat, swallow

6.4. _____ phag/o   D. cancer

6.5. _____ -lytic   E. immature, embryonic

Matching Word Parts—2

Write the letter of the correct answer on the line provided in the left column.

6.6. _____ immun/o   A. formation

6.7. _____ onc/o   B. flesh

6.8. _____ -plasm   C. protected, safe

6.9. _____ sarc/o   D. spleen

6.10. _____ splen/o   E. tumor

Matching Types of Pathogens

Write the letter of the correct answer on the line provided in the left column.

6.11. _____ parasite   A. bacteria capable of movement

6.12. _____ spirochete   B. chain-forming bacteria

6.13. _____ staphylococci   C. cluster-forming bacteria

6.14. _____ streptococci   D. live only by invading cells

6.15. _____ viruses   E. lives on or within another organism

Definitions

Circle the letter next to the correct answer.

6.16. The spleen _____ .

     a. is hemolytic

     b. contains lymphocytes

     c. stores red blood cells

     d. a, b, and c

6.17. Which medical term means an inflammation of the lymph nodes?

     a. adenoiditis

     b. lymphadenitis

     c. lymphoma

     d. mononucleosis

6.18. An immunosuppressant is _____ .

     a. a type of complex protein found in serum

     b. formed by B cells

     c. formed by T cells

     d. used to prevent the rejection of donor tissue

6.19. T cells are responsible for _____ .

a. creating antibodies

b. producing complement

c. producing immunoglobulins

d. producing interferon

6.20. Which structure is composed largely of lymphatic tissue yet plays an important role in the endocrine system?

a. bone marrow

b. liver

c. spleen

d. thymus

6.21. Which structures form a protective ring of lymphatic tissue surrounding the nose and mouth?

a. lacteals

b. lymph nodes

c. Peyer's patches

d. tonsils

6.22. Lymph vessels return intercellular fluid to the _____ .

a. arteries

b. cells

c. spleen

d. veins

6.23. Where are the lacteals located?

a. arm pits

b. groin

c. neck

d. small intestine

6.24. Which of the following occurs in the immune response?

a. Antibodies are produced find and to destroy antigens.

b. Antigens are produced to find and destroy antibodies.

c. Specialized erythrocytes are formed.

d. Specialized platelets are formed.

6.25. The thymus is located _____ to the heart.

a. anterior

b. inferior

c. posterior

d. superior

● Matching Structures

Write the letter of the correct answer on the line provided in the left column.

6.26. _____ lymph nodes

6.27. _____ skin

6.28. _____ spleen

6.29. _____ thymus

6.30. _____ vermiform appendix

A. acts as a physical barrier

B. filter harmful substances from lymph

C. has roles in lymphatic and endocrine systems

D. lymphatic tissue hanging from the lower portion of the cecum

E. stores extra erythrocytes

● Which Word?

Circle the correct term in each sentence.

6.31. The cells that protect the body by ingesting invading bacteria are *lymphokines* / *macrophages.*

6.32. A drug that blocks the growth of neoplasms and is used to treat cancer is an *antineoplastic* / *cytotoxic* drug.

6.33. Plasma cells develop from transformed *B cells* / *T cells.*

6.34. When created in the laboratory *immunoglobulin* / *interferon* is used in the treatment of hepatitis B and C and in some cancers.

6.35. Infectious mononucleosis is a *bacterial* / *viral* infection.

Spelling Counts

Find the misspelled word in each sentence. Then write that word, spelled correctly, on the line provided.

6.36.   A sarquoma is a malignant tumor that arises from connective tissue. _____

6.37.   The nasopharyngeal tonsils are also known as the adenods. _____

6.38.   Reubella is also known as 3-day measles. _____

6.39.   Antiobiotics are used to combat bacterial infections. _____

6.40.   Herpes soster is also known as shingles. _____

Matching Abbreviations

Write the letter of the correct answer on the line provided in the left column.

6.41. _____ CA, Ca   A. invasive ductal carcinoma

6.42. _____ HL   B. Kaposi's sarcoma

6.43. _____ IDC   C. invasive lobular carcinoma

6.44. _____ ILC   D. carcinoma

6.45. _____ KS   E. Hodgkin's lymphoma

Term Selection

Circle the letter next to the correct answer.

6.46.   Which term means not recurring and with a favorable chance for recovery?

a. benign

b. in situ

c. malignant

d. neoplasm

6.47.   Which of these conditions is frequently associated with an HIV infection?

a. lymphoma

b. Hodgkin's disease

c. Kaposi's sarcoma

d. myoma

6.48.   Which type of pathogen causes malaria?

a. parasites

b. rickettsia

c. spirochetes

d. viruses

6.49.   Which condition is caused by a bacillus?

a. aspergillosis

b. Lyme disease

c. Rocky Mountain spotted fever

d. tuberculosis

6.50.   Which condition is characterized by Koplik's spots in the mouth?

a. measles

b. mumps

c. shingles

d. rubella

Sentence Completion

Write the correct term on the line.

6.51.   The term that describes a serious system allergic reaction in which the patient can die within minutes is _____ .

6.52.   In _____ radioactive materials are implanted into the tissues to be treated.

6.53.   The _____ blot test is used to confirm a seropositive ELISA test for HIV.

6.54.   A/An _____ is a benign abnormal collection of lymphatic vessels forming a mass.

6.55.   Persistent generalized _____ is the continued presence of diffuse enlargement of lymph nodes.

True/False

If the statement is true, write T on the line. If the statement is false, write F on the line.

6.56.   _____ Lymph fluid always flows toward the thoracic cavity.

6.57.   _____ Splenomegaly means abnormal softening of the spleen.

6.58. _____ Lymphedema is an abnormal accumulation of fluid primarily in the legs and ankles.

6.59. _____ Acquired immunity is passed from the mother to child after birth.

6.60. _____ Reed-Sternberg cells are present in non-Hodgkin's lymphoma.

6.61. _____ Ductal carcinoma in situ accounts for the majority of all breast cancers.

6.62. _____ Teletherapy uses 3-dimensional computer imaging to aim radiation doses more precisely.

6.63. _____ Hodgkin's disease at stage I has a better cure rate than at stage IV.

6.64. _____ An osteosarcoma usually involves the bones of the sacrum.

6.65. _____ Breast cancer cannot occur in males because they do not have breast tissue.

● Clinical Conditions

Write the correct answer on the line.

6.66. Dr. Wei diagnosed her patient as having an enlarged spleen. The medical term for this condition is _____ .

6.67. The cause of Roger Thompson's infection was the _____ . This is caused by a group of large herpes-type viruses with a wide variety of disease effects.

6.68. Mr. Grossman was treated with a _____ drug. This is a hormone-like preparation used primarily as an anti-inflammatory and as an immunosuppressant.

6.69. Soon after her breast cancer was diagnosed, Dorothy Mullins' doctor performed a/an _____ . In this procedure the tumor and a margin of healthy tissue are removed.

6.70. Since his kidney transplant, it is necessary that Mr. Lanning take a/an _____ to prevent rejection of the donor organ.

6.71. Jose Sanchez received a poliomyelitis _____ to ensure his immunity to this disease.

6.72. Inglis complained that the glands in her neck were swollen. Dr. Neilson explained that these are the _____ lymph nodes.

6.73. Because he had chickenpox as a child, Rob Harris now has natural _____ immunity to this disease.

6.74. As a child, John Fogelman had a viral disease in which the parotid glands were swollen. John's doctor said he had the _____ .

6.75. Jane Doe is infected with HIV. One of her medications is acyclovir, which is a/an _____ drug.

● Which is the correct medical term?

Circle the letter next to the correct answer

6.76. Which condition is caused by the Epstein-Barr virus?

a. chickenpox

b. infectious mononucleosis

c. mumps

d. rubella

6.77. Which form of cancer starts in the milk glands of the breast?

a. ductal carcinoma in situ

b. invasive ductal carcinoma

c. invasive lobular carcinoma

d. non-Hodgkin's lymphoma

6.78. Which of the following is *not* a form of bacteria?

a. bacilli

b. parasites

c. rickettsia

d. spirochetes

6.79. Which medication is required to prevent rejection of a transplanted organ?

a. immunoglobulins

b. immunosuppressant

c. interferon

d. monoclonal antibodies

6.80. Which type of pathogen causes Lyme disease?

a. staphylococci

b. streptococci

c. spirochete

d. virus

● **Challenge Word Building**

These terms are *not* found in this chapter; however, they are made up of these familiar word parts. You may want to look in the glossary or use a medical dictionary to check your answers!

adenoid/o	-ectomy
aden/o	-itis
ang/o	-ology
immun/o	-oma
lymph/o	
splen/o	
tonsill/o	
thym/o	

6.81. The study of the immune system is known as _____ .

6.82. The medical term meaning the surgical removal of the spleen is a/an _____ .

6.83. The medical term meaning an inflammation of the thymus is _____ .

6.84. The medical term meaning an inflammation of the lymph vessels is _____ .

6.85. The medical term meaning to suture the spleen is _____ .

6.86. The medical term meaning the surgical removal of the adenoids is a/an _____ .

6.87. The medical term meaning the surgical removal of a lymph node is a/an _____ .

6.88. The medical term meaning a tumor originating in the thymus is _____ .

6.89. The medical term meaning an inflammation of the tonsils is _____ .

6.90. The medical term meaning an inflammation of the spleen is _____ .

● **Labeling Exercises**

Identify the numbered items on this diagram.

6.91. Tonsils and _____

6.92. Bone _____

6.93. Appendix and _____
_____

6.94. _____

6.95. _____

6.96. _____ lymphatic duct

6.97. _____ lymph nodes

6.98. _____ duct

6.99. _____ lymph nodes

6.100. _____ lymph nodes

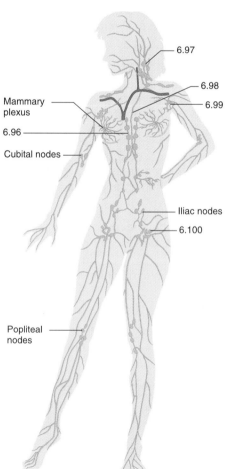

The Human Touch: Critical Thinking Exercise

The following story and questions are designed to stimulate critical thinking through class discussion or as a brief essay response. There are no easy or right-wrong answers to these questions.

Hernani Fermin, a 35-year-old married father, was diagnosed HIV positive 2 years ago. As a sales representative for a nationally recognized pharmaceutical company, Hernani's hectic travel schedule was beginning to take a toll on his health. A few weeks ago his doctor suggested he rethink his career goals. "You know stress and this disease don't mix," Dr. Wettstein had reminded him. "Why don't you look for something closer to home?"

That evening over lasagna his wife Emily suggested teaching. Hernani had enjoyed sharing the challenging concepts of math and science with 7th graders during the 6 years he had taught in a rural school upstate. It was only the financial demands of Kim and Kili's birth 7 years ago that had tempted him into the better paying field of pharmaceuticals.

He sent out resumes for the next 5 weeks. Finally one was well received by South Hills Middle School. They had an opening in their math department, plus a need for someone to coach after-school athletics, and they wanted to meet with him. He hadn't interviewed since the twins were born. He thought about the questions normally asked — would there be some about his health? Being HIV positive shouldn't have any bearing on his ability to teach, but parents might be concerned. And it might disqualify him for the school's health insurance policy. Hernani believed in honesty, but what would happen to his family if he revealed his HIV status?

Suggested Discussion Topics:

1. Do you think Hernani should reveal his HIV status to South Hills Middle School? If so, why? If not, why not?

2. Do you think South Hills Middle School would hire Hernani if they knew he was HIV positive? Why or why not?

3. How would you feel if your child was on one of the teams Mr. Fermin will be coaching? Why?

4. Discuss the insurance problems Hernani might encounter by changing jobs.

5. Confidentiality is an important physician-patient issue. Discuss whether it would be Dr. Wettstein's duty to reveal Hernani's HIV status if asked about it.

7 The Respiratory System

● **Overview of Structures, Word Parts, and Functions of the Respiratory System**

MAJOR STRUCTURES	RELATED WORD ROOTS	PRIMARY FUNCTIONS
Nose	nas/o	Exchange air during inhaling and exhaling; warms, moisturizes, and filters inhaled air.
Sinuses	sinus/o	Provide mucus, make bones of the skull lighter, aid in sound production.
Epiglottis	epiglott/o	Close off the trachea during swallowing.
Pharynx	pharyng/o	Transport air to and from the nose to the trachea.
Larynx	laryng/o	Make speech possible.
Trachea	trache/o	Transport air to and from the pharynx to the bronchi.
Bronchi	bronch/o, bronchi/o	Transport air from the trachea into the lungs.
Alveoli	alveol/o	Air sacs that exchange gases with the pulmonary capillary blood.
Lungs	pneum/o, pneumon/o	Bring oxygen into the body and remove carbon dioxide and some water waste from the body.

● VOCABULARY   Related to the Respiratory System

Check the box as you master each word part or term. Terms marked with the ❖ symbol are pronounced on the optional student audiotape.

Key Word Parts

- ☐ atel/o
- ☐ bronch/o, bronchi/o
- ☐ cyan/o
- ☐ -ectasis
- ☐ laryng/o
- ☐ ox/i, ox/o, ox/y
- ☐ pharyng/o
- ☐ phon/o
- ☐ pleur/o
- ☐ -pnea
- ☐ pneum/o, pneumon/o, pneu-
- ☐ pulm/o, pulmon/o
- ☐ tachy-
- ☐ thorac/o, -thorax
- ☐ trache/o

Key Medical Terms

- ☐ anoxia (ah-NOCK-see-ah)
- ☐ anthracosis (an-thrah-KOH-sis)
- ☐ aphonia (ah-FOH-nee-ah)
- ☐ apnea (AP-nee-ah *or* ap-NEE-ah) ❖
- ☐ asbestosis (ass-beh-STOH-sis)
- ☐ asphyxia (ass-FICK-see-ah)
- ☐ asphyxiation (ass-fick-see-AY-shun) ❖
- ☐ asthma (AZ-mah) ❖
- ☐ atelectasis (at-ee-LEK-tah-sis) ❖
- ☐ bradypnea (brad-ihp-NEE-ah *or* brad-ee-NEE-ah) ❖
- ☐ bronchiectasis (brong-kee-ECK-tah-sis) ❖
- ☐ bronchoconstrictor (brong-koh-kon-STRICK-tor)
- ☐ bronchodilator (brong-koh-dye-LAY-tor)
- ☐ bronchopneumonia (brong-koh-new-MOH-nee-ah) ❖
- ☐ bronchorrhagia (brong-koh-RAY-jee-ah) ❖
- ☐ bronchorrhea (brong-koh-REE-ah) ❖
- ☐ bronchoscopy (brong-KOS-koh-pee) ❖
- ☐ Cheyne-Stokes respiration (CHAYN-STOHKS) ❖
- ☐ croup (KROOP) ❖
- ☐ cystic fibrosis (SIS-tick figh-BROH-sis) ❖
- ☐ diphtheria (dif-THEE-ree-ah) ❖
- ☐ dysphonia (dis-FOH-nee-ah) ❖
- ☐ dyspnea (DISP-nee-ah) ❖
- ☐ emphysema (em-fih-SEE-mah) ❖
- ☐ empyema (em-pye-EE-mah) ❖
- ☐ endotracheal intubation (en-doh-TRAY-kee-al in-too-BAY-shun)
- ☐ epiglottis (ep-ih-GLOT-is) ❖
- ☐ epistaxis (ep-ih-STACK-sis) ❖

- ☐ hemoptysis (hee-MOP-tih-sis) ❖
- ☐ hemothorax (hee-moh-THOH-racks) ❖
- ☐ hyperpnea (high-perp-NEE-ah) ❖
- ☐ hyperventilation (high-per-ven-tih-LAY-shun) ❖
- ☐ hypopnea (high-poh-NEE-ah) ❖
- ☐ hypoxia (high-POCK-see-ah) ❖
- ☐ influenza (in-flew-EN-zah) ❖
- ☐ inhalation (in-hah-LAY-shun)
- ☐ laryngectomy (lar-in-JECK-toh-mee) ❖
- ☐ laryngitis (lar-in-JIGH-tis) ❖
- ☐ laryngoplasty (lah-RING-goh-plas-tee) ❖
- ☐ laryngoplegia (lar-ing-goh-PLEE-jee-ah) ❖
- ☐ laryngoscopy (lar-ing-GOS-koh-pee) ❖
- ☐ laryngospasm (lah-RING-goh-spazm) ❖
- ☐ mediastinum (mee-dee-as-TYE-num)
- ☐ mycoplasma pneumonia (my-koh-PLAZ-mah new-MOH-nee-ah) ❖
- ☐ nasopharyngitis (nay-zoh-far-in-JIGH-tis) ❖
- ☐ otolaryngologist (oh-toh-lar-in-GOL-oh-jist) ❖
- ☐ otorhinolaryngologist (oh-toh-rye-noh-lar-in-GOL-oh-jist) ❖
- ☐ pertussis (per-TUS-is) ❖
- ☐ pharyngitis (far-in-JIGH-tis)
- ☐ pharyngoplasty (fah-RING-goh-plas-tee)
- ☐ pharyngorrhagia (far-ing-goh-RAY-jee-ah) ❖
- ☐ pharyngorrhea (far-ing-goh-REE-ah) ❖
- ☐ pleuralgia (ploor-AL-jee-ah) ❖
- ☐ pleurectomy (ploor-ECK-toh-mee) ❖
- ☐ pleurisy (PLOOR-ih-see) ❖
- ☐ pneumoconiosis (new-moh-koh-nee-OH-sis) ❖
- ☐ *Pneumocystis carinii* pneumonia (new-moh-SIS-tis kah-RYE-nee-eye new-MOH-nee-ah) ❖
- ☐ pneumonectomy (new-moh-NECK-toh-mee) ❖
- ☐ pneumorrhagia (new-moh-RAY-jee-ah) ❖
- ☐ pneumothorax (new-moh-THOR-racks) ❖
- ☐ pulmonologist (pull-mah-NOL-oh-jist) ❖
- ☐ pyothorax (pye-oh-THOH-racks) ❖
- ☐ rhinorrhea (rye-noh-REE-ah)
- ☐ sinusitis (sigh-nuh-SIGH-tis) ❖
- ☐ sinusotomy (sigh-nuhs-OT-oh-mee) ❖
- ☐ spirometry (spy-ROM-eh-tree) ❖
- ☐ tachypnea (tack-ihp-NEE-ah) ❖
- ☐ thoracentesis (thoh-rah-sen-TEE-sis) ❖
- ☐ thoracostomy (thoh-rah-KOS-toh-mee) ❖
- ☐ thoracotomy (thoh-rah-KOT-toh-mee) ❖
- ☐ tracheitis (tray-kee-EYE-tis) ❖
- ☐ tracheoplasty (TRAY-kee-oh-plas-tee) ❖
- ☐ tracheostomy (tray-kee-OS-toh-mee) ❖
- ☐ tracheotomy (tray-kee-OT-oh-mee) ❖
- ☐ tuberculosis (too-ber-kew-LOH-sis)

● OBJECTIVES

On completion of this chapter, you should be able to:

1 Identify and describe the major structures and functions of the respiratory system.

2 Recognize, define, spell, and pronounce terms related to the pathology and diagnostic and treatment procedures of the respiratory system.

Functions of the Respiratory System

The functions of the respiratory system are to:

- Bring oxygen-rich air into the body for delivery to the blood cells.

- Expel waste products (carbon dioxide and water) that have been returned to the lungs by the blood.

- Produce the air flow through the larynx that makes speech possible.

Structures of the Respiratory System

For descriptive purposes the respiratory system is divided into upper and lower tracts (Figure 7.1).

- The **upper respiratory tract** consists of the nose, mouth, pharynx, epiglottis, larynx, and trachea (Figure 7.2).

- The **lower respiratory tract** consists of the bronchial tree and lungs. These structures are protected by the thoracic cavity.

The Nose

- Air enters the body through the nose and passes through the **nasal cavity**.

- The **nasal septum** (NAY-zal SEP-tum) is a wall of cartilage that divides the nose into two equal sections.

- **Mucous membrane** (MYOU-kus) is the specialized form of epithelial tissue that lines the nose and respiratory system.

- **Mucus** (MYOU-kus), which is secreted by the mucous membranes, helps to moisten, warm, and filter the air as it enters the nose. (Notice the different spellings: mucous is the name of the tissue; mucus is the secretion that flows from the tissue.)

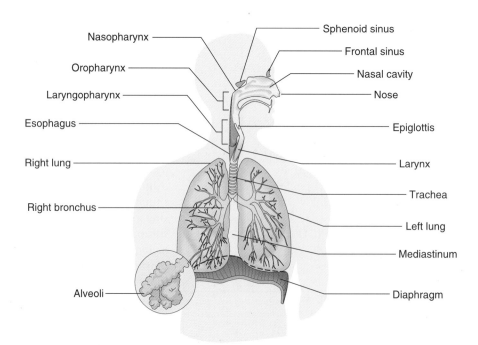

Nasopharynx

Oropharynx

Laryngopharynx

Esophagus

Right lung

Right bronchus

Alveoli

Sphenoid sinus

Frontal sinus

Nasal cavity

Nose

Epiglottis

Larynx

Trachea

Left lung

Mediastinum

Diaphragm

Respiratory System

FIGURE 7.1 Structures of the respiratory system.

Frontal sinus

Nasal cavity

Sphenoid sinus

Nasopharynx

Pharyngeal tonsil

Palatine tonsil

Oropharynx

Lingual tonsil

Epiglottis

Laryngopharynx

Vocal cords

Esophagus

Trachea

Tracheal cartilages

FIGURE 7.2 Structures of the upper respiratory tract.

- **Cilia** (**SIL**-ee-ah), the thin hairs located just inside the nostrils, filter incoming air to remove debris.
- The **olfactory receptors** (ol-**FACK**-toh-ree), the receptors for the sense of smell, are nerve endings located in the mucous membrane in the upper part of the nasal cavity.

The Tonsils

- The **tonsils**, which have an important function in protecting the body from invading organisms, form a protective circle around the entrance to the respiratory system. Tonsils, which are a type of lymphatic tissue, are discussed in Chapter 6.

The Sinuses

- A **sinus** is an air-filled cavity within a bone that is lined with mucous membrane.
- The functions of sinuses are (1) to make the bones of the skull lighter, (2) to help produce sound by giving resonance to the voice, and (3) to produce mucus that drains into the nasal cavity.
- The **paranasal sinuses** are located in the bones of the skull (**para** means near, **nas** means nose, and **al** means

pertaining to). Short ducts connect these sinuses to the nasal cavity.

- The sinuses are named for the bones in which they are located. The paranasal sinuses are summarized in Table 7.1.

Table 7.1

PARANASAL SINUSES

Maxillary sinuses (**MACK**-sih-**ler**-ee), located in the maxillary bones, are the largest of the paranasal sinuses.	**Frontal sinuses** are located in the frontal bone just above the eyebrows.
The **ethmoid sinuses** (**ETH**-moid), located in the ethmoid bones, are irregularly shaped air cells, separated from the orbital (eye) cavity only by a thin layer of bone.	The **sphenoid sinuses** (**SFEE**-noid), located in the sphenoid bone, are close to the optic nerves. An infection here can damage vision.

The Pharynx

- After passing through the nasal cavity, the air reaches the **pharynx** (**FAR**-inks) that is commonly known as the **throat** (see Figure 7.2). The pharynx has three divisions:

- The **nasopharynx** (**nay**-zoh-**FAR**-inks), the first division, is posterior to the nasal cavity and continues downward to behind the mouth.

- The **oropharynx** (**oh**-roh-**FAR**-inks), the second division, is the portion that is visible when looking into the mouth (see Figure 8.2). The oropharynx is shared by the respiratory and digestive systems.

- The **laryngopharynx** (lah-**ring**-goh-**FAR**-inks) is the third division, continues downward to the openings of the esophagus and trachea.

Protective Swallowing Mechanisms

The respiratory and digestive systems share part of the pharynx. During swallowing there is the risk of a blocked airway or pneumonia caused by something entering the lungs instead of traveling into the esophagus.

- Two protective mechanisms act automatically during swallowing to ensure that *only* air goes into the lungs.

- During swallowing the soft palate, which is the muscular posterior portion of the roof of the mouth, moves up and backward to close off the nasopharynx. This prevents food from going up into the nose. (Structures of the mouth are discussed in Chapter 8.)

- At the same time, the **epiglottis** (**ep**-ih-**GLOT**-is), which is a lidlike structure located at the base of the tongue, swings downward and closes off the laryngopharynx so food does not enter the trachea and the lungs.

The Larynx

- The **larynx** (**LAR**-inks), also known as the **voice box**, is a triangular chamber located between the pharynx and the trachea (Figure 7.3).

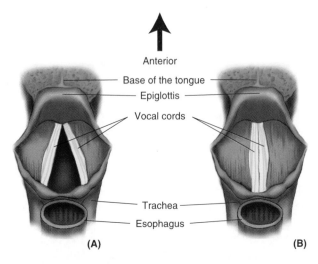

FIGURE 7.3 View of the larynx and vocal cords from above. (A) The vocal cords are open during breathing. (B) The vocal cords vibrate together during speech.

- The larynx is protected and held open by a series of nine separate cartilages. The **thyroid cartilage** is the largest and its prominent projection is commonly known as the **Adam's apple**.

- The larynx contains the **vocal cords**. While breathing the cords are separated to let air pass. During speech they are together and sound is produced as air expelled from the lungs causes the cords to vibrate against each other.

The Trachea

- Air passes from the larynx into the **trachea** (**TRAY**-kee-ah), which is commonly known as the **windpipe** (Figure 7.4).

- The trachea extends from the neck into the chest, directly in front of the esophagus and is held open by a series of C-shaped cartilage rings. The wall between these rings is elastic, enabling the trachea to adjust to different body positions.

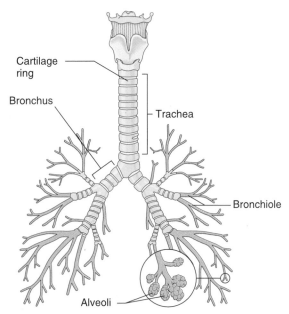

FIGURE 7.4 The trachea, bronchial tree, and alveoli.

The Bronchial Tree

- The trachea divides into two branches called **bronchi** (**BRONG**-kye). A branch goes into each lung (singular, **bronchus**).

- Within the lung the bronchus divides and subdivides into increasingly smaller bronchi. **Bronchioles** (**BRONG**-kee-ohlz) are the smallest branches of the bronchi.

- Because of the similarity of these branching structures to a tree, this is referred to as the **bronchial tree** (see Figure 7.4).

The Alveoli

- **Alveoli** (al-VEE-oh-lye), also known as **air sacs**, are the very small grapelike clusters found at the end of each bronchiole (see Figures 7.1 and 7.4). (Singular, **alveolus**.)
- The thin flexible walls of the alveoli are surrounded by a network of microscopic pulmonary capillaries.
- During respiration the gas exchange between the alveolar air and the pulmonary capillary blood occurs through the walls of the alveoli.

The Lungs

- A **lobe** is a division of the lungs (Figure 7.5).
- The **right lung** has three lobes: the superior, middle, and inferior.
- The **left lung** has two lobes: the superior and inferior.

The Mediastinum

- The **mediastinum** (**mee**-dee-as-**TYE**-num), also called the **interpleural space**, is located between the lungs (see Figure 7.1)
- This space contains the thoracic viscera including the heart, aorta, esophagus, trachea, bronchial tubes, and thymus gland.

The Pleura

- The **pleura** (PLOOR-ah) is a multilayered membrane that surrounds each lung with its blood vessels and nerves (plural, **pleurae**).
- The **parietal pleura** (pah-RYE-eh-tal PLOOR-ah) is the outer layer of pleura. It lines the thoracic cavity and forms the sac containing each lung.
- The **visceral pleura** (VIS-er-al PLOOR-ah) is the inner layer of pleura. It closely surrounds the lung tissue.
- The **pleural space**, also known as the **pleural cavity**, is the airtight space between the folds of the pleural membranes. It contains a watery lubricating fluid that prevents friction when the membranes rub together during respiration.

The Diaphragm

- The **diaphragm** (DYE-ah-fram) is the muscle that separates the thoracic cavity from the abdomen (see Figures 7.1 and 7.6). It is the contraction and relaxation of this muscle that makes breathing possible.
- The **phrenic nerve** (FREN-ick) stimulates the diaphragm and causes it to contract (**phren** means diaphragm or mind, and **ic** means pertaining to).

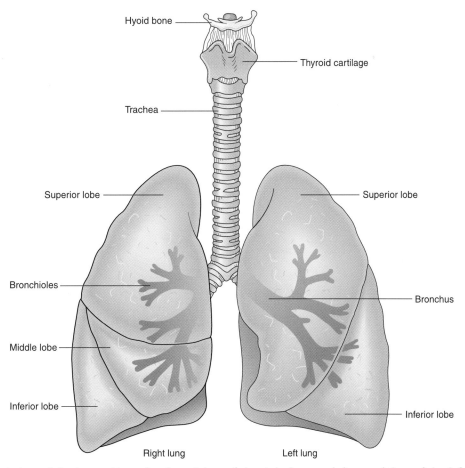

Hyoid bone

Thyroid cartilage

Trachea

Superior lobe

Superior lobe

Bronchioles

Bronchus

Middle lobe

Inferior lobe

Inferior lobe

Right lung

Left lung

FIGURE 7.5 External view of the lungs. Note the three lobes of the right lung and the two lobes of the left lung.

Respiration

Respiration is the exchange of gases that are essential to life. This occurs in the lungs as external respiration and on a cellular level as internal respiration.

External Respiration

- **Breathing** is the act of bringing air into and out of the lungs.
- **Inhalation** (**in**-hah-**LAY**-shun), also known as **inhaling**, is the act of taking in air as the diaphragm contracts and pulls downward. This causes the thoracic cavity to expand. This produces a vacuum within the thoracic cavity that draws air into the lungs (Figure 7.6A).
- **Expiration** (**ecks**-pih-**RAY**-shun), also known as **exhaling**, is the act of breathing out as the diaphragm relaxes and moves upward causing the thoracic cavity to become narrower. This action forces air out of the lungs (Figure 7.6B).

The Exchange of Gases Within the Lungs

As air moves in and out there is an **exchange of gases** within the lungs (Figure 7.7A).

- As air is **inhaled** into the alveoli, oxygen (O_2) immediately passes into the surrounding capillaries and is carried by the erythrocytes to all body cells.
- At the same time, the waste product carbon dioxide (CO_2) passes from the capillaries into the airspaces of the lungs to be **exhaled**.

Internal Respiration

- Internal respiration is the exchange of gases within the cells of all the body organs and tissues (Figure 7.7B).

- In this process, oxygen passes from the bloodstream into the tissue cells. At the same time, carbon dioxide passes from the tissue cells into the bloodstream.

Medical Specialties Related to the Respiratory System

- An **otolaryngologist** (**oh**-toh-**lar**-in-**GOL**-oh-jist), also known as an **otorhinolaryngologist** (**oh**-toh-**rye**-noh-**lar**-in-**GOL**-oh-jist), specializes in diagnosing and treating diseases and disorders of the ears, nose, and throat.
- A **pulmonologist** (**pull**-mah-**NOL**-oh-jist) is a physician who specializes in diagnosing and treating diseases and disorders of the lungs and associated tissues (**pulmon** means lung and **ologist** means specialist).
- A **respiratory therapist** (RT) provides treatment to ease or correct breathing problems.

Pathology of the Respiratory System

Chronic Obstructive Pulmonary Diseases

- **Chronic obstructive pulmonary disease**, also known as **COPD**, is a general term used to describe a group of respiratory conditions characterized by chronic airflow limitations.
- **Asthma** (**AZ**-mah) is a chronic allergic disorder characterized by episodes of severe breathing difficulty, coughing, and wheezing (Figure 7.8). Breathing difficulty during an asthma attack is caused by several factors (1) swelling and inflammation of the lining of the airways, (2) the production of thick mucus, and (3)

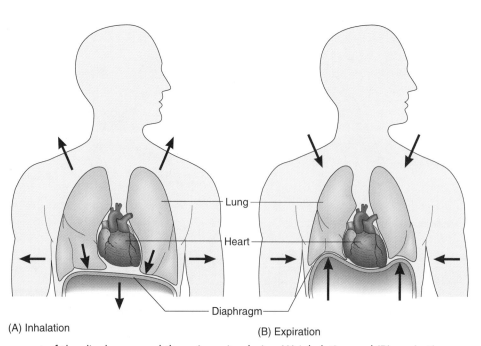

Lung

Heart

Diaphragm

(A) Inhalation   (B) Expiration

FIGURE 7.6 Movement of the diaphragm and thoracic cavity during (A) inhalation and (B) expiration.

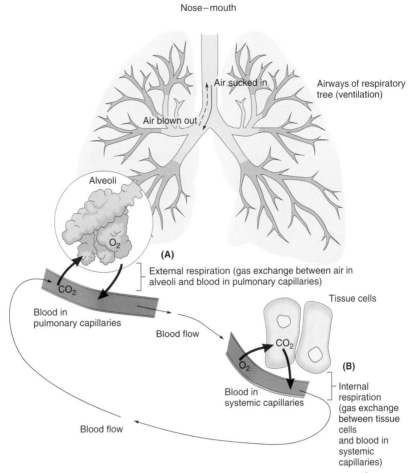

Nose–mouth

Air sucked in

Air blown out

Airways of respiratory tree (ventilation)

Alveoli

O₂

(A)

CO₂

Blood in pulmonary capillaries

Blood flow

External respiration (gas exchange between air in alveoli and blood in pulmonary capillaries)

Tissue cells

CO₂

O₂

(B)

Blood in systemic capillaries

Blood flow

Internal respiration (gas exchange between tissue cells and blood in systemic capillaries)

FIGURE 7.7 External and internal respiration compared. (A) External respiration with the exchange of gases between the lungs and capillaries. (B) Internal respiration with the exchange between the blood and tissues.

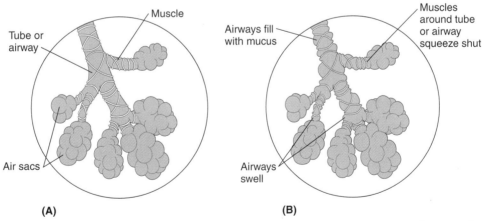

Muscle

Tube or airway

Air sacs

(A)

Airways fill with mucus

Muscles around tube or airway squeeze shut

Airways swell

(B)

FIGURE 7.8 Changes in the airways during an asthma episode. (A) Before the episode the muscles are relaxed and the airways are open. (B) During the episode the muscles tighten and the airways fill with mucus.

tightening of the muscles that surround the airways. (For treatment, see Bronchodilator.)

- **Bronchiectasis** (**brong**-kee-**ECK**-tah-sis) is chronic dilation (enlargement) of bronchi or bronchioles resulting from an earlier lung infection that was not cured (**bronchi** means bronchi and **ectasis** means enlargement). (Figure 7.9).

- **Emphysema** (**em**-fih-**SEE**-mah) is the progressive loss of lung function due a decrease in the total number of alveoli, the enlargement of the remaining alveoli, and then the progressive destruction of their walls (Figure 7.10A). As the alveoli are destroyed, breathing becomes increasingly rapid, shallow, and difficult. In an effort to compensate for the loss of capacity, the lungs expand

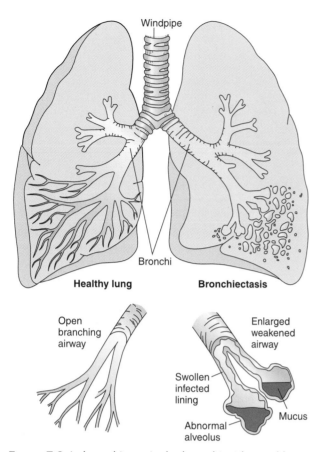

FIGURE 7.9 In bronchiectasis the bronchi widen and lose their elasticity. This allows mucus to accumulate in the alveoli.

and the chest assumes an enlarged barrel shape (Figure 7.10B).

- **Smoker's respiratory syndrome**, also known as **SRS**, is a group of symptoms seen in smokers. These chronic conditions include (1) a cough, (2) wheezing, (3) vocal hoarseness, (4) pharyngitis (sore throat), (5) difficult breathing, and (6) a susceptibility to respiratory infections.

Upper Respiratory Diseases

- **Allergic rhinitis** (rye-NIGH-tis), commonly referred to as an **allergy**, is an allergic reaction to airborne allergens that causes an increased flow of mucus (**rhin** means nose and **itis** means inflammation).
- **Croup** (KROOP) is an acute respiratory syndrome in children and infants characterized by obstruction of the larynx, hoarseness, and a barking cough.
- **Diphtheria** (dif-THEE-ree-ah) is an acute infectious disease of the throat and upper respiratory tract caused by the presence of diphtheria bacteria. Diphtheria can be prevented through immunization.
- **Epistaxis** (ep-ih-STACK-sis), also known as a **nosebleed**, is bleeding from the nose, usually caused by an injury, excessive use of blood thinners, or bleeding disorders.
- **Influenza** (in-flew-EN-zah), also known as **flu**, is an acute, highly contagious viral respiratory infection, spread by respiratory droplets, that occurs most commonly during the colder months. Some strains of influenza can be prevented by annual immunization.
- **Pertussis** (per-TUS-is), also known as **whooping cough**, is a contagious bacterial infection of the upper respiratory tract that is characterized by a paroxysmal cough.

(A)

(B)

FIGURE 7.10 Emphysema. (A) Changes in the alveoli. (B) Lateral x-ray shows lung enlargement and abnormal barrel chest in emphysema.

Paroxysmal (**par**-ock-**SIZ**-mal) means sudden or spasm-like. Pertussis can be prevented through immunization.

- **Rhinorrhea** (**rye**-noh-**REE**-ah), also known as a **runny nose**, is an excessive flow of mucus from the nose (**rhino** means nose and **rrhea** means abnormal flow).

- **Sinusitis** (**sigh**-nuh-**SIGH**-tis) is an inflammation of the sinuses (**sinus** means sinus and **itis** means inflammation).

- **Upper respiratory infection** (URI) and **acute nasopharyngitis** (nay-zoh-**far**-in-**JIGH**-tis) are among the terms used to describe the **common cold**.

Pharynx and Larynx

- **Pharyngitis** (**far**-in-**JIGH**-tis), also known as a **sore throat**, is an inflammation of the pharynx (**pharyng** means pharynx and **itis** means inflammation).

- **Pharyngorrhagia** (**far**-ing-goh-**RAY**-jee-ah) is bleeding from the pharynx (**pharyngo** means pharynx and **rrhagia** means bleeding).

- **Pharyngorrhea** (**far**-ing-goh-**REE**-ah) is a discharge of mucus from the pharynx (**pharyngo** means pharynx and **rrhea** means abnormal discharge).

- **Laryngoplegia** (**lar**-ing-goh-**PLEE**-jee-ah) is paralysis of the larynx (**laryngo** means larynx and **plegia** means paralysis).

- A **laryngospasm** (lah-**RING**-goh-spazm) is a sudden spasmodic closure of the larynx (**laryngo** means larynx and **spasm** means a sudden involuntary contraction).

Voice Disorders

- **Aphonia** (ah-**FOH**-nee-ah) is the loss of the ability to produce normal speech sounds (**a** means without, **phon** means voice or sound, and **ia** means abnormal condition).

- **Dysphonia** (dis-**FOH**-nee-ah) is any voice impairment including hoarseness, weakness, or loss of voice (**dys** means bad, **phon** means voice or sound, and **ia** means abnormal condition).

- **Laryngitis** (**lar**-in-**JIGH**-tis) is an inflammation of the larynx (**laryng** means larynx and **itis** means inflammation). This term is commonly used to describe voice loss caused by the inflammation.

Trachea and Bronchi

- **Tracheitis** (**tray**-kee-**EYE**-tis) is an inflammation of the trachea (**trache** means trachea and **itis** means inflammation).

- **Tracheorrhagia** (**tray**-kee-oh-**RAY**-jee-ah) is bleeding from the trachea (**tracheo** means trachea and **rrhagia** means bleeding).

- **Bronchitis** (brong-**KYE**-tis) is an inflammation of the bronchial walls (**bronch** means bronchus and **itis** means inflammation). Bronchitis is usually caused by an infection; however, it may also be caused by irritants such as smoking.

- **Bronchorrhagia** (**brong**-koh-**RAY**-jee-ah) is bleeding from the bronchi (**broncho** means bronchus and **rrhagia** means bleeding).

- **Bronchorrhea** (**brong**-koh-**REE**-ah) means an excessive discharge of mucus from the bronchi (**broncho** means bronchus and **rrhea** means abnormal flow).

Pleural Cavity

- **Pleurisy** (**PLOOR**-ih-see) is an inflammation of the visceral and parietal pleura in the thoracic cavity.

- **Pleuralgia** (ploor-**AL**-jee-ah) is pain in the pleura or in the side (**pleur** means pleura and **algia** means pain).

- **Pneumothorax** (**new**-moh-**THOR**-racks) is an accumulation of air or gas in the pleural space causing the lung to collapse (**pneumo** means lung or air, and **thorax** means chest). This may have an external cause such as a stab wound that perforates the chest wall. It may be caused internally by a perforation in the pleura surrounding the lung that allowed air to leak into the pleural space (Figure 7.11).

- **Pleural effusion** (eh-**FEW**-zhun) is the abnormal escape of fluid into the pleural cavity that prevents the lung from fully expanding. (**Effusion** is the escape of fluid from blood or lymphatic vessels into the tissues or a cavity.) (Figure 7.12).

- **Empyema** (**em**-pye-**EE**-mah), also known as **pyothorax** (**pye**-oh-**THOH**-racks), is an accumulation of pus in the pleural cavity. This is usually the result of a primary infection of the lungs. (Empyema is also used to describe pus in other body cavities.)

- **Hemothorax** (**hee**-moh-**THOH**-racks) is an accumulation of blood in the pleural cavity (**hemo** means blood and **thorax** means chest).

- **Hemoptysis** (hee-**MOP**-tih-sis) is spitting of blood or blood-stained sputum derived from the lungs or

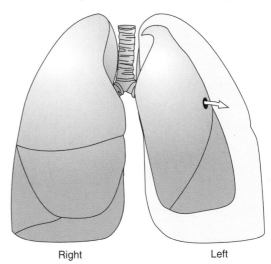

Right   Left

FIGURE 7.11 Pneumothorax is an accumulation of air or gas in the pleural space that causes the lung to collapse. In the left lung a perforation in the pleura allowed air to escape into the pleural space.

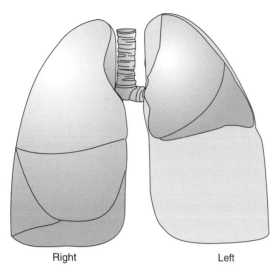

FIGURE 7.12 In pleural effusion fluid in the pleural cavity prevents the lung from fully expanding.

bronchial tubes as the result of a pulmonary or bronchial hemorrhage (**hemo** means blood and **ptysis** means spitting).

Lungs

- **Acute respiratory distress syndrome**, also known as **ARDS**, is a type of lung failure resulting from many different disorders that cause pulmonary edema. There are many causes of ARDS including severe infection, shock, pneumonia, burns, and injuries.

- **Pulmonary edema** (eh-DEE-mah) is an accumulation of fluid in lung tissues. (**Edema** means swelling.)

- **Pneumorrhagia** (new-moh-RAY-jee-ah) is bleeding from the lungs (**pneumo** means lungs and **rrhagia** means bleeding).

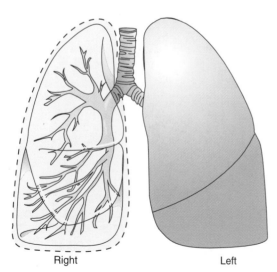

FIGURE 7.13 In atelectasis, as shown in the right lung, the lung fails to expand because air cannot pass blockage in the bronchioles.

- **Atelectasis** (at-ee-LEK-tah-sis), also known as a **collapsed lung**, is a condition in which the lung fails to expand because air cannot pass beyond the bronchioles that are blocked by secretions (**atel** means incomplete and **ectasis** means stretching). (Figure 7.13).

Tuberculosis

- **Tuberculosis** (too-ber-kew-LOH-sis), also known as **TB**, is an infectious disease caused by *Mycobacterium tuberculosis*. TB usually attacks the lungs; however, it may also affect other parts of the body. A healthy individual may carry TB but not get the disease. TB most commonly occurs when the immune system is weakened by another condition such as infection with human immunodeficiency virus (HIV).

- **Multidrug-resistant tuberculosis**, also known as **MDR-TB**, is a dangerous form of tuberculosis because the germs have become resistant to the effect of most TB drugs. This may occur if a TB infection has not been adequately treated. MDR-TB can be spread to others just like regular TB.

Pneumonia

- **Pneumonia** (new-MOH-nee-ah) is an inflammation of the lungs in which the air sacs fill with pus and other liquid (**pneumon** means lung or air and **ia** means abnormal condition). This fluid is known as an **exudate** (ECKS-you-dayt), which means accumulated fluid in a cavity that has penetrated through vessel walls into the adjoining tissue.

- The **main causes of pneumonia** are bacteria, viruses, fungi, or inhaled substances such as chemical irritants or vomit.

- **Bacterial pneumonia**, which is commonly caused by *Streptococcus pneumoniae*, is the only form of pneumonia that can be prevented through vaccination.

- **Viral pneumonia** accounts for approximately half of all pneumonias and may be complicated by an invasion of bacteria with all of the symptoms of bacterial pneumonia.

- **Lobar pneumonia** affects one or more lobes of a lung (Figure 7.14A).

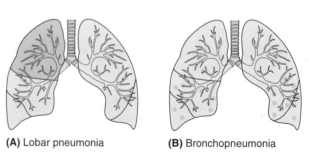

(A) Lobar pneumonia   **(B)** Bronchopneumonia

☐ Affected areas

FIGURE 7.14 Types of pneumonia. (A) Lobar pneumonia affects one or more lobes of a lung. (B) Bronchopneumonia affects the bronchioles.

- **Bronchopneumonia** (**brong**-koh-new-**MOH**-nee-ah) is a form of pneumonia that begins in the bronchioles (Figure 7.14B).

- **Double pneumonia** involves both lungs.

- **Aspiration pneumonia** may occur when a foreign substance, such as vomit, is inhaled into the lungs. (As used here, **aspiration** (**ass**-pih-**RAY**-shun) means inhaling or drawing a foreign substance, such as food, into the upper respiratory tract. Aspiration also means withdrawal by suction of fluids or gases from a body cavity.)

- **Mycoplasma pneumonia** (**my**-koh-**PLAZ**-mah new-**MOH**-nee-ah), also known as **mycoplasmal** or **walking pneumonia**, is a milder but longer lasting form of the disease caused by the fungi *Mycoplasma pneumoniae*.

- *Pneumocystis carinii* **pneumonia** (new-moh-**SIS**-tis kah-**RYE**-nee-eye new-**MOH**-nee-ah), also known as **PCP**, is caused by an infection with the parasite *Pneumocystis carinii*. PCP is an opportunistic infection that frequently occurs when the immune system is weakened by an HIV infection.

Environmental and Occupational Lung Diseases

- **Pneumoconiosis** (**new**-moh-**koh**-nee-**OH**-sis) is an abnormal condition caused by dust in the lungs that usually develops after years of environmental or occupational contact. This causes cell death and fibrosis (hardening) of the lung tissues. These disorders are named for the causative agents.

- **Anthracosis** (**an**-thrah-**KOH**-sis), also known as **black lung disease**, is caused by coal dust in the lungs (**anthrac** means coal dust and **osis** means condition).

- **Asbestosis** (**ass**-beh-**STOH**-sis) is caused by asbestos particles in the lungs and is found in workers from the ship building and construction trades.

- **Byssinosis** (**biss**-ih-**NOH**-sis), also known as **brown lung disease**, is caused by cotton, flax, or hemp dust in the lungs.

- **Silicosis** (**sill**-ih-**KOH**-sis), also known as **grinder's disease**, is caused by silica dust or glass in the lungs.

Pulmonary Fibrosis

- **Pulmonary fibrosis** (figh-**BROH**-sis) is the formation of scar tissue that replaces the pulmonary alveolar walls. (**Fibrosis** means the abnormal formation of fibrous tissue.) This condition may be caused by autoimmune disorders, infections, dust, gases, toxins, and some drugs. This destruction of lung tissue results in decreased lung capacity and increased difficulty in breathing.

- **Idiopathic pulmonary fibrosis**, also known as **IPF**, is a type of pulmonary fibrosis for which a cause cannot be identified. (**Idiopathic** [id-ee-oh-**PATH**-ick] means without known cause.)

Cystic Fibrosis

- **Cystic fibrosis** (**SIS**-tick figh-**BROH**-sis), also known as **CF**, is a genetic disorder in which the lungs are clogged with large quantities of abnormally thick mucus. Antibiotics are administered to control lung infections and daily physical therapy, known as **postural drainage**, is performed to remove excess mucus from the lungs.

- In CF the digestive system is also impaired by thick gluelike mucus that interferes with digestive juices. Digestive enzymes are administered to aid the digestive system

Breathing Disorders

Eupnea (youp-**NEE**-ah) means easy or normal breathing (**eu** means good and **pnea** means breathing). This is the baseline for judging some breathing disorders (Figure 7.15A).

- **Tachypnea** (**tack**-ihp-**NEE**-ah) is an abnormally rapid rate of respiration usually of more than 20 breaths per minute (**tachy** means rapid and **pnea** means breathing). (Figure 7.15B).

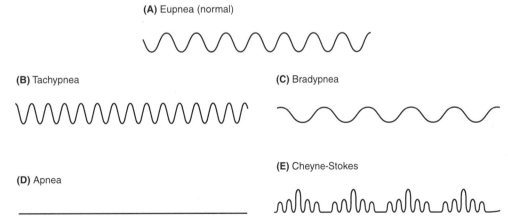

(A) Eupnea (normal)

(B) Tachypnea

(C) Bradypnea

(D) Apnea

(E) Cheyne-Stokes

Figure 7.15 Respiratory patterns. (A) Eupnea, also known as normal breathing. (B) Tachypnea, also known as abnormally rapid breathing. (C) Bradypnea, also known as abnormally slow breathing. (D) Apnea, is the absence of breathing. (E) Cheyne-Stokes is an alternating series of abnormal patterns.

- **Bradypnea** (**brad**-ihp-**NEE**-ah *or* **brad**-ee-**NEE**-ah) is an abnormally slow rate of respiration usually of less than 10 breaths per minute (**brady** means slow and **pnea** means breathing). (Figure 7.15C).

- **Apnea** (**AP**-nee-ah *or* ap-**NEE**-ah) is the absence of spontaneous respiration (**a** means without and **pnea** means breathing). (Figure 7.15D).

- **Sleep apnea syndromes**, also known as **SAS**, are a group of potentially deadly disorders in which breathing repeatedly stops during sleep for long enough periods to cause a measurable decrease in blood oxygen levels.

- In **Cheyne-Stokes respiration** (**CHAYN-STOHKS**), also known as **CSR**, there is a pattern of alternating periods of hyperpnea (rapid breathing), hypopnea (slow breathing), and apnea (the absence of breathing). (Figure 7.15E).

- **Dyspnea** (**DISP**-nee-ah), also known as **shortness of breath**, is difficult or labored breathing (**dys** means painful and **pnea** means breathing).

- **Hyperpnea** (**high**-perp-**NEE**-ah) is an abnormal increase in the depth and rate of the respiratory movements (**hyper** means excessive and **pnea** means breathing).

- **Hypopnea** (**high**-poh-**NEE**-ah) is shallow or slow respiration (**hypo** means decreased and **pnea** means breathing).

- **Hyperventilation** (**high**-per-**ven**-tih-**LAY**-shun) is abnormally rapid deep breathing, resulting in decreased levels of carbon dioxide at the cellular level.

Lack of Oxygen

- In an **airway obstruction** food or a foreign object blocks the airway and prevents air from entering or leaving the lungs. This is a life-threatening emergency requiring immediate action usually by the abdominal (Heimlich) maneuver.

- **Anoxia** (ah-**NOCK**-see-ah) is the absence or almost complete absence of oxygen from inspired gases, arterial blood, or tissues (**an** means without, **ox** means oxygen, and **ia** means abnormal condition). If anoxia continues for more than 4 to 6 minutes, irreversible brain damage may occur.

- **Asphyxia** (ass-**FICK**-see-ah) describes the pathologic changes caused by a lack of oxygen in air that is breathed in. This produces anoxia and hypoxia.

- **Asphyxiation** (ass-**fick**-see-**AY**-shun), also known as **suffocation**, is any interruption of breathing resulting in the loss of consciousness or death. Asphyxiation may be caused by an airway obstruction, drowning, smothering, choking, or inhaling gases such as carbon monoxide.

- **Cyanosis** (**sigh**-ah-**NOH**-sis) is a bluish discoloration of the skin caused by a lack of adequate oxygen (**cyan** means blue and **osis** means abnormal condition).

- **Hypoxia** (high-**POCK**-see-ah) is the condition of having subnormal oxygen levels in the cells that is less severe than anoxia (**hypo** means deficient, **ox** means oxygen, and **ia** means abnormal condition).

- **Respiratory failure** is a condition in which the level of oxygen in the blood becomes dangerously low or the level of carbon dioxide becomes dangerously high.

Sudden Infant Death Syndrome

- **Sudden infant death syndrome**, also known as **SIDS** and **crib death**, is the sudden and unexplainable death of an apparently healthy infant, between the ages of 2 weeks and 1 year, that typically occurs while the infant is sleeping. This happens more often among babies who sleep on their stomach. For this reason, it is recommended that infants be put down to sleep on the back or side.

Diagnostic Procedures of the Respiratory System

- **Respiratory rate**, also known as **RR**, is an important diagnostic sign. The RR is counted as the number of respirations per minute. A single **respiration** (breath) consists of one inhalation and one expiration. The normal range for adults is 15 to 20 respirations per minute.

- **Pulmonary function tests**, also known as **PFTs**, are a group of tests used to measure the capacity of the lungs to hold air as well as their ability to move air in and out and to exchange oxygen and carbon dioxide.

- **Phlegm** (**FLEM**) is the thick mucus secreted by the tissues lining the respiratory passages. When phlegm is ejected through the mouth, it is called **sputum** (**SPYOU**-tum). Sputum may be used for diagnostic purposes.

- **Bronchoscopy** (brong-**KOS**-koh-pee) is the visual examination of the bronchi using a **bronchoscope** (**broncho** means bronchus and **scopy** means direct visual examination). This may also be used for operative procedures such as tissue repair or the removal of a foreign object (Figure 7.16).

- **Laryngoscopy** (lar-ing-**GOS**-koh-pee) is the visual examination of the larynx using a **laryngoscope** (**laryngo** means larynx and **scopy** means a direct visual examination). This may also be used for operative procedures such as tissue repair or the removal of a foreign object.

- **Spirometry** (spy-**ROM**-eh-tree) is a testing method that uses a spirometer to record the volume of air inhaled or exhaled and the length of time each breath takes (**spiro** means to breathe and **metry** means to measure).

- **Tuberculin skin testing** (**TST**), which is a screening test to detect tuberculosis, can be performed by the **Mantoux method** or the **PPD** (purified protein derivative). In performing the test the skin of the arm is injected with a small amount of harmless tuberculin protein. A **negative result** (no response) indicates that TB is not present. A **positive result** (hardness within the testing area within 2 to 3 days) indicates the possibility of disease and should be followed by additional testing such as a chest x-ray and sputum testing.

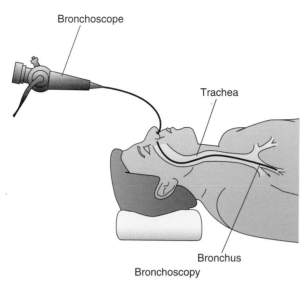

Bronchoscope

Trachea

Bronchus

Bronchoscopy

FIGURE 7.16 Bronchoscopy is the visual examination of the bronchi with the use of a bronchoscope.

- **Chest imaging**, also known as **chest x-rays**, is a valuable tool to show pneumonia, lung tumors, pneumothorax, pleural effusion, tuberculosis, and emphysema (see Figure 7.10B).

Treatment Procedures of the Respiratory System

Medications

- A **bronchoconstrictor** (**brong**-koh-kon-**STRICK**-tor) is an agent that narrows the opening of the passages into the lungs.
- A **bronchodilator** (**brong**-koh-dye-**LAY**-tor) is an agent that expands the opening of the passages into the lungs. At the first sign of an asthma attack, the patient uses an inhaler to self-administer a bronchodilator.

Nose and Throat

- **Septoplasty** (**SEP**-toh-**plas**-tee) is the surgical reconstruction of the nasal septum (**septo** means septum and **plasty** means surgical repair).
- A **sinusotomy** (**sigh**-nuhs-**OT**-oh-mee) is a surgical incision into a sinus (**sinus** means sinus and **otomy** means surgical incision). This procedure is used in the treatment of chronic sinusitis.
- **Functional endoscopic sinus surgery**, also known as **FSS**, is the surgical enlargement of the opening between the nose and sinus that is used to treat chronic sinusitis.
- **Pharyngoplasty** (fah-**RING**-goh-**plas**-tee) is the surgical repair of the pharynx (**pharyngo** means pharynx and **plasty** means surgical repair).
- A **pharyngostomy** (**far**-ing-**GOSS**-toh-mee) is the surgical creation of an artifical opening into the pharynx

(**pharyng** means pharynx and **ostomy** means surgically creating an opening). The resulting opening is called a **pharyngostoma** (**pharyngo** means pharynx and **stoma** means artificial mouth or opening).

- A **pharyngotomy** (**far**-ing-**GOT**-oh-mee) is a surgical incision of the pharynx (**pharyng** means pharynx and **otomy** means a surgical incision).
- A **laryngectomy** (**lar**-in-**JECK**-toh-mee) is the surgical removal of the larynx (**laryng** means larynx and **ectomy** means surgical removal).
- **Laryngoplasty** (lah-**RING**-goh-**plas**-tee) is the surgical repair of the larynx (**laryngo** means larynx and **plasty** means surgical repair).
- **Endotracheal intubation** (**en**-doh-**TRAY**-kee-al **in**-too-**BAY**-shun) is the passage of a tube through the nose or mouth into the trachea to establish an airway. (**Intubation** is the insertion of a tube, usually for the passage of air or fluids.)

Trachea and Bronchi

- **Tracheoplasty** (**TRAY**-kee-oh-**plas**-tee) is the surgical repair of the trachea (**tracheo** means trachea and **plasty** means surgical repair).
- **Tracheorrhaphy** (**tray**-kee-**OR**-ah-fee) means suturing of the trachea (**tracheo** means trachea and **rrhaphy** means to suture).
- A **tracheotomy** (**tray**-kee-**OT**-oh-mee) is usually an emergency procedure in which an incision is made into the trachea to gain access to the airway below a blockage (**trache** means trachea and **otomy** means surgical incision).
- A **tracheostomy** (**tray**-kee-**OS**-toh-mee) is creating an opening into the trachea and inserting a tube to facilitate the passage of air or the removal of secretions (**trache** means trachea and **ostomy** means surgically creating an opening). Placement of this tube may be temporary or permanent. The resulting opening is called a stoma (Figure 7.17).
- A **stoma** (**STOH**-mah) is an opening on a body surface. A stoma can occur naturally (for example, a pore in the skin), or may be created surgically.

Lungs, Pleura, and Thorax

- A **pneumonectomy** (**new**-moh-**NECK**-toh-mee) is the surgical removal of all or part of a lung (**pneumon** means lung and **ectomy** means surgical removal).
- A **lobectomy** (loh-**BECK**-toh-mee) is the surgical removal of a lobe of the lung. This term also is used to describe the removal of a lobe of the liver, brain, or thyroid gland (**lob** means lobe and **ectomy** means surgical removal).
- A **pleurectomy** (ploor-**ECK**-toh-mee) is the surgical removal of part of the pleura (**pleur** means pleura and **ectomy** means surgical removal).
- **Thoracentesis** (**thoh**-rah-sen-**TEE**-sis) is the puncture of the chest wall with a needle to obtain fluid from the

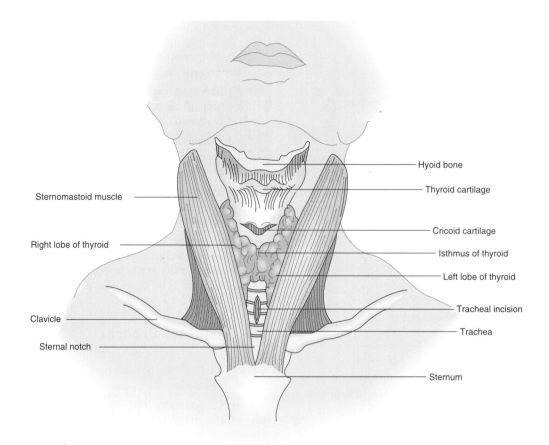

Sternomastoid muscle

Right lobe of thyroid

Clavicle

Sternal notch

Hyoid bone

Thyroid cartilage

Cricoid cartilage

Isthmus of thyroid

Left lobe of thyroid

Tracheal incision

Trachea

Sternum

FIGURE 7.17 A tracheostomy is performed to create an opening into the trachea to facilitate the passage of air or removal of secretions.

pleural cavity for diagnostic purposes, to drain pleural effusions, or to reexpand a collapsed lung (Figure 7.18). (Notice the spelling of this term. It is *not* a simple combination of familiar word parts.)

- A **thoracotomy** (**thoh**-rah-**KOT**-toh-mee) is a surgical incision into the wall of the chest (**thorac** means thorax or chest and **otomy** means surgical incision).

FIGURE 7.18 Fluid being removed from the pleural cavity by means of thorancentesis.

- A **thoracostomy** (**thoh**-rah-**KOS**-toh-mee) is the surgical creation of an opening into the chest (**thorac** means thorax or chest and **ostomy** means the surgical creation of an opening).

Respiratory Therapy

- **Supplemental oxygen** may be administered through a nasal canula or rebreather mask to add more oxygen to the air taken in as the patient breathes.
- **Postural drainage** is a procedure in which the patient is tilted and propped at different angles to drain secretions from the lungs.
- A **ventilator** is a mechanical device for artificial ventilation of the lungs that is used to replace or supplement the patient's natural breathing function. The goal is to wean the patient from the ventilator and to resume breathing on his own.
- A **respirator** is a machine used for prolonged artificial respiration. As an example, when a spinal cord injury destroys the natural breathing mechanism, the patient can continue to breathe through the use of a respirator.

Learning Exercises

Matching Word Parts—1

Write the letter of the correct answer on the line provided in the left column.

7.1. _____ atel/o

7.2. _____ bronch/o, bronchi/o

7.3. _____ cyan/o

7.4. _____ -ectasis

7.5. _____ laryng/o

A. stretching, dilation, enlargement

B. voice box

C. bronchial tube, wind pipe, a bronchus

D. blue

E. incomplete

Matching Word Parts—2

Write the letter of the correct answer on the line provided in the left column.

7.6. _____ ox/i, ox/o, ox/y

7.7. _____ pharyng/o

A. lung, air

B. oxygen

7.8. _____ phon/o

7.9. _____ pleur/o

7.10. _____ pneum/o, pneumon/o, pneu-

C. multilayered membrane

D. throat

E. voice

Matching Word Parts—3

Write the letter of the correct answer on the line provided in the left column.

7.11. _____ -pnea

7.12. _____ pulm/o, pulmon/o

7.13. _____ tachy-

7.14. _____ thorac/o, -thorax

7.15. _____ trache/o

A. windpipe

B. rapid

C. lung

D. chest or thorax

E. breathing

● **Definitions**

Circle the letter next to the correct answer.

7.16. The mediastinum _____ .

   a. contains the heart, aorta, esophagus, and trachea

   b. contains the lungs

   c. divides the chest and abdominal cavities

   d. is the central portion of the sternum (breastbone)

7.17. The epiglottis _____ .

   a. acts as a lid over the entrance to esophagus

   b. acts as a lid over the entrance to the trachea

   c. is commonly known as the Adam's apple

   d. is also known as the voice box

7.18. The pleura is _____ .

   a. a multilayered membrane surrounding each lung

   b. the lining of the thorax

   c. the nerve that causes the diaphragm to contract

   d. the site of external respiration

7.19. Which sinuses are located just above the eyes?

   a. ethmoid

   b. frontal

   c. maxillary

   d. sphenoid

7.20. The alveoli are _____ .

   a. branches of the bronchial tree

   b. flexible air sacs

   c. major divisions of the lungs

   d. the sacs that surround the lungs

7.21. The trachea divides into two branches called _____ .

   a. alveoli

   b. bronchi

   c. bronchus

   d. bronchioles

7.22. Which term means spitting blood or blood-stained sputum?

   a. effusion

   b. epistaxis

   c. hemoptysis

   d. hemothorax

7.23. What does pneumothorax mean?

   a. an abnormal lung condition caused by dust

   b. an accumulation of air or gas in the pleural space

   c. inflammation of the thorax

   d. inhalation of air into the thoracic cavity

7.24. Which term means an abnormally rapid rate of respiration (more than 20 breaths per minute)?

   a. apnea

   b. bradypnea

   c. dyspnea

   d. tachypnea

7.25. Which term means any voice impairment?

   a. aphonia

   b. dysphonia

   c. laryngitis

   d. laryngoplegia

● **Matching Structures**

Write the letter of the correct answer on the line provided in the left column.

7.26. _____ laryngopharynx   A. first division of the pharynx

7.27. _____ larynx   B. second division of the pharynx

7.28. _____ nasopharynx   C. third division of the pharynx

7.29. _____ oropharynx   D. voice box

7.30. _____ trachea   E. windpipe

Which Word?

Circle the correct term in each sentence.

7.31. The exchange of gases within the cells of the body is known as *external / internal* respiration.

7.32. The medical term to describe the lung disease caused by cotton, flax, or hemp dust is *anthracosis / byssinosis*.

7.33. The form of pneumonia that can be prevented through vaccination is *bacterial / viral*.

7.34. The medical term commonly known as shortness of breath is *dyspnea / eupnea*.

7.35. The term meaning an emergency procedure to gain access below a blocked airway is *tracheostomy / tracheotomy*.

Spelling Counts

Find the misspelled word in each sentence. Then write the word, spelled correctly, on the line provided.

7.36. The thick mucus secreted by the tissues that line the respiratory passages is called phlem.
_____

7.37. The medical term meaning an accumulation of pus in the pleural cavity is emphyema.
_____

7.38. The medical name for the disease commonly known as whooping cough is pertussosis.
_____

7.39. The medical term for the condition commonly known a TB is tuberculiosis.
_____

7.40. One of the terms used to describe the common cold is nasiopharyngitis.
_____

Matching Abbreviations

Write the letter of the correct answer on the line provided in the left column.

7.41. _____ ARDS   A. upper respiratory infection

7.42. _____ COPD   B. sudden infant death syndrome

7.43. _____ SIDS   C. smoker's respiratory syndrome

7.44. _____ SRS   D. chronic obstructive pulmonary disease

7.45. _____ URI   E. acute respiratory distress syndrome

Term Selection

7.46. Which term means the act of drawing a foreign substance into the upper respiratory tract?
a. aspiration
b. inhalation
c. inspiration
d. respiration

7.47. Which term means abnormally rapid deep breathing?
a. dyspnea
b. hyperpnea
c. hypopnea
d. hyperventilation

7.48. Which term means the surgical repair of the trachea?
a. tracheoplasty
b. tracheorrhaphy
c. tracheostomy
d. tracheotomy

7.49. When counting respiratory rate, a single respiration consists of _____ .
a. a single inhalation
b. a single expiration
c. one inhalation and one expiration
d. one external respiration and one internal respiration

7.50. Which technique is used in the routine treatment of cystic fibrosis?
a. a respirator
b. a ventilator
c. postural drainage
d. supplemental oxygen

● Sentence Completion

Write the correct term on the line.

7.51. The medical term meaning an absence of spontaneous respiration is _____ .

7.52. The sudden spasmodic closure of the larynx is a/an _____ .

7.53. The medical term meaning the escape of fluid into a body cavity is _____ .

7.54. The medical term meaning pain in the pleura or in the side is _____ .

7.55. The medical term meaning bleeding from the lungs is _____ .

● True/False

If the statement is true, write T on the line. If the statement is false, write F on the line.

7.56. _____ Tracheorrhagia is an inflammation of the trachea.

7.57. _____ The left lung has three lobes.

7.58. _____ Internal respiration is the exchange of gases within the cells of all the body organs and tissues.

7.59. _____ Hypoxia is the condition of having inadequate oxygen in the cells.

7.60. _____ Atelectasis is the incomplete expansion of a lung.

7.61. _____ Sudden infant death syndrome (SIDS) typically occurs between the ages of 6 to 12 months.

7.62. _____ The trachea divides into two branches called bronchioles.

7.63. _____ Croup is an allergic reaction to airborne allergens.

7.64. _____ A bronchoconstrictor is an agent that enlarges the opening of the passages into the lungs.

7.65. _____ Emphysema is a chronic obstructive pulmonary disease.

● Clinical Condition

Write the correct answer on the line.

7.66. Mrs. Jamison has a runny nose caused by an allergy to airborne allergens. Her condition is diagnosed as allergic _____ .

7.67. Dr. Timkins surgically removed a portion of the pleura. This procedure is known as a/an _____ .

7.68. Wendy Barlow required the surgical repair of her larynx. This procedure is known as a/an _____ .

7.69. During his asthma attacks Danny uses an inhaler containing a _____ . This medication expands the opening of the passages into Danny's lungs.

7.70. Mr. Partin received an immunization that is commonly known as a flu shot to prevent _____ .

7.71. When hit during the fight, Marvin Roper's nose started to bleed. The medical term for this condition is _____ .

7.72. The doctor's examination revealed that Jean Marshall has an accumulation of blood in the pleural cavity. This diagnosis is recorded on her chart as a/an _____ .

7.73. Duncan McCloud had a/an _____ performed to correct damage to the septum of his nose.

7.74. Susanne Holderman is suffering from an inflammation of the bronchial walls. Susanne's condition is _____ .

7.75. Because of an obstruction in his windpipe Ted Coleman required an emergency _____ .

● Which is the Correct Medical Term?

7.76. Which term means a chronic enlargement of the lower bronchial tree?

a. atelectasis

b. bronchiectasis

c. emphysema

d. pleurisy

7.77. Which substance is ejected through the mouth and used for diagnostic purposes in respiratory disorders?

a. phlegm

b. pleural effusion

c. saliva

d. sputum

7.78. Which term means a bluish discoloration of the skin caused by a lack of adequate oxygen?

a. asphyxia

b. cyanosis

c. epistaxis

d. hypoxia

7.79. Which statement applies to tuberculosis?

a. It is a bacterial infection.

b. It is a bloodborne pathogen.

c. It is a disease of the upper respiratory system.

d. It is a viral infection.

7.80. Which term means paralysis of the vocal bands?

a. aphonia

b. dysphonia

c. laryngitis

d. laryngoplegia

● **Challenge Word Building**

These terms are *not* found in this chapter; however, they are made up of these familiar word parts. You may want to look in the glossary or use a medical dictionary to check your answers!

bronch/o	-itis
epiglott/o	-ologist
laryng/o	-plasty
pharyng/o	-plegia
pneumon/o	-rrhagia
trache/o	-rrhea
	-scopy
	-stenosis

7.81. The medical term meaning an abnormal discharge from the pharynx is

_____ .

7.82. The medical term meaning inflammation of the lungs is _____ .

7.83. The medical term meaning a specialist in the study of the larynx is a/an

_____ .

7.84. The medical term meaning bleeding from the larynx is _____ .

7.85. The medical term meaning inflammation of both the pharynx and the larynx is

_____ .

7.86. The medical term meaning the abnormal narrowing of the lumen of the trachea

_____ .

7.87. The medical term meaning the surgical repair of a bronchial defect _____ .

7.88. The medical term meaning an inflammation of the epiglottis is _____ .

7.89. The medical term meaning the inspection of both the trachea and bronchi through a bronchoscope _____ .

7.90. The medical term meaning paralysis of the walls of the bronchi is _____ .

● Labeling Exercises

Identify the parts of numbered items on this diagram.

7.91. _____

7.92. Right _____

7.93. _____

7.94. _____

7.95. _____ sinus

7.96. _____ cavity

7.97. _____

7.98. _____

7.99. _____

7.100. _____

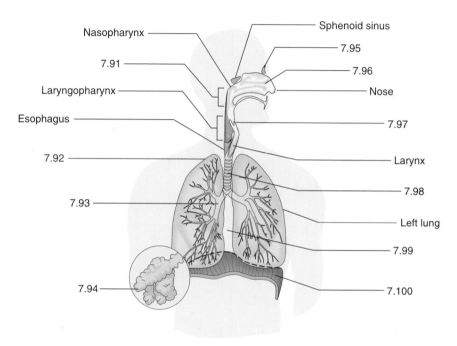

Respiratory System

The Human Touch: Critical Thinking Exercise

The following story and questions are designed to stimulate critical thinking through class discussion or as a brief essay response. There are no easy or right-wrong answers to these questions.

Sylvia Gaylord works as a legal aid on the 12th floor of an 18-story glass and steel monument to modern architectural technology in the center of the city. On clear days the views are spectacular. From her cubicle, Sylvia's eye catches the edge of a beautiful blue and white skyscape as she reaches for her medi-haler. This is the third attack since she returned from lunch 4 hours ago — her asthma is really bad today. But if she leaves work early again her boss will write her up. Sylvia concentrates on breathing normally.

Her roommate Kelly is a respiratory therapist at the county hospital. Kelly says Sylvia's asthma attacks are probably triggered by the city's high level of air pollution. That can't be true. They both run in the park every morning before work, and Sylvia rarely needs to use her inhaler. The problems start when she gets to work. The wheezing and coughing were so bad today that by the time she got up the elevator and into her cubicle she could hardly breathe.

Last night the cable news ran a story on the unhealthy air found in some buildings. They called it "sick building syndrome" and reported that certain employees developed allergic reactions just by breathing the air. "Hmmm," she thought, "it seems like more and more people are getting sick in our office. John has had the flu twice. Sid's bronchitis turned into bronchopneumonia and Nging complains of sinusitis. Could this building have an air quality problem?"

Suggested Discussion Topics:

1. Discuss which environmental factors might cause an asthma attack.
2. Discuss what Sylvia might do to find out if her building has an air quality problem.
3. Use proper medical terminology to describe what happens to Sylvia's airways during an asthma attack and how medications affect the symptoms.
4. Asthmatic medications, similar to Sylvia's inhaler, are easily available in drugstores without a prescription. Discuss the pros and cons of this practice.
5. If Sylvia's inhaler does not control her attack and her condition worsens, what steps should be taken promptly? Why?

CHAPTER

8 The Digestive System

● Overview of Structures, Word Parts, and Functions of the Digestive System

MAJOR STRUCTURES	RELATED WORD ROOTS	PRIMARY FUNCTIONS
Mouth	or/o	Begins preparation of food for digestion.
Pharynx	pharyng/o	Transports food from the mouth to the esophagus.
Esophagus	esophag/o	Transports food from the pharynx to the stomach.
Stomach	gastr/o	Breaks down food and mixes it with digestive juices.
Small intestines	enter/o	Completes digestion and absorption of most nutrients.
Large intestines	col/o	Absorbs excess water and prepares solid waste for elimination.
Rectum and anus	an/o, proct/o, rect/o	Controls the excretion of solid waste.
Liver	hepat/o	Secretes bile and enzymes to aid in the digestion of fats.
Gallbladder	cholecyst/o	Stores bile and releases it to the small intestine as needed.
Pancreas	pancreat/o	Secretes digestive juices and enzymes into small intestine as needed.

VOCABULARY   Related to the Digestive System

Check the box as you master each word part or term. Terms marked with the ❖ symbol are pronounced on the optional student audiotape.

Key Word Parts

- [ ] an/o
- [ ] cec/o
- [ ] chol/e
- [ ] col/o, colon/o
- [ ] enter/o
- [ ] esophag/o
- [ ] gastr/o
- [ ] hepat/o
- [ ] cholecyst/o
- [ ] -lithiasis
- [ ] pancreat/o
- [ ] -pepsia
- [ ] proct/o
- [ ] rect/o
- [ ] sigmoid/o

Key Medical Terms

- [ ] achlorhydria (ah-klor-HIGH-dree-ah) ❖
- [ ] aerophagia (ay-er-oh-FAY-jee-ah)
- [ ] amebic dysentery (ah-MEE-bik DIS-en-ter-ee) ❖
- [ ] anastomosis (ah-nas-toh-MOH-sis) ❖
- [ ] anoplasty (AY-noh-plas-tee)
- [ ] anorexia (an-oh-RECK-see-ah) ❖
- [ ] anoscopy (ah-NOS-koh-pee) ❖
- [ ] aphthous ulcers (AF-thus UL-serz) ❖
- [ ] bilirubin (bill-ih-ROO-bin) ❖
- [ ] borborygmus (bor-boh-RIG-mus) ❖
- [ ] botulism (BOT-you-lizm) ❖
- [ ] bruxism (BRUCK-sizm) ❖
- [ ] bulimia (byou-LIM-ee-ah or boo-LEE-mee-ah) ❖
- [ ] cholecystalgia (koh-lee-sis-TAL-jee-ah) ❖
- [ ] cholecystectomy (koh-lee-sis-TECK-toh-mee) ❖
- [ ] cholecystitis (koh-lee-sis-TYE-tis) ❖
- [ ] choledocholithotomy (koh-led-oh-koh-lih-THOT-oh-mee) ❖
- [ ] cholelithiasis (koh-lee-lih-THIGH-ah-sis) ❖
- [ ] cholera (KOL-er-ah)
- [ ] cirrhosis (sih-ROH-sis) ❖
- [ ] colitis (koh-LYE-tis) ❖
- [ ] colonoscopy (koh-lun-OSS-koh-pee) ❖
- [ ] colostomy (koh-LAHS-toh-mee) ❖
- [ ] diverticulectomy (dye-ver-tick-you-LECK-toh-mee) ❖
- [ ] diverticulitis (dye-ver-tick-you-LYE-tis) ❖
- [ ] duodenal ulcers (dew-oh-DEE-nal or dew-ODD-eh-nal UL-serz) ❖
- [ ] dyspepsia (dis-PEP-see-ah) ❖
- [ ] dysphagia (dis-FAY-jee-ah)
- [ ] emesis (EM-eh-sis) ❖

- [ ] emetic (eh-MET-ick) ❖
- [ ] enteritis (en-ter-EYE-tis)
- [ ] eructation (eh-ruk-TAY-shun) ❖
- [ ] esophageal reflux (eh-sof-ah-JEE-al REE-flucks) ❖
- [ ] esophageal varices (eh-sof-ah-JEE-al VAYR-ih-seez) ❖
- [ ] esophagoplasty (eh-SOF-ah-go-plas-tee)
- [ ] gastroduodenostomy (gas-troh-dew-oh-deh-NOS-toh-mee) ❖
- [ ] gastroenteritis (gas-troh-en-ter-EYE-tis) ❖
- [ ] gastrorrhagia (gas-troh-RAY-jee-ah) ❖
- [ ] gastrorrhea (gas-troh-REE-ah) ❖
- [ ] gastrorrhexis (gas-troh-RECK-sis) ❖
- [ ] gastrostomy (gas-TROS-toh-mee) ❖
- [ ] gingivectomy (jin-jih-VECK-toh-mee)
- [ ] gingivitis (jin-jih-VYE-tis)
- [ ] hematemesis (hee-mah-TEM-eh-sis or hem-ah-TEM-eh-sis) ❖
- [ ] hemoccult (HEE-moh-kult) ❖
- [ ] hemorrhoidectomy (hem-oh-roid-ECK-toh-mee) ❖
- [ ] hepatitis (hep-ah-TYE-tis) ❖
- [ ] hepatomegaly (hep-ah-toh-MEG-ah-lee) ❖
- [ ] hepatorrhaphy (hep-ah-TOR-ah-fee) ❖
- [ ] hepatorrhexis (hep-ah-toh-RECK-sis) ❖
- [ ] hepatotomy (hep-ah-TOT-oh-mee)
- [ ] herpes labialis (HER-peez lay-bee-AL-iss)
- [ ] hiatal hernia (high-AY-tal HER-nee-ah) ❖
- [ ] hyperemesis (high-per-EM-eh-sis) ❖
- [ ] ileectomy (ill-ee-ECK-toh-mee) ❖
- [ ] ileitis (ill-ee-EYE-tis)
- [ ] ileocecal (ill-ee-oh-SEE-kull)
- [ ] ileostomy (ill-ee-OS-toh-mee) ❖
- [ ] ileus (ILL-ee-us) ❖
- [ ] inguinal hernia (ING-gwih-nal HER-nee-ah) ❖
- [ ] intussusception (in-tus-sus-SEP-shun) ❖
- [ ] jaundice (JAWN-dis) ❖
- [ ] maxillofacial (mack-sill-oh-FAY-shul)
- [ ] melena (meh-LEE-nah or MEL-eh-nah) ❖
- [ ] nasogastric intubation (nay-zoh-GAS-trick in-too-BAY-shun)
- [ ] orthodontist (or-thoh-DON-tist) ❖
- [ ] periodontitis (pehr-ee-oh-don-TYE-tis) ❖
- [ ] peristalsis (pehr-ih-STAL-sis)
- [ ] pica (PYE-kah) ❖
- [ ] proctoplasty (PROCK-toh-plas-tee) ❖
- [ ] pyrosis (pye-ROH-sis) ❖
- [ ] regurgitation (ree-gur-jih-TAY-shun) ❖
- [ ] salmonella (sal-moh-NEL-ah) ❖
- [ ] sigmoidoscopy (sig-moi-DOS-koh-pee) ❖
- [ ] volvulus (VOL-view-lus) ❖

On completion of this chapter, you should be able to:

1 Identify and describe the major structures and functions of the digestive system.

2 Describe the processes of digestion, absorption, and metabolism.

3 Recognize, define, spell, and pronounce terms related to the pathology and diagnostic and treatment procedures of the digestive system.

Functions of the Digestive System

The digestive system is also known as the **alimentary canal** (al-ih-**MEN**-tar-ee) (**aliment** means to nourish and **ary** means pertaining to). This system is responsible for

- The intake and digestion of food
- The absorption of nutrients from digested food
- The elimination of solid waste products

Structures of the Digestive System

The **major structures** of the digestive system include the **oral cavity** (mouth), **pharynx** (throat), **esophagus**, **stomach**, **small intestine**, **large intestine**, and the **rectum** and **anus**.

Accessory organs related to the digestive system include the **liver**, **gallbladder**, and **pancreas** (Figure 8.1).

The Gastrointestinal Tract

The structures of the digestive system are also described as the **gastrointestinal** (gas-troh-in-**TESS**-tih-nal) or **GI tract** (**gastro** means stomach, **intestin** means intestine, and **al** means pertaining to).

- The **upper GI tract** consists of the mouth, esophagus, and stomach.
- The **lower GI tract** is made up of the small intestine, large intestines, rectum, and anus. The intestines are sometimes referred to as the **bowels**.
- When these terms are used to describe diagnostic procedures, the small intestine is usually included with the upper GI tract.

The Oral Cavity

The major structures of the oral cavity, also known as the **mouth**, are the lips, hard and soft palates, salivary glands, tongue, teeth, and the periodontium (Figure 8.2).

The Lips

The **lips**, also known as **labia** (**LAY**-bee-ah), form the opening to the oral cavity (singular, **labium**). (Labia are

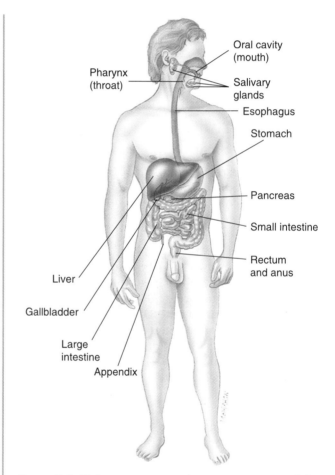

FIGURE 8.1 Major structures and accessory organs of the digestive system.

also part of the female genitalia.) Another word part relating to the lips of the mouth is **cheil/o**.

The Palate

The **palate** (**PAL**-at), which forms the roof of the mouth, consists of two parts: the hard and soft palates.

- The **hard palate** forms the bony anterior portion of the palate which is covered with a specialized mucous membrane.

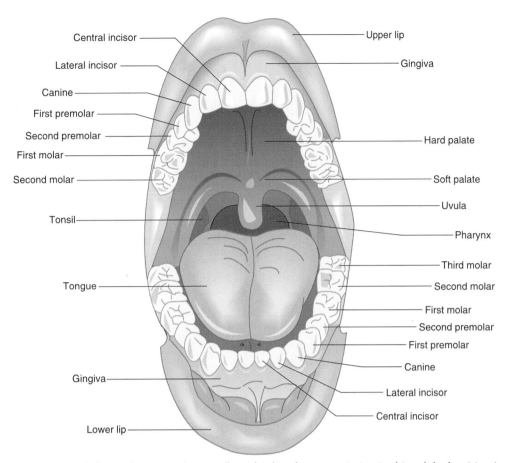

Central incisor — Upper lip

Lateral incisor — Gingiva

Canine

First premolar

Second premolar — Hard palate

First molar

Second molar — Soft palate

— Uvula

Tonsil — Pharynx

— Third molar

— Second molar

Tongue — First molar

— Second premolar

— First premolar

— Canine

Gingiva — Lateral incisor

— Central incisor

Lower lip

FIGURE 8.2 Major structures of the oral cavity. (The maxillary third molars are missing in this adult dentition.)

- **Rugae** (**ROO**-gay), which are irregular ridges or folds in the mucous membrane, cover the anterior portion of the hard palate. Rugae are also found in the stomach (singular, **ruga**).

- The **soft palate** forms the flexible posterior portion of the palate. It has the important role of closing off the nasal passage during swallowing so food does not move upward into the nasal cavity.

- The **uvula** (**YOU**-view-lah), which hangs from the free edge of the soft palate, helps in producing sounds and speech.

The Tongue

The **tongue**, which is very strong and flexible, aids in speech and moves food during chewing and swallowing.

- The upper surface of the tongue has a tough protective covering and contains the **papillae**, which are also known as the **taste buds**.

- The underside of the tongue is highly vascular and covered with delicate tissue. **Highly vascular** means containing many blood vessels. It is this structure that makes it possible for medications placed under the tongue to be quickly absorbed into the bloodstream.

Terms Related to the Teeth

- The term **dentition** (den-**TISH**-un) refers to the natural teeth arranged in the **maxillary** (upper) and **mandibular** (lower) arches.

- **Edentulous** (ee-**DEN**-too-lus) means without teeth. This term is used after the natural teeth have been lost.

- Human dentition includes four types of teeth: **incisors** and **canines** (also known as **cuspids**) that are used for biting and tearing; plus **premolars** (also known as **bicuspids**) and **molars** that are used for chewing and grinding.

- The **primary dentition**, also known as the **deciduous dentition** (dee-**SID**-you-us) or **baby teeth**, consists of 20 teeth (eight incisors, four canines, eight molars, and no premolars). The primary teeth are lost normally and replaced by the permanent teeth.

- The **permanent dentition** consists of 32 teeth (eight incisors, four canines, eight premolars, and twelve molars). These teeth are designed to last a lifetime.

- As used in dentistry, **occlusion** (ah-**KLOO**-zhun) is any contact between the chewing surfaces of the maxillary (upper) and mandibular (lower) teeth. **Malocclusion** (**mal**-oh-**KLOO**-zhun) is any deviation from a normal occlusion.

Structures and Tissues of the Teeth

- The **crown** of the tooth is the portion that is visible in the mouth. It is covered with **enamel**, the strongest tissue in the body (Figure 8.3).

- The **root** of the tooth holds the tooth securely in place within the dental arch. The root is protected by **cementum**. The crown and root meet at the **neck** of the tooth.

- **Dentin** makes up the bulk of the tooth and is protected by the enamel and cementum.

- The **pulp chamber** is the inner area of the crown of the tooth that runs downward to form the **root canals**. The **pulp** is made up of a rich supply of blood vessels and nerves.

The Periodontium

The **periodontium** (**pehr**-ee-oh-**DON**-shee-um) consists of the bone and soft tissues that surround and support the teeth (**peri** means surrounding, **odonti** means the teeth and **um** is the noun ending).

- The **gingiva** (**JIN**-jih-vah), also known as the **gums**, is the specialized mucous membrane that surrounds the teeth, covers the bone of the dental arches, and continues to form the lining of the cheeks.

The Salivary Glands

The **salivary glands** (**SAL**-ih-ver-ee) secrete **saliva** that moistens food, begins the digestive process, and cleanses the mouth (see Figure 8.1).

- There are three pairs of salivary glands: **parotid glands** (pah-**ROT**-id) located on the face in front of and slightly lower than each ear, **sublingual glands** located on the underside of the tongue, and **submandibular glands** located on the floor of the mouth.

The Pharynx

The **pharynx** (**FAR**-inks), also known as the **throat**, is the common passageway for both respiration and digestion (see Chapter 7).

- During swallowing food is prevented from moving from the pharynx into the lungs by the **epiglottis** (ep-ih-**GLOT**-is) that closes off the entrance to the trachea (windpipe). This allows food to move safely into the esophagus.

The Esophagus

The **esophagus** (eh-**SOF**-ah-gus), also known as the **gullet**, is a collapsible tube that leads from the pharynx to the stomach (see Figure 8.1).

- The **lower esophageal sphincter** (**SFINK**-ter), also known as the **cardiac sphincter**, is a ringlike muscle that controls the flow between the esophagus and the stomach. When this functions normally, stomach contents do not flow back into the esophagus.

The Stomach

The stomach is a saclike organ composed of the **fundus** (upper, rounded part), **body** (main portion), and **antrum** (lower part) (Figure 8.4).

- **Rugae** are the folds in the mucosa lining the stomach. Glands located within these folds produce the gastric juices that aid in digestion and mucus that forms the protective coating of the lining of the stomach.

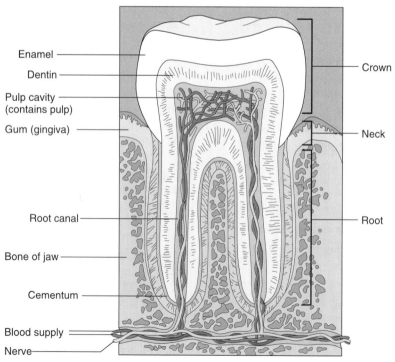

Enamel
Dentin
Pulp cavity (contains pulp)
Gum (gingiva)
Crown
Neck
Root canal
Bone of jaw
Cementum
Root
Blood supply
Nerve

FIGURE 8.3 Structures and tissues of the tooth.

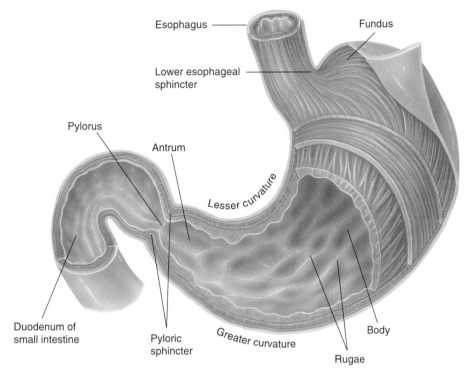

FIGURE 8.4 Structures of the stomach.

- The **pylorus** (pye-**LOR**-us) is the narrow passage connecting the stomach with the small intestine.
- The **pyloric sphincter** is the muscle ring that controls the flow from the stomach to the duodenum of the small intestine.

The Small Intestine

The **small intestine** extends from the pyloric sphincter to the first part of the large intestine. It is here that the nutrients from food are absorbed into the bloodstream.

The small intestine is a coiled organ up to 20 feet in length; however, it is known as the small intestine because it is smaller in diameter than the large intestine (see Figure 8.1).

Parts of the Small Intestine

The small intestine consists of the following three parts.

- The **duodenum** (dew-oh-**DEE**-num *or* dew-**ODD**-eh-num), the first portion of the small intestine, extends from the pylorus to the jejunum.
- The **jejunum** (jeh-**JOO**-num), the middle portion of the small intestine, extends from the duodenum to the ileum.
- The **ileum** (**ILL**-ee-um), the last portion of the small intestine, extends from the jejunum to the cecum of the large intestine.
- The **ileocecal sphincter** (ill-ee-oh-**SEE**-kull) controls the flow from the ileum of the small intestine into the cecum of the large intestine.

The Large Intestine

The large intestine extends from the end of the small intestine to the anus. The waste products of digestion are processed in the large intestine and then excreted through the anus (Figure 8.5).

- The three major parts of the large intestine are the **cecum**, **colon**, **rectum** and **anus**.

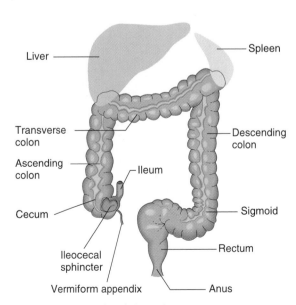

FIGURE 8.5 Structures of the colon.

The Cecum

The **cecum** (**SEE**-kum) is a pouch that lies on the right side of the abdomen. It extends from the end of the ileum to the beginning of the colon.

- The **vermiform appendix**, commonly called the **appendix**, hangs from the lower portion of the cecum (the name vermiform refers to its wormlike shape). The appendix serves no known function in the digestive system.

The Colon

The colon is subdivided into four parts:

- The **ascending colon** travels upward from the cecum to the undersurface of the liver.
- The **transverse colon** passes horizontally from right to left toward the spleen.
- The **descending colon** travels down the left side of the abdominal cavity to the sigmoid colon.
- The **sigmoid colon** (**SIG**-moid) is an S-shaped structure that continues from the descending colon above and joins with the rectum below.

The Rectum and Anus

- The **rectum**, which is the last division of the large intestine, ends at the anus.

- The **anus** is the lower opening of the digestive tract. The flow of waste through the anus is controlled by the two **anal sphincter muscles**.
- The term **anorectal** (**ah**-noh-**RECK**-tal) refers to the anus and rectum as a single unit (**ano** means anus, **rect** means rectum, and **al** means pertaining to).

Accessory Digestive Organs

The following organs are referred to as accessory organs because they play a key role in the digestive process but are not part of the gastrointestinal tract (Figure 8.6).

The Liver

The liver is located in the right upper quadrant of the abdomen and has several important functions. The term **hepatic** (heh-**PAT**-ick) means pertaining to the liver (**hepat** means liver and **ic** means pertaining to).

- The liver removes excess **glucose** (**GLOO**-kohs), also known as **blood sugar**, from the bloodstream and stores it as **glycogen** (**GLYE**-koh-jen) (a form of starch). When the blood sugar level is low, the liver converts glycogen back into glucose and releases it for use by the body.
- The liver destroys old erythrocytes (red blood cells), removes poisons from the blood, and manufactures some blood proteins.

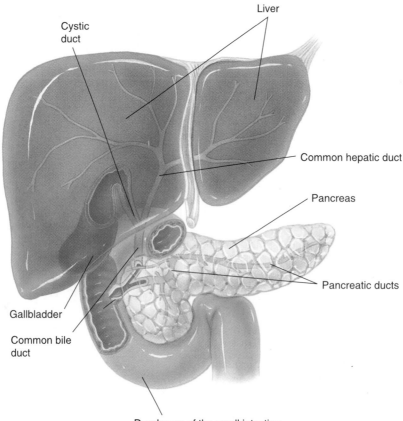

FIGURE 8.6 Accessory digestive organs: the liver, gallbladder, and pancreas.

- **Bilirubin** (bill-ih-**ROO**-bin), a pigment produced from the destruction of hemoglobin, is released by the liver in bile. Excess bilirubin in the blood is associated with jaundice.

- The liver secretes **bile**, which is a digestive juice containing enzymes that break down fat. The term **biliary** (**BILL**-ee-air-ee), as in the biliary system, means pertaining to bile.

- Bile travels down the **common hepatic duct** to the **cystic duct** that leads to the gallbladder where the bile is stored.

The Gallbladder

The **gallbladder** is a pear-shaped sac located under the liver. It stores and concentrates the bile for later use. The term **cholecystic** (**koh**-lee-**SIS**-tick) means pertaining to the gallbladder (**cholecyst** means gallbladder and **ic** means pertaining to).

- When bile is needed, the gallbladder contracts, forcing the bile out through the **cystic duct** and into the **common bile** duct that carries it into the duodenum of the small intestine.

The Pancreas

The **pancreas** (**PAN**-kree-as) is a feather-shaped organ located posterior to (behind) the stomach. It has important roles in both the digestive and endocrine systems. The endocrine functions plus the pathology and procedures related to the pancreas are discussed in Chapter 13.

- The pancreas synthesizes and secretes **pancreatic juices**. These juices are made up of sodium bicarbonate (to help neutralize stomach acids) and digestive enzymes (to process the protein, carbohydrates, and fats in food).

- The pancreatic juices leave the pancreas through the **pancreatic ducts** that join the **common bile duct** just before the entrance to the duodenum.

Digestion

Digestion is the process by which complex foods are broken down into nutrients in a form the body can use. The flow of food through the digestive system is shown in Figure 8.7.

- **Enzymes** (**EN**-zimes) are responsible for the chemical changes that break foods down into simpler forms of nutrients for use by the body.

- A **nutrient** is a substance, usually from food, that is necessary for normal functioning of the body.

Metabolism

- **Metabolism** (meh-**TAB**-oh-lizm) is the sum of anabolism and catabolism. That is, this term includes *all* of the processes involved in the body's use of these nutrients (**metabol** means change and **ism** means the condition).

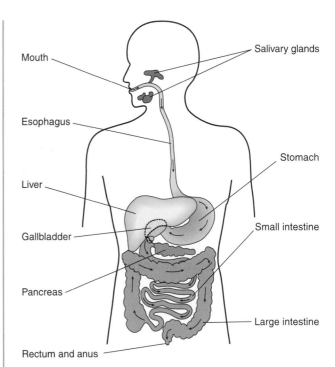

FIGURE 8.7 Schematic diagram showing the pathway of food through the digestive system.

- **Anabolism** (an-**NAB**-oh-lizm) is the building up of body cells and substances from nutrients.

- **Catabolism** (kah-**TAB**-oh-lizm), which is the opposite of anabolism, is the breaking down of body cells or substances, releasing energy and carbon dioxide (**catabol** means breaking down and **ism** means condition).

Absorption

Absorption (ab-**SORP**-shun) is the process by which completely digested nutrients are taken into the circulatory system by passing through the capillaries located in the walls of the small intestine.

- Fats and fat-soluble vitamins are absorbed into the lymphatic system through **villi** (**VILL**-eye), the tiny hairlike projections that line the walls of the small intestine (singular, **villus**).

The Role of the Mouth, Salivary Glands, and Esophagus

- **Mastication** (mass-tih-**KAY**-shun), also known as **chewing**, breaks food down into smaller pieces and mixes it with saliva. Saliva contains an enzyme that begins the chemical breakdown to convert starches into sugar.

- During swallowing food travels from the mouth into the pharynx and on into the **esophagus**.

- In the esophagus food moves downward through the action of gravity and peristalsis. **Peristalsis** (pehr-ih-

STAL-sis) is a series of wavelike contractions of the smooth muscles in a single direction.

The Role of the Stomach

- The **gastric juices** of the stomach contain **hydrochloric acid** and digestive enzymes.
- Few nutrients enter the bloodstream through the walls of the stomach. Instead, the churning action of the stomach works with the gastric juices to convert the food to chyme.
- **Chyme** (**KYM**) is the semifluid mass of partly digested food that passes from the stomach, through the pyloric sphincter, and into the small intestine.

The Role of the Small Intestine

Food is moved through the intestines by peristaltic action and digestion is completed in the duodenum after the chyme has been mixed with bile and pancreatic juice.

- Bile breaks apart large fat globules into smaller particles so enzymes in the pancreatic juices can digest the fats. This action is called **emulsification** and must be completed before the nutrients can be absorbed into the body.

The Role of the Large Intestine

The role of the entire large intestine is to receive the solid waste products of digestion and store them until they are eliminated from the body.

- Excess water is absorbed from the food waste through the walls of the large intestine and solid feces are formed. **Feces** (**FEE**-seez), also known as **stools**, are solid body wastes expelled through the rectum and anus.
- **Defecation** (**def**-eh-**KAY**-shun), also known as a **bowel movement**, is the evacuation or emptying of the large intestines.
- Gas is frequently produced by the normal, friendly bacteria in the colon, which helps to further break down food. The gas that is passed out of the body through the rectum is known as **flatulence** or **flatus**.
- **Borborygmus** (**bor**-boh-**RIG**-mus) is the rumbling noise caused by the movement of gas in the intestine.

Medical Specialties Related to the Digestive System

- A **dentist** holds a Doctor of Dental Surgery (DDS) or Doctor of Medical Dentistry degree (DMD) and specializes in diagnosing and treating diseases and disorders of teeth and tissues of the oral cavity (**dent** means teeth **ist** means specialist).
- A **gastroenterologist** (**gas**-troh-**en**-ter-**OL**-oh-jist) specializes in diagnosing and treating diseases and disorders of the stomach and intestines (**gastro** means stomach, **enter** means intestine, and **ologist** means specialist).

- An **internist** specializes in diagnosing and treating diseases and disorders of the internal organs.
- An **orthodontist** (**or**-thoh-**DON**-tist) is a dental specialist in the prevention or correction of abnormalities in the positioning of the teeth and related facial structures (**orth** means straight, **odont** means teeth, and **ist** mean a specialist).
- A **periodontist** (**pehr**-ee-oh-**DON**-tist) is a dental specialist who prevents or treats disorders of the tissues surrounding the teeth (**peri** means surrounding, **odont** means teeth, and **ist** mean a specialist).
- A **proctologist** (prock-**TOL**-oh-jist) specializes in disorders of the colon, rectum, and anus (**proct** means anus and rectum and **ologist** means specialist).

Pathology of The Digestive System

Tissues of the Oral Cavity

- **Aphthous ulcers** (**AF**-thus), also known as **canker sores**, are recurrent blister-like sores that break and form lesions on the soft tissues lining the mouth. Although the exact cause is known, the appearance of these sores is associated with stress, certain foods, or fever.
- **Herpes labialis** (**HER**-peez lay-bee-**AL**-iss), also known as **cold sores** or **fever blisters**, are blister-like sores caused by the herpes simplex virus that occur on the lips and adjacent tissue.
- A **cleft lip**, also known as a **harelip**, is a congenital defect resulting in a deep fissure of the lip running upward to the nose. (As used here, a **fissure** is a deep groove or opening.)
- A **cleft palate** is a congenital fissure of the palate that involves the upper lip, hard palate, and/or soft palate. If not corrected, this opening between the nose and mouth makes it difficult for the child to eat and speak.

Dental Diseases

- **Bruxism** (**BRUCK**-sizm) is involuntary grinding or clenching of the teeth that usually occurs during sleep and is associated with tension or stress. Bruxism wears away tooth structure, damages periodontal tissues, and injures the temporomandibular joint.
- **Dental calculus** (**KAL**-kyou-luhs) is hardened dental plaque on the teeth that irritates the surrounding tissues. The term **calculus** also describes hard deposits, commonly known as **stones**, formed in any part of the body.
- **Dental caries** (**KAYR**-eez), also known as **tooth decay** or a **cavity**, is an infectious disease that destroys the enamel and dentin of the tooth. If the decay process is not arrested, the pulp can be exposed and become infected.
- **Dental plaque** (**PLACK**) is a soft deposit consisting of bacteria and bacterial by-products that builds up on the teeth and is a major cause of dental caries and peri-

odontal disease. (**Plaque** also means a patch or small differentiated area on a body surface or the buildup of deposits of cholesterol in blood vessels.)

- **Periodontal disease**, also known as **periodontitis** (**pehr**-ee-oh-don-**TYE**-tis) is an inflammation of the tissues that surround and support the teeth (**peri** means surrounding, **odont** means tooth or teeth, and **itis** means inflammation). This is a progressive disease classified according to the degree of tissue involvement.

- **Gingivitis** (**jin**-jih-**VYE**-tis), an inflammation of the gums, is the earliest stage of periodontal disease (**gingiv** means gums and **itis** means inflammation).

- **Halitosis** (hal-ih-**TOH**-sis), also known as **bad breath**, may be caused by dental diseases or respiratory or gastric disorders (**halit** means breath and **osis** means condition of).

- **Temporomandibular disorders** (**tem**-poh-roh-man-**DIB**-you-lar), also known as **TMD** or **myofascial pain dysfunction** (**MPD**), are a group of complex symptoms including pain, headache, or difficulty in chewing that are related to the functioning of the temporomandibular joint.

Esophagus

- **Dysphagia** (dis-**FAY**-jee-ah) is difficulty in swallowing (**dys** means difficult and **phagia** means swallowing).

- **Esophageal reflux** (eh-**sof**-ah-**JEE**-al **REE**-flucks), also known as **gastroesophageal reflux disease** or **GERD**, is the upward flow of stomach acid into the esophagus. (**Reflux** means a backward or return flow.)

- **Esophageal varices** (eh-**sof**-ah-**JEE**-al **VAYR**-ih-seez) are enlarged and swollen veins at the lower end of the esophagus. Severe bleeding occurs if one of these veins ruptures.

- A **hiatal hernia** (high-**AY**-tal **HER**-nee-ah) is a protrusion of part of the stomach through the esophageal sphincter in the diaphragm (Figure 8.8). This condition may cause esophageal reflux and pyrosis.

- **Pyrosis** (pye-**ROH**-sis), also known as **heartburn**, is the burning sensation caused by the return of acidic stomach contents into the esophagus (**pyr** means fever or fire and **osis** means abnormal condition).

Stomach

- **Gastritis** (gas-**TRY**-tis) is an inflammation of the stomach (**gastr** means stomach and **itis** means inflammation).

- **Gastroenteritis** (**gas**-troh-en-ter-**EYE**-tis) is an inflammation of the stomach and intestines, especially the small intestine (**gastro** means stomach, **enter** means within, and **itis** means inflammation).

- **Gastrorrhagia** (gas-troh-**RAY**-jee-ah) is bleeding from the stomach (**gastro** means stomach and **rrhagia** means bleeding).

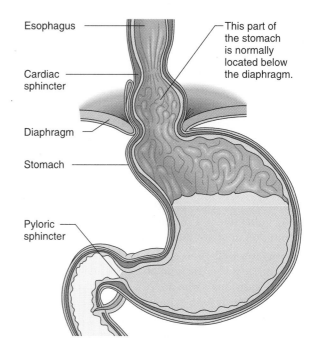

FIGURE 8.8 In a hiatal hernia part of the stomach protrudes through the esophageal opening in the diaphragm.

- **Gastrorrhea** (gas-troh-**REE**-ah) is the excessive flow of gastric secretions (**gastro** is stomach and **rrhea** means abnormal flow).

- **Gastrorrhexis** (gas-troh-**RECK**-sis) is a rupture of the stomach (**gastro** means stomach and **rrhexis** means rupture).

Peptic Ulcers

A **peptic ulcer**, also known as **PU**, is a lesion of the mucous membranes of the digestive system (**pept** means digestion and **ic** means pertaining to). These ulcers, which are frequently caused by the bacterium *Helicobacter pylori*, may occur in the lower end of the esophagus, the stomach, or the duodenum.

- **Gastric ulcers** are peptic ulcers that occur in the stomach.

- **Duodenal ulcers** (dew-oh-**DEE**-nal *or* dew-**ODD**-eh-nal **UL**-serz) are peptic ulcers that occur in the upper part of the small intestine and are the most common form of peptic ulcer.

- A **perforating ulcer** involves erosion through the entire thickness of the organ wall.

Eating Disorders

- **Anorexia** (an-oh-**RECK**-see-ah) is the lack or loss of appetite for food.

- **Anorexia nervosa** is an eating disorder characterized by a refusal to maintain a minimally normal body weight and an intense fear of gaining weight. Compulsive dieting and excessive exercising often cause the patient to become emaciated. **Emaciated** (ee-MAY-shee-ayt-ed) means abnormally thin.

- **Bulimia** (byou-LIM-ee-ah *or* boo-LEE-mee-ah), also known as **bulimia nervosa**, is an eating disorder characterized by episodes of binge eating followed by inappropriate compensatory behavior such as self-induced vomiting or misuse of laxatives, diuretics, or other medications.

- **Dehydration** is a condition in which fluid loss exceeds fluid intake and disrupts the body's normal electrolyte balance.

- **Malnutrition** is a lack of proper food or nutrients in the body, either due to a shortage of food or the improper absorption or distribution of nutrients.

- **Obesity** (oh-BEE-sih-tee) is an excessive accumulation of fat in the body. The term **obese** is usually used to refer to individuals who are 20% to 30% over the established standards for height, age, sex, and weight.

- **Pica** (PYE-kah) is an eating disorder in which there is persistent eating of nonnutritional substances such as clay. These abnormal cravings are sometimes associated with pregnancy.

Digestion and Vomiting

- **Achlorhydria** (ah-klor-HIGH-dree-ah) is the absence of hydrochloric acid from gastric secretions.

- **Aerophagia** (ay-er-oh-FAY-jee-ah) is the spasmodic swallowing of air followed by eructations (**aero** means air and **phagia** means swallowing).

- **Eructation** (eh-ruk-TAY-shun) is the act of belching or raising gas orally from the stomach.

- **Dyspepsia** (dis-PEP-see-ah), also known as **indigestion**, is an impairment of digestion (**dys** means painful and **pepsia** means digestion).

- **Emesis** (EM-eh-sis), also known as **vomiting**, means to expel the contents of the stomach through the esophagus and out of the mouth.

- **Hematemesis** (hee-mah-TEM-eh-sis *or* hem-ah-TEM-eh-sis) is vomiting blood (**hemat** means blood and **emesis** means vomiting).

- **Hyperemesis** (high-per-EM-eh-sis) means excessive vomiting (**hyper** means excessive and **emesis** means vomiting).

- **Nausea** (NAW-see-ah) is the sensation that leads to the urge to vomit.

- **Regurgitation** (ree-gur-jih-TAY-shun) is the return of swallowed food into the mouth.

Intestinal Disorders

- **Colorectal cancer** is a common form of cancer that often first manifests itself in polyps in the colon.

- **Diverticulitis** (dye-ver-tick-you-LYE-tis) is inflammation of one or more diverticulum (**diverticul** means diverticulum and **itis** means inflammation). A **divertic-**

ulum (dye-ver-TICK-you-lum) is a pouch or sac occurring in the lining or wall of a tubular organ including the intestines (plural, **diverticula**).

Inflammatory Bowel Disease

Chronic inflammatory diseases of the gastrointestinal tract are known as **inflammatory bowel disease** or IBD.

- **Colitis** (koh-LYE-tis) is an inflammation of the colon (**col** means colon and **itis** means inflammation).

- **Crohn's disease** is a chronic autoimmune disorder involving any part of the GI tract but most commonly resulting in scarring and thickening of the walls of ileum, colon or both.

- **Enteritis** (en-ter-EYE-tis) is an inflammation of the small intestines (**enter** means within and **itis** means inflammation).

- **Ileitis** (ill-ee-EYE-tis) is an inflammation of the ileum (**ile** means the ileum and **itis** means inflammation).

- **Spastic colon**, also known as **irritable bowel syndrome** or **IBS**, is a disorder of the motility (ability to move spontaneously) of the entire GI tract. It is characterized by abdominal pain, nausea, gas, constipation, and/or diarrhea.

Intestinal Obstructions

- **Ileus** (ILL-ee-us) is a temporary stoppage of intestinal peristalsis that may be accompanied by severe pain, abdominal distention, vomiting, absence of passage of stools, fever, and dehydration.

- **Intestinal adhesions** (ad-HEE-zhunz) abnormally hold together parts of the intestine where they normally should be separate. This condition, which is caused by inflammation or trauma, can lead to intestinal obstruction.

- **Intestinal obstruction** is a complete stoppage or serious impairment to the passage of the intestinal contents. A mechanical obstruction may result from a blockage that may be due to many causes including the presence of a tumor.

- In a **strangulating obstruction** the blood flow to a segment of the intestine is cut off. This may lead to gangrene and perforation.

- **Volvulus** (VOL-view-lus) is twisting of the intestine (bowel) on itself that causes an obstruction (Figure 8.9).

- **Intussusception** (in-tus-sus-SEP-shun) is the telescoping of one part of the intestine into the opening of an immediately adjacent part. This is typically a condition found in infants and young children (Figure 8.10).

- An **inguinal hernia** (ING-gwih-nal HER-nee-ah) is the protrusion of a small loop of bowel through a weak place in the lower abdominal wall or groin.

Infectious Diseases of the Intestines

Infectious diseases of the intestines may be transmitted through contaminated food and water or through poor

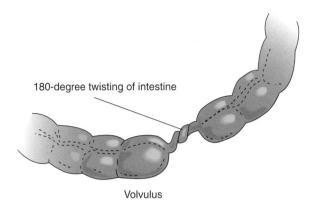

180-degree twisting of intestine

Volvulus

FIGURE 8.9 Volvulus is the twisting of the bowel on itself.

Telescoping of intestine

Intussusception

FIGURE 8.10 Intussusception is the telescoping of the bowel on itself.

sanitation practices. The more common of these diseases are discussed in Table 8.1.

Anorectal Disorders

- **Bowel incontinence** (in-KON-tih-nents) is the inability to control the excretion of feces. (Urinary incontinence refers to the inability to control urination and is discussed in Chapter 9.)
- **Constipation** is a decrease in frequency in the passage of stools, or difficulty in passing hard, dry stools.
- **Diarrhea** (**dye**-ah-**REE**-ah) is an abnormal frequency of loose or watery stools that may lead to dehydration (**dia** means through and **rrhea** means abnormal flow).
- **Hemorrhoids** (HEM-oh-roids), also known as **piles**, are enlarged veins in or near the anus that may cause pain and bleeding.
- **Melena** (meh-LEE-nah *or* MEL-eh-nah) is the passage of black stools containing digested blood.

Liver

- **Cirrhosis** (sih-ROH-sis) is a progressive degenerative disease of the liver characterized by disturbance of structure and function of the liver. It frequently results in jaundice and ultimately hepatic failure.
- **Hepatomegaly** (**hep**-ah-toh-**MEG**-ah-lee) is the enlargement of the liver (**hepato** means liver and **megaly** means enlargement).
- **Hepatorrhexis** (**hep**-ah-toh-**RECK**-sis) means rupture of the liver (**hepato** means liver and **rrhexis** means rupture).

Table 8.1

DISEASES OF THE INTESTINES

Name	Bacteria	Symptoms
Amebic dysentery (ah-**MEE**-bik **DIS**-en-**ter**-ee)	*Entamoeba histolytica* amoeba	Frequent, watery stools often with blood and mucus accompanied by pain, fever, and dehydration.
Botulism (**BOT**-you-lizm)	*Clostridium botulinum*	Food poisoning that is characterized by paralysis and is often fatal.
Cholera (**KOL**-er-ah)	*Vibrio cholerae*	Severe diarrhea, vomiting, and dehydration that can be fatal if not treated.
E. coli	*Escherichia coli*	Watery diarrhea that becomes bloody but is not usually accompanied by fever.
Salmonella (**sal**-moh-**NEL**-ah), nontyphoidal	*Salmonella*	Severe diarrhea, nausea, and vomiting accompanied by a high fever.
Typhoid fever (also known as **enteric fever**)	*Salmonella typhi*	Headache, delirium, cough, watery diarrhea, rash, and a high fever.

- Jaundice (JAWN-dis), also known as **icterus** (ICK-ter-us), is a yellow discoloration of the skin and other tissues caused by greater than normal amounts of bilirubin in the blood.

Hepatitis

Hepatitis (hep-ah-TYE-tis) is an inflammation of the liver that is usually caused by a virus but may also be caused by toxic substances (**hepat** means liver and **itis** means inflammation). The five varieties of hepatitis are shown in Table 8.2.

Table 8.2

HEPATITIS FROM A TO E

A	**Hepatitis virus A**, also known as **infectious hepatitis** or **HVA**, is transmitted by contaminated food and water.
B	**Hepatitis virus B**, also known as **serum hepatitis** or **HVB**, is bloodborne and can be prevented through vaccination. (**Bloodborne** means transmitted through direct contact with blood or body fluids contaminated with the virus.) Blood transfusions, sexual contact, and IV drug abuse are possible sources of contact with contaminated blood.
C	**Hepatitis virus C**, also known as **HVC**, is bloodborne and there is no vaccine to prevent this disease. HVC is a described as a silent epidemic because it can be present in the body for years and destroy the liver before any symptoms appear. This outcome is most likely to occur among individuals who received blood transfusions before 1992 when testing began to detect this virus.
D	**Hepatitis virus D**, also known as **HVD**, is bloodborne and there is no vaccine to prevent this disease.
E	**Hepatitis virus E**, also known as **HVE**, is transmitted through contaminated food and water.

Gallbladder

- Cholecystalgia (koh-lee-sis-TAL-jee-ah) is pain in the gallbladder (**cholecyst** means gallbladder and **algia** means pain).
- Cholecystitis (koh-lee-sis-TYE-tis) is inflammation of the gallbladder (**cholecyst** means gallbladder and **itis** means inflammation).

- A **gallstone**, also known as **biliary calculus**, is a hard deposit that forms in the gallbladder and bile ducts (plural, **calculi**). **Biliary** (BILL-ee-air-ee) means relating to bile. The formation of stones is discussed in Chapter 9.
- Cholelithiasis (koh-lee-lih-THIGH-ah-sis) is the presence of gallstones in the gallbladder or bile ducts (**chole** means bile or gall and **lithiasis** means presence of stones).

Diagnostic Procedures of the Digestive System

- **Abdominal CT**, or **CAT scan**, is a radiographic procedure that produces a detailed cross-section of the tissue structure within the abdomen, showing for example the presence of a tumor or obstruction. CT stands for **computed tomography** (**tomo** means slice or cut and **graphy** means recording).
- An **abdominal ultrasound** is a noninvasive test used to visualize internal organs by using very high frequency sound waves.
- **Anoscopy** (ah-NOS-koh-pee) is the visual examination of the anal canal and lower rectum using a short speculum called an **anoscope** (AY-no-skope). A **speculum** (SPECK-you-lum) is an instrument used to enlarge the opening of any body cavity to facilitate inspection of its interior.
- An **upper GI series**, or **barium swallow**, and **lower GI series**, or **barium enema** (BE), are radiographic studies to examine the digestive system. Barium is used as a contrast medium to make these structures visible.
- The term **enema** also describes a solution placed into the rectum and colon to empty the lower intestine through bowel activity. One purpose of an enema is to clear the bowels in preparation for an endoscopic examination.
- **Hemoccult** (HEE-moh-kult), also known as the **fecal occult blood test** or **FOBT**, is a laboratory test for hidden blood in the stools (**hemo** means blood, **occult** means hidden or difficult to see). A test kit may be used at home and the specimens are delivered to a laboratory or physician's office for evaluation.
- **Stool samples** are specimens of feces that are examined for content and characteristics. For example, fatty stools might indicate the presence of pancreatic problems. Cultures of the stool sample can be examined in the laboratory for the presence of bacteria or **O & P**, which are **ova** (parasite eggs) and **parasites**.

Endoscopic Procedures

An **endoscope** is an instrument used for visual examination of internal structures (**endo** means within and **scope** means an instrument for visual examination). Endoscopes are also used for obtaining biopsy samples, controlling bleeding, removing foreign objects, as well as other surgical and treatment procedures.

- **Colonoscopy** (**koh**-lun-**OSS**-koh-pee) is the direct visual examination of the inner surface of the colon, from the rectum to the cecum (**colono** means colon and **scopy** means visual examination).
- **Gastrointestinal endoscopy** is the endoscopic examination of the interior of the esophagus, stomach and duodenum.
- **Proctoscopy** is the endoscopic examination of the rectum and anus (**procto** means anus and rectum and **scopy** is the visual examination).
- **Sigmoidoscopy** (**sig**-moi-**DOS**-koh-pee) is the use of an endoscope for the direct visual examination of the interior of the entire rectum, sigmoid colon, and possibly a portion of the descending colon.

Treatment Procedures of the Digestive System

Medications

- **Acid blockers** taken before eating block the effects of histamine, which signals the stomach to produce acid.
- An **antiemetic** (**an**-tih-ee-**MET**-ick) prevents or relieves nausea and vomiting.
- An **emetic** (eh-**MET**-ick) produces vomiting.
- **Laxatives** are medications or foods given to stimulate bowel movements.
- **Oral rehydration therapy**, also known as **ORT**, is a treatment in which a solution of electrolytes is administered orally to counteract dehydration that may accompany severe diarrhea.

Oral Cavity and Esophagus

- **Esophagoplasty** (eh-**SOF**-ah-go-**plas**-tee) is the surgical repair of the esophagus (**esophago** means esophagus and **plasty** means surgical repair).
- An **extraction**, as the term is used in dentistry, is the surgical removal of a tooth.
- A **gingivectomy** (**jin**-jih-**VECK**-toh-mee) is the surgical removal of diseased gingival tissue (**gingiv** means gingival tissue and **ectomy** means surgical removal).
- **Maxillofacial surgery** (mack-**sill**-oh-**FAY**-shul) is specialized surgery of the face and jaws to correct deformities, treat diseases, and repair injuries.
- **Palatoplasty** (**PAL**-ah-toh-**plas**-tee) is surgical repair of a cleft palate (**palato** means palate and **plasty** means surgical repair).

Stomach

- A **gastrectomy** (gas-**TRECK**-toh-mee) is the surgical removal of all or a part of the stomach (**gastr** means stomach and **ectomy** means surgical removal).

- A **gastrotomy** (gas-**TROT**-oh-mee) is a surgical incision into the stomach (**gastr** means stomach and **otomy** means a surgical incision into).
- **Nasogastric intubation** (nay-zoh-**GAS**-trick in-too-**BAY**-shun) is the placement of a tube through the nose and into the stomach.

Intestines

- **Anoplasty** (**AY**-noh-**plas**-tee) is the surgical repair of the anus (**ano** means anus and **plasty** means surgical repair).
- A **colectomy** (koh-**LECK**-toh-mee) is the surgical removal of all or part of the colon (**col** means colon and **ectomy** means surgical removal).
- A **colotomy** (koh-**LOT**-oh-mee) is a surgical incision into the colon (**col** means colon and **otomy** means a surgical incision into).
- A **diverticulectomy** (**dye**-ver-**tick**-you-**LECK**-toh-mee) is the surgical removal of a diverticulum (**diverticul** means diverticulum and **ectomy** means surgical removal).
- A **gastroduodenostomy** (gas-troh-**dew**-oh-deh-**NOS**-toh-mee) is the removal of the pylorus of the stomach and the establishment of an anastomosis (connection) between the upper portion of the stomach and the duodenum (Figure 8.11). An **anastomosis** (ah-**nas**-toh-**MOH**-sis) is a surgical connection between two hollow or tubular structures (plural, **anastomoses**).
- A **hemorrhoidectomy** (**hem**-oh-roid-**ECK**-toh-mee) is the surgical removal of hemorrhoids (**hemorrhoid** means piles and **ectomy** means surgical removal).
- An **ileectomy** (ill-ee-**ECK**-toh-mee) is the surgical removal of the ileum (**ile** means the ileum and **ectomy** means surgical removal. Notice that this is term is spelled with two *e*s.)
- A **proctectomy** (prock-**TECK**-toh-mee) is the surgical removal of the rectum (**proct** means rectum and **ectomy** means surgical removal).

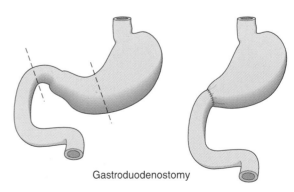

Gastroduodenostomy

FIGURE 8.11 In a gastroduodenostomy an anastomosis is formed where the stomach and duodenum are surgically joined.

- **Proctopexy** (**PROCK**-toh-**peck**-see) is the surgical fixation of the rectum to an adjacent tissue or organ (**proc-to** means rectum and **pexy** means surgical fixation).

- **Proctoplasty** (**PROCK**-toh-**plas**-tee) is the surgical repair of the rectum (**procto** means rectum and **plasty** means surgical repair).

Ostomies

An **ostomy** (**OSS**-toh-mee) is a surgical procedure to create an artificial opening between an organ and the body surface. This opening is called a **stoma** (**STOH**-mah). *Ostomy* can be used alone as a noun to describe a procedure or as a suffix with the word part that describes the organ involved.

- A **gastrostomy** (gas-**TROS**-toh-mee) is the surgical creation of an artificial opening into the stomach (**gastr** means stomach and **ostomy** means surgically creating an opening). This procedure is frequently performed for the placement of a permanent feeding tube.

- An **ileostomy** (**ill**-ee-**OS**-toh-mee) is the surgical creation of an opening between the ileum, at the end of the small intestine, and the abdominal wall (**ile** means small intestine and **ostomy** means surgically creating an opening).

- A **colostomy** (koh-**LAHS**-toh-mee) is the surgical creation of an opening between the colon and the body surface (**col** means colon and **ostomy** means surgically creating an opening). The entire segment of the intestine below the ostomy is usually removed and an effluent (moved discharge) flows from the stoma. A colostomy *may* be temporary, to divert feces from an area that needs to heal. Colostomies are named for the part of the colon where the stoma, or exit point, is located (Figure 8.12).

Ascending colostomy

Transverse colostomy

Descending colostomy

Sigmoid colostomy

FIGURE 8.12 Colostomy sites vary depending on the part of the bowel removed. The stoma is located at the end of the remaining intestine (shown in brown). The portion that has been removed is shown in blue.

Liver

- A **hepatectomy** (**hep**-ah-**TECK**-toh-mee) is the surgical removal of all or part of the liver (**hepat** means liver and **ectomy** means surgical removal).

- **Hepatotomy** (**hep**-ah-**TOT**-oh-mee) is a surgical incision into the liver (**hepat** means liver and **otomy** means surgical incision).

- **Hepatorrhaphy** (**hep**-ah-**TOR**-ah-fee) means to suture the liver (**hepato** means liver and **rrhaphy** means to suture).

- A **liver transplant** is an option for a patient whose liver has failed for a reason other than liver cancer. Because liver tissue regenerates, a partial transplant, in which only part of a liver is donated, may be adequate.

Gallbladder

- A **choledocholithotomy** (**koh**-**led**-oh-koh-lih-**THOT**-oh-mee) is an incision in the common bile duct for the removal of gallstones (**choledocho** means the common bile duct, **lith** means stone, and **otomy** means surgical incision).

- **Laparoscopic cholecystectomy** (**koh**-lee-sis-**TECK**-toh-mee), also known as a **lap choley**, is the surgical removal of the gallbladder using a laparoscope and other instruments while working through very small openings in the abdominal wall (Figure 8.13).

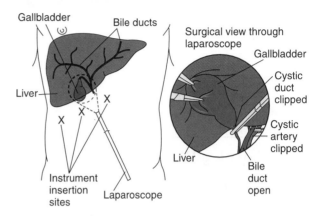

FIGURE 8.13 A lap choley is the surgical removal of the gallbladder using a laparoscope and other instruments.

CHAPTER

8

Learning Exercises

● Matching Word Parts—1

Write the letter of the correct answer on the line provided in the left column.

8.1. _____ enter/o   A. anus

8.2. _____ an/o   B. bile, gall

8.3. _____ cec/o   C. large intestine

8.4. _____ chol/e   D. cecum, blind gut

8.5. _____ col/o, colon/o   E. small intestine

● Matching Word Parts—2

Write the letter of the correct answer on the line provided in the left column.

8.6. _____ -lithiasis   A. stomach

8.7. _____ gastr/o   B. liver

8.8. _____ esophag/o   C. gallbladder

8.9. _____ hepat/o   D. esophagus

8.10. _____ cholecyst/o   E. presence of stones

● Matching Word Parts—3

Write the letter of the correct answer on the line provided in the left column.

8.11. _____ -pepsia   A. sigmoid colon

8.12. _____ pancreat/o   B. anus and rectum

8.13. _____ proct/o   C. digestion

8.14. _____ rect/o   D. pancreas

8.15. _____ sigmoid/o   E. rectum

● Definitions

Circle the letter next to the correct answer.

8.16. Which term means the visual examination of the anal canal and lower rectum performed using a speculum?

a. anoscopy

b. colonoscopy

c. proctoscopy

d. sigmoidoscopy

8.17. Which salivary glands are located on the face in front of, and slightly lower than, each ear?

a. maxillary

b. parotid

c. sublingual

d. submandibular

8.18. Which posterior teeth are used for grinding and chewing?

a. canines

b. cuspids

c. incisors

d. molars

8.19. The liver removes excess _____ from the bloodstream.

a. bilirubin

b. glucose

c. glycogen

d. lipase

8.20. Which substance is stored and concentrated by the gallbladder for later use?

a. bile

b. glycogen

c. hydrochloric acid

d. pepsin

8.21. The duodenum is part of the _____.

a. cecum

b. large intestine

c. small intestine

d. stomach

8.22. Which term describes the process of breaking down body cells or substances?

a. anabolism

b. catabolism

c. defecation

d. dentition

8.23. The receptors for the sense of taste are located on the _____.

a. hard palate

b. rugae

c. tongue

d. uvula

8.24. What specialized mucous membrane surrounds each tooth?

a. cementum

b. dentin

c. gingiva

d. pulp

8.25. Which medical condition is characterized by the telescoping of one part of the intestine into another?

a. borborygmus

b. flatus

c. intussusception

d. volvulus

Matching Structures

Write the letter of the correct answer on the line provided in the left column.

8.26. _____ cecum

8.27. _____ ileum

8.28. _____ jejunum

8.29. _____ rectum

8.30. _____ sigmoid colon

A. Pouch that lies on the right side of the abdomen and connects the small and large intestine.

B. Major part of the large intestine leading into the rectum.

C. Last division of the large intestine.

D. Middle portion of the small intestine.

E. Last portion of the small intestine.

Which Word?

Circle the correct term in each sentence.

8.31. The word that means vomiting blood is called *hematemesis / hyperemesis.*

8.32. *Hepatitis A / Hepatitis B* is transmitted by contaminated food and water.

8.33. An often fatal form of food poisoning is *bulimia / botulism.*

8.34. The medical term meaning an inflammation of the small intestine is *colitis / enteritis.*

8.35. The *vovulus / uvula* hangs from the free edge of the soft palate.

Spelling Counts

Find the misspelled word in each sentence. Then write that word, spelled correctly, on the line provided.

8.36. An ilectomy is the surgical removal of the last portion of the small intestine. _____

8.37. The cecum is connected to the ileum by the iliocecal sphincter. _____

8.38. Hepatarrhaphy means to suture the liver. _____

8.39. Proctoplexy is the surgical fixation of the rectum to some adjacent tissue or organ. _____

8.40. Hepatitus is an inflammation of the liver caused by a virus or by damage from toxic substances. _____

● Matching Abbreviations

Write the letter of the correct answer on the line provided in the left column.

8.41. _____ GI   A. irritable bowel syndrome

8.42. _____ DDS   B. ova and parasites

8.43. _____ IBS   C. gastrointestinal

8.44. _____ O & P   D. Doctor of Dental Surgery

8.45. _____ ORT   E. oral rehydration therapy

● Term Selection

Circle the letter next to the correct answer.

8.46. Which term means the surgical removal of all or part of the stomach?

     a. gastrectomy

     b. gastritis

     c. gastroenteritis

     d. gastrotomy

8.47. What term refers to difficulty in swallowing?

     a. anorexia

     b. dyspepsia

     c. dysphagia

     d. pyrosis

8.48. What term means a surgical incision into the colon?

     a. colectomy

     b. colostomy

     c. colotomy

     d. proctectomy

8.49. Which term refers to a disease that causes progressive degeneration of the liver?

     a. cirrhosis

     b. hepatomegaly

     c. hepatitis

     d. hepatorrhexis

8.50 Which term describes the pigment produced by the destruction of hemoglobin in the liver?

     a. bile

     b. bilirubin

     c. hydrochloric acid

     d. pancreatic juice

● Sentence Completion

Write the correct term on the line.

8.51. The folds in the mucosa lining the mouth and of the stomach are known as _____.

8.52. The return of swallowed food to the mouth is called _____ .

8.53. A yellow discoloration of the skin caused by greater than normal amounts of bilirubin in the blood is called _____.

8.54. The flow from the stomach to the duodenum is controlled by the _____ sphincter.

8.55. The medical term for the solid body wastes that are expelled through the rectum is/are _____.

● True/False

If the statement is true, write T on the line. If the statement is false, write F on the line.

8.56. _____ Amebic dysentery is an inflammation of the intestine caused by *Entamoeba histolytica*.

8.57. _____ Hepatitis B can be prevented through immunization.

8.58. _____ Bruxism means to be without natural teeth.

8.59. _____ Gastrorrhagia means the excessive flow of gastric secretions.

8.60. _____ Eructation is the act of belching or raising gas orally from the stomach.

8.61. _____ Cholelithiasis is the presence of stones in the large intestine.

8.62. _____ Fatty substances in a stool sample indicate a parasite problem.

8.63. _____ Periodontitis is the progressive destruction of dental enamel.

8.64. _____ Pica is a craving for nonnutritional substances such as clay.

8.65. _____ A choledocholithotomy is an incision in the common bile duct for the removal of gallstones.

● Clinical Conditions

Write the correct answer on the line.

8.66. James Ridgeview was treated for the temporary stoppage of intestinal peristalsis. The medical term for this condition is _____ .

8.67. Chang Hoon suffers from an inflammation of the stomach. The medical term for this condition is _____ .

8.68. Dr. Martinson described the patient as being _____ which means he was without natural teeth.

8.69. Baby Kilgore was vomiting almost continuously. The medical term for this excessive vomiting is _____ .

8.70. A/An _____ was performed on Mr. Gonzalez to create an opening between the colon and the body surface.

8.71. After eating Mr. Delahanty often suffers from heartburn. The medical term for this condition is _____ .

8.72. Catherine Baldwin's presenting symptom was the passage of black stools containing digested blood. The medical term for this condition is _____ .

8.73. Alberta Roberts was diagnosed as having an inflammation of one or more diverticulum. The medical term for this condition is _____ .

8.74. Jason Norton suffers from _____ labialis, which is also known as cold sores.

8.75. Lisa Wilson saw her dentist because she was concerned about bad breath. Her dentist refers to this condition as _____ .

● Which is the correct medical term?

Circle the letter next to the correct answer

8.76. Which term refers to a test for hidden blood in the stools?
a. anoscopy
b. colonoscopy
c. enema
d. hemoccult

8.77. In a patient with a colostomy the effluent flows from the _____ .
a. colon
b. ileus
c. rectum
d. stoma

8.78. What is the eating disorder characterized by binge eating followed by self-induced vomiting or the misuse of laxatives?
a. anorexia
b. bulimia
c. nervosa
d. pica

8.79. Which term describes the soft deposit of bacteria and bacterial by-products on the teeth that can lead to dental decay and periodontal disease?
a. calculus
b. caries
c. gingiva
d. plaque

8.80. Which medical term means the surgical repair of the rectum?
a. anoplasty
b. palatoplasty
c. proctopexy
d. proctoplasty

● Challenge Word Building

These terms are *not* found in this chapter; however, they are made up of these familiar word parts. You may want to look in the glossary or use a medical dictionary to check your answers!

co/o	-algia
enter/o	-ectomy
esophag/o	-itis
gastr/o	-megaly
hepat/o	-ic
proct/o	-pexy
sigmoid/o	-rrhexis

8.81. The medical term meaning to suture the injured stomach is _____ .

8.82. The medical term meaning pain in the esophagus is _____ .

8.83. The medical term meaning the surgical removal of all or part of the sigmoid colon is _____ .

8.84. The medical term meaning pain in and around the anus and rectum is _____ .

8.85. The medical term meaning the surgical fixation of the stomach to correct displacement is _____ .

8.86. The medical term meaning inflammation of the sigmoid colon is _____ .

8.87. The medical term meaning the surgical removal of all or part of the esophagus and stomach is _____ .

8.88. The medical term meaning referring to the liver and intestines is _____ .

8.89. The medical term meaning the abnormal enlargement of the liver is _____ .

8.90. The medical term meaning inflammation of the stomach, small intestine and large intestine is _____ .

● Labeling Exercises

Identify the numbered items on this diagram.

8.91. _____ glands

8.92. _____

8.93. _____

8.94. _____

8.95. _____

8.96. _____

8.97. _____ intestine

8.98. vermiform _____

8.99. _____ intestine

8.100. _____ and anus

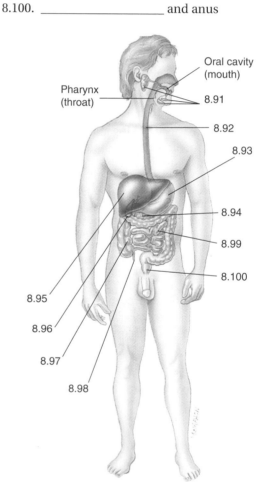

Oral cavity (mouth)

Pharynx (throat)

8.91
8.92
8.93
8.94
8.99
8.100
8.95
8.96
8.97
8.98

The Human Touch: Critical Thinking Exercise

The following story and questions are designed to stimulate critical thinking through class discussion or as a brief essay response. There are no easy or right-wrong answers to these questions.

"Stick the landing and our team walks away with the gold!" Coach Schaefer meant to be supportive as she squeezed Claire's shoulder. "What you mean is beat Leia's score for the Riverview team and we'll win," Claire thought sarcastically. She watched as Leia's numbers were shown from her last vault. A 6.8 out of a possible 7. "Great, just great! She chooses a less difficult vault, but with that toothpick body she gets more height than I ever will!" She wondered if Leia was naturally that thin, or did she use the secret method — you can't gain weight if the food doesn't stay in your stomach.

All season it had been that way. Everyone seemed to be watching the rivalry between West High's Claire and Riverview's "tiny-mighty" Leia. Claire was pretty sure that her 10-pound weight loss had improved both her floor routine and her tricky dismount off the beam. "I'm less than a half point behind, so coach should be happy," she thought. But just last week Coach Schaefer had a long talk with her when she got dizzy and fell off the balance beam. She asked Claire the one question she swore she'd never answer: "Just what have you been doing to lose the weight?"

Claire felt her hands sweat. "Just stick the landing," she told herself, but her body had a different agenda. Starved for fuel, her muscles failed, and the gold slipped out of reach.

Suggested Discussion Topics:

1. Who do you think sets the standards for how a person thinks he or she should look?

2. List several eating disorders. What personality traits do you think cause a person to develop eating disorders?

3. Discuss why anorexia and bulimia usually occur in young women between the ages of 12 and 28.

4. Athletes sometime abuse their bodies through dieting or drugs to achieve peak performances. What should the groups that oversee competitive athletics do about this?

5. Imagine you have a daughter. How would you know if she had an eating disorder? What kind of treatment might help her?

CHAPTER

9

The Urinary System

● **Overview of Structures, Word Parts, and Functions of the Urinary System**

Major Structures	Related Word Roots	Primary Functions
Kidneys	nephr/o, ren/o	Filter the blood to remove waste products, maintain electrolyte concentrations, and remove excess water to maintain the fluid volume within the body.
Renal pelvis	pyel/o	Collects urine produced by the kidney.
Urine	-uria, urin/o	Liquid waste products to be excreted.
Ureters	ureter/o	Transport urine from the kidneys to the bladder.
Urinary bladder	cyst/o, vesic/o	Store urine until it is excreted.
Urethra	urethr/o	Transports urine from bladder through the urethral meatus where it is excreted from the body.

● VOCABULARY   Related to the Urinary System

Check the box as you master each word part or term. Terms marked with the ❖ symbol are pronounced on the optional student audiotape.

Key Word Parts

- ☐ dia-
- ☐ -cele
- ☐ cyst/o
- ☐ -ectasis
- ☐ glomerul/o
- ☐ lith/o
- ☐ -lysis
- ☐ nephr/o
- ☐ -pexy
- ☐ pyel/o
- ☐ ren/o
- ☐ -tripsy
- ☐ ureter/o
- ☐ urethr/o
- ☐ -uria

Key Medical Terms

- ☐ **anuria** (ah-**NEW**-ree-ah) ❖
- ☐ **catheterization** (**kath**-eh-ter-eye-**ZAY**-shun) ❖
- ☐ **cystalgia** (sis-**TAL**-jee-ah) ❖
- ☐ **cystectomy** (sis-**TECK**-toh-mee) ❖
- ☐ **cystitis** (sis-**TYE**-tis) ❖
- ☐ **cystocele** (**SIS**-toh-seel) ❖
- ☐ **cystography** (sis-**TOG**-rah-fee) ❖
- ☐ **cystolith** (**SIS**-toh-lith) ❖
- ☐ **cystopexy** (**sis**-toh-**peck**-see) ❖
- ☐ **cystorrhagia** (**sis**-toh-**RAY**-jee-ah) ❖
- ☐ **cystorrhaphy** (sis-**TOR**-ah-fee) ❖
- ☐ **cystoscopy** (sis-**TOS**-koh-pee) ❖
- ☐ **diuresis** (**dye**-you-**REE**-sis) ❖
- ☐ **diuretics** (**dye**-you-**RET**-icks)
- ☐ **dysuria** (dis-**YOU**-ree-ah) ❖
- ☐ **enuresis** (**en**-you-**REE**-sis) ❖
- ☐ **epispadias** (**ep**-ih-**SPAY**-dee-as) ❖
- ☐ **glomerulonephritis** (gloh-**mer**-you-loh-neh-**FRY**-tis) ❖
- ☐ **glomerulus** (gloh-**MER**-you-lus)
- ☐ **hemodialysis** (**hee**-moh-dye-**AL**-ih-sis) ❖
- ☐ **homeostasis** (**hoh**-mee-oh-**STAY**-sis)
- ☐ **hydronephrosis** (**high**-droh-neh-**FROH**-sis) ❖
- ☐ **hydroureter** (**high**-droh-you-**REE**-ter)
- ☐ **hypospadias** (**high**-poh-**SPAY**-dee-as) ❖
- ☐ **incontinence** (in-**KON**-tih-nents)
- ☐ **interstitial cystitis** (in-ter-**STISH**-al sis-**TYE**-tis)
- ☐ **lithotomy** (lih-**THOT**-oh-mee)
- ☐ **lithotripsy** (**LITH**-oh-**trip**-see) ❖
- ☐ **meatotomy** (**mee**-ah-**TOT**-oh-mee) ❖

- ☐ **micturition** (**mick**-too-**RISH**-un)
- ☐ **nephrectasis** (neh-**FRECK**-tah-sis) ❖
- ☐ **nephritis** (neh-**FRY**-tis)
- ☐ **nephrolith** (**NEF**-roh-lith) ❖
- ☐ **nephrolithiasis** (**nef**-roh-lih-**THIGH**-ah-sis) ❖
- ☐ **nephrolithotomy** (**nef**-roh-lih-**THOT**-oh-mee) ❖
- ☐ **nephrologist** (neh-**FROL**-oh-jist)
- ☐ **nephrolysis** (neh-**FROL**-ih-sis) ❖
- ☐ **nephropathy** (neh-**FROP**-ah-thee)
- ☐ **nephropexy** (**NEF**-roh-**peck**-see) ❖
- ☐ **nephroptosis** (**nef**-rop-**TOH**-sis) ❖
- ☐ **nephropyosis** (**nef**-roh-pye-**OH**-sis) ❖
- ☐ **nephrosis** (neh-**FROH**-sis) v
- ☐ **nephrostomy** (neh-**FROS**-toh-me)
- ☐ **nephrotic syndrome** (neh-**FROT**-ick) ❖
- ☐ **nocturia** (nock-**TOO**-ree-ah) ❖
- ☐ **oliguria** (ol-ih-**GOO**-ree-ah) ❖
- ☐ **paraspadias** (**par**-ah-**SPAY**-dee-as) ❖
- ☐ **peritoneal dialysis** (**pehr**-ih-toh-**NEE**-al dye-**AL**-ih-sis) ❖
- ☐ **polyuria** (**pol**-ee-**YOU**-ree-ah) ❖
- ☐ **pyelitis** (**pye**-eh-**LYE**-tis) ❖
- ☐ **pyelogram** (**PYE**-eh-loh-**gram**) ❖
- ☐ **pyelonephritis** (**pye**-eh-loh-neh-**FRY**-tis) ❖
- ☐ **pyeloplasty** (**PYE**-eh-loh-**plas**-tee) ❖
- ☐ **pyelotomy** (**pye**-eh-**LOT**-oh-mee) ❖
- ☐ **suprapubic** (**soo**-prah-**PYOU**-bick)
- ☐ **uremia** (you-**REE**-mee-ah) ❖
- ☐ **ureterectasis** (you-**ree**-ter-**ECK**-tah-sis) ❖
- ☐ **ureterectomy** (**you**-ree-ter-**ECK**-toh-mee) ❖
- ☐ **ureterolith** (you-**REE**-ter-oh-**lith**) ❖
- ☐ **ureteroplasty** (you-**REE**-ter-oh-**plas**-tee) ❖
- ☐ **ureterorrhagia** (you-**ree**-ter-oh-**RAY**-jee-ah) ❖
- ☐ **ureterorrhaphy** (**you**-ree-ter-**OR**-ah-fee)
- ☐ **ureterostenosis** (you-**ree**-ter-oh-steh-**NOH**-sis) ❖
- ☐ **urethralgia** (**you**-ree-**THRAL**-jee-ah) ❖
- ☐ **urethritis** (**you**-reh-**THRIGH**-tis) ❖
- ☐ **urethropexy** (you-**REE**-throh-**peck**-see) ❖
- ☐ **urethroplasty** (you-**REE**-throh-**plas**-tee) ❖
- ☐ **urethrorrhagia** (you-**ree**-throh-**RAY**-jee-ah) ❖
- ☐ **urethrorrhaphy** (**you**-reh-**THROR**-ah-fee) ❖
- ☐ **urethrorrhea** (you-**ree**-throh-**REE**-ah) ❖
- ☐ **urethrostenosis** (you-**ree**-throh-steh-**NOH**-sis) ❖
- ☐ **urethrostomy** (**you**-reh-**THROS**-toh-mee) ❖
- ☐ **urethrotomy** (**you**-reh-**THROT**-oh-mee) ❖
- ☐ **urography** (you-**ROG**-rah-fee) ❖
- ☐ **vesicovaginal fissure** (**ves**-ih-koh-**VAG**-ih-nahl)

Functions of the Urinary System

The urinary system performs many functions that are important in maintaining **homeostasis** (hoh-mee-oh-**STAY**-sis), a state of equilibrium that produces a constant internal environment throughout the body (homeo means sameness and stasis means control). To achieve this, the urinary system

- Maintains the proper balance of water, salts, and acids in the body fluids by removing excess fluids from the body, or reabsorbing water as needed.

- Constantly filters the blood to remove urea and other waste materials from the bloodstream. **Urea** (you-**REE**-ah) is the major waste product of protein metabolism.

- Converts these waste products and excess fluids into **urine** in the kidneys and excretes them from the body via the urinary bladder.

Structures of the Urinary System

The urinary system consists of two kidneys, two ureters, one bladder, and a urethra (Figure 9.1). The adrenal glands, which are part of the endocrine system, are located on the top of the kidneys.

The Kidneys

The kidneys constantly filter the blood to remove waste products and excess water. These are excreted as urine, which is 95% water and 5% other wastes.

- The two kidneys are located retroperitoneally (behind the peritoneum, the membrane that lines the abdominal cavity) with one on each side of the vertebral column below the diaphragm.

- Each kidney consists of two layers that surround the **renal pelvis** (Figure 9.2A). **Renal** (**REE**-nal) means pertaining to the kidneys.

- The **renal cortex** (**KOR**-tecks) is the outer layer of the kidney. It contains over one million microscopic units called **nephrons**.

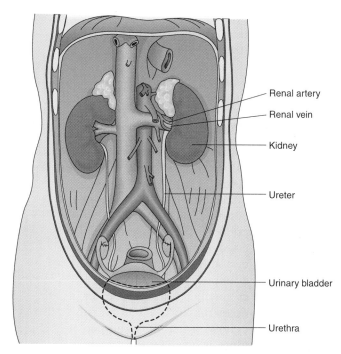

Renal artery
Renal vein
Kidney
Ureter
Urinary bladder
Urethra

FIGURE 9.1 Anterior view of the structures of the urinary system.

- The **medulla** (meh-**DULL**-ah) is the inner layer and it contains most of the urine-collecting tubules. (A **tubule** is a small tube.)

The Nephrons

Nephrons (**NEF**-rons) are the functional units of the kidneys. They form urine by the processes of filtration, reabsorption, and secretion (Figure 9.2B).

- Each nephron contains a **glomerulus** (gloh-**MER**-you-lus), which is a cluster of capillaries surrounded by a membrane called the Bowman's capsule (plural, **glomeruli**).

- Blood flows into the kidney through the renal artery. It is filtered in the capillaries of the glomerulus, and leaves the kidney through the renal vein.

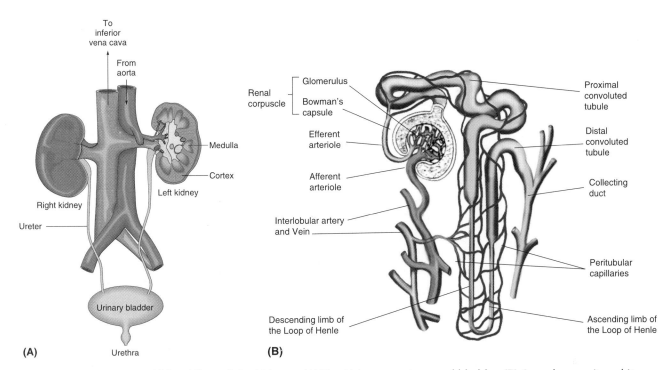

FIGURE 9.2 Structures and blood flow of the kidneys. (A) The kidneys, ureters, and bladder. (B) A nephron unit and its associated structures.

- Waste products pass through a series of urine-collecting tubules and are transported to the **renal pelvis** before entering the ureters.

- **Urochrome** (**YOU**-roh-krome) is the pigment that gives urine its normal yellow-amber or straw color (**uro** means urine and **chrome** means color). The color of urine can be influenced by normal factors such as the amount of liquid consumed or by diseases and medications.

The Ureters

The **ureters** (you-REE-ters) are narrow tubes, each about 10 to 12 inches long. Each ureter carries urine from a kidney to the urinary bladder.

The Urinary Bladder

The **urinary bladder** (Figure 9.3) is a hollow muscular organ that is a reservoir for urine. It is located in the anterior portion of the pelvic cavity behind the pubic symphysis and stores about 1 pint of urine. In a pregnant woman, the uterus resting on the bladder may decrease its capacity.

The Urethra

The **urethra** (you-REE-thrah) is the tube extending from the bladder to the outside of the body. ■ **Caution:** The spelling of *ureter* and *urethra* are very similar!

- Two **urinary sphincters**, one located at either end of the urethra, control the flow of urine from the bladder into the urethra and out of the urethra through the urethral meatus. (A **sphincter** is a ringlike muscle that closes a passageway.)

- The **urethral meatus** (you-REE-thrahl mee-**AY**-tus), also known as the **urinary meatus**, is the external opening of the urethra.

- The **female urethra** is approximately 1.5 inches long. The urethral meatus is located between the clitoris and the opening of the vagina. In the female, the urethra conveys only urine (see Figure 9.3).

- The **male urethra** is approximately 8 inches long and the urethral meatus is located at the tip of the penis. In the male, the urethra conveys both urine and semen. The neck of the urethra is surrounded by the prostate gland (see Figure 9.3) that is part of the reproductive system and is discussed in Chapter 14.

The Excretion of Urine

As the bladder fills up, pressure is placed on the base of the urethra, resulting in the urge to **urinate** or **micturate**.

- **Urination**, also known as **micturition** (**mick**-too-**RISH**-un) or **voiding**, is the normal process of excreting urine.

- Urination requires the coordinated contraction of the bladder muscles and relaxation of the sphincters. This forces the urine through the urethra and out through the urinary meatus.

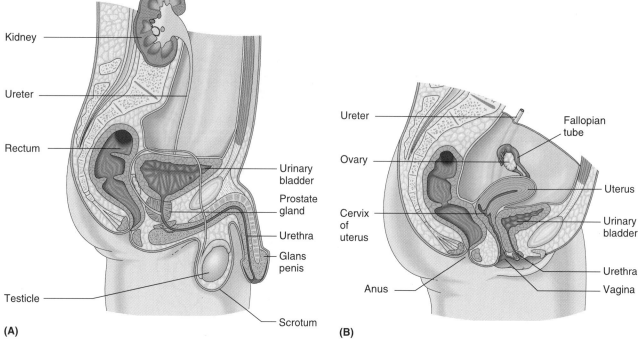

FIGURE 9.3 Cross-sectional view of the urinary structures. (A) Male. (B) Female.

Medical Specialties Related to the Urinary System

- A **nephrologist** (neh-**FROL**-oh-jist) specializes in diagnosing and treating diseases and disorders of the kidneys (**nephr** means kidney and **ologist** means specialist).

- A **urologist** (you-**ROL**-oh-jist) specializes in diagnosing and treating diseases and disorders of the urinary system of females and the genitourinary system of males (**ur** means urine and **ologist** means specialist).

Pathology of the Urinary System

Renal Failure

Renal failure, also known as **kidney failure**, is the inability of the kidney or kidneys to perform their functions. The body cannot replace damaged nephrons. When too many nephrons have been destroyed, the result is kidney failure.

- **Anuria** (ah-**NEW**-ree-ah), also known as **anuresis** (an-you-**REE**-sis), is the complete suppression (stopping) of urine formation by the kidneys (**an** means without and **uria** means urination).

- **Uremia** (you-**REE**-mee-ah), also known as **uremic poisoning**, is a toxic condition caused by excessive amount of urea and other waste products in the bloodstream (**ur** means urine and **emia** means blood condition).

- **Acute renal failure**, also known as **ARF**, has sudden onset and is characterized by uremia. ARF may be caused by many factors, including a drop in blood volume or blood pressure due to injury or surgery.

- **Chronic renal failure**, also known as **CRF**, is a progressive disease that may be caused by a variety of conditions. When kidney function is insufficient, dialysis or transplantation is required.

- **End-stage renal disease**, also known as **ESRD**, refers to the late stages of chronic renal failure.

Nephrotic Syndrome

Nephrotic syndrome (neh-**FROT**-ick), also known as **NS**, is a general group of kidney diseases (**nephro** means kidney and **tic** means pertaining to). The following are characteristics of kidney malfunction diseases:

- Edema (excessive fluid in the body tissue)

- Hyperproteinuria (abnormally *high* concentrations of protein (albumin) in the urine)

- Hypoproteinemia (abnormally *low* concentrations of protein (albumin) in the blood)

- Hyperlipidemia (abnormally *large* amount of lipids in the blood)

Nephrosis

- **Nephrosis** (neh-**FROH**-sis) and **nephropathy** (neh-**FROP**-ah-thee) both mean diseases of the kidney and these terms are used interchangeably with nephrotic syndrome (**nephr/o** means kidney and **osis** means abnormal condition).

- **Diabetic nephropathy** is a result of the damage to the kidney's capillary blood vessels that is caused by long-term diabetes mellitus (**nephr/o** means kidney and **pathy** means disease).

Kidneys

- **Glomerulonephritis** (gloh-**mer**-you-loh-neh-**FRY**-tis) is an inflammation of the kidney involving primarily the glomeruli (**glomerulo** means glomeruli, **nephr** means kidney, and **itis** means inflammation). In acute glomerulonephritis, the urine is dark brown or black in color. This condition is often related to an autoimmune problem.

- **Hydronephrosis** (**high**-droh-neh-**FROH**-sis) is the dilation (enlargement) of the renal pelvis of one or both kidneys (**hydro** means water, **nephr** means kidney, and **osis** means abnormal condition). This is the result of an obstruction of the flow of urine (Figure 9.4).

- **Nephrectasis** (neh-**FRECK**-tah-sis) is the distention of a kidney (**nephr** means kidney and **ectasis** means enlargement or stretching. **Distended** means enlarged).

- **Nephritis** (neh-**FRY**-tis) is an inflammation of the kidney (**nephr** means kidney and **itis** means inflammation).

- **Nephroptosis** (**nef**-rop-**TOH**-sis), also known as a **floating kidney**, is the downward displacement of the kidney (**nephro** means kidney and **ptosis** means drooping or dropping down).

- **Nephropyosis** (**nef**-roh-pye-**OH**-sis) is suppuration of the kidney (**nephro** means kidney, **py** means pus, and **osis** means condition). **Suppuration** means the formation or discharge of pus.

- **Pyelitis** (pye-eh-**LYE**-tis) is an inflammation of the renal pelvis (**pyel** means renal pelvis and **itis** means inflammation).

- **Pyelonephritis** (pye-eh-loh-neh-**FRY**-tis) is an inflammation of the renal pelvis and of the kidney (**pyeol** means renal pelvis, **nephr** means kidney, and **itis** means inflammation).

- **Renal colic** (**REE**-nal **KOLL**-ick) is an acute pain in the kidney area that is caused by blockage during the passage of a kidney stone.

Stones

A **stone**, also known as **calculus** (**KAL**-kyou-luhs), is an abnormal mineral deposit (plural, **calculi**). These stones vary in size from small sandlike granules to the size of marbles and are named for the organ or tissue where they are located (Figure 9.5 and Table 9.1).

- **Nephrolithiasis** (**nef**-roh-lih-**THIGH**-ah-sis) is a disorder characterized by the presence of stones in the kidney (**nephro** means kidney and **lithiasis** means the presence of stones).

Ureters

- **Hydroureter** (**high**-droh-you-**REE**-ter) is distention (stretching out) of the ureter with urine that cannot flow because the ureter is blocked (**hydro** means water and **ureter** means ureter). See Figure 9.4.

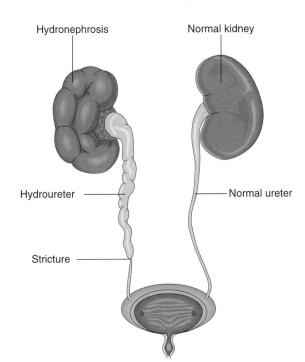

FIGURE 9.4 Hydroureter and hydronephrosis resulting from a urethral stricture.

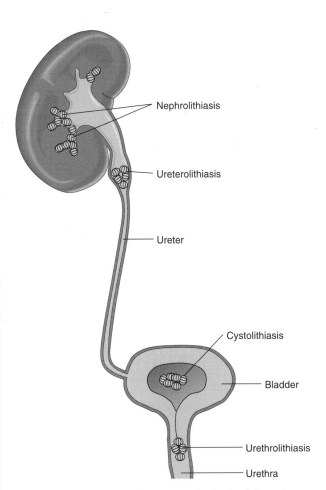

FIGURE 9.5 Names and locations of calculi of the urinary system.

Table 9.1

TYPES AND LOCATIONS OF URINARY STONES

Type of Stone	Word Parts	Location
Cystolith (**SIS**-toh-lith)	**cysto** means bladder **lith** means stone	Urinary bladder
Nephrolith (**NEF**-roh-lith), also known as **renal calculus** or a **kidney stone**	**nephro** means kidney **lith** means stone	Kidney
Ureterolith (you-**REE**-ter-oh-**lith**)	**uretero** means ureter **lith** means stone	Ureter

- **Ureterectasis** (you-**ree**-ter-ECK-tah-sis) means distention of a ureter (**ureter** means ureter and **ectasis** means enlargement).
- **Ureterorrhagia** (you-**ree**-ter-oh-RAY-jee-ah) is the discharge of blood from the ureter (**ureter** means ureter and **rrhagia** means bleeding).
- **Ureterostenosis** (you-**ree**-ter-oh-steh-NOH-sis) is a stricture of the ureter (**ureter** means ureter and **stenosis** means abnormal narrowing). A **stricture** is an abnormal band of tissue narrowing a body passage.

Urinary Bladder

- **Cystalgia** (sis-TAL-jee-ah) and **cystodynia** (sis-toh-DIN-ee-ah) both mean pain in the urinary bladder (**cyst** means bladder and **algia** means pain).
- **Cystitis** (sis-TYE-tis) is an inflammation of the bladder (**cyst** mean bladder and **itis** means inflammation).
- **Interstitial cystitis** (**in**-ter-STISH-al sis-TYE-tis) is an inflammation within the wall of the bladder. This is a chronic condition with symptoms similar to those of cystitis.
- A **cystocele** (SIS-toh-seel) is a hernia of the bladder through the vaginal wall (**cysto** means bladder and **cele** means hernia).
- **Cystorrhagia** (sis-toh-RAY-jee-ah) is bleeding from the bladder (**cysto** means bladder and **rrhagia** means bleeding).
- **Urinary tract infections**, also known as **UTIs**, usually begin in the bladder. These infections occur more frequently in women because of the shortness of the urethra and the proximity of its opening to the vagina and rectum.
- A **vesicovaginal fissure** (ves-ih-koh-VAG-ih-nahl) is an abnormal opening between the bladder and vagina

(**vesico** means bladder, **vagin** means vagina, and **al** means pertaining to).

Urethra

- Blockage of the urethra can cause urine to back up into the ureters, called **reflux**. This can eventually result in damage to the kidneys.
- **Urethralgia** (you-ree-THRAL-jee-ah) is pain in the urethra (**urethr** means uretha and **algia** means pain).
- **Urethritis** (you-reh-THRIGH-tis) is an inflammation of the urethra (**urethr** means urethra and **itis** means inflammation).
- **Urethrorrhagia** (you-ree-throh-RAY-jee-ah) is bleeding from the urethra (**urethro** means urethra and **rrhagia** means bleeding).
- **Urethrorrhea** (you-ree-throh-REE-ah) is an abnormal discharge from the urethra (**urethro** means urethra and **rrhea** means abnormal flow).
- **Urethrostenosis** (you-ree-throh-steh-NOH-sis) is the stricture or stenosis of the urethra (**urethr** means urethra and **stenosis** means tightening or narrowing).

Abnormal Urethral Openings

- **Epispadias** (ep-ih-SPAY-dee-as) in the male is a congenital abnormality in which the urethral opening is located on the dorsal (upper surface) of the penis (**epi** means over). In the female with epispadias, the urethral opening is in the region of the clitoris.
- **Hypospadias** (high-poh-SPAY-dee-as) in the male is a congenital abnormality in which the urethral opening is on the undersurface of the penis (**hypo** means below). In the female with hypospadias the urethral opening is into the vagina.
- **Paraspadias** (par-ah-SPAY-dee-as) is a congenital abnormality in males in which the urethral opening is on one side of the penis (**para** means beside).

Urination

- **Diuresis** (dye-you-REE-sis) is the increased excretion of urine (**diur** means increasing the output of urine and **esis** means an abnormal condition).
- **Dysuria** (dis-YOU-ree-ah) is difficult or painful urination (**dys** means painful and **uria** means urination). This condition is frequently associated with UTIs.
- **Enuresis** (en-you-REE-sis) is the involuntary discharge of urine. **Nocturnal enuresis**, which occurs during sleep, is also known as **bed-wetting**. (Nocturnal means night.)
- **Nocturia** (nock-TOO-ree-ah) is excessive urination during the night (**noct** means night and **uria** means urination).
- **Oliguria** (ol-ih-GOO-ree-ah) means scanty urination (**olig** means scanty and **uria** means urination).

- **Polyuria** (pol-ee-**YOU**-ree-ah) means excessive urination (**poly** means many and **uria** means urination).
- **Urinary retention** is the inability to void or empty the bladder.

Incontinence

- **Incontinence** (in-**KON**-tih-nents) means the inability to control excretory functions.
- **Urinary incontinence** is the inability to control the voiding of urine.
- **Urinary stress incontinence** is the inability to control the voiding of urine under physical stress such as running, sneezing, laughing, or coughing.
- **Urge incontinence** is when urination occurs involuntarily as soon as an urgent desire to urinate is felt. This urge may be triggered by a physical movement rather than by a full bladder.

Diagnostic Procedures of the Urinary System

- **Catheterization** (kath-eh-ter-eye-**ZAY**-shun) is the insertion of a sterile catheter through the urethra and into the urinary bladder. This is most commonly performed to withdraw urine, relieve urinary retention pressures, or prevent incontinence during surgical procedures. A catheter may also be used to place fluid, such as a chemotherapy solution, into the bladder.
- **Cystoscopy** (sis-**TOS**-koh-pee), which is also known as **cysto**, is the visual examination of the urinary bladder using a cystoscope (**cysto** means bladder and **scopy** means visual examination). A **cystoscope** (**SIS**-toh-skope) also is used for treatment procedures such as the removal of tumors (see Figure 9.6).
- An **intravenous pyelogram** (**PYE**-eh-loh-**gram**), referred to as an **IVP**, is a radiographic (x-ray) study of the kidneys and ureters in which iodine is injected into a vein as a contrast medium to define these structures more clearly (**pyelo** means renal pelvis and **gram** means record).
- A **KUB** (kidneys, ureters, bladder) is a radiographic study of these structures without the use of a contrast medium. This study is also referred to as a **flat-plate of the abdomen**.
- **Intravenous urography** (you-**ROG**-rah-fee) is the radiographic visualization of the urinary tract with the use of a contrast medium (Figure 9.7). The resulting record is called a **urogram** (**uro** means urine and **gram** means record).
- **Excretory urography** is so named because it traces the action of the kidney as it processes and excretes dye injected into the bloodstream.

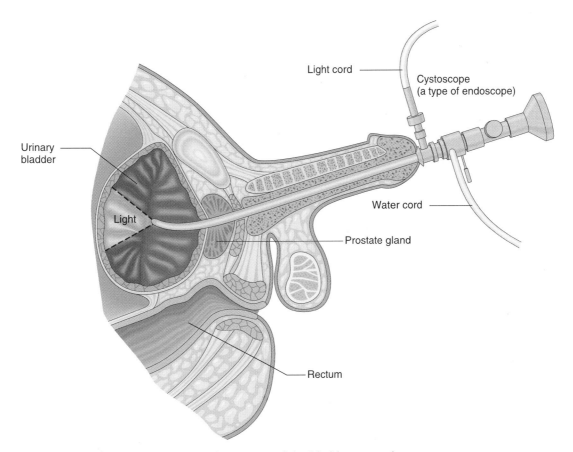

FIGURE 9.6 Use of a cystoscope to examine the interior of the bladder in a male.

Figure 9.7 An intravenous urogram showing the internal structures of the kidneys and ureters.

- **Retrograde urography** is a radiograph of the urinary system taken after dye has been placed in the urethra through a sterile catheter and caused to flow upward (backward) through the urinary tract.

- **Cystography** (sis-**TOG**-rah-fee) is a radiographic examination of the bladder after instillation of a contrast medium via a urethral catheter. The resulting film is called a **cystogram** (**cysto** means bladder and **gram** means record).

- **Voiding cystourethrography** (**sis**-toh-you-ree-**THROG**-rah-fee), also known as a **VCUG**, may be performed after cystography. In this diagnostic procedure a fluoroscope is used to examine the flow of urine from the bladder and through the urethra (**cysto** means bladder, **urethro** means urethra, and **graphy** means process of recording).

- **Urinalysis** (**you**-rih-**NAL**-ih-sis) is the examination of urine to determine the presence of abnormal elements. These tests are discussed in Chapter 15.

Treatment Procedures of the Urinary System

Medications

- **Diuretics** (**dye**-you-**RET**-icks) are medications administered to increase urine secretion to rid the body of excess sodium and water.

Dialysis

Dialysis (dye-**AL**-ih-sis) is a procedure to remove waste products from the blood of patients whose kidneys no longer function (**dia** means complete or through and **lysis** means separation). The two types of dialysis in common use are hemodialysis and peritoneal dialysis.

Hemodialysis

Hemodialysis (**hee**-moh-dye-**AL**-ih-sis), also known as **HD**, filters waste products from the patient's blood (**hemo** means blood, **dia** means complete or through, and **lysis** means separation). A shunt implanted in the patient's arm is connected to the artifical kidney machine and arterial blood flows through the filters. The filters contain **dialysate**, a solution made up of water and electrolytes, which removes excess fluids and waste from the blood. After these are removed the blood is returned to the body through a vein (Figure 9.8).

Figure 9.8 Hemodialysis filters waste from the patient's blood. Blood leaves the body via an artery, is filtered, and then returned into a vein.

Peritoneal Dialysis

In **peritoneal dialysis** (**pehr**-ih-toh-**NEE**-al dye-**AL**-ih-sis) the lining of the peritoneal cavity acts as the filter to remove waste from the blood. Dialysate solution is run into the peritoneal cavity and the fluid is exchanged through a catheter implanted in the abdominal wall. This type of dialysis is used for renal failure and also certain types of poisoning (Figure 9.9).

- **Continuous ambulatory peritoneal dialysis**, also known as **CAPD**, provides ongoing dialysis as the patient goes about his daily activities. In this procedure a dialysate solution is instilled from a plastic container worn under the patient's clothing. Every 6 to 8 hours the used solution is drained back into this bag and the bag discarded. A new bag is then attached, the solution is instilled, and the process continues.

- **Continuous cycling peritoneal dialysis**, also known as **CCPD**, uses a machine to cycle the dialysate fluid during the night while the patient sleeps.

FIGURE 9.9 Peritoneal dialysis removes waste through a fluid exchange in the peritoneal cavity.

Kidneys

- A **renal transplantation**, also known as a **kidney transplant**, is the grafting of a donor kidney into the body to replace the recipient's failed kidneys (Figure 9.10).
- **Nephrolysis** (neh-**FROL**-ih-sis) is the freeing of a kidney from adhesions (**nephro** means kidney and **lysis** means setting free). An **adhesion** (ad-**HEE**-zhun) is a band of fibers that holds structures together abnormally.
- *Note:* The suffix **-lysis** means setting free; however, it also means destruction. Therefore the term nephrolysis can also describe a pathologic condition in which there is the destruction of kidney substance.
- **Nephropexy** (**NEF**-roh-**peck**-see) is the surgical fixation of a floating kidney (**nephro** means kidney and **pexy** means surgical fixation).
- A **nephrostomy** (neh-**FROS**-toh-mee) is the establishment of an opening between the pelvis of the kidney through its cortex to the exterior of the body (**nephr** means kidney and **ostomy** means creating an opening).
- **Pyeloplasty** (**PYE**-eh-loh-**plas**-tee) is the surgical repair of the renal pelvis (**pyelo** means the renal pelvis and **plasty** means surgical repair).
- A **pyelotomy** (pye-eh-**LOT**-oh-mee) is a surgical incision into the renal pelvis (**pyel** means the renal pelvis and **otomy** means surgical incision).

Removal of Kidney Stones

- **Lithotripsy** (**LITH**-oh-**trip**-see), also known as **extracorporeal shock-wave lithotripsy** or ESWL, is the

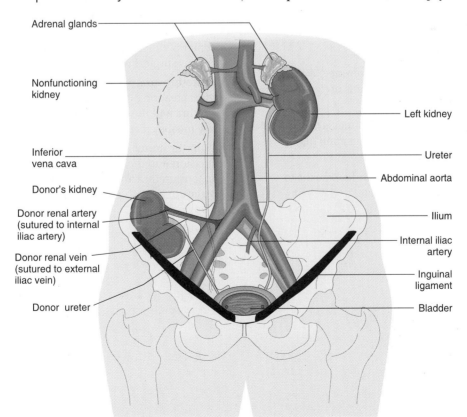

FIGURE 9.10 In a renal transplant the new kidney is placed lower in the abdomen.

destruction of a kidney stone with the use of ultrasonic waves traveling through water (**litho** means stone and **tripsy** means to crush). **Extracorporeal** means situated or occurring outside the body (Figure 9.11).

- A **nephrolithotomy** (**nef**-roh-lih-**THOT**-oh-mee) is the surgical removal of a kidney stone through an incision in the kidney (**nephro** means kidney, **lith** means stone, and **otomy** means surgical incision).

FIGURE 9.11 In extracorporeal lithotripsy the shock wave is transmitted through a water-filled cushion.

Ureters

- A **ureterectomy** (**you**-ree-ter-**ECK**-toh-mee) is the surgical removal of a ureter (**ureter** means ureter and **ectomy** means surgical removal).

- **Ureteroplasty** (you-**REE**-ter-oh-**plas**-tee) is the surgical repair of a ureter (**uretero** means ureter and **plasty** means surgical repair).

- **Ureterorrhaphy** (**you**-ree-ter-**OR**-ah-fee) means to suture a ureter (**uretero** means ureter and **rrhaphy** means to suture).

Urinary Bladder

- A **cystectomy** (sis-**TECK**-toh-mee) is the surgical removal of all or part of the urinary bladder (**cyst** means bladder and **ectomy** means surgical removal).

- **Cystopexy** (**SIS**-toh-**peck**-see) is the surgical fixation of the bladder to the abdominal wall (**cysto** means bladder and **pexy** means surgical fixation).

- **Cystorrhaphy** (sis-**TOR**-ah-fee) means suturing of the bladder (**cyst** means bladder and **rrhaphy** means to suture).

- A **lithotomy** (lih-**THOT**-oh-mee) is a surgical incision for the removal of a stone, usually from the bladder (**lith** means stone and **otomy** means surgical incision). This term also is used to describe a physical examination position, as discussed in Chapter 15.

- A **suprapubic catheter** (**soo**-prah-**PYOU**-bick) is an indwelling catheter placed into the bladder through a small incision made through the abdominal wall just *above* (**supra** means above) the pubic bone. (**Indwelling** means something that remains inside the body for a prolonged time.)

Urethra

- A **meatotomy** (**mee**-ah-**TOT**-oh-mee) is an incision of the urinary meatus to enlarge the opening (**meat** means meatus and **otomy** means surgical incision).

- **Urethropexy** (you-**REE**-throh-**peck**-see) is the surgical fixation of the urethra usually for the correction of urinary stress incontinence (**urethro** means urethra and **pexy** means surgical fixation).

- **Urethroplasty** (you-**REE**-throh-**plas**-tee) is the surgical repair of the urethra (**urethro** means urethra and **plasty** means surgical repair).

- A **urethrostomy** (you-reh-**THROS**-toh-mee) is the surgical creation of a permanent opening between the urethra and the skin (**urethro** means urethra and **ostomy** means creating an opening).

- A **urethrotomy** (**you**-reh-**THROT**-oh-mee) is a surgical incision into the urethra for relief of a stricture (**urethr** means urethra and **otomy** means surgical incision). A **stricture** is an abnormal band of tissue narrowing a body passage).

Learning Exercises

● Matching Word Parts—1

Write the letter of the correct answer on the line provided in the left column.

9.1. _____ -cele   A. bladder

9.2. _____ cyst/o   B. glomerulus

9.3. _____ glomerul/o   C. hernia, tumor, cyst

9.4. _____ lith/o   D. kidney

9.5. _____ nephr/o   E. stone, calculus

● Matching Word Parts—2

Write the letter of the correct answer on the line provided in the left column.

9.6. _____ -lysis   A. surgical fixation

9.7. _____ -pexy   B. setting free, separation

9.8. _____ pyel/o   C. kidney

9.9. _____ ren/o   D. renal pelvis

9.10. _____ -tripsy   E. to crush

● Matching Word Parts—3

Write the letter of the correct answer on the line provided in the left column.

9.11. _____ dia   A. urination

9.12. _____ ureter/o   B. ureter

9.13. _____ -ectasis   C. urethra

9.14. _____ -uria   D. complete, through

9.15. _____ urethr/o   E. enlargement, stretching

● Definitions

Circle the letter next to the correct answer.

9.16. The narrow tubes that carry urine from the kidneys to the urinary bladder are called _____.

   a. glomeruli

   b. nephrons

   c. urethras

   d. ureters

9.17. The term lithotomy means _____ .

   a. an examination position

   b. a surgical incision for the removal of a stone

   c. the presence of a stone

   d. a and b

9.18. The increased excretion of urine is known as _____ .

   a. anuria

   b. diuresis

   c. dysuria

   d. oliguria

9.19. Urine collects in the _____ before entering the ureters.

   a. glomeruli

   b. nephrons

   c. renal pelvis

   d. urinary bladder

9.20. The flow of urine from the bladder is controlled by _____ .

   a. glomeruli

   b. sphincters

   c. the urethral meatus

   d. the urinary meatus

9.21. Which structures form urine by the processes of filtration, reabsorption, and secretion?

   a. glomeruli

   b. nephrons

   c. renal pyramids

   d. renal tubules

9.22. In the male, which structure carries both urine and semen?

   a. nephron

   b. renal pelvis

   c. ureter

   d. urethra

9.23 The external opening of the urethra is known as the urethral _____ .

   a. capsule

   b. meatus

   c. pelvis

   d. sphincter

9.24. The suffix -lysis means _____ .

   a. binding together

   b. dissolution

   c. setting free

   d. synthesis

9.25. In _____ the urethral opening is on one side of the penis.

   a. epispadias

   b. hyperspadias

   c. hypospadias

   d. paraspadias

● Matching Structures

Write the letter of the correct answer on the line provided in the left column.

9.26. _____ glomerulus   A. The portion of a nephron active in filtering urine

9.27. _____ meatus   B. Carries urine from a kidney to the urinary bladder

9.28. _____ renal cortex   C. External opening of the urethra

9.29. _____ ureter   D. Outer layer of the kidney

9.30. _____ urethra   E. Tube from the bladder to the outside of the body

Which Word?

Circle the correct term in each sentence.

9.31. A surgical incision into the renal pelvis is *pyelotomy / pyeloplasty.*

9.32. A discharge of blood from the ureter is *ureterorrhagia / urethrorrhagia.*

9.33. The medical term meaning excessive urination is known as *incontinence / polyuria.*

9.34. The medical term meaning an inflammation of the bladder is *cystitis / pyelitis.*

9.35. The major waste product of protein metabolism is *urea / urine.*

Spelling Counts

Find the misspelled word in each sentence. Then write that word, spelled correctly, on the line provided.

9.36. Urinoalysis is the examination of the physical and chemical properties of urine to determine the presence of abnormal elements. _____

9.37. Incontinance means being unable to control excretory functions. _____

9.38. Catherozation is the process used to withdraw urine from the bladder. _____

9.39. Cystorhagia is bleeding from the bladder. _____

9.40. Glomeronephritis is an inflammation of the kidney involving primarily the glomeruli. _____

Matching Abbreviations

Write the letter of the correct answer on the line provided in the left column.

9.41. _____ ESWL   A. nephrotic syndrome

9.42. _____ CRF   B. hemodialysis

9.43. _____ HD   C. extracorporeal shock-wave lithotripsy

9.44. _____ NS   D. intravenous pyelogram

9.45. _____ IVP   E. chronic renal failure

Term Selection

Circle the letter next to the correct answer.

9.46. Which term means the complete suppression (stopping) of urine formation by the kidneys?

a. anuria

b. nocturia

c. oliguria

d. polyuria

9.47. Which term means suturing of the bladder?

a. cystorrhaphy

b. cystorrhagia

c. cystorrhexis

d. nephrorrhaphy

9.48. Which term means the freeing of a kidney from adhesions?

a. nephrolithiasis

b. nephrolysis

c. nephropyosis

d. pyelitis

9.49. Which term means scanty urination?

a. diuresis

b. dysuria

c. enuresis

d. oliguria

9.50. Which term means the process of artificially filtering waste products from the patient's blood?

a. diuresis

b. hemodialysis

c. homeostasis

d. hydroureter

● Sentence Completion

Write the correct term on the line.

9.51.   An incision of the urinary meatus to enlarge the opening is a/an _____.

9.52.   A stone lodged in a ureter is a/an

_____.

9.53.   The surgical creation of a permanent opening of the urethra is a/an _____.

9.54.   The surgical fixation of the bladder to the abdominal wall is a/an _____.

9.55.   Urination is also known as voiding or

_____.

● True/False

If the statement is true, write T on the line. If the statement is false, write F on the line.

9.56.   _____ The ureters are about 10 to 12 inches long.

9.57.   _____ The urinary bladder is located in the posterior portion of the pelvic cavity.

9.58.   _____ A glomerulus consists of a cluster of capillaries.

9.59.   _____ The medulla is the outer layer of the kidney.

9.60.   _____ Distention means enlarged.

9.61.   _____ The male urethra is approximately 1.5 inches long.

9.62.   _____ Urine is formed by the processes of filtration, reabsorption, and secretion.

9.63.   _____ The female urethra conveys both urine and the menstrual flow.

9.64.   _____ A cystolith is a hernia of the urinary bladder.

9.65.   _____ Hydronephrosis is the dilation of the pelvis and calices of one or both kidneys resulting from obstruction to the flow of urine.

● Clinical Conditions

Write the correct answer on the line.

9.66.   Mrs. Baldridge suffers from excessive urination during the night. The medical term for this is _____ .

9.67.   The surgery for Rosita LaPinta included the surgical repair of the urethra. This procedure is called _____ .

9.68.   Doris Volk has a chronic bladder condition involving inflammation within the wall of the bladder. This is known as _____ cystitis.

9.69.   John Danielson is being treated for abnormal narrowing of the ureter. This condition is known as _____ .

9.70.   Norman Smith was born with the opening of the urethra on the upper surface of the penis. This is called _____ .

9.71.   Ralph Clark's form of dialysis involves the removal of waste from the blood through a fluid exchange in the _____ cavity.

9.72.   Roberta Gridley is scheduled for surgical repair of damage to the ureter. This procedure is a/an _____ .

9.73.   Letty Harding's physician ordered an IVP. The full name of this diagnostic x-ray study is an intravenous _____ .

9.74.   Mr. Morita was diagnosed as having an inflammation of the kidney. The medical term for this condition is _____ .

9.75.   Mrs. Franklin has a kidney stone. Rather than operate, the doctor used _____ to destroy the stone.

● Which is the correct medical term?

Circle the letter next to the correct answer

9.76.   Which term refers to a hernia of the bladder through the vaginal wall?

a. cystocele

b. cystolith

c. cystopexy

d. vesicovaginal fissure

9.77. Which term refers to the inability to empty the bladder?

a. incontinence

b. dysuria

c. enuresis

d. urinary retention

9.78. Which term refers to the distention of the ureter with urine due to blockage from any cause?

a. hydroureter

b. ureterolith

c. ureterostenosis

d. homeostasis

9.79. Which term refers to pain in the urethra?

a. cystitis

b. nephritis

c. urethralgia

d. urethritis

9.80. Which term refers to a doctor who specializes in diagnosing and treating diseases and disorders of the kidneys?

a. gastroenterologist

b. nephrologist

c. proctologist

d. urologist

● Challenge Word Building

These terms are *not* found in this chapter; however, they are made up of these familiar word parts. You may want to look in the glossary or use a medical dictionary to check your answers!

cyst/o	-cele
nephr/o	-itis
pyel/o	-lysis
ureter/o	- malacia
urethr/o	- ostomy
	- otomy
	-plasty
	-ptosis
	-rrhexis
	-sclerosis

9.81. The creation of an artifical opening between the urinary bladder and the exterior of the body is a/an _____ .

9.82. A surgical incision into the kidney is a/an _____ .

9.83. The medical term meaning abnormal hardening of the kidney is _____ .

9.84. The medical term meaning prolapse of the bladder into the urethra is _____ .

9.85. A hernia in the urethral wall is a/an _____ .

9.86. The procedure to separate adhesions around a ureter is _____ .

9.87. The medical term meaning abnormal softening of the kidney is _____ .

9.88. The medical term meaning an inflammation of the renal pelvis and kidney is _____ .

9.89. The medical term meaning rupture of the bladder is _____ .

9.90. The medical term meaning surgical repair of the bladder is _____ .

● Labeling Exercises

Identify the numbered items on this diagram.

9.91. _____ gland

9.92. right _____

9.93. inferior _____
_____

9.94. renal _____

9.95. renal _____

9.96. abdominal _____

9.97. _____

9.98. urinary _____

9.99. _____

9.100. urethral _____

The Human Touch: Critical Thinking Exercise

The following story and questions are designed to stimulate critical thinking through class discussion or as a brief essay response. There are no easy or right-wrong answers to these questions.

"Guess what — my baby sister is getting married, and she wants me to give her away!" Cody Gantry let out a whoop as he read the e-mail out loud to his wife. He could imagine his sister's smiling face as she sat at her computer on the other side of the Atlantic. Cody and Billie Jean were only 2 years apart, and she had followed her big brother's footsteps and joined the Army when she graduated from high school. Stationed in Germany, she worked on sensitive computerized targeting systems. Now he knew why she so often mentioned a fellow officer named Jon Vorheese.

Cody's mind drifted back to his own military career in South Korea. It had been cut short when a nephrolith led to hydronephrosis. Severe nephropyosis developed and the Army doctors were forced to perform a nephrectomy. He had received a medical discharge and been sent stateside just 3 days shy of his 25th birthday.

Back at home, Cody married his high school sweetheart and went to work in the local garage. Now Cody was almost 30 and needed dialysis weekly as the result of kidney failure. He was on a waiting list for a kidney transplant — but there was a chronic shortage of donor organs.

Cody certainly felt well enough to make a short trip to Germany for Billie Jean's wedding. What if a donor kidney finally became available right before he was scheduled to leave or while he was away? Would his urologist approve of him leaving the country while on dialysis? He was certain there were hospitals in Berlin with dialysis facilities, but he'd heard that in some countries, a shortage of dialysis equipment meant that the procedure was only available to residents. He'd do almost anything for the chance to walk his sister down the aisle on her big day . . .

Suggested Discussion Topics:

1. Explain the two types of dialysis procedures in terms your mother or father would understand.
2. Discuss what could happen to Cody if he skipped one or more of his dialysis treatments.
3. Dialysis is not as common in many countries as it is in the United States. Discuss possible reasons for this.
4. Cody is a veteran with a medical discharge. Is his health care covered as a veteran's benefit or by a private insurance company? Would a private insurance company pay for his treatment while overseas?
5. Cody needs a kidney transplant. Discuss your views on ethical ways in which recipients should be selected. What could be done to improve the supply of donor organs?

10 The Nervous System

● Overview of Structures, Word Parts, and Functions of the Nervous System

MAJOR STRUCTURES	RELATED WORD ROOTS	PRIMARY FUNCTIONS
Brain	**encephal/o**	Coordinates all activities of the body, receives and transmits messages throughout the body.
Spinal cord	**myel/o**	Transmits nerve impulses between the brain, limbs, and lower part of the body.
Nerves	**neur/i, neur/o**	Receive and transmit messages to and from all parts of the body.
Sensory organs ■ Ears (hearing) ■ Eyes (sight) ■ Nose (smell) ■ Skin (touch) ■ Tongue (taste)		Receive external stimulation and transmit it to the sensory neurons. The eyes and ears are discussed in Chapter 11.

● VOCABULARY   Related to the Nervous System

Check the box as you master each word part or term. Terms marked with the ❖ symbol are pronounced on the optional student audiotape.

Key Word Parts

☐ ambul/o
☐ cephal/o
☐ concuss/o
☐ contus/o
☐ ech/o
☐ encephal/o
☐ -esthesia
☐ klept/o
☐ mening/o
☐ myel/o
☐ narc/o
☐ neur/i, neur/o
☐ -phobia
☐ psych/o
☐ somn/o

Key Medical Terms

☐ **acrophobia** (ack-roh-**FOH**-bee-ah) ❖
☐ **Alzheimer's disease** (**ALTZ**-high-merz) ❖
☐ **amnesia** (am-**NEE**-zee-ah) ❖
☐ **amobarbital** (**am**-oh-**BAR**-bih-tal) ❖
☐ **amyotrophic lateral sclerosis** (ah-**my**-oh-**TROH**-fick) ❖
☐ **analgesic** (an-al-**JEE**-zick) ❖
☐ **anesthesia** (an-es-**THEE**-zee-ah) ❖
☐ **anesthesiologist** (an-es-**thee**-zee-**OL**-oh-jist) ❖
☐ **anesthetic** (an-es-**THET**-ick) ❖
☐ **anesthetist** (ah-**NES**-theh-tist) ❖
☐ **anxiety state**
☐ **aphasia** (ah-**FAY**-zee-ah) ❖
☐ **autistic** (aw-**TISS**-tick) ❖
☐ **barbiturate** (bar-**BIT**-you-rayt)
☐ **Bell's palsy**
☐ **catatonic** (kat-ah-**TON**-ick)
☐ **cerebral** (**SER**-eh-bral *or* seh-**REE**-bral) ❖
☐ **cerebral palsy** (**SER**-eh-bral *or* seh-**REE**-bral **PAWL**-zee) ❖
☐ **cerebrovascular accident** (ser-eh-broh-**VAS**-kyou-lar) ❖
☐ **claustrophobia** (klaws-troh-**FOH**-bee-ah) ❖
☐ **cognition** (kog-**NISH**-un)
☐ **comatose** (**KOH**-mah-tohs)
☐ **concussion** (kon-**KUSH**-un) ❖
☐ **contusion** (kon-**TOO**-zhun) ❖
☐ **cranial hematoma** (**hee**-mah-**TOH**-mah) ❖
☐ **craniocele** (**KRAY**-nee-oh-**seel**) ❖
☐ **delirium** (dee-**LIR**-ee-um) ❖
☐ **delirium tremens** (dee-**LIR**-ee-um **TREE**-mens)
☐ **delusion** (dee-**LOO**-zhun) ❖
☐ **dementia** (dee-**MEN**-shee-ah) ❖

☐ **dyslexia** (dis-**LECK**-see-ah) ❖
☐ **echoencephalography** (**eck**-oh-en-**sef**-ah-**LOG**-rah-fee) ❖
☐ **electroconvulsive therapy** (ee-**leck**-troh-kon-**VUL**-siv) ❖
☐ **electroencephalography** (ee-**leck**-troh-en-**sef**-ah-**LOG**-rah-fee) ❖
☐ **empathy** (**EM**-pah-thee) ❖
☐ **encephalitis** (en-sef-ah-**LYE**-tis) ❖
☐ **encephalography** (en-**sef**-ah-**LOG**-rah-fee) ❖
☐ **epidural anesthesia** (ep-ih-**DOO**-ral **an**-es-**THEE**-zee-ah) ❖
☐ **grand mal epilepsy** (**GRAN MAHL EP**-ih-**lep**-see) ❖
☐ **Guillain-Barré syndrome** (gee-**YAHN**-bah-**RAY**) ❖
☐ **hallucination** (hah-**loo**-sih-**NAY**-shun) ❖
☐ **hemorrhagic** (**hem**-oh-**RAJ**-ick) ❖
☐ **hydrocephalus** (high-droh-**SEF**-ah-lus) ❖
☐ **hyperesthesia** (**high**-per-es-**THEE**-zee-ah) ❖
☐ **hypochondriasis** (**high**-poh-kon-**DRY**-ah-sis) ❖
☐ **kleptomania** (klep-toh-**MAY**-nee-ah) ❖
☐ **malingering** (mah-**LING**-ger-ing)
☐ **meningitis** (men-in-**JIGH**-tis) ❖
☐ **meningocele** (meh-**NING**-goh-**seel**) ❖
☐ **migraine headache** (**MY**-grayn) ❖
☐ **multiple sclerosis** (skleh-**ROH**-sis) ❖
☐ **Munchausen syndrome** (**MUHN**-chow-zen) ❖
☐ **myelitis** (my-eh-**LYE**-tis) ❖
☐ **myelography** (my-eh-**LOG**-rah-fee) ❖
☐ **myelosis** (my-eh-**LOH**-sis) ❖
☐ **narcissistic** (nahr-sih-**SIS**-tick) ❖
☐ **narcolepsy** (**NAR**-koh-**lep**-see) ❖
☐ **neurologist** (new-**ROL**-oh-jist) ❖
☐ **paresthesia** (par-es-**THEE**-zee-ah) ❖
☐ **Parkinson's disease**
☐ **peripheral neuropathy** (new-**ROP**-ah-thee) ❖
☐ **petit mal epilepsy** (peh-**TEE MAHL EP**-ih-**lep**-see) ❖
☐ **poliomyelitis** (**poh**-lee-oh-**my**-eh-**LYE**-tis) ❖
☐ **posttraumatic stress disorder**
☐ **psychiatrist** (sigh-**KYE**-ah-trist) ❖
☐ **psychologist** (sigh-**KOL**-oh-jist) ❖
☐ **pyromania** (pye-roh-**MAY**-nee-ah) ❖
☐ **schizophrenia** (skit-soh-**FREE**-nee-ah) ❖
☐ **sciatica** (sigh-**AT**-ih-kah) ❖
☐ **seizure** (**SEE**-zhur)
☐ **syncope** (**SIN**-koh-pee) ❖
☐ **tetanus** (**TET**-ah-nus)
☐ **thalamotomy** (thal-ah-**MOT**-oh-mee) ❖
☐ **tic douloureux** (**TICK** doo-loo-**ROO**) ❖
☐ **transient ischemic attack** (iss-**KEE**-mick) ❖

● OBJECTIVES

On completion of this chapter, you should be able to:

1 Describe the functions and structures of the nervous system.

2 Identify the major divisions of the nervous system and describe the structures of each by location and function.

3 Identify the medical specialists who treat disorders of the nervous system.

4 Recognize, define, spell, and pronounce terms related to the pathology and diagnostic and treatment procedures of the nervous system.

5 Recognize, define, spell, and pronounce terms related to the pathology and diagnostic and treatment procedures of mental health disorders.

Functions of the Nervous System

The nervous system, with the brain as its center, coordinates and controls all bodily activities. When the brain ceases functioning, the body dies.

Structures of the Nervous System

The major structures of the nervous system are the brain, spinal cord, nerves, and sensory organs. For descriptive purposes the nervous system is divided into three parts: the central, peripheral, and autonomic nervous systems (Figure 10.1).

- The **central nervous system**, also known as the **CNS**, includes the brain and spinal cord.

- The **peripheral nervous system**, also known as the **PNS**, includes the 12 pairs of cranial nerves extending from the brain, and the 31 pairs of spinal nerves extending from the spinal cord.

- The **autonomic nervous system**, also known as the **ANS**, includes peripheral nerves and ganglia on either side of the spinal cord. (*Note:* Some textbooks include the ANS as a division of the peripheral nervous system. Both ways are correct.)

The Nerves

A **nerve** is one or more bundles of neuron cells (impulse carrying fibers) that connect the brain and the spinal cord with other parts of the body.

- A **tract** is a bundle or group of nerve fibers located within the brain or spinal cord. **Ascending tracts** carry nerve impulses *toward* the brain. **Descending tracts** carry nerve impulses *away from* the brain.

- A **ganglion** (GANG-glee-on) is a knotlike mass or group of nerve cell bodies located outside the CNS (plural, **ganglia** or **ganglions**).

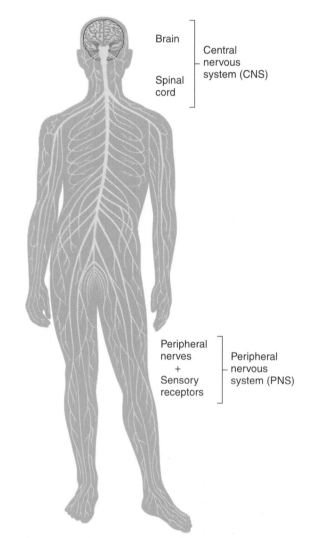

FIGURE 10.1 Structural organization of the central and peripheral nervous systems.

- A **plexus** (**PLECK**-sus) is a network of intersecting nerves and blood or lymphatic vessels (see Figure 10.10).
- **Innervation** (**in**-err-**VAY**-shun) is the supply of nerves to a body part. It also means the stimulation of a body part through the action of nerves.
- **Receptors** are sites in the sensory organs (eyes, ears, skin, nose, and taste buds) that receive external stimulation. The receptors send the stimulus through the sensory neurons to the brain for interpretation. Eyes and ears are discussed in Chapter 11.
- A **stimulus** is anything that excites or activates a nerve and causes an impulse (plural, **stimuli**).
- An **impulse** is a wave of excitation transmitted through nerve fibers and neurons.

The Reflexes

A **reflex** (**REE**-flecks) is an automatic, involuntary response to some change, either inside or outside the body. Deep tendon reflexes are discussed in Chapter 4.

- Maintenance of the heart rate, breathing rate, and blood pressure are reflex actions. Coughing, sneezing, and reactions to painful stimuli are also reflex actions.

The Neurons

A **neuron** (**NEW**-ron) is the basic cell of the nervous system.

- The three types of neurons are described according to their function. These are summarized in Table 10.1 and illustrated in Figure 10.2.
- The mnemonic **ACE** can help you remember the types of neurons and their roles: **A**fferent (sending), **C**onnecting (associative), **E**fferent (motor). (A **mnemonic** is a device intended to aid memory.)

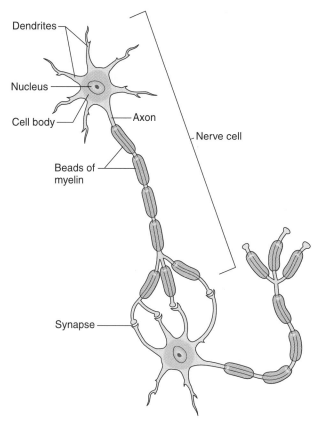

FIGURE 10.2 Structures of a neuron.

Neuron Parts

- Each neuron consists of a cell body, several dendrites, a single axon, and terminal end fibers.
- The **dendrites** (**DEN**-drytes) are rootlike structures that receive impulses and conduct them to the cell body.
- The **axon** (**ACK**-son) extends away from the cell body and conducts impulses away from the nerve cell. Some axons, but not all, are protected by a white fatty tissue covering called **myelin** (**MY**-eh-lin).
- **Terminal end fibers** are the branching fibers of the neuron that lead the nervous impulse away from the axon and toward the synapse.

Synapses

A **synapse** (**SIN**-apps) is the space between two neurons or between a neuron and a receptor organ.

Neurotransmitters

- A **neurotransmitter** (**new**-roh-trans-**MIT**-er) is a chemical messenger that transmits messages between nerve cells by making it possible for the nerve impulse to jump across the synapse from one neuron to another.
- At least 30 neurotransmitters have been identified. Each neurotransmitter is located within a specific group of neurons and has specific functions. Examples are shown in Table 10.2

Neuroglia

The **neuroglia** (new-**ROG**-lee-ah), also known as **glial cells**, are the supportive and connective cells of the ner-

Table 10.1

TYPES OF NEURONS	
Afferent neurons (**AF**-er-ent)	Also known as **sensory neurons**, they emerge from the skin or sense organs and carry impulses *toward* the brain and spinal cord.
Connecting neurons	Also known as **associative neurons**, they carry impulses from one neuron to another.
Efferent neurons (**EF**-er-ent)	Also known as **motor neurons**, they carry impulses *away from* the brain and spinal cord and toward the muscles and glands.

Table 10.2

EXAMPLES OF NEUROTRANSMITTERS AND THEIR FUNCTIONS	
Acetylcholine (**ass**-eh-til-**KOH**-leen)	Released at some synapses in the spinal cord and at neuromuscular junctions, acetylcholine influences muscle action.
Dopamine (**DOH**-pah-meen)	Released within the brain, dopamine is thought to cause some forms of psychosis and abnormal movement disorders such as Parkinson's disease.
Endorphins (en-**DOR**-fins)	Released within the spinal cord in the pain condition pathway, endorphins inhibit the conduction of pain impulses and act as natural pain relievers.
Serotonin (**sehr**-oh-**TOH**-nin or **seer**-oh-**TOH**-nin)	Released in the brain, serotonin has roles in sleep and pleasure recognition.

vous system. **Glial** means pertaining to glue and neuroglia is sometimes referred to as nerve glue.

Myelin Sheath

A **myelin sheath** is the white protective covering over some nerve cells including parts of the spinal cord, white matter of the brain, and most peripheral nerves (Figure 10.3).

- **White matter**. The myelin sheath gives nerve fibers a white color and myelinated axons of nerves are

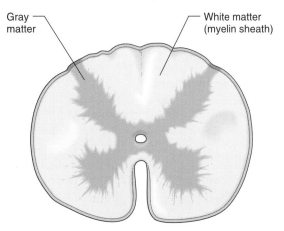

Gray matter

White matter (myelin sheath)

FIGURE 10.3 Cross section of the spinal cord shows white matter and gray matter.

referred to as *white matter*. The term **myelinated** (MY-eh-lih-**nayt**-ed) means having a myelin sheath.
- **Gray matter**. Those portions of nerves that *do not* have a myelin sheath are gray and make up the *gray matter* of the brain and spinal cord.

The Central Nervous System

The CNS is made up of the brain and spinal cord. These structures are protected externally by the bones of the cranium and spinal column (see Chapter 3). Within these bony structures, the brain and spinal cord are protected by the meninges and cerebrospinal fluid.

The brain parts are shown in Figure 10.4. The body functions controlled by these brain parts are summarized in Table 10.3. Notice that the functions vital to life support are located in the most protected portion of the brain.

The Meninges

The **meninges** (meh-**NIN**-jeez) are three layers of connective tissue membrane that enclose the brain and spinal cord (singular, **meninx**). These are the dura mater, arachnoid membrane, and the pia mater (Figure 10.5).

Table 10.3

WHERE IS IT CONTROLLED?	
Brain Part	**Controls**
Cerebrum—Uppermost and least protected layer of the brain	Responsible for the highest level of thought including judgment, memory, association, and critical thinking.
Thalamus—Located below the cerebrum	Monitors sensory stimuli by suppressing some and magnifying others.
Hypothalamus—Located below the thalamus	Controls vital body functions (see Table 10.4).
Cerebellum—Located in the lower back of the cranium below the cerebrum	Coordinates muscular activity for smooth and steady movements.
Pons—Located in the brainstem at the base of the brain	Nerves cross over so that one side of the brain controls the opposite side of the body.
Medulla oblongata—Most protected part of the brain	Controls the basic vital functions of life.

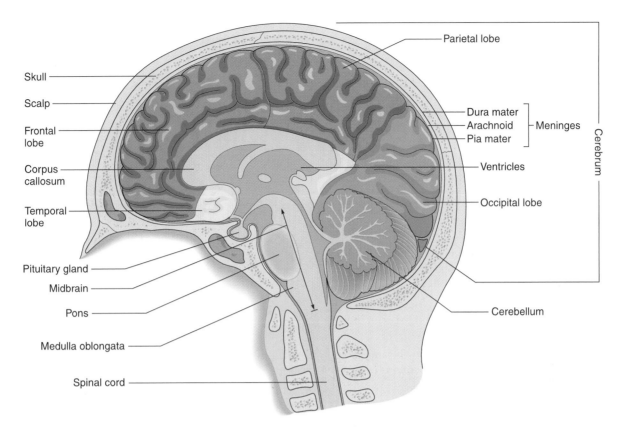

Skull

Scalp

Frontal
lobe

Corpus
callosum

Temporal
lobe

Pituitary gland

Midbrain

Pons

Medulla oblongata

Spinal cord

Parietal lobe

Dura mater
Arachnoid — Meninges
Pia mater

Ventricles

Occipital lobe

Cerebrum

Cerebellum

FIGURE 10.4 Cross section of the brain.

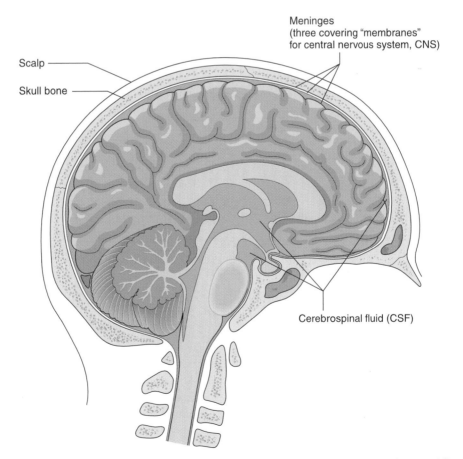

Scalp

Skull bone

Meninges
(three covering "membranes"
for central nervous system, CNS)

Cerebrospinal fluid (CSF)

FIGURE 10.5 The brain and its protective coverings. This is a lateral cross section with cerebrospinal fluid shown in pink.

Dura Mater

The **dura mater** (**DOO**-rah **MAY**-ter) is the thick, tough, outermost membrane of the meninges.

- The **epidural space** (ep-ih-**DOO**-ral) is located *above* the dura mater and within the surrounding bone walls (**epi** means above and **dural** means pertaining to dura mater). It contains fat and supportive connective tissues to cushion the dura mater.

- The **subdural space** (sub-**DOO**-ral) is located *below* the dura membrane and above the arachnoid membrane (**sub** means below and **dural** means pertaining to dura mater).

Arachnoid Membrane

The **arachnoid membrane** (ah-**RACK**-noid), which resembles a spider web, is the second layer surrounding the brain and spinal cord.

- The arachnoid membrane is loosely attached to the other meninges to allow space for fluid between the layers.

- The **subarachnoid space**, located below the arachnoid membrane and above the pia mater, contains cerebrospinal fluid.

Pia Mater

The **pia mater**, the third layer of the meninges, is located nearest to the brain and spinal cord. It consists of delicate connective tissue with a rich supply of blood vessels.

Cerebrospinal Fluid

Cerebrospinal fluid, also known as **CSF**, is a clear, colorless, watery fluid produced by special capillaries within the ventricles of the brain.

- The CSF flows throughout the brain and around the spinal cord, and its function is to nourish, cool, and cushion these organs from shock or injury.

The Cerebrum

The **cerebrum** (seh-**REE**-brum) is the largest and uppermost portion of the brain. It is responsible for all thought, judgment, memory, association, and discrimination.

- The term **cerebral** (**SER**-eh-bral *or* seh-**REE**-bral) means pertaining to the cerebrum or brain.

- The **cerebral cortex**, made up of gray matter, is the outer layer of the cerebrum and is arranged in folds.

Cerebral Hemispheres

- The cerebrum is divided into the **left hemisphere** and the **right hemisphere** (Figure 10.6). These are also referred to as the left and right brain.

- The two cerebral hemispheres are connected at the lower midpoint by the **corpus callosum** (**KOR**-pus kah-**LOH**-sum). (See Figures 10.4 and 10.8.)

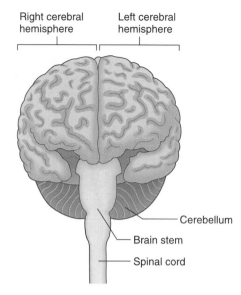

FIGURE 10.6 The brain is divided into right and left hemispheres.

Lobes

Each hemisphere is divided into four **lobes** and each lobe is named for the bone of the cranium covering it (Figure 10.7).

- The **frontal lobe** controls motor functions.

- The **parietal lobe** receives and interprets nerve impulses from the sensory receptors.

- The **occipital lobe** controls eyesight.

- The **temporal lobe** controls the senses of hearing and smell.

Ventricles

The four **ventricles** located within the middle region of the cerebrum contain CSF. (A **ventricle** is a small cavity, such as the ventricles of the brain and of the heart.)

The Thalamus

The **thalamus** (**THAL**-ah-mus), which is located below the cerebrum, produces sensations by relaying impulses to and from the cerebral cortex and the sense organs of the body (Figure 10.8).

The Hypothalamus

The **hypothalamus** (high-poh-**THAL**-ah-mus), located below the thalamus, has seven major regulatory functions. These are summarized in Table 10.4.

- The hypothalamus communicates with other parts of the body by secreting neurohormones. (A **neurohormone** is a hormone secreted by, or acting on, a part of the nervous system.)

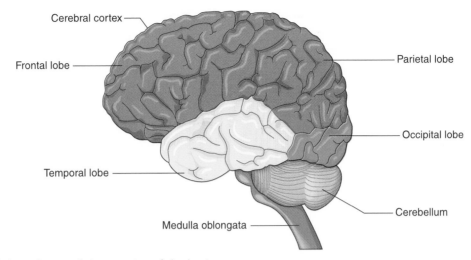

FIGURE 10.7 Left lateral view of the exterior of the brain.

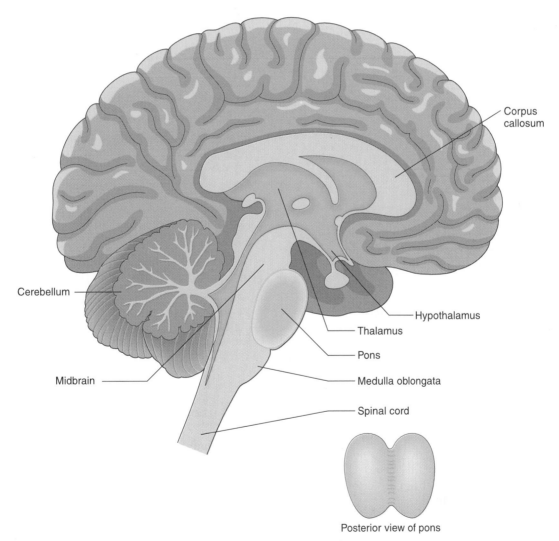

FIGURE 10.8 Schematic representation of the inner structures of the brain.

Table 10.4

REGULATORY FUNCTIONS OF THE HYPOTHALAMUS

1. Regulate and integrate the autonomic nervous system thereby controlling heart rate, blood pressure, respiratory rate, and digestive tract activity.

2. Regulate emotional responses and behavior.

3. Regulate body temperature.

4. Regulate food intake by controlling hunger sensations.

5. Regulate water balance and thirst.

6. Regulate sleep–wake cycles.

7. Regulate endocrine system activity.

The Cerebellum

The **cerebellum** (**ser**-eh-**BELL**-um) is the second largest part of the brain. It is located at the back of the head below the posterior part of the cerebrum.

- The cerebellum receives incoming messages regarding movement within joints, muscle tone, and positions of the body. From here messages are relayed to the different parts of the brain that control skeletal muscles.

The Brainstem

The **brainstem** is the stalklike portion of the brain that connects the cerebral hemispheres with the spinal cord. It is made up of the midbrain, pons, and medulla oblongata.

The Midbrain

The **midbrain** extends from the lower surface of the cerebrum to the pons. It is a short narrow segment that provides conduction pathways to and from higher and lower centers.

The Pons

The **pons** (**PONZ**), which means bridge, is situated at the base of the brain. It is here that nerve cells cross from one side of the brain to control the opposite side of the body.

- The nerves that control the left side of the body are found in the right side of the brain. Because the nerves cross at the pons, an injury to the right side of the brain affects the left side of the body.

- The nerves that control the right side of the body are found in the left side of the brain. Because the nerves cross at the pons, an injury to the left side of the brain affects the right side of the body.

The Medulla Oblongata

The **medulla oblongata** (meh-**DULL**-ah ob-long-**GAH**-tah) is located at the lowest part of the brainstem. It controls basic life functions including the muscles of respiration, heart rate, and blood pressure.

The Spinal Cord

The **spinal cord**, also known as the **SC**, is the pathway for impulses going to and from the brain.

- The spinal cord contains all the nerves that affect the limbs and lower part of the body.

- The spinal cord is protected by CSF and is surrounded by the three meninges.

- The gray matter in the spinal cord, which is not protected by a myelin sheath, is located in the internal section. The myelinated white matter composes the outer portion of the spinal cord (see Figure 10.3).

The Peripheral Nervous System

The **peripheral nervous system** (PNS) consists of the cranial nerves (extending from the brain) and the spinal nerves (extending from the spinal cord).

The Cranial Nerves

The 12 pairs of **cranial nerves** originate from the undersurface of the brain. Each nerve of a pair serves half of the body and both nerves are identical in function and structure.

- The cranial nerves are identified by Roman numerals and named for the area or function they serve (Figure 10.9).

The Spinal Nerves

The 31 pairs of **spinal nerves** are usually named for the artery they accompany or the body part they innervate (Figure 10.10).

- As an example, the femoral nerve innervates muscles associated with the femur (the bone of the upper leg).

The Autonomic Nervous System

The **autonomic nervous system** (ANS) controls the involuntary actions of the body (Figure 10.11).

- The ANS is subdivided into two divisions: the **sympathetic** and **parasympathetic nervous systems**.

- As shown in Table 10.5, one division balances the activity of the other to maintain homeostasis. **Homeostasis** (hoh-mee-oh-**STAY**-sis) is the process of maintaining the constant internal environment of the body.

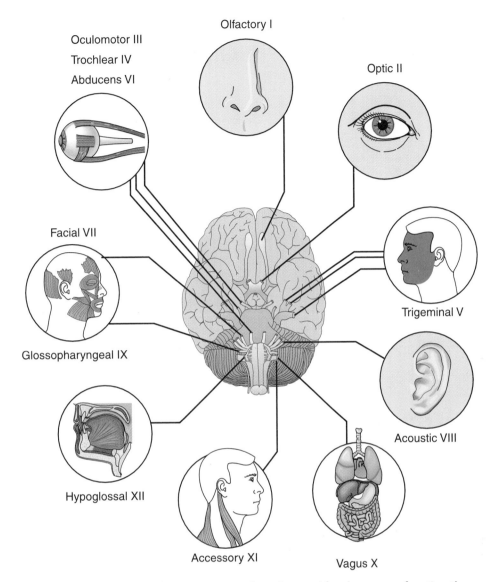

FIGURE 10.9 Cranial nerves are identified with Roman numerals and named for the area or function they serve.

Table 10.5

DIVISIONS OF THE AUTONOMIC NERVOUS SYSTEM AND THEIR CONTRASTING ACTIONS

Sympathetic Nervous System	Parasympathetic Nervous System
Prepares the body for emergency and stressful situations by increasing the breathing rate, heart rate, and blood flow to muscles.	Returns the body to normal after a stressful response. It also maintains normal body functions during ordinary circumstances that are not emotionally or physically stressful.

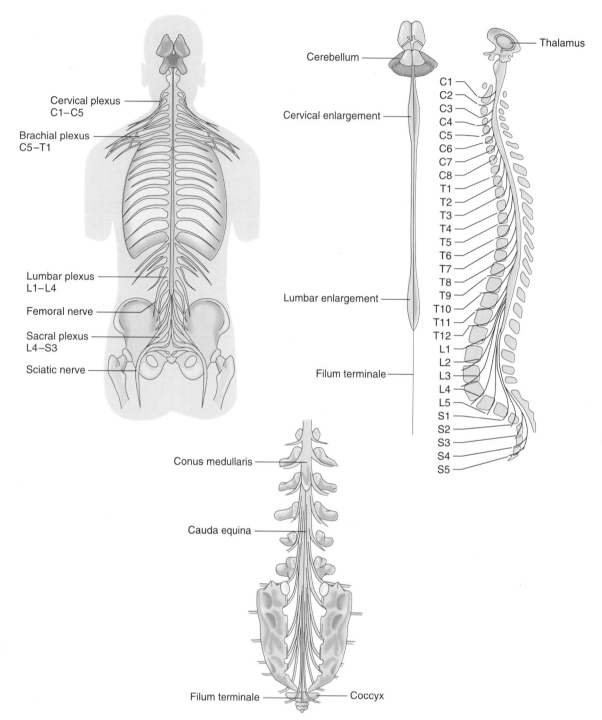

FIGURE 10.10 The spinal cord and nerves. Most spinal nerves are named for the corresponding vertebrae.

Medical Specialties Related to the Nervous System

- An **anesthesiologist** (an-es-thee-zee-OL-oh-jist) is a physician who specializes in administering anesthetic agents before and during surgery (**an** means without, **esthesi** means feeling, and **ologist** means specialist).

- An **anesthetist** (ah-NES-theh-tist) is a person trained in administering anesthesia but who is not necessarily a physician, for example, a nurse anesthetist (**an** means without, **esthet** means feeling, and **ist** means specialist).

- A **neurologist** (new-ROL-oh-jist) specializes in diagnosing and treating diseases and disorders of the ner-

Special senses
(controls pupil size)

Respiratory system
(controls respiratory rate)

Cardiovascular system
(controls heart rate and blood flow)

Digestive system
(controls functions of stomach and small intestine)

Digestive system
(controls flow of pancreatic juices)

Endocrine system
(adrenal glands stimulate the sympathetic nervous system)

Digestive system
(controls functions of large intestine)

FIGURE 10.11 The autonomic nervous system controls the involuntary actions of the body. Shown here are examples of the major body systems involved.

vous system (**neur** means nerve and **ologist** means specialist).

- A **neurosurgeon** is a physician who specializes in surgery of the nervous system.

- A **psychiatrist** (sigh-**KYE**-ah-trist) holds a Medical Doctor (MD) degree and specializes in diagnosing and treating chemical dependencies, emotional problems, and mental illness (**psych** means mind and **iatrist** means specialist).

- A **psychologist** (sigh-**KOL**-oh-jist) holds other than a medical degree and specializes in evaluating and treat-

ing emotional problems (**psych** means mind and **ologist** means specialist).

Pathology of the Nervous System

Head and Meninges

- **Cephalalgia** (**sef**-ah-**LAL**-jee-ah), also known as a **headache**, is pain in the head (**cephal** means head and **algia** means pain). It is also known as **cephalodynia** (**sef**-ah-loh-**DIN**-ee-ah).

- A **migraine headache** (**MY**-grayn) is a syndrome characterized by sudden, severe, sharp headache usually present only on one side.

- An **encephalocele** (en-**SEF**-ah-loh-**seel**), also known as a **craniocele** (**KRAY**-nee-oh-**seel**), is a congenital gap in the skull with herniation of brain substance (**encephalo** means brain and **cele** means hernia). Compare this with a meningocele.

- **Hydrocephalus** (high-droh-**SEF**-ah-lus) is an abnormally increased amount of CSF within the brain (**hydro** means water, **cephal** means head, and **us** is a singular noun ending).

- A **meningocele** (meh-**NING**-goh-**seel**) is the protrusion of the membranes of the brain or spinal cord through a defect in the skull or spinal column (**meningo** means meninges and **cele** means hernia). Compare this with an encephalocele.

- **Meningitis** (**men**-in-**JIGH**-tis) is an inflammation of the meninges of the brain or spinal cord (**mening** means meninges and **itis** means inflammation). (Plural, **meningitides**.) Compare with encephalitis.

Disorders of the Brain

- **Alzheimer's disease** (**ALTZ**-high-merz), also known as **AD**, is a group of disorders associated with degenerative changes in the brain structure leading to characteristic symptoms including progressive memory loss, impaired cognition, and personality changes.

- **Cognition** (kog-**NISH**-un) describes the mental activities associated with thinking, learning, and memory.

- **Encephalitis** (en-sef-ah-**LYE**-tis) is an inflammation of the brain (**encelphal** means brain and **itis** means inflammation). (Plural, **encephalitides**.) Compare with meningitis.

- **Parkinson's disease**, also known as **PD**, is a chronic slowly progressive, degenerative, CNS disorder. It is characterized by fine muscle tremors, a masklike facial expression, and a shuffling gait. (**Gait** means manner of walking.)

- **Tetanus** (**TET**-ah-nus), also known as **tet** or **lockjaw**, is an acute and potentially fatal bacterial infection of the CNS caused by the tetanus bacillus. Tetanus can be prevented through immunization.

Brain Injuries

- **Amnesia** (am-**NEE**-zee-ah) is a disturbance in the memory marked by total or partial inability to recall past experiences. The cause may be a brain injury, illness, or psychological disturbance.

- A **concussion** (kon-**KUSH**-un), also called a **cerebral concussion**, is a violent shaking up or jarring of the brain (**concuss** means shaken together and **ion** means condition). (Figure 10.12)

FIGURE 10.12 A concussion is the violent shaking up or jarring of the brain.

- A **cerebral contusion** (kon-**TOO**-zhun) is the bruising of brain tissue as a result of a head injury (**contus** means bruise and **ion** means condition).

- A **cranial hematoma** (hee-mah-**TOH**-mah *or* hem-ah-**TOH**-mah) is a collection of blood trapped in the tissues of the brain (**hemat** means blood and **oma** means tumor). Named for their location, the types of cranial hematomas include **epidural hematoma**, **subdural hematoma**, and **intracerebral hematoma** (Figure 10.13).

Altered States of Consciousness

- **Conscious**, also known as being **alert**, means awake, aware, and responding appropriately.

- **Syncope** (**SIN**-koh-pee), also known as **fainting**, is the brief loss of consciousness caused by brief lack of oxygen in the brain.

- **Lethargy** (**LETH**-ar-jee) is a lowered level of consciousness marked by listlessness, drowsiness, and apathy. As used here, **apathy** means indifference and a reduced level of activity.

- A **stupor** (**STOO**-per) is a state of impaired consciousness marked by a lack of responsiveness to environmental stimuli.

- A **coma** (**KOH**-mah) is a profound (deep) state of unconsciousness marked by the absence of spontaneous eye movements, no response to painful stimuli, and no vocalization (speech). **Comatose** (**KOH**-mah-tohs) refers to one who is in a coma.

Delirium and Dementia

- **Delirium** (dee-**LIR**-ee-um) is a potentially reversible condition often associated with a high fever that comes on suddenly in which the patient is confused, disoriented, and unable to think clearly.

- **Dementia** (dee-**MEN**-shee-ah) is a slowly progressive decline in mental abilities including memory, thinking, judgment, and the ability to pay attention.

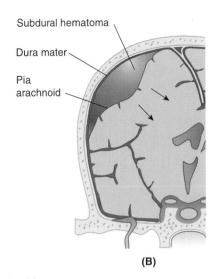

Subdural hematoma

Dura mater

Pia
arachnoid

Dura mater

Hematoma

(A)

(B)

FIGURE 10.13 Cranial hematomas. (A) Epidural hematoma. (B) Subdural hematoma.

Brain Tumors

A **brain tumor** is an abnormal growth within the brain that may be either benign (not life-threatening) or malignant (life-threatening). A malignant brain tumor may originate in the brain as the primary site, or it may spread from a secondary site in another part of the body.

- Any abnormal growth in the brain can cause damage in two ways. First if the tumor is invasive, it destroys brain tissue. Second because the skull is hard, the tumor can damage the brain by causing pressure on it (Figure 10.14).

FIGURE 10.14 A brain tumor visualized by magnetic resonance imaging.

Strokes

A **stroke**, also known as a **cerebrovascular accident** (ser-eh-broh-VAS-kyou-lar) or **CVA**, is damage to the brain that occurs when the blood flow to the brain is disrupted because a blood vessel supplying it is either blocked or has ruptured (Figure 10.15).

Ischemic Attacks

- A **transient ischemic attack** (iss-KEE-mick), also known as a **TIA**, is the temporary interruption in the blood supply to the brain. Symptoms include weakness, dizziness, or loss of balance. These pass within a few minutes; however, a TIA may be a warning of an impending stroke.

- The most common type of stroke in older people is an **ischemic stroke** in which the carotid artery is narrowed and the flow of blood in the brain is blocked, or a **cerebral thrombosis** in which a thrombus (clot) blocks the artery. This disruption of blood flow usually affects the cerebrum and damages the controls of movement, language, and senses.

- **Aphasia** (ah-**FAY**-zee-ah) is the loss of the ability to speak, write, or comprehend the written or spoken word (**a** means without and **phasia** means speech). Aphasia is often due to brain damage associated with a stroke.

- A carotid endarterectomy, described in Chapter 5, may be performed to prevent an ischemic stroke by opening a blocked artery before a stroke occurs.

Hemorrhagic Stroke

In a **hemorrhagic stroke** (**hem**-oh-**RAJ**-ick), also known as a **bleed**, a blood vessel in the brain leaks or ruptures. This type of stroke is less common but more deadly. A hemorrhagic stroke affects the area of the brain damaged by the leaking blood (Figure 10.16).

FIGURE 10.15 Stroke damage reflects the affected area of the brain. (A) Ischemic stroke. (B) Hemorrhagic stroke. *(By permission of Mayo Foundation; from June 1995 Medical Essay, Supplement to Mayo Clinic Health Letter.)*

FIGURE 10.16 Magnetic resonance image of a brain with the area of a bleed visible in the lower right.

Sleep Disorders

- **Insomnia** is the prolonged or abnormal inability to sleep. This condition is usually a symptom of another problem such as depression, pain, or excessive caffeine.

- **Narcolepsy** (**NAR**-koh-**lep**-see) is a syndrome characterized by recurrent uncontrollable seizures of drowsiness and sleep (**narco** means stupor and **lepsy** means seizure).

- **Somnambulism** (som-**NAM**-byou-lizm), also known as **noctambulism** or **sleepwalking**, is the condition of walking without awakening (**somn** means sleep, **ambul** means to walk, and **ism** means condition of).

- **Somnolence** (**SOM**-noh-lens) is a condition of unnatural sleepiness or semiconsciousness approaching coma; however, a somnolent person can usually be aroused by verbal stimuli.

Spinal Cord

- **Myelitis** (**my**-eh-**LYE**-tis) is an inflammation of the spinal cord (**myel** means spinal cord and **itis** means inflammation). Myelitis also means inflammation of bone marrow (**myel** means bone marrow and **itis** means inflammation).

- A **myelosis** (my-eh-**LOH**-sis) is a tumor of the spinal cord (**myel** means spinal cord and **osis** means abnormal condition). Myelosis also means an abnormal proliferation of bone marrow tissue (**myel** means bone marrow and **osis** means abnormal condition).

- **Multiple sclerosis** (skleh-**ROH**-sis), also known as **MS**, is a progressive autoimmune disorder characterized by scattered patches of demyelination of nerve fibers of the brain and spinal cord. Demyelination, which is the loss of this protective myelin covering, disrupts the transmission of nerve impulses and causes symptoms including tremors, paralysis, and speech disturbances.

- **Poliomyelitis** (**poh**-lee-oh-**my**-eh-**LYE**-tis), also known as **polio**, is a viral infection of the gray matter of the spinal cord that may result in paralysis. This can be prevented through immunization (**polio** means gray, **myel** means spinal cord, and **itis** means inflammation).
- **Postpolio syndrome** is the recurrence later in life of some polio symptoms in individuals who have had poliomyelitis and have recovered from it.
- **Radiculitis** (rah-**dick**-you-**LYE**-tis), also known as a **pinched nerve**, is an inflammation of the root of a spinal nerve (**radicul** means root, nerve root and **itis** means inflammation). This term usually applies to that portion of the root that lies between the spinal cord and the intervertebral canal of the spinal column (see Figure 3.18B).
- **Spinal cord injuries**, also known as **SCI**, are discussed in Chapter 4 under Paralysis.

Nerves

- **Amyotrophic lateral sclerosis** (ah-**my**-oh-**TROH**-fick), also known as **ALS** or **Lou Gehrig's disease**, is a degenerative disease of the motor neurons in which patients become progressively weaker until they are completely paralyzed. Intellect, eye motion, bladder function, and sensations are spared.
- **Bell's palsy** is paralysis of the facial (seventh cranial) nerve that causes drooping only on the affected side of the face. Compare with tic douloureux.
- **Guillain-Barré syndrome** (gee-**YAHN**-bah-**RAY**), also known as **GBS** or **acute ascending polyneuritis**, is characterized by rapidly worsening muscle weakness that may lead to temporary paralysis. GBS is presumed to be an autoimmune reaction that may occur after a mild infection, surgery, or an immunization.
- **Peripheral neuropathy** (new-**ROP**-ah-thee), also known as **peripheral neuritis** (new-**RYE**-tis), is a painful condition of the nerves of the hands and feet due to peripheral nerve damage to that may be caused by disease such as diabetes, alcoholism, autoimmune diseases, and exposure to toxic substances.
- **Tic douloureux** (**TICK** doo-loo-**ROO**), also known as **trigeminal neuralgia**, is inflammation of the trigeminal (fifth cranial) nerve. It is characterized by sudden, intense, sharp pain on one side of the face. Compare with Bell's palsy.
- **Sciatica** (sigh-**AT**-ih-kah) is inflammation of the sciatic nerve that results in pain along the course of the nerve through the thigh and leg.

Abnormal Sensations

- **Causalgia** (kaw-**ZAL**-jee-ah) is an intense burning pain after an injury to a sensory nerve (**caus** means burning and **algia** means pain).
- **Hyperesthesia** (**high**-per-es-**THEE**-zee-ah) means a condition of excessive sensitivity to stimuli (**hyper** means excessive and **esthesia** means sensation or feeling).
- **Paresthesia** (par-es-**THEE**-zee-ah) is an abnormal sensation, such as burning, tingling, or numbness, for no apparent reason (**par** means abnormal and **esthesia** means sensation or feeling).

Cerebral Palsy

Cerebral palsy (**SER**-eh-bral *or* seh-**REE**-bral **PAWL**-zee), also known as **CP**, is a condition characterized by poor muscle control, spasticity, and other neurologic deficiencies caused by an injury to the part of the brain that controls muscle movements. This injury occurs during pregnancy, birth or soon after birth. CP occurs more often in premature or low birthweight infants.

Convulsions and Seizures

The terms **convulsion** and **seizure** (**SEE**-zhur) are used interchangeably to describe a sudden, violent, involuntary contraction of a group of muscles caused by a disturbance in brain function. Convulsions have many causes including brain injury, lesions, or extreme high fever.

- A **generalized tonic-clonic seizure**, also known as a **generalized seizure**, is characterized by a loss of consciousness and tonic convulsions followed by clonic convulsions.
- A **tonic convulsion** is a state of continuous muscular contraction that results in rigidity and violent spasms.
- A **clonic convulsion** is a state marked by alternate contraction and relaxation of muscles resulting in jerking movements of the face, trunk, or extremities.
- A **localized seizure**, also known as a **partial seizure**, begins with specific motor, sensory, or psychomotor phenomena without loss of consciousness.

Epilepsy

Epilepsy (**EP**-ih-**lep**-see) is a group of neurologic disorders characterized by recurrent episodes of seizures.

- **Grand mal epilepsy** (**GRAN MAHL EP**-ih-**lep**-see), which is the more severe form, is characterized by generalized tonic-clonic seizures.
- **Petit mal epilepsy** (peh-**TEE MAHL EP**-ih-**lep**-see), also known as **absence epilepsy**, is the milder form in which there is a sudden, temporary loss of consciousness, lasting only a few seconds. These are very mild, do not include convulsive movements, and may not be noticed.
- An **epileptic aura** is a manifestation, such as a particular smell or light, that may be experienced just before a seizure.

Mental Health

Although described as mental disorders these conditions are often caused by physical changes, substance abuse, medications, or any combination of these factors.

Developmental Disorders

- **Mental retardation** is significantly below average general intellectual functioning that is accompanied by significant limitation in adaptive functioning.

- An **autistic disorder** (aw-TISS-tick), also known as **autism** (AW-tizm), is a disorder in which a young child cannot develop normal social relationships, behaves in compulsive and ritualistic ways, and frequently has poor communication skills.

- **Attention deficit disorder**, also known as **ADD**, is a short attention span and impulsiveness that are inappropriate for the child's developmental age.

- An **attention deficit/hyperactivity disorder**, also known as **ADHD**, is a pattern of inattention and hyperactivity that is inappropriate for the child's developmental age. This condition may persist into adulthood.

- **Dyslexia** (dis-LECK-see-ah), also known as a **reading disorder**, is a learning disability characterized by reading achievement that falls substantially below that expected given the individual's chronological age, measured intelligence, and age-appropriate education.

Substance-Related Disorders

- An **addiction** is the compulsive and overwhelming involvement with a specific activity despite the fact that it causes significant health hazards plus recurrent legal and social problems. The addiction may be to actions such as gambling or smoking. Abused substances include alcohol, medications, or illegal drugs.

- As an example, **alcoholism** (AL-koh-hol-izm) is chronic alcohol dependence or abuse with specific signs and symptoms of withdrawal. **Withdrawal** is a psychological or physical syndrome (or both) caused by the abrupt cessation (stopping) of the use of a drug in a habituated individual.

- **Delirium tremens** (dee-LIR-ee-um TREE-mens), also known as **DTs**, is a form of acute organic brain syndrome due to alcohol withdrawal and is characterized by sweating, tremor, restlessness, anxiety, mental confusion, and hallucinations.

Schizophrenia and Other Psychotic Disorders

- A **psychotic disorder** (sigh-KOT-ick) is characterized by the derangement of personality, loss of contact with reality, and deterioration of normal social functioning.

- **Schizophrenia** (skit-soh-FREE-nee-ah) is a psychotic disorder characterized by delusions, hallucinations, disorganized speech that is often incoherent, and disruptive or catatonic behavior.

- A **delusion** (dee-LOO-zhun) is a false personal belief that is maintained despite obvious proof or evidence to the contrary.

- A **hallucination** (hah-loo-sih-NAY-shun) is a sense perception (sight, touch, sound, smell, or taste) that has no basis in external stimulation.

- **Catatonic behavior** (kat-ah-TON-ick) is marked by a lack of responsiveness, stupor, and a tendency to remain in a fixed posture.

Mood Disorders

- A **manic episode** is a distinct period during which there is an abnormally, and persistently elevated, expansive and irritable mood.

- A **major depressive episode** is a prolonged period during which there is either a depressed mood or the loss of interest or pleasure in nearly all activities.

- A **bipolar disorder**, also known as a **manic-depressive episode**, is a clinical course characterized by the occurrence of manic episodes alternating with depressive episodes.

Panic Disorders

- **Panic disorders** are characterized by the sudden, unanticipated recurrence of a group of symptoms known as a panic attack. Once a person has experienced a panic attack, he or she will go to great lengths to avoid having it happen again.

- A **panic attack** includes intense feelings of apprehension, fearfulness, terror, and impending doom. Physical symptoms include shortness of breath, profuse sweating, heart palpitations, chest pain, and choking sensations.

Anxiety Disorders

- An **anxiety state** is a feeling of apprehension, tension, or uneasiness that stems from the anticipation of danger, the source of which is largely unknown or unrecognized.

- An **obsessive-compulsive disorder** is a pattern of specific behaviors such as repeated handwashing. **Obsessions** are persistent ideas, thoughts, or images that cause the individual anxiety or distress. **Compulsions** are repetitive behaviors the goal of which is to prevent or reduce anxiety or stress.

- **Posttraumatic stress disorder**, also known as **PTSD**, is the development of characteristic symptoms after a psychologically traumatic event such as witnessing a shooting, surviving a natural disaster, or being held as a hostage. Symptoms include numbed responsiveness to external stimuli, anxiety, sleep disorders, restlessness, difficulty concentrating, and depression.

Phobias

- A **phobia** (FOH-bee-ah) is a persistent irrational fear of a specific thing or situation. This fear is strong enough to cause avoidance of that thing or situation.

- **Acrophobia** (ack-roh-FOH-bee-ah) is an excessive fear of being in high places (**acro** means top and **phobia** means abnormal fear).

- **Agoraphobia** (ag-oh-rah-FOH-bee-ah) is an overwhelming and irrational fear of leaving the familiar setting of home or venturing into the open (**agora** means market place and **phobia** means abnormal fear).

- **Claustrophobia** (**klaws**-troh-**FOH**-bee-ah) is an abnormal fear of being in narrow or enclosed spaces (**claustro** means barrier and **phobia** means abnormal fear).

Somatoform Disorders

- **Somatoform** (soh-**MAT**-oh-**form**) is the term used to describe the presence of physical symptoms that suggest general medical conditions not explained by the patient's actual medical condition.
- A **conversion disorder**, such as paralysis of an arm or disturbance of vision, is characterized by a change in function that suggests a physical disorder but has no physical cause. Apparently these symptoms are an expression of the patient's psychological problems that he has converted into physical symptoms.
- **Hypochondriasis** (**high**-poh-kon-**DRY**-ah-sis) is characterized by a preoccupation with fears of having, or the idea that one has, a serious disease based on misinterpretation of one or more bodily signs or symptoms.

Impulse-Control Disorders

- **Kleptomania** (**klep**-toh-**MAY**-nee-ah) is a disorder characterized by a recurrent failure to resist impulses to steal objects not for immediate use or their monetary value (**klepto** means to steal and **mania** means madness).
- **Pyromania** (**pye**-roh-**MAY**-nee-ah) is a disorder characterized by a recurrent failure to resist impulses to set fires (**pyro** means fire and **mania** means madness).

Personality Disorders

- A **personality disorder** is an enduring pattern of inner experience and behavior that deviates markedly from the expectations of the individual's culture. This pattern is pervasive and inflexible, has an onset in adolescence or early adulthood, is stable over time, and leads to distress or impairment.
- An **antisocial personality disorder** is a pattern of disregard for, and violation of, the rights of others. This pattern brings the individual into continuous conflict with society.
- A **narcissistic personality disorder** (**nahr**-sih-**SIS**-tick) is a pattern of an exaggerated need for admiration and complete lack of empathy. **Empathy** (**EM**-pah-thee) is the ability to understand another person's mental and emotional state without becoming personally involved.

Other Conditions

- **Malingering** (mah-**LING**-ger-ing) is characterized by the intentional creation of false or grossly exaggerated physical or psychological symptoms, motivated by external incentives such as avoiding work.
- **Munchausen syndrome** (**MUHN**-chow-zen), named for a German nobleman in the 1700s, is a condition in which the "patient" repeatedly makes up clinically convincing simulations of disease for the purpose of gaining medical attention.
- **Munchausen syndrome by proxy** is a form of child abuse. Although seeming very concerned about the child's well-being, the abusive parent will falsify an illness in a child by making up or creating symptoms and then seeking medical treatment.

Diagnostic Procedures of the Nervous System

- **Computed tomography**, also known as a **CAT scan**, and **magnetic resonance imaging** (MRI) are important diagnostic tools of the nervous system because they can image the soft tissue structures of the brain and spinal cord (see Figures 10.14 and 10.16). These diagnostic techniques are discussed further in Chapter 15.
- **Echoencephalography** (eck-oh-en-**sef**-ah-**LOG**-rah-fee) is the use of ultrasound imaging to diagnose a shift in the midline structures of the brain (**echo** means sound, **encephalo** means brain, and **graphy** means the process of recording).
- **Electroencephalography** (ee-**leck**-troh-en-**sef**-ah-**LOG**-rah-fee), also known as an **EEG**, is the process of recording electrical brain wave activity (**electro** means electric, **encephalo** means brain, and **graphy** means the process of recording). The resulting record is called an **electroencephalogram**. These brain waves may also be displayed on a monitor.
- **Encephalography** (en-**sef**-ah-**LOG**-rah-fee) is a radiographic study demonstrating the intracranial fluid-containing spaces of the brain (**encephalo** means brain and **graphy** means the process of recording). The resulting record is called an **encephalogram**.
- **Myelography** (**my**-eh-**LOG**-rah-fee) is a radiographic study of the spinal cord after the injection of a contrast medium (**myelo** means spinal cord and **graphy** means the process of recording). The resulting record is called a **myelogram**.
- Determining the patient's **level of consciousness**, also known as **LOC**, is an important part of a neurologic evaluation. This is established by observing the patient and evaluating his reactions to stimuli.

Treatment Procedures of the Nervous System

Medications to Treat Mental Disorders

- **Tranquilizers**, also known as **antianxiety drugs**, suppress anxiety and relax muscles.
- An **antidepressant** prevents or relieves depression.
- An **antipsychotic** (**an**-tih-sigh-**KOT**-ick) is used to treat symptoms of severe psychiatric disorders.

- **Psychotropic drugs** (**sigh**-koh-**TROP**-pick) are capable of affecting the mind, emotions, and behavior and are used in the treatment of mental illnesses.

Pain Control

- **Transcutaneous electronic nerve stimulation**, also known as **TENS**, is a method of pain control by the application of electronic impulses to the nerve endings through the skin.
- An **analgesic** (**an**-al-**JEE**-zick) is a drug that relieves pain without affecting consciousness.
- **Nonnarcotic analgesics** such as aspirin are used for mild to moderate pain.
- **Narcotic analgesics** such as morphine, Demerol, and codeine are used to relieve severe pain; however, they may cause physical dependence or addiction.

Sedative and Hypnotic Medications

- A **sedative** depresses the CNS and produces calm and diminished responsiveness without producing sleep. **Sedation** is the effect produced by a sedative.
- A **hypnotic** depresses the CNS and usually produces sleep.
- A **barbiturate** (bar-**BIT**-you-rayt) is a class of drugs whose major action is a calming or depressed effect on the CNS.
- **Amobarbital** (**am**-oh-**BAR**-bih-tal) is a barbiturate used as a sedative and hypnotic.
- **Phenobarbital** (**fee**-noh-**BAR**-bih-tal) is a barbiturate used as a sedative and as an anticonvulsant.
- An **anticonvulsant** (**an**-tih-kon-**VUL**-sant) prevents seizures and convulsions.

Anesthesia

Anesthesia (**an**-es-**THEE**-zee-ah) is the absence of normal sensation, especially sensitivity to pain (**an** means without and **esthesia** means feeling).

- An **anesthetic** (**an**-es-**THET**-ick) is the medication used to induce anesthesia. The anesthetic may be topical, local, regional, or general (Figure 10.17).
- **Topical anesthesia** numbs only the tissue surface and is applied as a liquid, ointment, or spray.
- **Local anesthesia** is the loss of sensation in a limited area and is produced by injecting an anesthetic solution near that area.
- **Regional anesthesia**, the temporary interruption of nerve conduction, is produced by injecting an anesthetic solution near the nerves to be blocked.
- **Epidural anesthesia** (ep-ih-**DOO**-ral **an**-es-**THEE**-zee-ah) is regional anesthesia produced by injecting a local anesthetic into the epidural space of the lumbar or sacral region of the spine.
- **Spinal anesthesia** is produced by injecting an anesthetic into the subarachnoid space, which is located

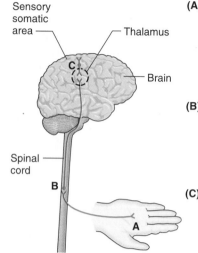

(A) Pain messages are picked up by free nerve endings in the skin. Local anesthetic blocks this.

(B) Message is carried into the spinal cord. Spinal anesthetic blocks this.

(C) Message is then carried to the cortex of the brain. General anesthetic blocks this.

Figure 10.17 Pain may be blocked through the action of anesthetics at points A, B, or C.

below the arachnoid membrane and above the pia mater that surrounds the spinal cord.

- **General anesthesia** involves the total loss of body sensation and consciousness as induced by various anesthetic agents, given primarily by inhalation or intravenous injection.

Brain and Head

- **Electroshock therapy**, also known as **electroconvulsive therapy** (ee-**leck**-troh-kon-**VUL**-siv), also known as **ECT**, is a controlled convulsion produced by the passage of an electric current through the brain. ECT is used primarily in the treatment of depression and mental disorders that do not respond to other forms of therapy.
- A **lobectomy** (loh-**BECK**-toh-mee) is surgical removal of a portion of the brain to treat brain cancer or seizure disorders that cannot be controlled with medication.
- **Thalamotomy** (thal-ah-**MOT**-oh-mee) is a surgical incision into the thalamus (**thalam** means thalamus and **otomy** means surgical incision). This procedure, which destroys brain cells, is performed to quiet the tremors of Parkinson's disease, to treat some psychotic disorders, or to stop intractable pain.

Nerves

- A **neurectomy** (new-**RECK**-toh-mee) is the surgical removal of a nerve (**neur** means nerve and **ectomy** means surgical removal).
- **Neuroplasty** (**NEW**-roh-**plas**-tee) is the surgical repair of a nerve or nerves (**neur** means nerve and **plasty** means surgical repair).
- **Neurorrhaphy** (new-**ROR**-ah-fee) means to suture the ends of a severed nerve (**neuro** means nerve and **rrhaphy** means to suture).
- A **neurotomy** (new-**ROT**-oh-mee) is a surgical incision or the dissection of a nerve (**neur** means nerve and **otomy** means a surgical incision).

Learning Exercises

● Matching Word Parts—1

Write the letter of the correct answer on the line provided in the left column.

10.1. _____ ambul/o   A. brain

10.2. _____ concuss/o   B. bruise

10.3. _____ contus/o   C. shaken together

10.4. _____ ech/o   D. sound

10.5. _____ encephal/o   E. to walk

● Matching Word Parts—2

Write the letter of the correct answer on the line provided in the left column.

10.6. _____ -esthesia   A. meninges

10.7. _____ cephal/o   B. sensation, feeling

10.8. _____ klept/o   C. spinal cord

10.9. _____ mening/o   D. to steal

10.10. _____ myel/o   E. head

● Matching Word Parts—3

Write the letter of the correct answer on the line provided in the left column.

10.11. _____ narc/o   A. abnormal fear

10.12. _____ neur/i, neur/o   B. mind

10.13. _____ -phobia   C. nerve

10.14. _____ psych/o   D. sleep

10.15. _____ somn/o   E. stupor

● Definitions

Circle the letter next to the correct answer.

10.16. Which term describes the space between two neurons or between a neuron and a receptor?

a. dendrite

b. ganglion

c. plexus

d. synapse

10.17. Which term describes the protective covering over some nerve cells that is known as white matter?

a. myelin sheath

b. neuroglia

c. neurotransmitter

d. pia mater

10.18. Which term describes the rootlike structures of a nerve that receive impulses and conducts them to the cell body?

a. dendrites

b. ganglions

c. impulses

d. terminal end fibers

10.19. Which term describes the layer of the meninges that is located nearest the brain and spinal cord?

a. arachnoid membrane

b. dura mater

c. meninx

d. pia mater

10.20. Which portion of the brain controls seven vital body functions?

a. cerebral cortex

b. cerebellum

c. hypothalamus

d. thalamus

10.21. Which division of the autonomic nervous system is concerned with body functions under stress?

a. cranial

b. parasympathetic

c. peripheral

d. sympathetic

10.22. Which term describes a network of intersecting nerves and blood or lymphatic vessels?

a. ganglion

b. plexus

c. synapse

d. tract

10.23. Which part of the nervous system includes the cranial nerves?

a. autonomic

b. central

c. cranial

d. peripheral

10.24. Which lobe of the cerebrum controls motor functions?

a. frontal

b. occipital

c. parietal

d. temporal

10.25. Which neurons carry impulses *away from* the brain and spinal cord and toward the muscles and glands?

a. afferent

b. associative

c. connecting

d. efferent

● Matching Structures

Write the letter of the correct answer on the line provided in the left column.

10.26. _____ cerebellum

A. where nerves cross over

10.27. _____ cerebrum

B. uppermost layer of the brain

10.28. _____ hypothalamus

C. most protected part of the brain

10.29. _____ medulla oblongata

D. coordinates muscular activity

10.30. _____ pons

E. controls vital body functions

Which Word?

Circle the correct term in each sentence.

10.31. A physician who specializes in administering anesthetic agents is an *anesthetist / anesthesiologist.*

10.32. A lowered level of consciousness marked by listlessness and drowsiness is described as *apathy / stupor.*

10.33. A disturbance in the memory marked by the inability to recall past experiences is known as *amnesia / aphasia.*

10.34. A sense perception that has no basis in external stimulation is a/an *delusion / hallucination.*

10.35. An excessive fear of heights is *acrophobia / agoraphobia.*

Spelling Counts

Find the misspelled word in each sentence. Then write that word, spelled correctly, on the line provided.

10.36. A miagraine headache is characterized by sudden, severe, sharp headache that is usually present only on one side.

_____

10.37. Altzheimer's disease is a group of disorders associated with degenerative changes including progressive memory loss, impaired thinking, and personality changes.

_____

10.38. An anesthethic is the medication administered to block the normal sensation of pain.

_____

10.39. Epalepsy is a group of neurologic disorders characterized by recurrent episodes of convulsive seizure. _____

10.40. Schiatica is a nerve inflammation that may result in pain through the thigh and leg.

_____

Matching Abbreviations

Write the letter of the correct answer on the line provided in the left column.

10.41. _____ CP   A. Parkinson's disease

10.42. _____ CVA   B. multiple sclerosis

10.43. _____ MS   C. cerebral palsy

10.44. _____ PD   D. tetanus

10.45. _____ tet   E. cerebrovascular accident

Term Selection

Circle the letter next to the correct answer.

10.46. Which term describes a potentially reversible condition, often associated with a high fever, in which the patient is confused, disoriented, and unable to think clearly?

a. delirium

b. dementia

c. lethargy

d. stupor

10.47. Which term describes an inflammation of the spinal cord?

a. encephalitis

b. myelitis

c. myelosis

d. radiculitis

10.48. Which condition is also known as sleep walking?

a. narcolepsy

b. somnambulism

c. somnolence

d. sleep apnea

10.49. Which condition is also known as acute ascending polyneuritis?

a. Bell's palsy

b. Guillain-Barré syndrome

c. Lou Gehrig's disease

d. tic douloureux

10.50. Which term describes a reading disorder?

a. attention deficit disorder

b. autism

c. dyslexia

d. mental retardation

Sentence Completion

Write the correct term on the line.

10.51. The general term used to describe bruising of brain tissue as a result of a head injury is a cerebral _____ .

10.52. A feeling of apprehension, tension, or uneasiness that stems from the anticipation of danger, the source of which is largely unknown or unrecognized is a/an _____ state.

10.53. The term used to describe a disorder characterized by a recurrent failure to resist impulses to set fires is _____ .

10.54. _____ syndrome by proxy is a form of child abuse.

10.55. Medication that is administered to prevent or relieve depression is known as a/an _____ .

True/False

If the statement is true, write T on the line. If the statement is false, write F on the line.

10.56. _____ Causalgia is an intense burning pain following an injury to a sensory nerve.

10.57. _____ A cephalocele is the rupture of the membranes of the brain and spinal cord.

10.58. _____ Postpolio syndrome occurs in older patients who have had poliomyelitis.

10.59. _____ The nerves that control the left side of the body are found in the right side of the brain.

10.60. _____ Electroencephalography produces a picture of the structures of the brain.

10.61. _____ In a hemorrhagic stroke a blood vessel in the brain leaks or ruptures.

10.62. _____ Demyelination is the destruction or loss of the myelin sheath from myelinated fibers.

10.63. _____ A sedative depresses the CNS and produces sleep.

10.64. _____ A pattern of repeated handwashing is a bipolar disorder.

10.65. _____ Tic douloureux is an inflammation of the trigeminal nerve.

Clinical Conditions

Write the correct answer on the line.

10.66. Harvey Ikeman's chart listed him as being _____ . This means that he is in a coma.

10.67. After the auto accident, Anthony DeNatali required _____ to suture the ends of a severed nerve in his hand.

10.68. George Houghton suffered a transient _____ attack (TIA). Sometimes this is a warning of a stroke.

10.69. Ted Duncan had Parkinson's disease. To control the tremors, his doctor performed a/an _____ . This is a surgical incision into the thalamus.

10.70. Mary Beth Cawthorn was diagnosed as having _____ _____ , which is also known as MS. This autoimmune disease is characterized by patches of demyelinated nerve fibers.

10.71. Joanne Ladner suffers from recurrent uncontrollable seizures of drowsiness and sleep. Her doctor diagnosed this condition as _____ .

10.72. After her stroke Mildred Carson was unable to understand written or spoken words. This condition is called _____ .

10.73. Jill Beck said she fainted. The medical term for this brief loss of consciousness caused by a lack of oxygen in the brain is _____ .

10.74. The Baily baby was born with _____ . This condition is an abnormally increased amount of cerebrospinal fluid within the brain.

10.75. After the accident, the MRI indicated that Juan Ramirez had a collection of blood trapped in the tissues of the brain. This condition is called a cranial _____ .

Which is the correct medical term?

Circle the letter next to the correct answer.

10.76. Which medical term describes an intense burning pain after an injury to a sensory nerve?

a. causalgia

b. hyperesthesia

c. hypoesthesia

d. paresthesia

10.77. Which disorder is characterized by generalized tonic-clonic seizures?

a. autism

b. grand mal epilepsy

c. petit mal epilepsy

d. schizophrenia

10.78. Which condition is likely to develop after witnessing a shooting?

a. a conversion disorder

b. an anxiety state

c. panic attacks

d. posttraumatic stress disorder

10.79. Which form of anesthesia affects only the surface of the tissues?

a. epidural

b. local

c. regional

d. topical

10.80. Which medication, or treatment, is administered to control convulsions?

a. amobarbital

b. electroconvulsive therapy

c. phenobarbital

d. transcutaneous electronic nerve stimulation

● Challenge Word Building

These terms are *not* found in this chapter; however, they are made up of these familiar word parts. You may want to look in the glossary or use a medical dictionary to check your answers!

poly-	encephal/o	-algia
	mening/o	-itis
	myel/o	-malacia
	neur/o	-oma
		-pathy

10.81. The medical term meaning pain in a nerve or nerves is _____ .

10.82. The medical term meaning abnormal softening of the meninges is known as _____ .

10.83. The medical term used to describe benign neoplasms made up of neurons and nerve fibers is a/an _____ .

10.84. The medical term meaning any degenerative disease of the brain is _____ .

10.85. The medical term meaning an inflammation affecting many nerves is _____ .

10.86. The medical term meaning abnormal softening of nerve tissue is known as _____ .

10.87. The medical term meaning inflammation of the meninges and the brain is _____ .

10.88. The medical term meaning any pathological condition of the spinal cord is _____ .

10.89. The medical term meaning abnormal softening of the brain is _____ .

10.90. The medical term meaning inflammation of the meninges, brain, and spinal cord is _____ .

● Labeling Exercises

Identify the numbered items on these diagrams.

10.91. _____ cortex

10.92. _____ lobe

10.93. _____ lobe

10.94. _____ lobe

10.95. _____ lobe

10.96. _____

10.97. _____ callosum

10.98. _____

10.99. _____ oblongata

10.100. _____ cord

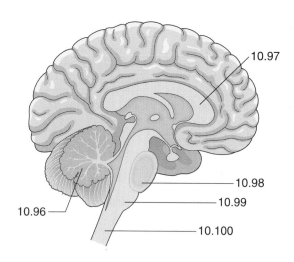

The Human Touch: Critical Thinking Exercise

The following story and questions are designed to stimulate critical thinking through class discussion or as a brief essay response. There are no easy or right-wrong answers to these questions.

Calle Washington read the information Dr. Thakker gave her with numb disbelief. "Multiple sclerosis is a neurological disorder characterized by demyelination of nerve fibers in the brain and spinal column. This disease may be progressively debilitating with symptoms that could include numbness, paralysis, ataxia, pain, and blindness. Some patients do experience life-threatening complications. This disease attacks young adults. It affects more women than men."

"Well, I sure fit the profile," thought Calle bitterly. She took a deep breath, trying to quiet the fluttering in her stomach. How could this happen now? Everything was so perfect. Her wedding gown was getting its last alterations, and the tickets for her honeymoon in Jamaica were in the desk drawer. Gabe was putting the final touches on the house where they planned on raising their family. Suddenly her fairy tale life was turning into a nightmare.

She couldn't expect Gabe to waste his future caring for someone in a wheelchair, could she? And what would happen once her fellow teachers at the day care center noticed that her balance was sometimes off? She couldn't risk hurting one of the children, but if she lost her job she'd lose her health insurance. Dr. Thakker had said there were new drugs for MS, but he'd mentioned that they were very expensive. And what about the children that she and Gabe both wanted? Could she still have a baby, and take care of it?

"Maybe I should take out an ad that says 'Twenty-five year old female seeks cure for deadly disease before marrying Prince Charming'," she thought, trying to laugh through her tears . . .

Possible Discussion Topics:

1. Discuss whether or not Calle and Gabe should go ahead with the wedding.

2. How might Calle's condition effect her job? Should she be asked to resign?

3. If Calle loses her job at the day care center and she tries to find work elsewhere, should she disclose the fact that she has MS?

4. Insurance companies want the people they insure to have physicals and provide information about previous illnesses and diseases. Discuss whether or not you think this is an ethical practice? If you think it is not ethical, why do you think the insurance companies do it?

5. What Federal legislation is designed to help disabled individuals? Do you think this law would apply to Calle's situation?

Special Senses: The Eyes and Ears

● **Overview of Structures, Word Parts, and Functions of the Eyes and Ears**

MAJOR STRUCTURES	RELATED WORD ROOTS	PRIMARY FUNCTIONS
Eyes	opt/i, opt/o, optic/o, ophthalm/o	Receptor organs for the sense of sight.
Adnexa of the eye		Accessory structures that provide external protection and movement for the eyes.
Lacrimal apparatus	lacrim/o, dacry/o	Produces, stores, and removes tears.
Iris	ir/i, ir/o, irid/o, irit/o	Controls the amount of light entering the eye.
Lens	phac/o	Focuses rays of light on the retina.
Retina	retin/o	Converts light images into electrical impulses and transmits them to the brain.
Ears	acous/o, acout/o, audi/o, audit/o, ot/o	Receptor organs for the sense of hearing; also help to maintain balance.
Outer ear	pinn/i	Transmits sound waves to the middle ear.
Middle ear	myring/o, tympan/o	Transmits sound waves to the inner ear.
Inner ear	labyrinth/o	Receives sound vibrations and transmits them to the brain.

● VOCABULARY   Related to the Special Senses

Check the box as you master each word part or term. Terms marked with the ❖ symbol are pronounced on the optional student audiotape.

Key Word Parts

- ☐ blephar/o
- ☐ -cusis
- ☐ dacryocyst/o
- ☐ irid/o
- ☐ kerat/o
- ☐ -metry
- ☐ ophthalm/o
- ☐ -opia
- ☐ ot/o
- ☐ presby/o
- ☐ pseud/o
- ☐ retin/o
- ☐ scler/o
- ☐ trop/o
- ☐ tympan/o

Key Medical Terms

- ☐ **accommodation** (ah-**kom**-oh-**DAY**-shun) ❖
- ☐ **adnexa** (ad-NECK-sah) ❖
- ☐ **amblyopia** (am-blee-OH-pee-ah) ❖
- ☐ **ametropia** (am-eh-TROH-pee-ah) ❖
- ☐ **anisocoria** (an-ih-so-KOH-ree-ah) ❖
- ☐ **astigmatism** (ah-STIG-mah-tizm) ❖
- ☐ **audiologist** (aw-dee-OL-oh-jist)
- ☐ **blepharoptosis** (blef-ah-roh-TOH-sis *or* blef-ah-rop-TOH-sis) ❖
- ☐ **cataract** (KAT-ah-rakt) ❖
- ☐ **chalazion** (kah-LAY-zee-on) ❖
- ☐ **conjunctivitis** (kon-**junk**-tih-VYE-tis) ❖
- ☐ **conjunctivoplasty** (kon-junk-TYE-voh-**plas**-tee)
- ☐ **convergence** (kon-VER-jens)
- ☐ **dacryocystitis** (**dack**-ree-oh-sis-TYE-tis) ❖
- ☐ **diplopia** (dih-PLOH-pee-ah) ❖
- ☐ **ectropion** (eck-TROH-pee-on) ❖
- ☐ **emmetropia** (em-eh-TROH-pee-ah) ❖
- ☐ **entropion** (en-TROH-pee-on) ❖
- ☐ **esotropia** (es-oh-TROH-pee-ah) ❖
- ☐ **eustachitis** (you-stay-KYE-tis) ❖
- ☐ **exotropia** (eck-soh-TROH-pee-ah) ❖
- ☐ **fenestration** (fen-es-TRAY-shun) ❖
- ☐ **glaucoma** (glaw-KOH-mah) ❖
- ☐ **hemianopia** (hem-ee-ah-NOH-pee-ah) ❖
- ☐ **hordeolum** (hor-DEE-oh-lum) ❖
- ☐ **hyperopia** (high-per-OH-pee-ah) ❖
- ☐ **intravenous fluorescein angiography** (flew-oh-RES-ee-in) ❖
- ☐ **iridectomy** (ir-ih-DECK-toh-mee) ❖
- ☐ **iritis** (eye-RYE-tis) ❖
- ☐ **keratitis** (ker-ah-TYE-tis) ❖

- ☐ **keratotomy** (**ker**-ah-TOT-oh-mee) ❖
- ☐ **labyrinthectomy** (**lab**-ih-rin-THECK-toh-mee) ❖
- ☐ **labyrinthitis** (**lab**-ih-rin-THIGH-tis) ❖
- ☐ **mastoidectomy** (**mas**-toy-DECK-toh-mee)
- ☐ **mastoiditis** (**mas**-toy-DYE-tis)
- ☐ **Menière's syndrome** (**men**-ee-AYRZ *or* men-YEHRS) ❖
- ☐ **monochromatism** (**mon**-oh-KROH-mah-tizm) ❖
- ☐ **myopia** (my-OH-pee-ah) ❖
- ☐ **myringectomy** (**mir**-in-JECK-toh-mee) ❖
- ☐ **myringitis** (**mir**-in-JIGH-tis) ❖
- ☐ **myringotomy** (**mir**-in-GOT-oh-mee) ❖
- ☐ **nyctalopia** (**nick**-tah-LOH-pee-ah) ❖
- ☐ **nystagmus** (nis-TAG-mus) ❖
- ☐ **ophthalmologist** (ahf-thal-MOL-oh-jist) ❖
- ☐ **optometrist** (op-TOM-eh-trist) ❖
- ☐ **otitis media** (oh-TYE-tis MEE-dee-ah) ❖
- ☐ **otomycosis** (**oh**-toh-my-KOH-sis) ❖
- ☐ **otoplasty** (OH-toh-**plas**-tee) ❖
- ☐ **otopyorrhea** (oh-toh-**pye**-oh-REE-ah) ❖
- ☐ **otorrhagia** (oh-toh-RAY-jee-ah) ❖
- ☐ **otosclerosis** (**oh**-toh-skleh-ROH-sis)
- ☐ **papilledema** (**pap**-ill-eh-DEE-mah) ❖
- ☐ **patulous** (PAT-you-lus)
- ☐ **phacoemulsification** (fay-koh-ee-**mul**-sih-fih-KAY-shun *or* fack-koh-ee-**mul** sih-fih-KAY-shun) ❖
- ☐ **presbycusis** (**pres**-beh-KOO-sis) ❖
- ☐ **presbyopia** (**pres**-bee-OH-pee-ah) ❖
- ☐ **purulent otitis media** (PYOU-roo-lent oh-TYE-tis MEE-dee-ah)
- ☐ **retinopexy** (RET-ih-noh-**peck**-see) ❖
- ☐ **scleritis** (skleh-RYE-tis) ❖
- ☐ **scotoma** (skoh-TOH-mah) ❖
- ☐ **stapedectomy** (**stay**-peh-DECK-toh-mee)
- ☐ **strabismus** (strah-BIZ-mus) ❖
- ☐ **synechia** (sigh-NECK-ee-ah) ❖
- ☐ **tarsectomy** (tahr-SECK-toh-mee) ❖
- ☐ **tarsorrhaphy** (tahr-SOR-ah-fee) ❖
- ☐ **tinnitus** (tih-NIGH-tus) ❖
- ☐ **tonometry** (toh-NOM-eh-tree) ❖
- ☐ **trabeculoplasty** (trah-BECK-you-loh-**plas**-tee) ❖
- ☐ **tympanectomy** (**tim**-pah-NECK-toh-mee) ❖
- ☐ **tympanocentesis** (**tim**-pah-noh-sen-TEE-sis)
- ☐ **tympanometry** (**tim**-pah-NOM-eh-tree) ❖
- ☐ **tympanoplasty** (**tim**-pah-noh-PLAS-tee)
- ☐ **tympanostomy tubes** (**tim**-pan-OSS-toh-mee)
- ☐ **vertigo** (VER-tih-go)
- ☐ **xerophthalmia** (**zeer**-ahf-THAL-mee-ah) ❖

● OBJECTIVES

On completion of this chapter, you should be able to:

1 Describe the functions and structures of the eyes and adnexa.

2 Recognize, define, spell, and pronounce terms related to the pathology and diagnostic and treatment procedures of eye disorders.

3 Describe the functions and structures of the ears.

4 Recognize, define, spell, and pronounce terms related to the pathology and diagnostic and treatment procedures of ear disorders.

Medical Specialties Related to the Eyes and Ears

- An **audiologist** (**aw**-dee-**OL**-oh-jist) specializes in the measurement of hearing function and the rehabilitation of persons with hearing impairments (**audi** means hearing and **ologist** means specialist).

- An **ophthalmologist** (ahf-thal-**MOL**-oh-jist) specializes in diagnosing and treating diseases and disorders of the eye (**ophthalm** means eye and **ologist** means specialist).

- An **optometrist** (op-**TOM**-eh-trist) holds a Doctor of Optometry (OD) degree and specializes in measuring the accuracy of vision to determine if corrective lenses or eyeglasses are needed (**opto** means vision and **metrist** means one who measures).

- An **otolaryngologist** (**oh**-toh-**lar**-in-**GOL**-oh-jist) is a physician who specializes in the care of the ears, nose, and throat (**oto** means ear, **laryng** means larynx, and **ologist** means specialist).

Functions of the Eyes and Ears

The eyes and ears are sensory receptor organs. Abbreviations used to describe these sensory organs are listed in Table 11.1.

Table 11.1

COMPARISON OF ABBREVIATIONS RELATING TO THE EYES AND EARS			
Eyes		**Ears**	
OD	right eye	**AD**	right ear
OS	left eye	**AS**	left ear
OU	each eye or both eyes	**AU**	each ear or both ears

Functions of the Eyes

The function of the eyes is to receive images and transmit them to the brain.

- The term **optic** means pertaining to the eye or sight (**opt** means sight and **ic** means pertaining to).

- **Ocular** (**OCK**-you-lar) means pertaining to the eye (**ocul** means eye and **ar** means pertaining to).

- **Extraocular** (**eck**-strah-**OCK**-you-lar) means outside the eyeball (**extra** means on the outside, **ocul** means eye, and **ar** means pertaining to).

- **Intraocular** (**in**-trah-**OCK**-you-lar) means within the eyeball (**intra** means within, **ocul** means eye, and **ar** means pertaining to).

Functions of the Ears

The functions of the ears are to receive sound impulses and transmit them to the brain. The inner ear also helps to maintain balance.

- The term **auditory** (**AW**-dih-**tor**-ee) means pertaining to the sense of hearing (**audit** means hearing or sense of hearing and **ory** means pertaining to).

- **Acoustic** (ah-**KOOS**-tick) means relating to sound or hearing (**acous** means hearing or sound and **tic** means pertaining to).

Structures of the Eyes

Adnexa of the Eyes

The **adnexa of the eye**, also known as **adnexa oculi**, include the orbit, eye muscles, eyelids, eyelashes, conjunctiva, and lacrimal apparatus. (Figure 11.1). **Adnexa** (ad-**NECK**-sah) means the appendages or accessory structures of an organ.

The Orbit

The **orbit**, also known as the **eye socket**, is the bony cavity of the skull that contains and protects the eyeball and its associated muscles, blood vessels, and nerves.

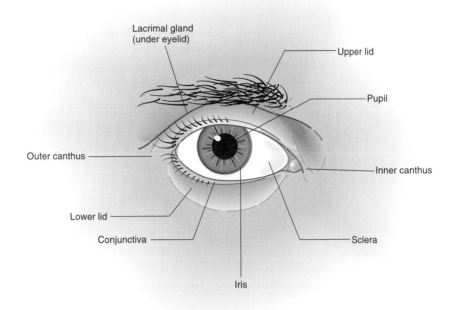

Figure 11.1 Major structures and adnexa of the right eye.

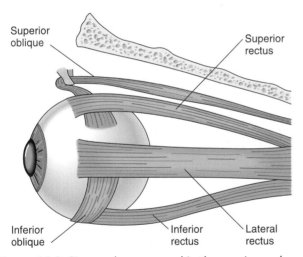

Figure 11.2 Six muscles, arranged in three pairs, make major eye movement possible. These are superior and inferior rectus, superior and inferior oblique, and lateral and medial rectus (not visible here).

The Eye Muscles

The six major muscles attached to each eye make possible a wide range of movement (Figure 11.2).

- The muscles of both eyes work together in coordinated movements that enable normal binocular vision. **Binocular** refers to the use of both eyes working together.

The Eyelids

The **upper and lower eyelids** of each eye protect the eyeball from foreign matter, excessive light, and impact.

- The **canthus** (**KAN**-thus) is the angle where the upper and lower eyelids meet (plural, **canthi**).

- The **inner canthus** is where the eyelids meet nearest the nose. The **epicanthus** (**ep**-ih-**KAN**-thus) is a vertical fold of skin on either side of the nose. In some people this covers the inner canthus.

- The **tarsus** (**TAHR**-suhs), also known as the **tarsal plate**, is the platelike framework within the upper and lower eyelids that provides stiffness and shape. ■ **Caution:** Tarsus also refers to the seven tarsal bones of the instep (plural, **tarsi**).

The Eyebrows and Eyelashes

The **eyebrows and eyelashes** prevent foreign matter from reaching the eyes.

- The edges of the eyelids contain **cilia** (**SIL**-ee-ah), also known as **eyelashes**, and oil-producing sebaceous glands.

The Conjunctiva

The **conjunctiva** (kon-junk-**TYE**-vah) is the mucous membrane that lines the underside of each eyelid and continues to form a protective covering over the exposed surface of the eyeball (plural, **conjunctivae**).

The Lacrimal Apparatus

The **lacrimal apparatus** (**LACK**-rih-mal), also known as the **tear apparatus**, consists of the structures that produce, store, and remove tears.

- The **lacrimal glands** are located above the outer corner of each eye. These glands secrete **lacrimal fluid**, also known as **tears**, that maintains moisture on the anterior surface of the eyeball.

- **Lacrimation** (lack-rih-**MAY**-shun) is the normal continuous secretion of tears by the lacrimal glands.
- The **lacrimal canaliculi** (**LACK**-rih-mal kan-ah-**LICK**-you-lye) are the ducts at the inner corner of each eye. These ducts collect tears and drain them into the lacrimal sac (singular, **canaliculus**).
- The **lacrimal sac**, also known as the **dacryocyst** (**DACK**-ree-oh-sist) or **tear sac**, is an enlargement of the upper portion of the lacrimal duct.
- The **lacrimal duct**, also known as the **nasolacrimal duct**, is the passageway that drains lacrimal fluid into the nose.

The Eyeball

The eyeball, also known as the **globe**, is a 1-inch sphere with walls made up of three layers: the sclera, choroid, and retina (Figure 11.3). The interior of the eye is divided into anterior and posterior segments.

The Sclera

The **sclera** (**SKLEHR**-ah), also known as the **white of the eye**, is the fibrous tissue outer layer of the eye. It maintains the shape of the eye and protects the delicate inner layers of tissue. ■ **Caution:** The word part **scler/o** means both the white of the eye and it means hard.

- The **cornea** (**KOR**-nee-ah) is the transparent anterior portion of the sclera. It is the cornea that provides most of the optical power of the eye.

The Uveal Tract

The **uveal tract** (**YOU**-vee-ahl), also known as the **uvea** (**YOU**-vee-ah) is the vascular layer of the eye. It includes the choroid, iris, and ciliary body (Figure 11.4).

The Choroid

The **choroid** (**KOH**-roid), also known as the **choroid layer** or **choroid coat**, is the opaque middle layer of the eyeball. **Opaque** (oh-**PAYK**) means that light cannot pass through this substance.

- The choroid contains many blood vessels and provides the blood supply for the entire eye.

The Iris, Pupil, and Lens

- The **iris** is the pigmented (colored) muscular layer that surrounds the pupil.
- The **pupil** is the black circular opening in the center of the iris that permits light to enter the eye.
- Muscles within the iris control the amount of light that is allowed to enter.
- To **decrease** the amount of light, these circular muscles contract and make the opening smaller.

FIGURE 11.4 The uveal tract includes the choroid, iris, and ciliary body.

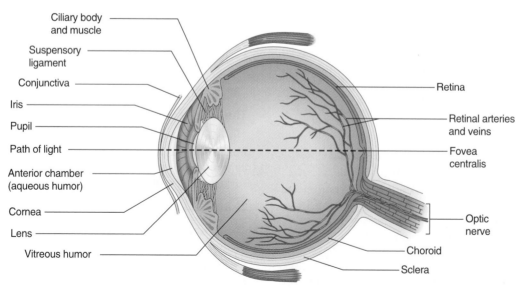

FIGURE 11.3 Structures of the eyeball shown in cross section.

- To **increase** the amount of light, the muscles dilate (relax) and make the opening larger.
- The **lens**, also known as the **crystalline lens**, is the clear, flexible, and curved structure that focuses images on the retina. It is held in place by the suspensory ligaments from the ciliary body. It is contained within a clear capsule and is located behind the iris and pupil.

The Ciliary Body

The **ciliary body** (**SIL**-ee-ehr-ee), which is located within the choroid, is a set of muscles and suspensory ligaments that adjust the lens to refine the focus of light rays on the retina.

- To focus on nearby objects, these muscles adjust the lens to make it thicker. To focus on distant objects, these muscles stretch the lens so it is thinner.

The Retina

The **retina** (**RET**-ih-nah) is the sensitive inner nerve layer of the eye located between the posterior chamber and the choroid layer at the back of the eye.

- The retina contains specialized light-sensitive cells called **rods** (black and white receptors) and **cones** (color receptors).
- These rods and cones receive images and convert them into nerve impulses.

The Macula Lutea and Fovea Centralis

- The **macula lutea** (**MACK**-you-lah **LOO**-tee-ah) is a clearly defined yellow area in the center of the retina (*macula* means spot and *lutea* means yellow). This is the area of sharpest central vision.
- The **fovea centralis** (**FOH**-vee-ah sen-**TRAH**-lis) is a pit in the middle of the macula lutea. Color vision is best in this area because it contains a high concentration of cones.

The Optic Disk and Nerve

- The **optic disk**, also known as the **blind spot**, is the region in the eye where the nerve endings of the retina gather to form the optic nerve. It is called the blind spot because it does not contain any rods or cones.
- The **optic nerve**, also known as the **II cranial nerve**, transmits the nerve impulses from the retina to the brain.

Segments of the Eye

The eye is divided into anterior and posterior segments.

Anterior Segment of the Eye

The front one-third of the eyeball, known as the **anterior segment**, is divided into anterior and posterior chambers (Figure 11.5).

- The **anterior chamber** is located behind the inner surface of the cornea and in front of the iris. The **posterior chamber** is located between the back of the iris and the front of the lens.

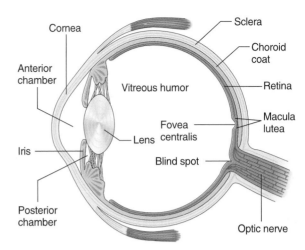

FIGURE 11.5 The anterior portion of the eye (in front of the lens) contains aqueous humor. The posterior portion (behind the lens capsule) is filled with vitreous humor.

- These chambers are filled with **aqueous fluid**, also known as **aqueous humor**. A **humor** is any clear body liquid or semifluid substance.
- This fluid nourishes the intraocular structures and is constantly filtered and drained through the **trabecular meshwork** and the **canal of Schlemm** (Figure 11.6).
- This constant drainage regulates **intraocular pressure** (IOP), which normally is between 12 and 21 mm Hg (see Diagnostic Procedures).

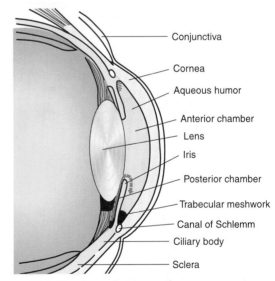

FIGURE 11.6 The flow of aqueous humor.

Posterior Segment of the Eye

- The **posterior** two-thirds of the eyeball is filled with **vitreous humor** (**VIT**-ree-us), which is also known as **vitreous gel**. This soft, clear, jelly-like mass aids the eye in maintaining its shape.
- The posterior portion of the eye is lined with the retina and its related structures.

Normal Action of the Eyes

- **Accommodation** (ah-**kom**-oh-**DAY**-shun) is the process whereby the eyes make adjustments for seeing objects at various distances. These adjustments include constriction (narrowing) or dilation (widening) of the pupil, movement of the eyes, and changes in the shape of the lens.

- **Convergence** (kon-**VER**-jens) is the simultaneous inward movement of both eyes (toward each other), usually in an effort to maintain single binocular vision as an object comes nearer.

- **Emmetropia** (em-eh-**TROH**-pee-ah), also known as **EM**, is the normal relationship between the refractive power of the eye and the shape of the eye that enables light rays to focus correctly on the retina (**emmetr** means in proper measure and **opia** means vision condition). Compare this with hyperopia and myopia.

- **Refraction** is the ability of the lens to bend the light rays to help them focus on the retina (see Figure 11.9A).

Visual Acuity

Visual acuity is the ability to distinguish object details and shape at a distance. Normal vision stated as 20/20.

- A **Snellen chart** is used to measure visual acuity. The results are recorded as two numbers in fraction form (Figure 11.7).

- The **first number** indicates the distance from the chart which is standardized at 20 feet. The **second number** indicates the deviation from the norm based on the ability to read lines of letters on the chart.

- As an example, a person with 20/40 vision can read at 20 feet what someone with normal vision could read at 40 feet.

Pathology of the Eyes

The Eyelids

- **Blepharoptosis** (**blef**-ah-roh-**TOH**-sis *or* **blef**-ah-rop-**TOH**-sis) is drooping of the upper eyelid (**blepharo** means eyelid and **ptosis** means drooping or sagging) (Figure 11.8A).

- **Ectropion** (eck-**TROH**-pee-on) is the eversion (turning outward) of the edge of the eyelid (**ec** mean out, **trop** means turn, and **ion** means condition) (Figure 11.8B).

- **Entropion** (en-**TROH**-pee-on) is the inversion (turning inward) of the edge of the eyelid (**en** means in, **trop** means turn, and **ion** means condition) (Figure 11.8C).

- A **hordeolum** (hor-**DEE**-oh-lum), also known as a **stye**, is an infection of one or more glands at the border of the eyelid (Figure 11.8D).

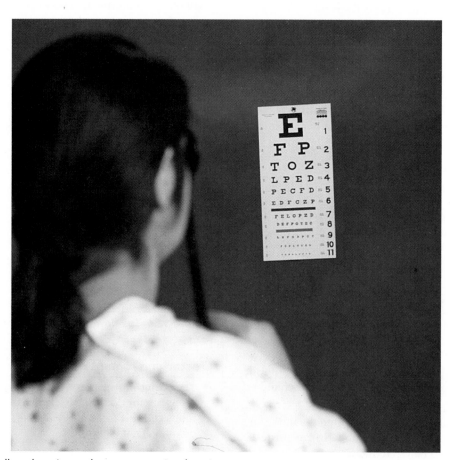

Figure 11.7 A Snellen chart is used to measure visual acuity.

(A)

(C)

(B)

(D)

FIGURE 11.8 Disorders of the eyelid. (A) Blepharoptosis. (B) Ectropion. (C) Entropion. (D) Hordeolum.

- A **chalazion** (kah-LAY-zee-on), also known as an **internal hordeolum**, is a localized swelling of the eyelid resulting from obstruction of one of the sebaceous (oil-producing) glands of the eyelid.

Additional Adnexa Pathology

- **Dacryocystitis** (**dack**-ree-oh-sis-TYE-tis) is an inflammation of the lacrimal sac and is associated with faulty tear drainage (**dacryocyst** means tear sac and **itis** means inflammation).

- **Conjunctivitis** (kon-**junk**-tih-VYE-tis), also known as **pinkeye**, is an inflammation of the conjunctiva (**conjunctiv** means conjunctiva and **itis** means inflammation).

- **Xerophthalmia** (**zeer**-ahf-THAL-mee-ah), also known as **dry eye**, is drying of eye surfaces characterized by the loss of luster of the conjunctiva and cornea (**xer** means dry, **ophthalm** means eye and **ia** means abnormal condition).

Sclera, Cornea, and Iris

- **Scleritis** (skleh-RYE-tis) is an inflammation of the sclera (**scler** means white of eye and **itis** means inflammation). *Note:* **scler/o** also means hard.

- **Keratitis** (ker-ah-TYE-tis) is an inflammation of the cornea (**kerat** means cornea and **itis** means inflammation). *Note:* **kerat/o** also means hard.

- A **corneal abrasion** is an injury, such as a scratch or irritation, to the outer layers of the cornea.

- A **corneal ulcer** is a pitting of the cornea caused by an infection or injury. These ulcers heal with treatment; however, they may leave a cloudy scar that impairs vision.

- **Iritis** (eye-RYE-tis) is an inflammation of the iris (**irit** means iris and **itis** means inflammation).

- **Synechia** (sigh-NECK-ee-ah) is an adhesion that binds the iris to any adjacent structure (plural, **synechiae**). An **adhesion** (ad-HE-zhun) holds structures together abnormally.

Eye

- **Anisocoria** (an-ih-so-KOH-ree-ah) is a condition in which the pupils are unequal in size (**aniso** means unequal, **cor** means pupil, and **ia** means abnormal condition). This may be congenital (present at birth) or caused by a head injury, aneurysm, or pathology of the central nervous system.

- A **cataract** (**KAT**-ah-rakt) is the loss of transparency of the lens. This may be congenital (present at birth) or caused by trauma (injury) or disease; however, the formation of most cataracts is associated with ageing (Figure 11.9B).

- **Choked disk**, also known as **papilledema** (pap-ill-eh-DEE-mah), is swelling and inflammation of the optic nerve at the point of entrance through the optic disk. This swelling is caused by increased intracranial pressure and may be due to a tumor pressing on the optic nerve.

- **Floaters**, also known as **vitreous floaters**, are particles that float in the vitreous fluid and cast shadows on the retina. Floaters occur normally with aging or in association with vitreous detachments, retinal tears, or intraocular inflammations.

- **Nystagmus** (nis-TAG-mus) is an involuntary, constant, rhythmic movement of the eyeball.

- In a **retinal detachment**, also known as a **detached retina**, the retina is pulled away from its normal position of being attached to the choroid in the back of the eye. A **retinal tear** occurs if the retina tears (develops a hole) as it is pulled away from its normal position.

- **Uveitis** (you-vee-EYE-tis) is an inflammation anywhere in the uveal tract (**uve** means uveal tract and **itis** means inflammation). It may affect the choroid, iris, or ciliary body and has many possible causes including diseases elsewhere in the body. Uveitis can rapidly damage the eye and produce complications including cataracts, detached retina, and glaucoma.

Glaucoma

Glaucoma (glaw-KOH-mah) is characterized by increased intraocular pressure (IOP). If untreated this pressure damages the optic nerve and causes the loss of peripheral vision and eventually blindness (Figure 11.9C).

(A)

(C)

(B)

(D)

FIGURE 11.9 Pathology causes vision changes. (A) Normal vision. (B) Vision reduced by cataracts. (C) The loss of peripheral vision caused by untreated glaucoma. (D) The loss of central vision due to macular degeneration.

- In **open-angle glaucoma**, which is the most common form of glaucoma, the trabecular meshwork becomes blocked.

- In **closed-angle glaucoma** the opening between the cornea and iris narrows so that fluid cannot reach the trabecular meshwork. This may cause a sudden increase in pressure and produce severe pain, nausea, redness of the eye, and blurred vision. Without immediate treatment blindness may occur in as little as 2 days.

- Glaucoma does not produce symptoms noticed by the patient until the optic nerve has been damaged; however, it can be detected before damage occurs through regular eye examinations including tonometry and visual field testing.

Macular Degeneration

Macular degeneration (**MACK**-you-lar) is a gradually progressive condition that results in the loss of central vision but not in total blindness (Figure 11.9D). This condition, which most frequently affects older people, is also known as **age-related macular degeneration** or **AMD**.

- **Dry-type macular degeneration**, which accounts for 90% of cases, is caused by the atrophy (deterioration) of the macula.

- **Wet-type macular degeneration** is associated with the formation of new blood vessels that produce small hemorrhages.

Functional Defects

- **Diplopia** (dih-**PLOH**-pee-ah), also known as **double vision**, is the perception of two images of a single object (**dipl** means double and **opia** means vision condition).

- **Hemianopia** (**hem**-ee-ah-**NOH**-pee-ah) is blindness in one half of the visual field.

- **Monochromatism** (**mon**-oh-**KROH**-mah-tizm), also known as **color blindness**, is the lack of the ability to distinguish colors (**mono** means one, **chromat** means color, and **ism** means condition).

- **Nyctalopia** (**nick**-tah-**LOH**-pee-ah), also known as **night blindness**, is a condition in which the individual has difficulty seeing at night (**nyctal** means night and **opia** means vision condition).

- **Presbyopia** (**pres**-bee-**OH**-pee-ah) describes the changes in the eyes that occur with aging (**presby** means old age and **opia** means vision condition). With aging the lens becomes less flexible and the muscles of the ciliary body become weaker. The result is that the eyes are no longer able to focus the image properly on the retina.

Strabismus

- **Strabismus** (strah-**BIZ**-mus), also known as a **squint**, is a disorder in which the eyes cannot be directed in a parallel manner toward the same object (Figure 11.10).

- **Esotropia** (**es**-oh-**TROH**-pee-ah), also known as **cross-eyes**, is strabismus characterized by an inward deviation

FIGURE 11.10 Strabismus is a disorder in which the eyes cannot be directed in a parallel manner toward the same object.

of one eye in relation to the other (**eso** means inward, **trop** means turn, and **ia** means abnormal condition).

- **Exotropia** (**eck**-soh-**TROH**-pee-ah), also known as **wall-eye**, is strabismus characterized by the outward deviation of one eye relative to the other (**exo** means outward, **trop** means turn, and **ia** means abnormal condition).

Refractive Disorders

A **refractive disorder** is a condition in which the lens and cornea do not bend light so that it focuses properly on the retina. Normal refraction is shown in Figure 11.11A.

(A) Normal eye
Light rays focus on the retina

(B) Hyperopia (farsightedness)
Light rays focus beyond the retina

(C) Myopia (nearsightedness)
Light rays focus in front of the retina

FIGURE 11.11 Refraction. (A) Normal eye. (B) Hyperopia (farsightedness).(C) Myopia (nearsightedness).

- **Ametropia** (am-eh-**TROH**-pee-ah) is an error of refraction in which only objects located a finite distance from the eye are focused on the retina (**ametr** means out of proportion and **opia** means vision condition).

- **Astigmatism** (ah-**STIG**-mah-tizm) is a condition in which the eye does not focus properly because of unequal curvatures of the cornea.

- **Hyperopia** (**high**-per-**OH**-pee-ah), also known as **farsightedness**, is a defect in which light rays focus beyond the retina. This condition occurs most commonly after age 40 (Figure 11.11B).

- **Myopia** (my-**OH**-pee-ah), also known as **nearsightedness**, is a defect in which light rays focus in front of the retina. This condition occurs most commonly in school-aged children (Figure 11.11C).

Blindness

- **Amblyopia** (am-blee-**OH**-pee-ah) is a dimness of vision or the partial loss of sight without detectable disease of the eye (**ambly** means dim or dull and **opia** means vision condition).

- **Blindness** is the inability to see. Although some sight remains, **legal blindness** is the point at which, under law, an individual is considered to be blind. A commonly used standard is that a person is legally blind when his best-corrected vision is reduced to 20/200 or less (see Normal Action of the Eyes).

- **Scotoma** (skoh-**TOH**-mah), also known as **blind spot**, is an abnormal area of absent or depressed vision surrounded by an area of normal vision.

Diagnostic Procedures of the Eyes

Routine Diagnostic Procedures

- **Visual acuity measurement** (ah-**KYOU**-ih-tee) is an evaluation of the eye's ability to distinguish object details and shape (see Normal Action of the Eyes).

- **Refraction** is an examination procedure to determine an eye's refractive error and the best corrective lenses to be prescribed. A **diopter** (dye-**AHP**-tur) is a unit of measurement of lens refractive power.

- **Tonometry** (toh-**NOM**-eh-tree) measures **intraocular pressure** (IOP). Abnormally high pressure may be an indication of glaucoma.

- In preparation for an examination of the interior of the eye, it is necessary to **dilate** (**DYE**-layt) the pupils. This is accomplished by administering **mydriatic drops** (**mid**-ree-**AT**-ick) that produce temporary paralysis, which forces the pupils to remain wide open even in the presence of bright light.

Specialized Diagnostic Procedures

- **Fluorescein staining** (**flew**-oh-**RES**-ee-in) is used to visualize a corneal abrasion (injury). When the stain is applied, corneal abrasions are stained bright green.

- In **intravenous fluorescein angiography** (**flew**-oh-**RES**-ee-in **an**-jee-**OG**-rah-fee), also known as **IVFA**, a dye is injected into the arm and pictures are taken as the dye passes through the blood vessels in the retina. This test allows the doctor to detect leaking blood vessels within the eye.

- A **visual field test** is used to determine losses in peripheral vision. Such a loss is characteristic of glaucoma.

Treatment Procedures of the Eyes

The Orbit and Eyelids

- **Orbitotomy** (or-bih-**TOT**-oh-mee) is a surgical incision into the orbit for biopsy, abscess drainage, and removal of a tumor mass or foreign object (**orbit** means bony socket and **otomy** means surgical incision).

- A **tarsectomy** (tahr-**SECK**-toh-mee) is the surgical removal of a segment of the tarsal plate of the upper or lower eyelid (**tars** means eyelid and **ectomy** means surgical removal).

- **Tarsorrhaphy** (tahr-**SOR**-ah-fee) is partially or completely suturing together the upper and lower eyelids (**tars** means eyelid and **rrhaphy** means to suture). This procedure is performed to provide protection to the eye when the lids are paralyzed and unable to close normally.

- Cosmetic procedures relating to the eyelids are discussed in Chapter 12.

Conjunctiva, Cornea, and Iris

- **Conjunctivoplasty** (kon-junk-**TYE**-voh-**plas**-tee) is the surgical repair of the conjunctiva (**conjunctivo** means conjunctiva and **plasty** means surgical repair).

- A **corneal transplant**, also known as **keratoplasty** (**KER**-ah-toh-**plas**-tee), is the surgical replacement of scarred or diseased cornea with clear corneal tissue from a donor (**kerato** means cornea and **plasty** means surgical repair).

- An **iridectomy** (ir-ih-**DECK**-toh-mee) is the surgical removal of a portion of the iris tissue (**irid** means iris and **ectomy** means surgical removal).

- **Radial keratotomy** (ker-ah-**TOT**-oh-mee), also known as **RK**, is used to correct myopia (**kerat** means cornea and **otomy** means surgical incision). During the surgery partial incisions are made in the cornea causing it to flatten.

Cataract Surgery

- **Lensectomy** (len-**SECK**-toh-mee) is the general term used to describe the surgical removal of a cataract-clouded lens.

- **Extracapsular cataract extraction**, also known as **ECCE**, is the removal of a cloudy lens that leaves the posterior lens capsule intact (Figure 11.12).

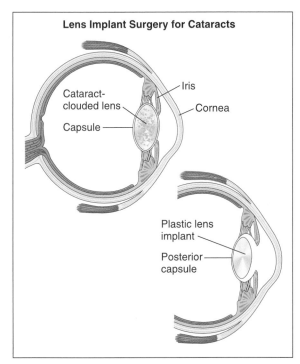

Lens Implant Surgery for Cataracts

Cataract-clouded lens
Iris
Cornea
Capsule

Plastic lens implant
Posterior capsule

FIGURE 11.12 In an extracapsular extraction, the lens is removed, the posterior lens capsule is left intact, and an intraocular lens (IOL) is placed.

- **Intracapsular cataract extraction**, also known as **ICCE**, is the removal of a cloudy lens including the surrounding capsule.
- **Phacoemulsification** (**fay**-koh-ee-**mul**-sih-fih-**KAY**-shun *or* **fack**-koh-ee-**mul**-sih-fih-**KAY**-shun) is the use of ultrasonic vibration to shatter and break up a cataract, making it easier to remove.
- An **intraocular lens**, also known as an **IOL**, is a plastic lens surgically implanted to replace the natural lens.
- **Aphakia** (ah-**FAY**-kee-ah) is the absence of the lens of an eye after cataract extraction (**a** means without, **phak** means lens, and **ia** means abnormal condition).
- **Pseudophakia** (**soo**-doh-**FAY**-kee-ah) is an eye in which the natural lens is replaced with an IOL (**pseudo** means false, **phak** means lens, and **ia** means abnormal condition).

Laser Treatments

Lasers have a wide range of applications in the treatment of eye disorders. (For more details on how lasers work, see Chapter 12.) In the treatment of eye disorders lasers are used for the following reasons.

- Treat **open-angle glaucoma** by creating an opening that allows fluid to drain properly to prevent pressure buildup within the eye. This procedure is known as **laser trabeculoplasty** (trah-**BECK**-you-loh-**plas**-tee).

- Treat **closed-angle glaucoma** by creating an opening in the iris to allow proper drainage. This procedure is known as **laser iridotomy** (ir-ih-**DOT**-oh-mee).
- Treat some forms of **macular degeneration** by sealing leaking or damaged blood vessels.
- Treat **retinal tears** by sealing the torn portion.
- Reattach a **detached retina**. This procedure is also known as **retinopexy** (**RET**-ih-noh-**peck**-see).
- Correct **refraction disorders** by reshaping of the top layer of the cornea. This procedure is known as **photorefractive keratectomy** (**ker**-ah-**TECK**-toh-mee) or **PRK**.
- Remove **clouded tissue** that may form in the posterior portion of the lens capsule after cataract extraction.

Structures of the Ears

The ear is divided into three separate regions: the outer ear, middle ear, and inner ear (Figure 11.13).

The Outer Ear

- The **pinna** (**PIN**-nah), also known as the **auricle**, is the external portion of the ear. This structure catches sound waves and transmits them into the external auditory canal.
- The **external auditory canal** transmits sound waves from the pinna to the middle ear.
- **Cerumen** (seh-**ROO**-men), also known as **earwax**, is secreted by ceruminous glands that line the auditory canal. This sticky yellow-brown substance has protective functions because it traps small insects, dust, debris, and certain bacteria to prevent them from entering the middle ear.

The Middle Ear

- The **tympanic membrane** (tim-**PAN**-ick), also known as the **TM** or **eardrum**, is located between the outer and middle ear (Figure 11.14). (The word parts **myring/o** and **tympan/o** both mean tympanic membrane.)
- When sound waves reach it, this membrane transmits the sound by vibrating.
- The middle ear is surrounded by the **mastoid cells** that are hollow air spaces located in the mastoid process of the temporal bone. An infection in the middle ear can rapidly spread to these cells.

The Auditory Ossicles

The **auditory ossicles** (**OSS**-ih-kulz) are three small bones found in the middle ear. These bones transmit the sound waves from the eardrum to the inner ear by vibration. These bones, which are named for their shapes, are the:

- **Malleus** (**MAL**-ee-us) also known as the **hammer**.
- **Incus** (**ING**-kus) also known as the **anvil**.
- **Stapes** (**STAY**-peez) also known as the **stirrup**.

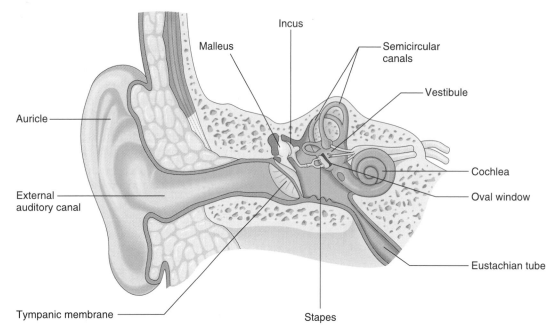

FIGURE 11.13 Structures of the ear shown in cross section.

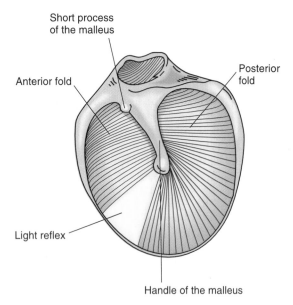

FIGURE 11.14 Schematic of the normal tympanic membrane as viewed from the auditory canal.

The Eustachian Tubes

The **eustachian tubes** (you-STAY-shun *or* you-STAY-kee-an) are also known as the **auditory tubes**. These narrow tubes, which lead from the middle ear to the nasopharynx, equalize the air pressure in the middle ear with that of the outside atmosphere.

- The **oval window**, located under the base of the stapes, is the membrane that separates the middle ear from the inner ear.

The Inner Ear

The **inner ear**, also known as the **labyrinth** (**LAB**-ih-rinth), contains the sensory receptors for hearing and balance.

- The **cochlea** (**KOCK**-lee-ah) is the spiral-shaped passage that leads from the oval window.
- The **cochlear duct**, located within the cochlea, is filled with fluid that vibrates when the sound waves strike it.
- The **organ of Corti**, also located within the cochlea, is the receptor site that receives these vibrations and relays them to the **auditory nerve fibers** that transmit them to the auditory center of the cerebral cortex, where they are interpreted and heard.
- The three **semicircular canals**, also located within the inner ear, contain **endolymph** (a liquid) and sensitive hairlike cells. The bending of these hairlike cells in response to the movements of the head sets up impulses in nerve fibers to help maintain equilibrium. **Equilibrium** is the state of balance.
- The **acoustic nerves**, cranial nerve VIII, transmit this information to the brain and the brain sends messages to muscles in all parts of the body to ensure that equilibrium is maintained.

Normal Action of the Ears

- Sound waves enter the ear through the pinna, travel down the auditory canal, and strike the TM between the outer and middle ear. This is called **air conduction**.
- As the eardrum vibrates, it moves the auditory ossicles and these conduct sound waves through the middle ear. This is called **bone conduction**.

- Sound vibrations reach the inner ear via the oval window. The structures of the inner ear receive the sound waves and relay them to the brain. This is called **sensorineural conduction**.

Pathology of the Ears

Outer Ear

- **Impacted cerumen** is an accumulation of cerumen that forms a solid mass adhering to the walls of the external auditory canal. (**Impacted** means lodged or wedged firmly in place.)
- **Otalgia** (oh-**TAL**-gee-ah), also known as an earache, is pain in the ear (**oto** means ear and **algia** means pain).
- **Otitis** (oh-**TYE**-tis) means any inflammation of the ear (**oto** means ear and **itis** means inflammation). The second term gives the location of the inflammation.
- **Otitis externa** is an inflammation of the outer ear.
- **Otomycosis** (oh-toh-my-**KOH**-sis), also known as **swimmer's ear**, is a fungal infection of the external auditory canal (**oto** means ear, **myc** means fungus, and **osis** means abnormal condition).
- **Otopyorrhea** (oh-toh-**pye**-oh-**REE**-ah) is the flow of pus from the ear (**oto** means ear, **pyo** means pus, and **rrhea** means abnormal flow).
- **Otorrhagia** (oh-toh-**RAY**-jee-ah) is bleeding from the ear (**oto** means ear and **rrhagia** means bleeding).

Middle Ear

- **Eustachitis** (**you**-stay-**KYE**-tis) is an inflammation of the eustachian tube (**eustach** means eustachian tube and **itis** means inflammation).
- **Mastoiditis** (mas-toy-**DYE**-tis) is an inflammation of any part of the mastoid process (**mastoid** means mastoid process and **itis** means inflammation).
- **Myringitis** (mir-in-**JIGH**-tis) is an inflammation of the tympanic membrane (**myring** means eardrum and **itis** means inflammation).
- **Otosclerosis** (oh-toh-skleh-**ROH**-sis) is ankylosis of the bones of the middle ear resulting in a conductive hearing loss (**oto** means ear and **sclerosis** means abnormal hardening). **Ankylosis** (ang-kih-**LOH**-sis) means fused together.
- **Patulous eustachian tube** (**PAT**-you-lus) is distention of the eustachian tube. (**Patulous** means extended, spread wide open.)

Otitis Media

- **Acute otitis media** (oh-**TYE**-tis **MEE**-dee-ah), also known as **AOM**, is an inflammation of the middle ear usually associated with an upper respiratory infection that is most commonly seen in young children.

- **Serous otitis media** (**SEER**-us oh-**TYE**-tis **MEE**-dee-ah), also known as **SOM**, is a fluid buildup in the middle ear that may follow acute otitis media or be caused by obstruction of the eustachian tube (Figure 11.15A).
- SOM is also known as **otitis media with effusion**. **Effusion** (eh-**FEW**-zhun) is the escape of fluid from blood or lymphatic vessels into the tissues or a cavity.
- **Purulent otitis media** (**PYOU**-roo-lent oh-**TYE**-tis **MEE**-dee-ah) is a buildup of pus within the middle ear (Figure 11.15B).

Inner Ear

- **Labyrinthitis** (lab-ih-rin-**THIGH**-tis) is an inflammation of the labyrinth resulting in vertigo. **Vertigo** (**VER**-tih-goh) is a sense of whirling, dizziness, and the loss of balance.
- **Menière's syndrome** (men-ee-**AYRZ** *or* men-**YEHRS**) is a chronic disease of the inner ear characterized by three main symptoms: attacks of vertigo (dizziness), a fluctuating hearing loss (usually in one ear), and tinnitus.
- **Tinnitus** (tih-**NIGH**-tus) is a ringing, buzzing, or roaring sound in the ears.

Hearing Loss

- **Deafness** is the complete or partial loss of the ability to hear. It may range from the inability to hear sounds of a certain pitch or intensity to a complete loss of hearing.

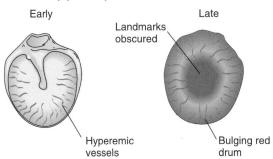

(A) Serous otitis media

Hairline air-fluid level

Air bubbles

Fluid (amber-colored)

(B) Acute purulent otitis media

Early

Late

Landmarks obscured

Hyperemic vessels

Bulging red drum

FIGURE 11.15 The tympanic membrane in the presence of otitis media. (A) Serous otitis media. (B) Acute purulent otitis media. Hyperemic means increased blood within these vessels.

- A **conductive hearing loss** is one in which the outer or middle ear does not conduct sound vibrations to the inner ear normally.

- A **noise-induced hearing loss** is the result of the loss of sensitive hairlike cells of the inner ear. This damage is most commonly caused by repeated exposure to very intense noise such as aircraft engines, noisy equipment, and loud music.

- A **sensorineural hearing loss**, also known as **nerve deafness**, is a symptom of problems affecting the inner ear.

- **Presbycusis** (**pres**-beh-**KOO**-sis) is a progressive hearing loss occurring in old age (**presby** means old age and **cusis** means hearing).

Diagnostic Procedures of the Ears

- **Audiometry** (**aw**-dee-**OM**-eh-tree) is the use of an audiometer to measure hearing (**audio** means hearing and **metry** means to measure).

- An **audiometer** (**aw**-dee-**OM**-eh-ter) is an electronic device that produces acoustic stimuli of a known frequency and intensity (**audio** means hearing and **meter** means to measure).

- **Speech audiometry** measures the threshold of speech reception (hearing speech sounds) and speech discrimination (understanding speech sounds).

- An **evoked potential audiometer** is an instrument that detects response to sound stimuli by changes in the electroencephalogram (record of brain wave activity).

- **Tympanometry** (**tim**-pah-**NOM**-eh-tree) is the indirect measurement of acoustical energy absorbed or reflected by the middle ear (**tympano** means eardrum and **metry** means to measure). In a conductive hearing loss, the middle ear absorbs relatively less sound and reflects relatively more sound. This test is used to test for middle ear effusion (fluid buildup) or eustachian tube obstruction. The resulting record is a **tympanogram**.

- **Monaural** (mon-**AW**-rahl) testing involving one ear (**mon** means one, **aur** means hearing, and **al** means pertaining to).

- **Binaural** (bye-**NAW**-rul *or* bin-**AW**-rahl), testing involving both ears (**bi** means two, **aur** means hearing, and **al** means pertaining to).

Treatment Procedures of the Ears

Outer Ear

- **Otoplasty** (**OH**-toh-**plas**-tee) is the surgical repair of the pinna of the ear (**oto** means ear and **plasty** means surgical repair).

Middle Ear

- A **mastoidectomy** (mas-toy-**DECK**-toh-mee) is the surgical removal of mastoid cells (**mastoid** means mastoid process and **ectomy** means surgical removal).

- A **myringectomy** (mir-in-**JECK**-toh-mee), also known as a **tympanectomy** (tim-pah-**NECK**-toh-me), is the surgical removal of all or part of the tympanic membrane (**myring** means eardrum and **ectomy** means surgical removal).

- A **myringotomy** (mir-in-**GOT**-oh-mee) is the surgical incision of the eardrum to create an opening for the placement of tympanostomy tubes (**myring** means eardrum and **otomy** means surgical incision).

- **Tympanocentesis** (tim-pah-noh-sen-**TEE**-sis) is the surgical puncture the tympanic membrane with a needle to remove fluid from the middle ear (**tympano** means eardrum and **centesis** means a surgical puncture to remove fluid).

- **Tympanoplasty** (tim-pah-noh-**PLAS**-tee) is the surgical correction of a damaged middle ear (**tympano** means eardrum and **plasty** means a surgical repair).

- **Tympanostomy tubes** (tim-pan-**OSS**-toh-mee) are tiny ventilating tubes placed through the eardrum to provide ongoing drainage for fluids and to relieve pressure that can build up after ear infections.

- A **stapedectomy** (stay-peh-**DECK**-toh-mee) is the surgical removal of the stapes.

Inner Ear

- A **fenestration** (fen-es-**TRAY**-shun) is a surgical procedure in which a new opening is made in the labyrinth of the inner ear to restore hearing.

- A **labyrinthectomy** (lab-ih-rin-**THECK**-toh-mee) is the surgical removal of the labyrinth (**labyrinth** means labyrinth and **ectomy** means surgical removal).

- A **labyrinthotomy** (lab-ih-rin-**THOT**-oh-mee) is a surgical incision into the labyrinth (**labyrinth** means labyrinth and **otomy** means a surgical incision).

Learning Exercises

Matching Word Parts—1

Write the letter of the correct answer on the line provided in the left column.

11.1. _____ blephar/o   A. cornea, hard

11.2. _____ -cusis   B. to measure

11.3. _____ kerat/o   C. eyelid

11.4. _____ dacryocyst   D. hearing

11.5. _____ -metry   E. tear sac

Matching Word Parts—2

Write the letter of the correct answer on the line provided in the left column.

11.6. _____ pseud/o   A. eye, vision

11.7. _____ irid/o   B. false

11.8. _____ -opia   C. iris of the eye

11.9. _____ opthalm/o   D. old age

11.10. _____ presby/o   E. vision condition

Matching Word Parts—3

Write the letter of the correct answer on the line provided in the left column.

11.11. _____ ot/o   A. retina

11.12. _____ retin/o   B. hard, white of eye

11.13. _____ scler/o   C. turn

11.14. _____ tympan/o   D. ear

11.15. _____ trop/o   E. eardrum

● Definitions

Circle the letter next to the correct answer.

11.16. Which structure maintains the shape of the eye and protects the delicate inner tissues?

a. choroid

b. conjunctiva

c. cornea

d. sclera

11.17. Which structure is a spiral-shaped passage that leads from the oval window of the inner ear?

a. cochlea

b. eustachian tube

c. organ of Corti

d. semicircular canal

11.18. Which structure is also known as the blind spot?

a. fovea centralis

b. macula lutea

c. optic disk

d. optic nerve

11.19. Which structure lies between the outer ear and the middle ear?

a. mastoid process

b. oval window

c. pinna

d. tympanic membrane

11.20. Which structure separates the middle ear from the inner ear?

a. eustachian

b. inner canthus

c. oval window

d. tympanic membrane

11.21. Which of the auditory ossicles is also known as the anvil?

a. incus

b. labyrinth

c. malleus

d. stapes

11.22. What does the term patulous mean?

a. abnormal hardening

b. abnormal narrowing

c. closed, filled with fluid

d. extended, spread wide open

11.23. Which term means the lessening of the accommodation of the lens occurring normally with aging?

a. ametropia

b. amblyopia

c. presbyopia

d. presbycusis

11.24. Which term describes reattachment of a detached retina using a laser?

a. keratoplasty

b. laser trabeculoplasty

c. photorefractive keratectomy

d. retinopexy

11.25. Which form of otitis media involves a buildup of pus in the middle ear?

a. acute otitis media

b. otitis media with effusion

c. purulent otitis media

d. serous otitis media

● Matching Conditions

Write the letter of the correct answer on the line provided in the left column.

11.26. _____ diplopia   A. squint

11.27. _____ esotropia   B. nearsightedness

11.28. _____ hyperopia   C. farsightedness

11.29. _____ myopia   D. double vision

11.30. _____ strabismus   E. cross-eyes

● Which Word?

Circle the correct term in each sentence.

11.31. The turning inward of an eyelid is called *ectropion* / *entropion*.

11.32. The term meaning bleeding from the ears is
otorrhagia / otorrhea.

11.33. The surgical placement of a ventilating tube
through the eardrum to drain fluid is a
myringotomy / tympanostomy.

11.34. A visual field test to determine losses in
peripheral vision is used to diagnose *cataracts
/ glaucoma.*

11.35. A hearing test that involves both ears is *binaural / binocular.*

● **Spelling Counts**

Find the misspelled word in each sentence. Then write
that word, spelled correctly, on the line provided.

11.36. The euctachian tubes lead from the middle
ear to the pharynx. _____

11.37. Cerunem, which is also known as earwax, is
secreted by glands that line the external auditory canal. _____

11.38. An astegmatism is a condition in which the
eye does not focus properly because of
unequal curvatures of the cornea.
_____

11.39. The surgical procedure in which a new opening is made in the labyrinth of the inner ear is
known as a fenistration.
_____

11.40. A Snellen chart is used to measure visual acuity. _____

● **Matching Abbreviations**

Write the letter of the correct answer on the line provided in the left column.

11.41. _____ AD   A. both eyes

11.42. _____ AS   B. left ear

11.43. _____ OD   C. left eye

11.44. _____ OS   D. right ear

11.45. _____ OU   E. right eye

● **Term Selection**

Circle the letter next to the correct answer.

11.46. Which condition may be treated by radial keratotomy?

a. astigmatism

b. cataracts

c. hyperopia

d. myopia

11.47. Which term describes a condition in which
the pupils are unequal in size?

a. anisocoria

b. choked disk

c. macular degeneration

d. synechia

11.48. Which term describes the surgical repair of
the pinna of the ear?

a. keratoplasty

b. myringoplasty

c. otoplasty

d. tympanoplasty

11.49. Which term describes a condition that results
in the loss of central vision?

a. glaucoma

b. macular degeneration

c. presbyopia

d. uveitis

11.50. Which term describes a condition that is also
known as a stye?

a. blepharoptosis

b. chalazion

c. dacryocystitis

d. hordeolum

● Sentence Completion

Write the correct term on the line.

11.51. The ability of the lens to bend light rays to help them focus on the retina is known as _____ .

11.52. A sense of whirling, dizziness, and the loss of balance is called _____ .

11.53. A specialist in measuring the accuracy of vision is a/an _____ .

11.54. The medical term meaning an inflammation of the cornea is _____ .

11.55. The medical term for color blindness is _____ .

● True/False

If the statement is true, write T on the line. If the statement is false, write F on the line.

11.56. _____ Dacryocystitis is associated with faulty tear drainage.

11.57. _____ A sensorineural hearing loss is also known as nerve deafness.

11.58. _____ A tarsorrhaphy is the surgical repair of the eyelids.

11.59. _____ Binaural refers to hearing in both ears.

11.60. _____ Open-angle glaucoma causes severe pain and a sudden increase in eye pressure.

11.61. _____ Rods in the retina are the receptors for color.

11.62. _____ Aqueous fluid is drained through the canal of Schlemm.

11.63. _____ Scotoma is an area of absent or depressed vision surrounded by an area of normal vision.

11.64. _____ Synechia is an adhesion of the cornea to the surrounding structures.

11.65. _____ Tympanometry is a diagnostic test to measure hearing.

● Clinical Conditions

Write the correct answer on the line.

11.66. Following the boxing match, Jack Lawson required _____ to repair the pinna of his injured ear.

11.67. Sheila McClelland suffers from a/an _____ hearing loss because the middle ear does not conduct sound vibrations to the inner ear normally.

11.68. Edward Cooke was treated for an inflammation of mastoid cells. The medical term for this condition is _____ .

11.69. Margo Wilkins was diagnosed as having deterioration of the macula lutea of the retina. The medical term for this condition is _____ _____ .

11.70. Mr. Eisner suffers from a progressive hearing loss that occurs in old age. The medical term for this condition is _____ .

11.71. Juan Ramirez has an earache caused by a buildup of fluid in the middle ear. His doctor referred to this condition as serous _____ _____ .

11.72. Adrienne Jacobus says she suffers from night blindness. The medical term for this condition is _____ .

11.73. Maude Colson is troubled by _____ , which is a ringing sound in her ears.

11.74. Paul Ogelthorpe is color blind. This condition is listed on his chart as _____ .

11.75. Mrs. Liu's hearing loss was diagnosed as being caused by ankylosis of the bones of the middle ear. The medical term for this condition is _____ .

● Which is the correct medical term?

Circle the letter next to the correct answer.

11.76. Which medical term describes a chronic disease of the inner ear characterized mainly by dizziness, a fluctuating hearing loss, and tinnitus?

    a. eustachitis

    b. Menière's syndrome

    c. papilledema

    d. xerophthalmia

11.77. Which medical term describes an adhesion that binds the iris to an adjacent structure?

    a. blepharoptosis

    b. convergence

    c. scleritis

    d. synechia

11.78. Which medical term describes the condition commonly known as double vision?

    a. ametropia

    b. diplopia

    c. esotropia

    d. hemianopia

11.79. Which medical term describes the condition commonly known as farsightedness?

    a. amblyopia

    b. exotropia

    c. hyperopia

    d. myopia

11.80. Which medical term describes an accumulation of earwax in the auditory canal?

    a. conjunctivitis

    b. impacted cerumen

    c. otitis externa

    d. pseudophakia

● Challenge Word Building

These terms are *not* found in this chapter; however, they are made up of these familiar word parts. You may want to look in the glossary or use a medical dictionary to check your answers!

blephar/o	-algia
irid/o	-ectomy
lacrim/o	-edema
ophthalm/o	-itis
labyrinth/o	-ology
retin/o	-otomy
	-pathy

11.81. The medical term meaning pain felt in the iris is _____ .

11.82. The medical term meaning inflammation of the eyelid is _____ .

11.83. The medical term meaning an incision into the iris is known as a/an

_____ .

11.84. The medical term meaning any disease of the retina is _____ .

11.85. The medical term meaning the study of the eye is _____ .

11.86. The medical term meaning swelling of the eyelid is _____ .

11.87. The medical term meaning a surgical incision into the lacrimal duct is a/an

_____ .

11.88. The medical term meaning the surgical removal of the labyrinth of the inner ear is a/an _____ .

11.89. The medical term meaning any disease of the iris is _____ .

11.90. The medical term meaning inflammation of the retina is _____ .

● Labeling Exercises

Identify the numbered items on these diagrams.

11.91. _____

11.92. _____ chamber

11.93. crystalline _____

11.94. _____

11.95. _____ centralis

11.96. _____ or _____

11.97 external _____ canal

11.98. _____ membrane

11.99. _____ tube

11.100. _____

11.91 — Sclera · Choroid coat · Vitreous humor · Retina · 11.95 · 11.92 · 11.93 · 11.94 · Blind spot · Optic nerve

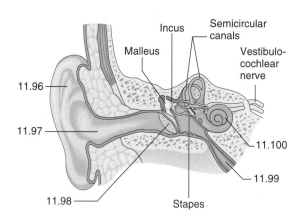

Incus · Semicircular canals · Malleus · Vestibulo-cochlear nerve · 11.96 · 11.97 · 11.100 · 11.99 · 11.98 · Stapes

The Human Touch: Critical Thinking Exercise

The following story and questions are designed to stimulate critical thinking through class discussion or as a brief essay response. There are no easy or right-wrong answers to these questions.

William Davis is 62 years old. He was employed as a postal worker until his declining eyesight forced him into early retirement a few months ago. His wife Mildred died last year of complications from diabetes after a prolonged and expensive hospitalization. Mr. Davis does not trust the medical community; because of this, he has not been to a doctor since his wife's death.

Mr. Davis is not considered legally blind, but his presbyopia and the advancing cataract in his right eye are starting to interfere with his ability to take care of himself. He still drives to the market once a week, but angry drivers honk and yell at him. He pays for his groceries with a credit card because he is afraid the checker will cheat him if he accidentally gives her the wrong bill. He complains that the cleaning lady hides things from him and deliberately leaves the furniture out of place. When she leaves he can't find his slippers, or an ashtray. Yesterday he put his lit pipe down in a wooden bowl by accident.

His son insists on taking him to see the ophthalmologist that treated his wife's diabetic retinopathy. Dr. Hsing believes Mr. Davis' sight can be improved in the right eye by performing phacoemulsification and pseudophakia. Mr. Davis listens in fear as the doctor explains. "Without this procedure your sight will only get worse."

Mr. Davis thinks about all the medical "procedures" that were tried on Mildred, and she died anyway. He doesn't want to go into the hospital, and he doesn't want any operations. But his son is talking about taking away his car if he doesn't do something about his failing sight. What more can be taken away from him, he thinks bitterly. First his wife, then his job, and now his independence . . .

Suggested Discussion Topics:

1. Discuss how Mr. Davis' loss of sight is affecting the way he treats and is treated by others.
2. Mr. Davis is a patient at the clinic where you work. Discuss the ways you would adjust your usual routine to accommodate his needs.
3. Close your eyes and keep them closed for 15 minutes while a classmate or friend leads you around. Discuss how you felt and what could have been done to make the experience less stressful.
4. Discuss why cataract surgery would be scary to Mr. Davis and what Dr. Hsing and his staff could do to ease his apprehension.
5. If he doesn't go ahead with the surgery, there are support groups that can help Mr. Davis cope with his vision loss. What groups might help him deal with his grief and depression?

Skin: The Integumentary System

- ## Overview of Structures, Word Parts, and Functions of the Integumentary System

Major Structures	Related Word Roots	Primary Functions
Skin	cutane/o, dermat/o, derm/o	Intact skin is the first line of defense for the immune system. Skin also waterproofs the body and is the major receptor for the sense of touch.
Sebaceous glands	seb/o	Secrete sebum (oil) to lubricate the skin and discourage the growth of bacteria on the skin.
Sweat glands	hidr/o	Secrete sweat to regulate body temperature and water content and excrete some metabolic waste.
Hair	pil/i, pil/o	Aids in controlling the loss of body heat.
Nails	onych/o, ungu/o	Protect the dorsal surface of the last bone of each finger and toe.

● VOCABULARY   Related to the Skin

Check the box as you master each word part or term. Terms marked with the ❖ symbol are pronounced on the optional student audiotape.

Key Word Parts

- ☐ albin/o
- ☐ bi/o
- ☐ derm/o, dermat/o
- ☐ erythr/o
- ☐ hidr/o
- ☐ kerat/o
- ☐ lip/o
- ☐ melan/o
- ☐ myc/o
- ☐ onych/o
- ☐ pedicul/o
- ☐ pil/o
- ☐ rhytid/o
- ☐ seb/o
- ☐ xer/o

Key Medical Terms

- ☐ **abrasion** (ah-**BRAY**-zhun)
- ☐ **actinic keratosis** (ack-**TIN**-ick **kerr**-ah-**TOH**-sis) ❖
- ☐ **albinism** (**AL**-bih-niz-um) ❖
- ☐ **alopecia** (al-oh-**PEE**-shee-ah) ❖
- ☐ **anhidrosis** (an-high-**DROH**-sis) ❖
- ☐ **blepharoplasty** (**BLEF**-ah-roh-**plas**-tee) ❖
- ☐ **bulla** (**BULL**-ah)
- ☐ **carbuncle** (**KAR**-bung-kul) ❖
- ☐ **cauterization** (kaw-ter-eye-**ZAY**-shun) ❖
- ☐ **cellulitis** (**sell**-you-**LYE**-tis) ❖
- ☐ **chloasma** (kloh-**AZ**-mah) ❖
- ☐ **cicatrix** (sick-**AY**-tricks) ❖
- ☐ **comedo** (**KOM**-eh-doh) ❖
- ☐ **contusion** (kon-**TOO**-zhun)
- ☐ **debridement** (day-breed-**MON**) ❖
- ☐ **decubitus ulcer** (dee-**KYOU**-bih-tus) ❖
- ☐ **dermabrasion** (der-mah-**BRAY**-zhun) ❖
- ☐ **dermatitis** (der-mah-**TYE**-tis) ❖
- ☐ **dermatomycosis** (**der**-mah-toh-my-**KOH**-sis) ❖
- ☐ **dermatoplasty** (**DER**-mah-toh-**plas**-tee)
- ☐ **diaphoresis** (dye-ah-foh-**REE**-sis)
- ☐ **dyschromia** (dis-**KROH**-mee-ah) ❖
- ☐ **dysplastic nevi** (dis-**PLAS**-tick **NEE**-vye) ❖
- ☐ **ecchymosis** (eck-ih-**MOH**-sis) ❖
- ☐ **eczema** (**ECK**-zeh-mah) ❖
- ☐ **epithelioma** (ep-ih-thee-lee-**OH**-mah)
- ☐ **erythema** (er-ih-**THEE**-mah) ❖
- ☐ **exfoliative cytology** (ecks-**FOH**-lee-**ay**-tiv sigh-**TOL**-oh-jee) ❖
- ☐ **furuncle** (**FYOU**-rung-kul) ❖
- ☐ **gangrene** (**GANG**-green) ❖

- ☐ **granuloma** (gran-you-**LOH**-mah) ❖
- ☐ **hemangioma** (hee-**man**-jee-**OH**-mah *or* heh-**man**-jee-**OH**-mah) ❖
- ☐ **hirsutism** (**HER**-soot-izm) ❖
- ☐ **hyperhidrosis** (**high**-per-high-**DROH**-sis) ❖
- ☐ **impetigo** (im-peh-**TYE**-go) ❖
- ☐ **keloid** (**KEE**-loid) ❖
- ☐ **keratosis** (kerr-ah-**TOH**-sis)
- ☐ **koilonychia** (koy-loh-**NICK**-ee-ah) ❖
- ☐ **lipectomy** (lih-**PECK**-toh-mee)
- ☐ **lipedema** (lip-eh-**DEE**-mah)
- ☐ **lipocytes** (**LIP**-oh-sights)
- ☐ **lipoma** (lih-**POH**-mah)
- ☐ **liposuction** (**LIP**-oh-**suck**-shun *or* **LYE**-poh-**suck**-shun) ❖
- ☐ **lupus erythematosus** (**LOO**-pus er-ih-**thee**-mah-**TOH**-sus) ❖
- ☐ **macule** (**MACK**-youl) ❖
- ☐ **melanoma** (mel-ah-**NOH**-mah) ❖
- ☐ **miliaria** (mill-ee-**AYR**-ee-ah)
- ☐ **onychia** (oh-**NICK**-ee-ah) ❖
- ☐ **onychocryptosis** (on-ih-koh-krip-**TOH**-sis) ❖
- ☐ **onychomycosis** (on-ih-koh-my-**KOH**-sis) ❖
- ☐ **papilloma** (pap-ih-**LOH**-mah)
- ☐ **papule** (**PAP**-youl)
- ☐ **paronychia** (**par**-oh-**NICK**-ee-ah) ❖
- ☐ **pediculosis** (pee-**dick**-you-**LOH**-sis) ❖
- ☐ **petechiae** (pee-**TEE**-kee-ee) ❖
- ☐ **pruritus** (proo-**RYE**-tus) ❖
- ☐ **psoriasis** (soh-**RYE**-uh-sis) ❖
- ☐ **purpura** (**PUR**-pew-rah) ❖
- ☐ **purulent** (**PYOU**-roo-lent) ❖
- ☐ **putrefaction** (pyou-treh-**FACK**-shun) ❖
- ☐ **rhinophyma** (rye-noh-**FIGH**-muh) ❖
- ☐ **rhytidectomy** (rit-ih-**DECK**-toh-mee) ❖
- ☐ **rosacea** (roh-**ZAY**-shee-ah) ❖
- ☐ **scabies** (**SKAY**-beez) ❖
- ☐ **scleroderma** (sklehr-oh-**DER**-mah *or* skleer-oh-**DER**-mah) ❖
- ☐ **seborrhea** (seb-oh-**REE**-ah) ❖
- ☐ **seborrheic keratosis** (seb-oh-**REE**-ick **kerr**-ah-**TOH**-sis) ❖
- ☐ **subungual hematoma** (sub-**UNG**-gwal **hee**-mah-**TOH**-mah)
- ☐ **tinea** (**TIN**-ee-ah) ❖
- ☐ **urticaria** (ur-tih-**KAR**-ree-ah) ❖
- ☐ **verrucae** (veh-**ROO**-see) ❖
- ☐ **vesicle** (**VES**-ih-kul) ❖
- ☐ **vitiligo** (vit-ih-**LYE**-goh) ❖
- ☐ **wheal** (**WHEEL**) ❖
- ☐ **xeroderma** (zee-roh-**DER**-mah) ❖

● **OBJECTIVES**

On completion of this chapter, you should be able to:

1 Identify and describe the functions and structures of the integumentary system.

2 Identify the medical specialists associated with the integumentary system.

3 Recognize, define, spell, and pronounce the terms used to describe the pathology and

diagnostic and treatment procedures related to the skin.

4 Recognize, define, spell, and pronounce terms used to describe the pathology and diagnostic and treatment procedures related to hair, nails, and sebaceous glands.

Functions of the Integumentary System

The **integumentary system** (in-**teg**-you-**MEN**-tah-ree), which makes up the outer covering of the body, serves many important functions beyond appearance.

Functions of the Skin

- The skin waterproofs the body and prevents fluid loss.
- Intact (unbroken) skin plays important roles in the immune system (see Chapter 6).
- Skin is the major receptor for the sense of touch.
- Skin helps the body synthesize (manufacture) vitamin D from the sun's ultraviolet light, while screening out harmful ultraviolet radiation.

Functions of Related Structures

- **Sebaceous glands** (seh-**BAY**-shus), also known as **oil glands**, secrete **sebum** (oil) that lubricates the skin and discourages the growth of bacteria on the skin.
- **Sweat glands** help regulate body temperature and water content by secreting sweat. Also, a small amount of metabolic waste is excreted through the sweat glands.
- **Hair** helps control the loss of body heat.
- **Nails** protect the dorsal surface of the last bone of each toe and finger.

Structures of the Integumentary System

The integumentary system consists of the skin and its related structures: sebaceous glands, sweat glands, hair, and nails (Figure 12.1).

The Skin

Skin covers the external surfaces of the body. The terms **derma** and **cutaneous** (kyou-**TAY**-nee-us) are both used

to describe the skin (**cutane** means skin and **ous** means pertaining to).

The skin is a complex system of specialized tissues and is made up of three strata (layers) of tissue (Figure 12.2). These three layers are the

- Epidermis
- Dermis
- Subcutaneous layer

The Epidermis

Epithelial tissues (ep-ih-**THEE**-lee-al) form a protective covering for *all* of the internal and external surfaces of the body. The **epidermis** (ep-ih-**DER**-mis), which is the outermost layer of the skin, is made up of several specialized epithelial tissues.

- **Squamous epithelial tissue**, which forms the upper layer, consists of flat, scaly cells that are continuously sloughed off (shed). **Squamous** (**SKWAY**-mus) means scalelike.
- The epidermis does not contain any blood vessels or connective tissue and is dependent on lower layers for nourishment.
- Cells are produced in the lower **basal layer** and pushed upward. When these cells reach the surface they die and become filled with keratin.
- **Keratin** (**KER**-ah-tin) is a fibrous, water-repellent protein. Soft keratin is a primary component of the epidermis. Hard keratin is found in the hair and nails.
- The basal cell layer also contains special cells called **melanocytes** (**MEL**-ah-noh-sights *or* meh-**LAN**-oh-sights). These cells produce and contain a dark brown to black pigment called **melanin** (**MEL**-ah-nin). The type and amount of melanin pigment determines the color of the skin.
- Melanin also protects the skin against some of the harmful ultraviolet rays of the sun. **Ultraviolet** (**UV**) refers to light that is beyond the visible spectrum at the violet end. Some UV rays help the skin produce vitamin D, but others can cause damage.

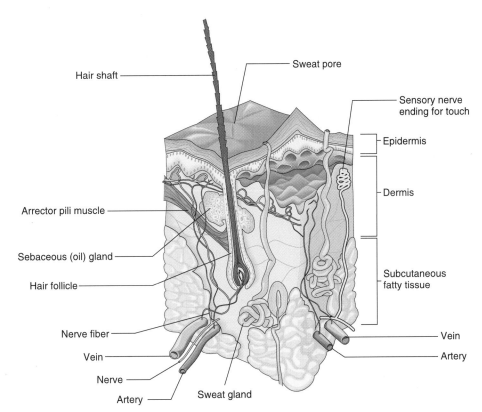

FIGURE 12.1 Structures of the skin.

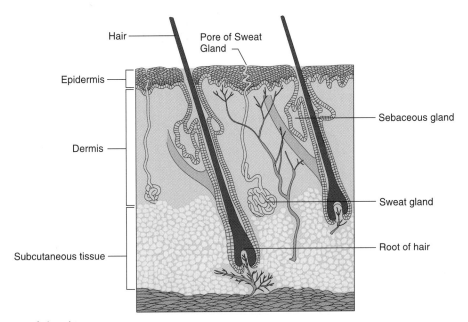

FIGURE 12.2 Layers of the skin.

The Dermis

The **dermis** (DER-mis) is the thick layer of living tissue directly below the epidermis. It contains connective tissue, blood and lymph vessels, nerve fibers, plus hair follicles and sebaceous and sweat glands.

Sensitive nerve endings in the dermis receive impulses that enable the body to recognize sensory stimuli such as touch, temperature, pain, and pressure.

- **Tactile** (TACK-til) means pertaining to touch.
- **Perception** is the ability to recognize sensory stimulus.

Tissues Within the Dermis

- **Collagen** (**KOL**-ah-jen), which means glue, is a tough, yet flexible, fibrous protein material. In addition to being found in the skin, collagen is also found in bone, cartilage, tendons, and ligaments. Some cosmetics contain artificially produced collagen protein, claiming it minimizes wrinkles.

- **Mast cells**, which are found in the connective tissue of the dermis, respond to injury or infection by producing and releasing substances including heparin and histamine.

- **Heparin** (**HEP**-ah-rin), which is released in response to injury, is an anticoagulant.

- **Histamine** (**HISS**-tah-meen), which is released in response to allergens, causes itching and increased mucous secretion.

The Subcutaneous Layer

The **subcutaneous layer**, located just below the skin, connects the skin to the surface muscles.

- This layer is made up of loose connective tissue and fatty **adipose tissue**. **Adipose** (**AD**-ih-pohs) means fat.

- **Cellulite** is a nontechnical term for the subcutaneous deposit of fat, especially in the thighs and buttocks.

- **Lipocytes** (**LIP**-oh-sights), also known as **fat cells**, are predominant in the subcutaneous layer where they manufacture and store large quantities of fat.

Associated Structures of the Integumentary System

The structures associated with the integumentary system (Figure 12.3) are the

- Sebaceous glands
- Sweat glands
- Hair
- Nails

The Sebaceous Glands

Sebaceous glands (seh-**BAY**-shus) are located in the dermis layer of the skin and are closely associated with hair follicles.

- These glands secrete **sebum** (**SEE**-bum), which is released through ducts opening into the hair follicles. From here the sebum moves onto the surface and lubricates the skin. Because sebum is slightly acidic it also discourages the growth of bacteria on the skin.

- The milk-producing **mammary glands**, which are modified sebaceous glands, are often classified with the integumentary system. However, they also are part of the reproductive system and are discussed in Chapter 14.

The Sweat Glands

Sweat glands are tiny, coiled glands found on almost all body surfaces. They are most numerous in the palms of

FIGURE 12.3 Glands of the skin.

the hands, the soles of the feet, the forehead, and the armpits. Ducts from sweat glands open on the surface of the skin through **pores**.

- **Sweat**, also known as **perspiration**, is secreted by sweat glands and is made up of 99% water plus some salt and metabolic waste products.

- **Perspiring**, or secreting sweat, is a means of excreting excess water. It also cools the body as the sweat evaporates into the air. Body odor associated with sweat comes from the interaction of the perspiration with bacteria on the skin's surface.

- **Hidrosis** (high-**DROH**-sis) means the production and excretion of sweat (**hidr** means sweat and **osis** means condition.)

The Hair

Hair fibers are rodlike structures composed of tightly fused, dead protein cells filled with hard keratin. The darkness of the hair color is determined by the amount of melanin produced by the melanocytes that surround the core of the hair shaft.

- **Hair follicles** are the sacs that hold the **root** of the hair fibers. The **arrector pili** (ah-**RECK**-tor **PYE**-lye), also known as the **erector muscles**, are tiny muscle fibers attached to the hair follicles that cause the hair to stand erect. In response to cold or fright, these muscles contract causing raised areas of skin known as goose bumps. This action reduces heat loss through the skin.

The Nails

A nail, also known as an **unguis** (**UNG**-gwis), is the keratin plate covering the dorsal surface of the last bone of each toe and finger (plural, **ungues**). Each nail consists of these parts (Figure 12.4):

- The **nail body**, which is translucent, is closely molded to the surface of the underlying tissues. It is made up of hard, keratinized plates of epidermal cells.

- The **nail bed**, which joins the nail body to the underlying connective tissue, nourishes the nail. The blood vessels here give the nail its characteristic pink color.

- The **free edge**, which is the portion of the nail not attached to the nail bed, extends beyond the tip of the finger or toe.

Free edge
Nail body
Lunula
Cuticle
Nail matrix (located under the nail body)
Root (located under the edge of the skin)

FIGURE 12.4 Structures of the finger or toenail.

- The **cuticle** is a narrow band of epidermis attached to the surface of the nail just in front of the root. (Cuticle means little skin.)

- The **lunula** (**LOO**-new-lah) is a pale half-moon-shaped region at the nail root and is generally found in the thumbnail and in varying degrees in other nails (plural, **lunulae**). (Lunula means little moon.)

- The **root** fastens the nail to the finger or toe by fitting into a groove in the skin.

Medical Specialties Related to the Integumentary System

- A **dermatologist** (**der**-mah-**TOL**-oh-jist) specializes in diagnosing and treating disorders of the skin (**dermat** means skin and **ologist** means specialist).

- A **cosmetic surgeon**, also known as a **plastic surgeon**, specializes in the surgical restoration and reconstruction of body structures. **Plastic** in this title refers to **-plasty** the word part meaning surgical repair.

Pathology of the Integumentary System

Sebaceous Gland Disorders

- **Acne vulgaris** (**ACK**-nee vul-**GAY**-ris) is a chronic inflammatory disease that is characterized by pustular eruptions of the skin in or near the sebaceous glands. Although common during puberty and adolescence, it also occurs in adults.

- A **comedo** (**KOM**-eh-doh) is a lesion formed by the buildup of sebum and keratin in a hair follicle. Often associated with acne vulgaris, when the sebum plug is exposed to air it oxidizes and becomes a **blackhead** (plural, **comedones**).

- A **sebaceous cyst** (seh-**BAY**-shus) is a cyst of a sebaceous gland, containing yellow, fatty material. (A **cyst** is a closed sac or pouch containing fluid or semisolid material.)

- **Seborrhea** (seb-oh-**REE**-ah) is any of several common skin conditions in which there is an overproduction of sebum (**sebo** means sebum and **rrhea** means flow).

- **Seborrheic dermatitis** (seb-oh-**REE**-ick **der**-mah-**TYE**-tis) is an inflammation of the upper layers of the skin, caused by seborrhea. This results in the scaling of the scalp known as **dandruff**. Mild dandruff may be caused only by overactive oil glands. In newborns this condition results in a scalp rash known as **cradle cap**.

- A **seborrheic keratosis** (seb-oh-**REE**-ick **kerr**-ah-**TOH**-sis) is a benign flesh-colored, brown or black skin tumor. These growths tend to occur most often in the elderly.

Sweat Gland Disorders

- **Anhidrosis** (an-high-**DROH**-sis) is the condition of lacking or being without sweat (**an** means without, **hidr** means sweat, and **osis** means abnormal condition).

- **Hyperhidrosis** (**high**-per-high-**DROH**-sis) is a condition of excessive sweating (**hyper** means excessive, **hidr** means sweat, and **osis** means abnormal condition).

- **Diaphoresis** (**dye**-ah-foh-**REE**-sis) means profuse, but not necessarily excessive, sweating.

- **Miliaria** (**mill**-ee-**AYR**-ee-ah), also known as **heat rash** and **prickly heat**, is an inflammation caused by trapped sweat. This produces a skin rash and itching. (Do not confuse this with *malaria*, an infectious disease.)

Hair

Excessive Hairiness

- **Hirsutism** (**HER**-soot-izm) means abnormal hairiness (**hirsut** means hairy and **ism** means condition). This term usually refers to the appearance of male body or facial hair patterns in the female.

Abnormal Hair Loss

- **Alopecia** (**al**-oh-**PEE**-shee-ah), also known as **baldness**, is the partial or complete loss of hair (**alopec** means baldness and **ia** means condition).

- **Alopecia areata** is an autoimmune disorder in which there are well-defined bald areas, usually on the scalp and face.

- **Alopecia capitis totalis** is an uncommon condition characterized by the loss of all the hair on the scalp.

- **Alopecia universalis** is the total loss of hair on all parts of the body.

- **Female pattern baldness** is a condition in which the hair thins in the front and on the sides, and sometimes on the crown. It rarely leads to total hair loss.

- **Male pattern baldness** is a common hair loss pattern in men, with the hairline receding from the front to the back until only a horseshoe shaped area of hair remains in the back and temples.

Nails

- **Clubbing** is abnormal curving and shine on the nails that is often accompanied by enlargement of the fingertips. This condition can be hereditary or can be caused by changes associated with oxygen deficiencies related to coronary or pulmonary disease.

- **Koilonychia** (**koy**-loh-**NICK**-ee-ah), also known as **spoon nail**, is a malformation of the nails in which the outer surface is concave or scooped out (**koil** means hollow or concave, **onych** means fingernail or toenail, and **ia** means condition). Koilonychia is often indicative of iron-deficiency anemia.

- **Onychia** (oh-**NICK**-ee-ah), also known as **onychitis** (on-ih-**KYE**-tis), is an inflammation of the matrix of the nail (**onych** means fingernail or toenail and **ia** means condition).

- **Onychocryptosis** (**on**-ih-koh-krip-**TOH**-sis) means ingrown toenail (**onycho** means fingernail or toenail, **crypt** means hidden, and **osis** means abnormal condition).

- **Onychomycosis** (**on**-ih-koh-my-**KOH**-sis) is any fungal infection of the nail (**onycho** means fingernail or toenail, **myc** means fungus, and **osis** means abnormal condition). This condition, which is difficult to treat, may cause the nails to turn yellow, brown or black and become thick or brittle, depending on what type of fungus is involved.

- **Onychophagia** (**on**-ih-koh-**FAY**-jee-ah) means nail-biting or eating (**onycho** means fingernail or toenail and **phagia** means eating).

- **Paronychia** (**par**-oh-**NICK**-ee-ah) is an acute or chronic infection of the skin fold at the margin of a nail (**par** means along side of, **onych** means fingernail or toenail, and **ia** means condition).

- A **subungual hematoma** (sub-**UNG**-gwal **hee**-mah-**TOH**-mah), which is usually caused by an injury, is a collection of blood trapped in the tissues under a nail. Eventually this blood is resorbed by the body.

Pigmentation

- **Albinism** (**AL**-bih-niz-um) is an inherited deficiency or absence of pigment in the skin, hair, and eyes due to an abnormality in production of melanin (**albin** means white and **ism** means condition).

- **Chloasma** (kloh-**AZ**-mah), also known as **melasma** or the **mask of pregnancy**, is a pigmentation disorder characterized by brownish colored spots on the face. This may occur during pregnancy and usually disappears after delivery.

- **Dyschromia** (dis-**KROH**-mee-ah) is any disorder of the pigmentation of the skin or hair (**dys** means bad, **chrom** means color, and **ia** means condition).

- **Melanosis** (**mel**-ah-**NOH**-sis) is any condition of unusual deposits of black pigment in different parts of the body (**melan** means black and **osis** means abnormal condition).

- **Vitiligo** (vit-ih-**LYE**-goh) is a condition in which a loss of melanocytes results in whitish areas of skin bordered by normally pigmented areas. The unpigmented skin is extremely sensitive to sunburn.

Surface Lesions

A **lesion** (**LEE**-zhun) is a pathologic change of the tissues due to disease or injury. Lesions are described by their appearance, location, color, and size as measured in centimeters (Figure 12.5).

FIGURE 12.5 Lesions are described by length in centimeters.

- A **contusion** (kon-**TOO**-zhun) is an injury that does not break the skin and is characterized by swelling, discoloration, and pain.

- A **crust** is a collection of dried serum and cellular debris (Figure 12.6).

- An **ecchymosis** (eck-ih-**MOH**-sis), also known as a **bruise**, is a purplish area caused by hemorrhaging (bleeding) within the skin (plural, **ecchymoses**).

- A **macule** (**MACK**-youl) is a discolored, *flat* spot that is *less than* 1 cm in diameter. Freckles or flat moles are macules.

- **Nevi** (**NEE**-vye), also known as **moles**, are small dark skin growths that develop from melanocytes in the skin. Normally these growths are benign. **Dysplastic nevi** (dis-**PLAS**-tick **NEE**-vye) are atypical moles that may develop into skin cancer.

- A **nodule** (**NOD**-youl) is a small *solid* bump. It may be felt within the skin or it may be raised as if it had formed below the surface of the skin and pushed upward. A cyst is a nodule.

- A **papule** (**PAP**-youl) is a small, solid, raised skin lesion that is *less than* 0.5 cm in diameter. Warts, insect bites, and skin tags are types of papules.

- **Petechiae** (pee-**TEE**-kee-ee), which are small pinpoint hemorrhages, are smaller versions of ecchymoses (bruises) (singular, **petechia**).

- A **plaque** (**PLACK**) is a solid raised area of skin that is different from the area around it and *greater than* 0.5 cm in diameter. The lesions of psoriasis are plaques. (The term plaque also has several other meanings.)

- A **scale** is a flaking or dry patch made up of excess dead epidermal cells. Some shedding of scales is normal. Excessive shedding of scales is associated with skin disorders such as psoriasis.

- **Verrucae** (veh-**ROO**-see), also known as **warts**, are skin lesions caused by the human papillomavirus (singular, **verruca**). **Plantar warts** develop on the sole of the foot.

- A **wheal** (**WHEEL**) is a smooth, *slightly elevated*, swollen area that is redder or paler than the surrounding skin that is usually accompanied by itching, for example, an insect bite or hives.

Fluid-Filled Lesions

- An **abscess** (**AB**-sess) is a localized collection of pus within a circumscribed area that is associated with tissue destruction. **Circumscribed** (**SER**-kum-skryebd) means contained within a limited area and **purulent** (**PYOU**-roo-lent) means producing or containing pus.

- A **bulla** (**BULL**-ah) is a large circumscribed elevation of skin containing fluid that is *more than* 0.5 cm in diameter (Figure 12.7) (plural, **bullae**). A large blister is a bulla.

- A **cyst** is a closed sac or pouch containing fluid or semisolid material. The most common type of cyst is one filled with sebaceous secretions.

- A **pustule** (**PUS**-tyoul) is a small, circumscribed elevation of the skin containing pus. Pus containing pimples, such as those associated with acne, are pustules.

- A **vesicle** (**VES**-ih-kul) is a circumscribed elevation of skin containing fluid that is *less than* 0.5 cm in diameter. A small blister is a vesicle.

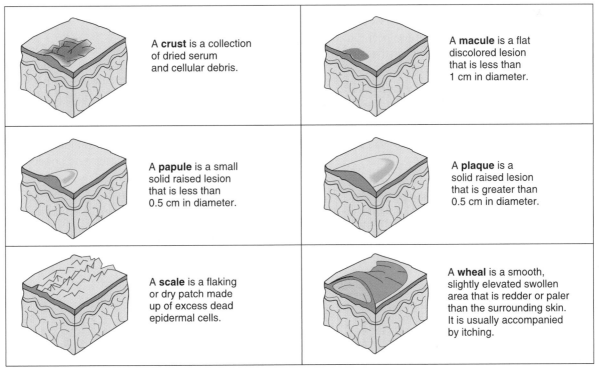

FIGURE 12.6 Surface lesions of the skin.

A **bulla** is a large vesicle that is more than 0.5 cm in diameter.

A **cyst** is a closed sack or pouch containing fluid or semisolid material.

A **pustule** is a small circumscribed elevation of the skin containing pus.

A **vesicle** is a circumscribed elevation of skin containing fluid that is less than 0.5 cm in diameter.

FIGURE 12.7 Fluid-filled lesions.

Lesions Through the Skin

- An **abrasion** (ah-**BRAY**-zhun) is an injury in which superficial layers of skin are scraped or rubbed away. The term abrasion also describes treatment involving scraping or rubbing away skin.

- A **fissure** of the skin is a groove or crack-like sore (Figure 12.8). The term fissure also describes normal folds in the contours of the brain.

- A **laceration** (**lass**-er-**AY**-shun) is a torn or jagged wound or an accidental cut.

- A **puncture wound** is a deep hole made by a sharp object such as a nail. The risk for infection, especially tetanus, is greater with this type of wound.

- An **ulcer** (**UL**-ser) is an open sore or erosion of the skin or mucous membrane resulting in tissue loss and usually with inflammation. *Note:* Ulcers also occur inside the body. Those associated with the digestive system are discussed in Chapter 8.

- A **decubitus ulcer**, also known as a **pressure ulcer** or **bedsore**, is an ulcerated area caused by prolonged pressure that cuts off circulation to a body part. (**Decubitus** [dee-**KYOU**-bih-tus] means lying down.)

Birthmarks

- A **port-wine stain** is a large reddish purple discoloration of the face or neck. This discoloration will not resolve without treatment (Figure 12.9). See Laser Treatments of Skin Conditions.

- A **strawberry hemangioma** (hee-**man**-jee-**OH**-mah *or* heh-**man**-jee-**OH**-mah) is a soft raised birthmark. This dark reddish purple growth is a benign tumor made up of newly formed blood vessels. These usually resolve without treatment by about age 7 years.

General Skin Conditions

- **Dermatitis** (**der**-mah-**TYE**-tis) is an inflammation of the upper layers of skin (**dermat** means skin and **itis** means inflammation).

- **Contact dermatitis** is a localized allergic response caused by contact with an irritant or allergen. Symptoms include erythroderma (redness), itching, and rash (Figure 12.10).

- **Dermatosis** (**der**-mah-**TOH**-sis) is a general term used to denote any skin lesion or group of lesions, or eruptions of any type that is *not* associated with inflammation (**dermat** means skin and **osis** means abnormal condition). (Plural, **dermatoses**.)

- **Eczema** (**ECK**-zeh-mah) is an acute or chronic skin inflammation characterized by erythema, papules, vesicles, pustules, scales, crusts, scabs, and possibly itching. These symptoms may occur alone or in combination.

- **Erythema** (er-ih-**THEE**-mah) is any redness of the skin such as a nervous blush, inflammation, or mild sunburn.

An **ulcer** is an open sore or erosion of the skin or mucous membrane resulting in tissue loss.

A **fissure** of the skin is a groove or crack-like sore.

FIGURE 12.8 Lesions through the skin.

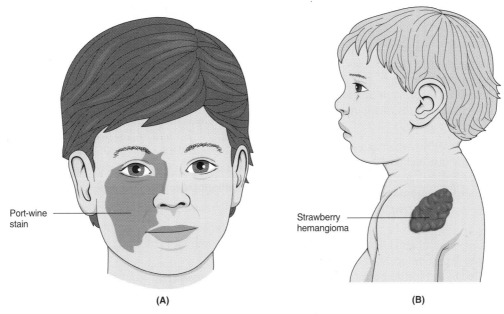

Figure 12.9 Types of birthmarks: (A) Port-wine stain; (B) Strawberry hemangioma

Figure 12.10 Contact dermatitis caused by poison oak. *(Courtesy of Timothy Berger, MD, Associate Clinical Professor, University of California, San Francisco)*

- **Lupus erythematosus** (**LOO**-pus er-ih-**thee**-mah-**TOH**-sus), also known as **LE** or **systemic lupus erythematosus** (SLE), is an autoimmune disorder characterized by a red, scaly rash on the face and upper trunk. In addition to the skin symptoms, LE also involves other body systems.
- **Lipedema** (lip-eh-**DEE**-mah) is an abnormal swelling due to the collection of fat and fluid under the skin, usually between the calf and ankle (**lip** means fat and **edema** means swelling). Compare with lymphedema in Chapter 6.

- **Pruritus** (proo-**RYE**-tus), also known as **itching**, is associated with most forms of dermatitis (**prurit** means itching and **us** is a singular noun ending).
- **Psoriasis** (soh-**RYE**-uh-sis) is a chronic autoimmune disorder of the skin characterized by red papules covered with silvery scales that occur predominantly on the elbows, knees, scalp, back, and buttocks (Figure 12.11).

Figure 12.11 Psoriasis is characterized by silvery scales. *(Courtesy of Robert A. Silverman, MD, Clinical Associate Professor, Department of Pediatrics, Georgetown University)*

- **Purpura** (**PUR**-pew-rah) is a condition characterized by hemorrhage into the skin that causes spontaneous bruising (**purpur** means purple and **a** is a noun ending).

- **Rosacea** (roh-**ZAY**-shee-ah) is a chronic condition of unknown cause that produces redness, tiny pimples, and broken blood vessels. It usually occurs on the central area of the face and appears more often in people with fair complexions.

- **Scleroderma** (**sklehr**-oh-**DER**-mah *or* **skleer**-oh-**DER**-mah) is an autoimmune disorder that causes abnormal tissue thickening usually starting on the hands, feet, or face (**sclero** means hard and **derma** means skin). Some forms of the disease spread to other body systems and can be fatal.

- **Urticaria** (**ur**-tih-**KAR**-ree-ah), also known as **hives**, is a skin condition characterized by localized areas of swelling accompanied by itching that is associated with an allergic reaction (**urtic** means rash and **aria** means connected with).

- **Xeroderma** (zee-roh-**DER**-mah) is excessively dry skin (**xero** means dry and **derma** means skin).

Bacterial Skin Infections

- A **carbuncle** (**KAR**-bung-kul) is a cluster of furuncles (boils) that result in extensive sloughing of skin and scar formation.

- **Cellulitis** (**sell**-you-**LYE**-tis) is a diffuse infection of connective tissue with severe inflammation within the layers of the skin. **Diffuse** means widespread.

- **Furuncles** (**FYOU**-rung-kuls), also known as **boils**, are large tender, swollen, areas caused by staphylococcal infection around hair follicles.

- **Gangrene** (**GANG**-green) is necrosis (tissue death) that is usually associated with a loss of circulation. The tissue death is followed by bacterial invasion that causes putrefaction. **Putrefaction** (**pyou**-treh-**FACK**-shun) is decay that produces foul-smelling odors.

- **Impetigo** (**im**-peh-**TYE**-goh) is a highly contagious bacterial skin infection characterized by isolated pustules that become crusted and rupture.

Fungal Skin Infections

- **Tinea** (**TIN**-ee-ah), also known as **ringworm**, is a fungus skin disease affecting different areas of the body. **Tinea capitis** is found on the scalps of children; **tinea pedis**, also known as **athlete's foot**, is found between the toes and on the feet; and **tinea cruris**, also known as **jock itch**, is found in the genital area.

- **Dermatomycosis** (**der**-mah-toh-my-**KOH**-sis), also known as **tinea versicolor**, is a fungal infection that causes white to light brown areas on the skin (**dermato** means skin, **myc** means fungus, and **osis** means abnormal condition).

Parasitic Skin Infestations

An **infestation** is the dwelling of a parasite on external surface tissue. Some parasites live on the skin temporarily, others lay eggs and reproduce there.

- **Scabies** (**SKAY**-beez) is a skin infection caused by an infestation with the itch mite.

- **Pediculosis** (pee-**dick**-you-**LOH**-sis) is an infestation with lice (**pedicul** means lice and **osis** means abnormal condition). There are three different types of lice, each attracted to a specific part of the body.

- **Pediculosis capitis** is an infestation with head lice.

- **Pediculosis corporis** is an infestation with body lice.

- **Pediculosis pubis** is an infestation with lice in the pubic hair and pubic region.

Skin Growths

- A **callus** (**KAL**-us) is a thickening of part of the skin on the hands or feet caused by repeated rubbing. (Compare with callus in Chapter 3.) A **clavus**, or **corn**, is a callus in the keratin layer of the skin covering the joints of the toes.

- A **cicatrix** (sick-**AY**-tricks) is a normal scar resulting from the healing of a wound (plural, **cicatrices**).

- **Granulation tissue** normally forms during the healing of a wound to create what will become scar tissue.

- **Granuloma** (gran-you-**LOH**-mah) is a general term used to describe small knotlike swellings of granulation tissue (**granul** meaning granular and **oma** means tumor). Granulomas may result from inflammation, injury, or infection.

- A **keloid** (**KEE**-loid) is an abnormally raised or thickened scar that is usually smooth and shiny.

- A **keratosis** (kerr-ah-**TOH**-sis) is any skin growth, such as a **wart** or **callus**, in which there is overgrowth and thickening of the skin (**kerat** means hard or horny and **osis** means abnormal condition. *Note:* **kerat/o** also refers to the cornea of the eye). (Plural, **keratoses**.)

- A **lipoma** (lih-**POH**-mah) is a benign fatty deposit under the skin, causing a bump (**lip** means fatty and **oma** means tumor).

- A **papilloma** (pap-ih-**LOH**-mah) is a benign epithelial tumor that projects from the surrounding surface (**papill** means resembling a nipple and **oma** means tumor.)

- **Polyp** (**POL**-ip) is a general term used most commonly to describe a mushroom-like growth from the surface of a mucous membrane such as a polyp in the nose. These growths have many causes and are not necessarily malignant.

- **Rhinophyma** (rye-noh-**FIGH**-muh), also known as **bulbous nose**, is hyperplasia (overgrowth) of the nose (**rhino** means nose and **phyma** means growth). This condition is often associated with rosacea (see Figure 12.16).

- **Skin tags** are small flesh-colored or light brown growths that hang from the body by fine stalks. Skin tags are benign and tend to enlarge with age.

Skin Cancer

Skin cancer is the most common form of cancer today, but fortunately most skin cancers are curable. Sun exposure is one of the main factors in predicting skin cancer.

- An **actinic keratosis** (ack-**TIN**-ick **kerr**-ah-**TOH**-sis) is a precancerous skin lesion caused by excessive exposure to the sun. Actinic keratoses are raised rough, dry, or scaly spots that are tan, brown, gray, or red in color.

- **Basal cell carcinoma** is a malignant tumor of the basal cell layer of the epidermis. Found mainly on the face, this is the most frequent and least harmful type of skin cancer. Basal cell carcinoma is slow growing and rarely spreads to other parts of the body. These lesions are smooth, raised with a depression in the center, pink in color, and tend to bleed easily (Figure 12.12).

- An **epithelioma** (**ep**-ih-thee-lee-**OH**-mah) is a benign or malignant tumor originating in the epidermis that may occur on the skin or mucous membranes (**epitheli** means epithelial tissue and **oma** means tumor).

- **Malignant melanoma** (mel-ah-**NOH**-mah), also known as **MM**, is skin cancer derived from cells capable of forming melanin. This cancer can occur in the skin of any part of the body and may metastasize to the lungs, liver, and brain. These lesions are usually asymmetrical (not evenly shaped), have irregular borders (ragged or blurred margins), are mixed colors (tan, brown, black, red, blue, and white), and larger in diameter than a pencil eraser (Figure 12.13). Moles with these characteristics may be signs of malignant melanoma.

- **Squamous cell carcinoma** begins as a malignant tumor of the squamous cells of the epithelium; however, it can quickly spread to other body systems. These cancers start as skin lesions that appear to be sores that will not heal or sores with a crusted, heaped-up look (Figure 12.14).

Burns

A **burn** is an injury to body tissues caused by heat, flame, electricity, sun, chemicals, or radiation. The severity of a burn is described according to the percentage of the total body skin surface affected (more than 15% is considered serious). It is also described according to the depth or layers of skin involved (Table 12.1 and Figure 12.15).

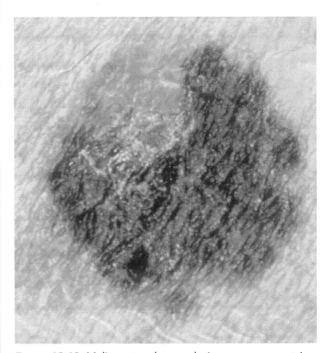

FIGURE 12.13 Malignant melanoma lesions are asymmetrical, have irregular borders, are mixed colors, and larger in diameter than a pencil eraser. *(Courtesy of the American Academy of Dermatology.)*

FIGURE 12.12 Basal cell carcinoma. *(Courtesy of Robert A. Silverman, MD, Clinical Associate Professor, Department of Pediatrics, Georgetown University)*

FIGURE 12.14 Squamous cell carcimoma. *(Courtesy of Robert A. Silverman, MD, Clinical Associate Professor, Department of Pediatrics, Georgetown University)*

Table 12.1

CLASSIFICATION OF BURN SEVERITY		
Type of Burn	**Also Known As**	**Layers of Skin Involved**
First-degree	**Superficial burns, sunburn**	No blisters, superficial damage to the epidermis
Second-degree	**Partial thickness burns**	Blisters; superficial damage to the epidermis
Third-degree	**Full thickness burns**	Damage to the epidermis, corium, and subcutaneous layers

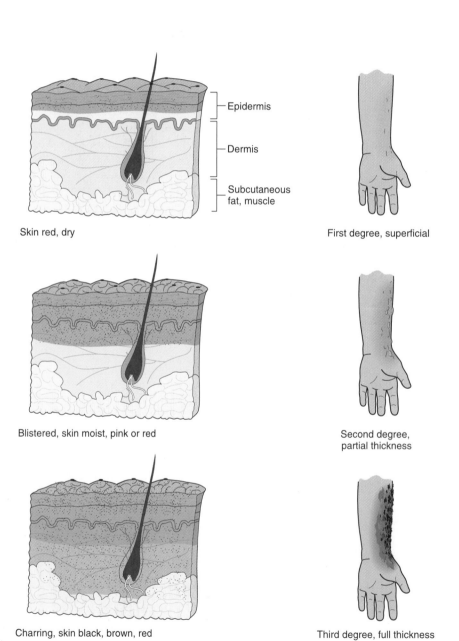

Skin red, dry

First degree, superficial

Blistered, skin moist, pink or red

Second degree, partial thickness

Charring, skin black, brown, red

Third degree, full thickness

FIGURE 12.15 The degree of a burn is determined by the layers of skin involved.

Diagnostic Procedures of the Integumentary System

A **biopsy** (**BYE**-op-see) is the removal of a small piece of living tissue for examination to confirm or establish a diagnosis (**bi** means pertaining to life and **opsy** means view of).

- In an **incisional biopsy** a piece, but not all, of the tumor or lesion is removed. (**Incision** means to cut into.)
- In an **excisional biopsy**, the entire tumor or lesion plus a margin of surrounding tissue are removed. **Excision** (eck-**SIH**-zhun) means the complete removal of a lesion or organ.
- In a **needle biopsy**, a hollow needle is used to remove a core of tissue for examination.
- **Exfoliative cytology** (ecks-**FOH**-lee-**ay**-tiv sigh-**TOL**-oh-jee) is a biopsy technique in which cells are scraped from the tissue and examined under a microscope.

Treatment Procedures of the Integumentary System

Transdermal Medications

The skin is able to absorb certain drugs and other chemical substances used to treat problems ranging from acne to angina attacks.

- A **topical** application is one that applies to a specific location. Topical medication is put on the skin to treat the area it is applied to.
- **Transdermal** refers to the application of medicine to unbroken skin so that it is absorbed continuously to produce a systemic effect. A transdermal patch may be used to convey medications such as nitroglycerin for angina pectoris, hormones for hormone replacement therapy, or scopolamine for motion sickness.

Preventive Measures

- **Sunscreen** that blocks out the harmful ultraviolet B (UVB) rays is sometimes measured in terms of the strength of the **sun protection factor** (SPF). Some sunscreens also give protection against ultraviolet A (UVA).

Tissue Removal

- **Cauterization** (**kaw**-ter-eye-**ZAY**-zhun) is the destruction of tissue by burning for therapeutic purposes. This technique is used in conjunction with **curettage** to remove and destroy basal cell tumors. (**Curettage** (**kyou**-reh-**TAHZH**) is the removal of material from the surface by scraping.)
- **Chemical peel**, also known as **chemabrasion** (keem-ah-**BRAY**-shun), is the use of chemicals to remove the outer layers of skin to treat acne scaring, fine wrinkling, and general keratoses.
- **Cryosurgery** is the destruction or elimination of abnormal tissue cells, such as warts or tumors, through the application of extreme cold, often by using liquid nitrogen.
- **Debridement** (day-breed-**MON**) is the removal of dirt, foreign objects, damaged tissue, and cellular debris from a wound to prevent infection and to promote healing.
- **Dermabrasion** (**der**-mah-**BRAY**-zhun) is a form of abrasion involving the use of revolving wire brushes or sandpaper.
- **Incision and drainage** (**I & D**) involves incision (cutting open) of a lesion, such as an abscess, and draining the contents.
- **Mohs' chemosurgery** is a zinc chloride paste used to remove recurrent tumors and scarlike basal cell carcinomas, with a minimum of normal tissue loss but complete removal of the tumor. As each layer is removed it is examined microscopically, and the procedure continues until it is determined that the entire tumor has been removed. This technique is especially useful in treating basal cell epitheliomas.

Laser Treatment of Skin Conditions

The term **laser** is an acronym for **l**ight **a**mplification by **s**timulated **e**mission of **r**adiation. An **acronym** (**ACK**-roh-nim) is a word formed from the initial letter or letters of the major parts of a compound term. Lasers are used to treat skin and many conditions affecting other body systems.

Each type of laser derives its name from the substance (solid, liquid, or gas) within the laser tube. This substance is stimulated to emit light that is strengthened to a specific wavelength. The wavelength and power of the beam are the keys to the laser's effect on tissue. Some wavelengths are capable of destroying all skin tissue; others target tissue of particular color.

- **Rhinophyma** is treated by using a carbon dioxide laser to reshape the nose by vaporizing the excess tissue (Figure 12.16).

FIGURE 12.16 Rhinophyma before laser treatment. (*Courtesy of Robert A. Silverman, MD, Clinical Associate Professor, Department of Pediatrics, Georgetown University*)

- **Port-wine stain** is treated using short pulses of laser light to remove the birthmark. Treatment may require many sessions because only a small section is treated at a time.
- **Tattoos** are removed by using lasers that target particular colors.
- Lasers are also used in the treatment of some skin cancers, precancer of the lip, and warts that recur around nails and on the soles of feet.

Cosmetic Procedures

- **Blepharoplasty** (**BLEF**-ah-roh-**plas**-tee), also known as a **lid lift**, is the surgical reduction of the upper and lower eyelids (**blepharo** means eyelid and **plasty** mean surgical repair).
- **Dermatoplasty** (**DER**-mah-toh-**plas**-tee), also known as a **skin graft**, is the replacement of damaged skin with tissue taken from a donor site on the patient's body (**dermato** means skin and **plasty** means surgical repair).
- **Lipectomy** (lih-**PECK**-toh-mee) is the surgical removal of fat beneath the skin (**lip** means fat and **ectomy** means surgical removal).
- **Liposuction** (**LIP**-oh-**suck**-shun *or* **LYE**-poh-**suck**-shun) is the surgical removal of fat beneath the skin with the aid of suction. It is also known as **suction-assisted lipectomy**.
- **Rhytidectomy** (**rit**-ih-**DECK**-toh-mee), also known as a **facelift**, is the surgical removal of excess skin for the elimination of wrinkles (**rhytid** means wrinkle and **ectomy** means surgical removal).
- **Sclerotherapy** (**sklehr**-oh-**THER**-ah-pee), used in the treatment of spider veins (small veins that can be seen through the skin), involves injecting a sclerosing solution (saline solution) into the vein being treated. This irritates the tissue, causes swelling, and eventually closes off the vein.

Learning Exercises

● Matching Word Parts—1

Write the letter of the correct answer on the line provided in the left column.

12.1. _____ albin/o   A. life

12.2. _____ rhytid/o   B. red

12.3. _____ erythr/o   C. wrinkle

12.4. _____ bi/o   D. sweat

12.5. _____ hidr/o   E. white

● Matching Word Parts—2

Write the letter of the correct answer on the line provided in the left column.

12.6. _____ derm/o,   A. black, dark skin
           dermat/o

12.7. _____ kerat/o   B. fat, lipid

12.8. _____ lip/o   C. lice

12.9. _____ melan/o   D. horny, hard

12.10. _____ pedicul/o   E. skin

● Matching Word Parts—3

Write the letter of the correct answer on the line provided in the left column.

12.11. _____ onych/o   A. dry

12.12. _____ pil/o   B. fungus

12.13. _____ seb/o   C. hair

12.14. _____ xer/o   D. nail

12.15. _____ myc/o   E. sebum

● Definitions

Circle the letter next to the correct answer.

12.16. Which term describes a diffuse infection of connective tissue?

    a. abscess

    b. cellulitis

    c. fissure

    d. ulcer

12.17. Heparin is a/an _____ .

    a. anticoagulant

    b. mast cell

    c. substance that produces itching

    d. tough flexible fibrous protein material

12.18. Pruritus is commonly known as _____ .

    a. baldness

    b. dry skin

    c. itching

    d. pus

12.19. An ecchymosis is commonly known as a/an _____ .

    a. abscess

    b. bruise

    c. scar

    d. ulcer

12.20. Which term means profuse sweating?

    a. anhidrosis

    b. diaphoresis

    c. hidrosis

    d. miliaria

12.21. Which term describes a normal scar left by a wound?

    a. cicatrix

    b. keloid

    c. keratosis

    d. papilloma

12.22. Which type of therapy is used to remove a port-wine stain?

    a. abrasion

    b. cryosurgery

    c. laser

    d. Mohs' chemosurgery

12.23. Which term describes the removal of dirt, foreign objects, damaged tissue and cellular debris from a wound?

    a. debridement

    b. drainage

    c. excision

    d. incision

12.24. Which degree of burn has no blisters and only superficial damage to the epidermis?

    a. fourth

    b. third

    c. second

    d. first

12.25. Also known as warts, which lesions are caused by the human papillomavirus?

    a. nevi

    b. petechiae

    c. scabies

    d. verrucae

● Matching Structures

Write the letter of the correct answer on the line provided in the left column.

12.26. _____ dermis — A. Secrete sebum to lubricate the skin.

12.27. _____ keratin — B. Finger and toenails.

12.28. _____ mammary glands — C. A fibrous protein found in hair, nails, and skin.

12.29. _____ sebaceous glands — D. The layer of skin below the epidermis.

12.30. _____ unguis — E. Milk-producing sebaceous glands.

Which Word?

Circle the correct term in each sentence.

12.31. The medical term for the condition commonly known as an ingrown toenail is *onychomycosis / onychocryptosis.*

12.32. A contagious, superficial skin infection usually seen in young children is *impetigo / xeroderma.*

12.33. A torn or jagged wound or an accidental cut wound is known as a *laceration / lesion.*

12.34. Found mainly on the face, a *basal cell / squamous cell* carcinoma is the most frequent but least harmful type of skin cancer.

12.35. Also known as warts, the medical term for this condition is *petechiae / verrucae.*

Spelling Counts

Find the misspelled word in each sentence. Then write that word, spelled correctly, on the line provided.

12.36. Soriasis is a chronic disease of the skin characterized by itching and by red papules covered with silvery scales. _____

12.37. Exema is an inflammatory skin disease with erythema, papules, and scabs. _____

12.38. An abcess is a localized collection of pus. _____

12.39. Onyochia is an inflammation of the nail bed, resulting in the loss of the nail. _____

12.40. Skleroderma is an autoimmune disorder that causes abnormal tissue thickening. _____

Matching Abbreviations

Write the letter of the correct answer on the line provided in the left column.

12.41. _____ I & D　　A. light amplification by stimulated emission of radiation

12.42. _____ LASER　　B. incision and draining

12.43. _____ UVA　　C. lupus erythematosus

12.44. _____ UVB　　D. ultraviolet B

12.45. _____ LE　　E. ultraviolet A

Term Selection

Circle the letter next to the correct answer.

12.46. Which term means a small knotlike swelling of granulation tissue that may result from inflammation, injury, or infection?

a. cicatrix
b. granuloma
c. keratosis
d. petechiae

12.47. Which term means an infestation of body lice?

a. pediculosis capitis
b. pediculosis corpus
c. pediculosis pubis
d. scabies

12.48. Which term means any redness of the skin?

a. cellulitis
b. ecchymosis
c. erythema
d. urticaria

12.49. Which term describes a dry patch made up of excessive dead epidermal cells?

a. bulla
b. macule
c. plaque
d. scale

12.50. Which term describes a cluster of boils that result in extensive sloughing of skin and scar formation?

a. acne vulgaris
b. carbuncle
c. comedo
d. furuncle

● **Sentence Completion**

Write the correct term on the line.

12.51. The term meaning producing or containing pus is _____ .

12.52. The medical term meaning a fungus infection of the nail is _____ .

12.53. Tissue death followed by bacterial invasion and putrefaction is known as _____ .

12.54. Any condition of unusual deposits of black pigment is known as _____ .

12.55. The medical term for the condition commonly known as hives is _____ .

● **True/False**

If the statement is true, write T on the line. If the statement is false, write F on the line.

12.56. _____ A carbon dioxide laser is used to remove tattoos.

12.57. _____ Diffuse means confined to a limited area.

12.58. _____ Dermatomycosis is a superficial fungal infection of the skin.

12.59. _____ Squamous cell carcinoma can spread quickly to other body systems.

12.60. _____ Dermatosis is any condition of the skin associated with inflammation.

12.61. _____ Putrefaction is decay that produces foul-smelling odors.

12.62. _____ A skin tag that enlarges in the elderly is malignant.

12.63. _____ The arrector pili is a tiny muscle that causes the hair to stand erect.

12.64. _____ An abnormally raised scar is known as a granuloma.

12.65. _____ A lipoma is a benign tumor made up of mature fat cells.

● **Clinical Conditions**

Write the correct answer on the line.

12.66. Robert Harris has a disease of unknown origin in which there are well-defined bald patches. Robert has a form of alopecia _____ .

12.67. Jordan Caswell has an inherited deficiency or absence of pigment in the skin, hair, and eyes due to an abnormality in production of melanin. This disorder is called _____ .

12.68. Mike Young hit his thumb with a hammer and soon there was a collection of blood beneath the nail. This is called a/an _____ _____ .

12.69. Mrs. Higachi fell and bruised her arm. The medical term for this condition is a/an _____ .

12.70. Rosita Chavez was diagnosed as suffering from a disorder with bleeding beneath the skin that causes spontaneous bruising. The medical term for this condition is _____ .

12.71. Henry Walton was treated for a skin infection caused by the itch mite. This was entered on his chart as treatment for _____ .

12.72. Dr. Liu found that Jeanette Isenberg had an abnormal skin lesion caused by excessive exposure to the sun. The medical term for this is _____ keratosis.

12.73. Mrs. Garrison had cosmetic surgery that is commonly known as a lid lift. The medical term for this treatment is a/an _____ .

12.74. Tammy's teacher sent home a note alerting Tammy's parent that many of the children in the class had head lice. The medical term for this condition is _____ capitis.

12.75. Agnes Farrington uses a patch to prevent motion sickness. This is known as _____ administration.

● Which is the correct medical term?

Circle the letter next to the correct answer.

12.76. Which term refers to an infection of the fold of skin at the margin of a nail?

    a. dyschromia

    b. onychia

    c. paronychia

    d. vitiligo

12.77. Which term refers to the procedure commonly known as a face lift?

    a. blepharoplasty

    b. debridement

    c. rhinoplasty

    d. rhytidectomy

12.78. Which form of biopsy removes the entire lesion?

    a. cauterization

    b. excisional

    c. incisional

    d. needle

12.79. Which term refers to a malformation of the nail also called spoon nail?

    a. clubbing

    b. koilonychia

    c. onychomycosis

    d. paronychia

12.80. Which term describes therapy used in the treatment of spider veins?

    a. chemical peel

    b. dermabrasion

    c. dermatoplasty

    d. sclerotherapy

● Challenge Word Building

These terms are *not* found in this chapter; however, they are made up of these familiar word parts. You may want to look in the glossary or use a medical dictionary to check your answers!

an-	py/o	-derma
hypo-	hidr/o	-ectomy
	dermat/o	-ia
	melan/o	-itis
	myc/o	-malacia
	onych/o	-oma
	rhin/o	-osis
		-pathy
		-plasty

12.81. The medical term meaning abnormal softening of the nails is _____ .

12.82. The medical term meaning an abnormal condition resulting in the diminished flow of perspiration is _____ .

12.83. The medical term meaning plastic surgery to change the shape or size of the nose is _____ .

12.84. The medical term meaning a tumor arising from the nail bed is _____ .

12.85. The medical term meaning any pus forming skin disease is _____ .

12.86. The medical term meaning the surgical removal of a finger or toenail is a/an _____ .

12.87. The medical term meaning pertaining to the absence of finger or toenails is _____ .

12.88. The medical term meaning any disease of the skin _____ .

12.89. The medical term meaning any disease caused by a fungus is _____ .

12.90. The medical term meaning that an excess of melanin is present in an area of inflammation of the skin _____ .

● Labeling Exercises

Identify the lesions:

12.91. _____

12.92. _____

12.93. _____

12.94. _____

12.95. _____

12.96. _____

12.97. _____

12.98. _____

12.99. _____

12.100. _____

 A **12.91** is a closed sack or pouch containing fluid or semisolid material.

 A **12.92** is a small circumscribed elevation of the skin containing pus.

 A **12.93** is a circumscribed elevation of skin containing fluid that is less than 0.5 cm in diameter.

 A **12.94** is a large vesicle that is more than 0.5 cm in diameter.

 A **12.95** is an open sore or erosion of the skin or mucous membrane resulting in tissue loss.

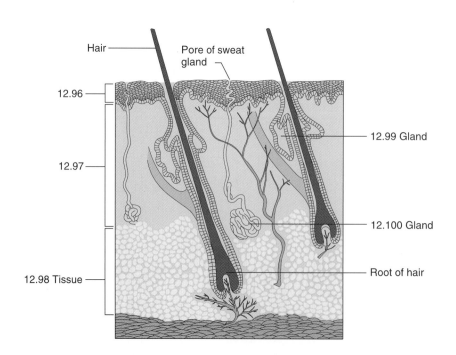

Hair | Pore of sweat gland

12.96

12.97

12.98 Tissue

12.99 Gland

12.100 Gland

Root of hair

The Human Touch: Critical Thinking Exercise

The following story and questions are designed to stimulate critical thinking through class discussion or as a brief essay response. There are no easy or right-wrong answers to these questions.

"OK, guys, we're late again." Shaylene Boulay calls out to her two older sons, Nathan, Jr., 10, and Carl, 12. Grabbing the lunches Nate Sr. packed, she walks out the back door. "Come on Michel, school time!" Shaylene peers under the porch for her 5-year-old. Their house is only a mile from the waterfront and he loves to race cars between their dog Bubba's big paws in the cool sand underneath the porch. "Look at you!" As Shaylene dusts him off and heads to the truck, she notices that the rash of blisters on his leg is still bright red. Must be ant bites, she thinks.

"Have a good day!" Shaylene hands Nathan and Carl their lunches as they hop out of the truck at the middle school. Next stop, Oak Creek Elementary. As Michel starts to get out, clutching his brown lunch bag tightly, his kindergarten teacher comes rushing over. "Michel, what are you doing here today? Didn't you give your mother the note from the nurse?"

"What note? Michel, honey, did you forget to give Mama something from school?" Michel smiles sheepishly and reaches into his shorts pocket for a wadded up piece of paper. The note says: "We believe Michel has impetigo on his leg. This condition is very contagious. Please consult your doctor as soon as possible. We will need a note from him before we can allow Michel to reenter class."

"Oh no," Shaylene thinks. "I'm due for my shift at the diner in 15 minutes. Nobody's home to watch Michel. We don't have the money to see Dr. Gaines again already. And what if this rash on my arm is that thing Michel has?" She sits clutching the wheel of the old pickup, asking herself over and over, "What am I gonna do?"

Suggested Discussion Questions:

1. Look up impetigo in a medical dictionary and read its description. Discuss how Shaylene could mistake the symptoms for something else.

2. You work in Dr. Gaines' office and the Boulays have an appointment today. What precautions would you take while seeing this family?

3. Shaylene is having difficulty understanding Dr. Gaines. She asks you to explain. Using information from a medical dictionary and terminology she can understand, describe the symptoms and treatment of impetigo.

4. Discuss Shaylene's responsibility to her children, job, and the school. Provide her with a solution to her question: "What am I gonna do."

5. What should Shaylene do to prevent her other children from getting impetigo?

13

The Endocrine System

● **Overview of Structures, Word Parts, and Functions of the Endocrine System**

Major Structures	Related Word Roots	Primary Functions
Adrenal glands (2)	adren/o	Regulate electrolyte levels, influence metabolism, and respond to stress.
Gonads ▪ Male testicles (2) ▪ Female ovaries (2)	gonad/o	Regulate development and maintenance of secondary sex characteristics.
Pancreatic islets	pancreat/o	Control blood sugar levels and glucose metabolism.
Parathyroid glands (4)	parathyroid/o	Regulate calcium levels throughout the body.
Pineal gland (1)	pineal/o	Influence the sleep–wakefulness cycle.
Pituitary gland (1)	pituit/o, pituitar/o	Controls the activity of the other endocrine glands.
Thymus (1)	thym/o	Plays a major role in the immune reaction.
Thyroid gland (1)	thyr/o, thyroid/o	Stimulates metabolism, growth, and activity of the nervous system.

VOCABULARY   Related to the Endocrine System

Check the box as you master each word part or term. Terms marked with the ❖ symbol are pronounced on the optional student audiotape.

Key Word Parts
- [ ] acr/o
- [ ] adren/o
- [ ] crin/o
- [ ] -dipsia
- [ ] gonad/o
- [ ] -ism
- [ ] pancreat/o
- [ ] parathyroid/o
- [ ] pineal/o
- [ ] pituit/o
- [ ] poly-
- [ ] somat/o
- [ ] thym/o
- [ ] thyr/o, thyroid/o
- [ ] -tropin

Key Medical Terms
- [ ] **acromegaly** (**ack**-roh-**MEG**-ah-lee) ❖
- [ ] **Addison's disease** (**AD**-ih-sonz) ❖
- [ ] **adrenalitis** (ah-**dree**-nal-**EYE**-tis) ❖
- [ ] **aldosteronism** (al-**DOSS**-teh-roh-**niz**-em *or* al-doh-**STER**-ohn-izm) ❖
- [ ] **chemical thyroidectomy** (**thigh**-roi-**DECK**-toh-mee) ❖
- [ ] **cretinism** (**CREE**-tin-izm) ❖
- [ ] **Cushing's syndrome** (**KUSH**-ingz **SIN**-drohm) ❖
- [ ] **diabetes insipidus** (**dye**-ah-**BEE**-teez in-**SIP**-ih-dus) ❖
- [ ] **diabetes mellitus** (**dye**-ah-**BEE**-teez mel-**EYE**-tus *or* **MEL**-ih-tus) ❖
- [ ] **diabetic ketoacidosis** (**kee**-toh-**ass**-ih-**DOH**-sis) ❖
- [ ] **diabetic retinopathy** (**ret**-ih-**NOP**-ah-thee) ❖
- [ ] **electrolytes** (ee-**LECK**-troh-lytes) ❖
- [ ] **endocrinopathy** (**en**-doh-krih-**NOP**-ah-thee) ❖
- [ ] **epinephrine** (**ep**-ih-**NEF**-rin)
- [ ] **estrogen** (**ES**-troh-jen)
- [ ] **exophthalmos** (**eck**-sof-**THAL**-mos) ❖
- [ ] **fructosamine test** (**fruck**-**TOHS**-ah-meen) ❖
- [ ] **gestational diabetes mellitus** (jes-**TAY**-shun-al **dye**-ah-**BEE**-teez mel-**EYE**-tus *or* **MEL**-ih-tus) ❖
- [ ] **gigantism** (jigh-**GAN**-tiz-em *or* **JIGH**-en-tiz-em) ❖
- [ ] **glucagon** (**GLOO**-kah-gon)
- [ ] **glycohemoglobin** (**glye**-koh-**hee**-moh-**GLOH**-bin) ❖
- [ ] **goiter** (**GOI**-ter) ❖
- [ ] **gonadotropic hormone** (**gon**-ah-doh-**TROHP**-ick)
- [ ] **Graves' disease** (**GRAYVZ**-dih-**ZEEZ**) ❖
- [ ] **growth hormone** (GH)
- [ ] **gynecomastia** (**guy**-neh-koh-**MAS**-tee-ah) ❖
- [ ] **Hashimoto's thyroiditis** (hah-shee-**MOH**-tohz **thigh**-roi-**DYE**-tis) ❖
- [ ] **hypercalcemia** (**high**-per-kal-**SEE**-mee-ah) ❖

- [ ] **hypercrinism** (**high**-per-**KRY**-nism) ❖
- [ ] **hyperglycemia** (**high**-per-glye-**SEE**-mee-ah) ❖
- [ ] **hypergonadism** (**high**-per-**GOH**-nad-izm) ❖
- [ ] **hyperinsulinism** (**high**-per-**IN**-suh-lin-izm) ❖
- [ ] **hyperparathyroidism** (**high**-per-**par**-ah-**THIGH**-roid-izm) ❖
- [ ] **hyperpituitarism** (**high**-per-pih-**TOO**-ih-tah-rizm) ❖
- [ ] **hyperthyroidism** (**high**-per-**THIGH**-roid-izm) ❖
- [ ] **hypocalcemia** (**high**-poh-kal-**SEE**-mee-ah) ❖
- [ ] **hypocrinism** (**high**-poh-**KRY**-nism) ❖
- [ ] **hypoglycemia** (**high**-poh-gly-**SEE**-mee-ah) ❖
- [ ] **hypogonadism** (**high**-poh-**GOH**-nad-izm) ❖
- [ ] **hypoparathyroidism** (**high**-poh-**par**-ah-**THIGH**-roid-izm) ❖
- [ ] **hypophysectomy** (high-**pof**-ih-**SECK**-toh-mee) ❖
- [ ] **hypopituitarism** (**high**-poh-pih-**TOO**-ih-tah-rizm) ❖
- [ ] **hypothyroidism** (**high**-poh-**THIGH**-roid-izm) ❖
- [ ] **insulin** (**IN**-suh-lin)
- [ ] **insulinoma** (in-suh-lin-**OH**-mah) ❖
- [ ] **laparoscopic adrenalectomy** (ah-**dree**-nal-**ECK**-toh-mee) ❖
- [ ] **lobectomy** (loh-**BECK**-toh-mee) ❖
- [ ] **metabolism** (meh-**TAB**-oh-**lizm**) ❖
- [ ] **myxedema** (**mick**-seh-**DEE**-mah) ❖
- [ ] **norepinephrine** (**nor**-ep-ih-**NEF**-rin)
- [ ] **oxytocin** (**ock**-sih-**TOH**-sin)
- [ ] **pancreatalgia** (**pan**-kree-ah-**TAL**-jee-ah) ❖
- [ ] **pancreatitis** (**pan**-kree-ah-**TYE**-tis) ❖
- [ ] **parathyroid hormone** (PTH)
- [ ] **parathyroidectomy** (**par**-ah-**thigh**-roi-**DECK**-toh-mee) ❖
- [ ] **pheochromocytoma** (fee-oh-**kroh**-moh-sigh-**TOH**-mah) ❖
- [ ] **pinealectomy** (pin-ee-al-**ECK**-toh-mee) ❖
- [ ] **pinealopathy** (pin-ee-ah-**LOP**-ah-thee) ❖
- [ ] **pituitarism** (pih-**TOO**-ih-tar-izm) ❖
- [ ] **pituitary adenoma** (pih-**TOO**-ih-**tair**-ee **ad**-eh-**NOH**-mah) ❖
- [ ] **polydipsia** (**pol**-ee-**DIP**-see-ah) ❖
- [ ] **polyuria** (**pol**-ee-**YOU**-ree-ah) ❖
- [ ] **progesterone** (proh-**JES**-ter-ohn)
- [ ] **prolactinoma** (proh-**lack**-tih-**NOH**-mah) ❖
- [ ] **steroid** (**STEHR**-oid)
- [ ] **testosterone** (tes-**TOS**-teh-rohn)
- [ ] **tetany** (**TET**-ah-nee) ❖
- [ ] **thymectomy** (thigh-**MECK**-toh-mee) ❖
- [ ] **thymitis** (thigh-**MY**-tis) ❖
- [ ] **thymoma** (thigh-**MOH**-mah) ❖
- [ ] **thymosin** (**THIGH**-moh-sin)
- [ ] **thyroid-stimulating hormone** (TSH)
- [ ] **thyromegaly** (**thigh**-roh-**MEG**-ah-lee) ❖
- [ ] **thyrotoxicosis** (**thy**-roh-**tock**-sih-**KOH**-sis) ❖
- [ ] **thyroxine** (thigh-**ROCK**-sin)

● OBJECTIVES

On completion of this chapter, you should be able to:

1 Describe the role of the hypothalamus and endocrine glands in maintaining homeostasis.

2 Name and describe the functions of the primary hormones secreted by each of the endocrine glands.

3 Recognize, define, spell, and pronounce terms relating to the pathology and diagnostic and treatment procedures of the endocrine glands.

Functions of the Endocrine System

The primary function of the endocrine system is to produce hormones. Because the hormones are secreted directly into the bloodstream they are able to reach cells and organs throughout the body.

A **hormone** is a chemical messenger with a specialized function. The major hormones, their sources, and functions are described in Table 13.1.

Steroid Hormones

Steroid hormones help control metabolism, inflammation, immune functions, salt and water balance, development of sexual characteristics, and the ability to withstand illness and injury.

- The term **steroid** (**STEHR**-oid) describes both hormones produced by the body and artificially produced hormones used in medications to duplicate the action of the naturally occurring steroids.

Anabolic Steroids

Anabolic steroids (**an**-ah-**BOL**-ick), which are chemically related to the male sex hormone testosterone, have been used illegally by athletes to increase strength and muscle mass. This use usually can be detected through urine and blood testing.

- Serious side effects of anabolic steroid use include liver damage, altered body chemistry, testicular shrinkage and breast development in males, plus unpredictable mood swings and violence.

- Steroid use in teenagers also stops long bone development, resulting in shortened stature.

Structures of the Endocrine System

The major glands of the endocrine system include (Figure 13.1):

- One **pituitary gland** (divided into two lobes)
- One **thyroid gland**
- Four **parathyroid glands**
- Two **adrenal glands**
- One **pancreas** (**pancreatic islets**)
- One **thymus**
- One **pineal gland**
- Two **gonads** (ovaries in females, testes in males)

Medical Specialties Related to the Endocrine System

- An **endocrinologist** (**en**-doh-krih-**NOL**-oh-jist) specializes in diagnosing and treating diseases and malfunctions of the glands of internal secretion (**endo** means within, **crin** means to secrete, and **ologist** means specialist).

Pathology of the Endocrine System

- **Endocrinopathy** (**en**-doh-krih-**NOP**-ah-thee) is any disease due to a disorder of the endocrine system (**endo** means within, **crino** means to secrete, and **pathy** means disease).

- **Hypercrinism** (**high**-per-**KRY**-nism) is a condition caused by excessive secretion of any gland, especially an endocrine gland (**hyper** means excessive, **crin** means to secrete, and **ism** means condition).

- **Hypocrinism** (**high**-poh-**KRY**-nism) is a condition caused by deficient secretion of any gland, especially an endocrine gland (**hypo** means deficient, **crin** means to secrete, and **ism** means condition).

Diagnostic Procedures Related to the Endocrine System

- Nuclear medicine and imaging techniques, which are described in Chapter 15, are used to diagnose and treat disorders affecting the endocrine system.

- Urine and blood testing are used to measure endocrine hormone levels and to detect the presence of anabolic steroids.

Table 13.1

HORMONES FROM A TO T		
Hormone	**Source**	**Functions**
Aldosterone	adrenal cortex	Aids in regulating the levels of salt and water in the body.
Androgens	adrenal cortex and gonads	Influence sex-related characteristics.
Adrenocorticotropic hormone (ACTH)	pituitary gland	Stimulates the growth and secretions of the adrenal cortex.
Antidiuretic hormone (ADH)	pituitary gland	Helps control blood pressure by reducing the amount of water that is excreted.
Calcitonin	thyroid gland	Works with the parathyroid hormone to regulate calcium levels in the blood and tissues.
Cortisol	adrenal cortex	Regulates the metabolism of carbohydrates, fats, and proteins in the body. Also has an anti-inflammatory action.
Epinephrine	adrenal medulla	Stimulates the sympathetic nervous system.
Estrogen	ovaries	Develops and maintains the female secondary sex characteristics and regulates the menstrual cycle.
Follicle-stimulating hormone (FSH)	pituitary gland	In the female, stimulates the secretion of estrogen and the growth of ova (eggs). In the male, stimulates the production of sperm.
Glucagon	pancreatic islets	Increases the level of glucose in the bloodstream.
Growth hormone (GH)	pituitary gland	Regulates the growth of bone, muscle and other body tissues.
Human chorionic gonadotropin (HCG)	placenta	Stimulates the secretion of the hormones required to maintain the pregnancy.
Insulin (In)	pancreatic islets	Regulates the transport of glucose to body cells and stimulates the conversion of excess glucose to glycogen for storage.
Lactogenic hormone (LTH)	pituitary gland	Stimulates and maintains the secretion of breast milk.
Luteinizing hormone (LH)	pituitary gland	In the female, stimulates ovulation. In the male, stimulates testosterone secretion.
Melatonin	pineal gland	Influences the sleep–wakefulness cycles.
Norepinephrine	adrenal medulla	Stimulates the sympathetic nervous system.
Oxytocin (OXT)	pituitary gland	Stimulates uterine contractions during childbirth. Causes milk to flow from the mammary glands after birth.
Parathyroid hormone (PTH)	parathyroid glands	Works with calcitonin to regulate calcium levels in the blood and tissues.
Progesterone	ovaries	Completes preparation of the uterus for possible pregnancy.
Testosterone	testicles	Stimulates the development of male secondary sex characteristics.
Thymosin	thymus	Plays an important role in the immune system.
Thyroid hormones (T_4 and T_3)	thyroid gland	Regulates the rate of metabolism.
Thyroid-stimulating hormone (TSH)	pituitary gland	Stimulates the secretion of hormones by the thyroid gland.

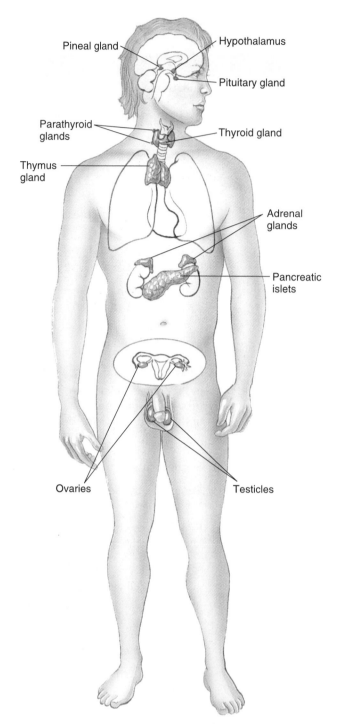

FIGURE 13.1 Structures of the endocrine system.

The Pituitary Gland

The pea-sized **pituitary gland** (pih-**TOO**-ih-**tair**-ee) is located at the base of the brain just below the hypothalamus and is composed of anterior and posterior lobes.

Functions of the Pituitary Gland

The primary function of the pituitary gland, also known as the **master gland**, is to control the activity of the other endocrine glands (Figure 13.2).

Thyroid feedback system

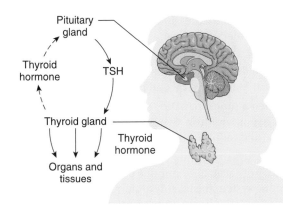

Figure 13.2 The pituitary gland secretes thyroid-stimulating hormone (TSH) that signals the thyroid gland to produce thyroid hormones. These hormones travel through the bloodstream to organs and tissues throughout the body.

- The pituitary acts in response to stimuli from the hypothalamus of the brain. This system of checks and balances maintains an appropriate blood level of each hormone.

Secretions of the Pituitary Gland: Anterior Lobe

- The **adrenocorticotropic hormone**, also known as **ACTH** or **adrenotropin**, stimulates the growth and secretions of the adrenal cortex (**adreno** means adrenal glands and **tropin** means stimulating).

- The **follicle-stimulating hormone**, also known as **FSH** or **follitropin**, in the female stimulates the secretion of estrogen and the growth of ova (eggs) in the ovaries. In the male it stimulates the production of sperm in the testicles.

- The **growth hormone**, also known as **GH** or **somatotropin** (**STH**), regulates the growth of bone, muscle, and other body tissues (**somato** means body and **tropin** means to stimulate).

- The **lactogenic hormone**, also known as **LTH** or **prolactin**, stimulates and maintains the secretion of breast milk after childbirth.

- The **luteinizing hormone**, also known as **LH** or **luteotropin**, stimulates ovulation in the female. In the male it stimulates testosterone secretion.

- The **melanocyte-stimulating hormone**, also known as **MSH** or **melanotropin**, increases pigmentation of the skin (**melano** means black and **tropin** means to stimulate).

- The **thyroid-stimulating hormone**, also known as **TSH** or **thyrotropin**, stimulates the growth and secretions of the thyroid gland (**thyro** means thyroid and **tropin** means stimulating).

Secretions of the Pituitary Gland: Posterior Lobe

- The **antidiuretic hormone**, also known as **ADH**, maintains the water balance within the body by promoting the reabsorption of water through the kidneys (see Chapter 9). When more ADH is secreted, less urine is produced. In contrast, when a **diuretic** (**dye**-you-**RET**-ick) is administered it increases urine secretion.

- **Oxytocin** (**ock**-sih-**TOH**-sin), also known as **OXT**, stimulates uterine contractions during childbirth. After birth, it stimulates the flow of milk from the mammary glands.

Pathology of the Pituitary Gland

- **Acromegaly** (**ack**-roh-**MEG**-ah-lee) is enlargement of the extremities (hands and feet) caused by excessive secretion of the growth hormone *after* puberty (**acro** means extremities and **megaly** means enlargement). Compare with gigantism.

- **Alcohol consumption** inhibits the secretion of ADH and results in increased urine output that can disrupt the body's fluid balance.

- **Gigantism** (jigh-**GAN**-tiz-em *or* **JIGH**-en-tiz-em) is abnormal overgrowth of the body caused by excessive secretion of the growth hormone *before* puberty. Compare with acromegaly.

- **Hyperpituitarism** (**high**-per-pih-**TOO**-ih-tah-rizm) is pathology that results in the excessive secretion by the anterior lobe of the pituitary gland (**hyper** means excessive, **pituitar** means pituitary, and **ism** means condition).

- **Hypopituitarism** (**high**-poh-pih-**TOO**-ih-tah-**rizm**) is a condition of reduced secretion due to the partial or complete loss of the function of the anterior lobe of the pituitary gland (**hypo** means deficient, **pituitar** means pituitary, and **ism** means condition).

- A **pituitary adenoma** (**ad**-eh-**NOH**-mah) is a benign tumor of the pituitary gland that causes the excess hormone secretion. An ACTH-secreting tumor stimulates the excess production of cortisol that causes most cases of Cushing's syndrome (see Pathology of the Adrenal Glands).

- **Pituitarism** (pih-**TOO**-ih-tar-izm) is any disorder of pituitary function (**pituitar** means pituitary and **ism** means condition).

- A **prolactin-producing adenoma**, also known as a **prolactinoma** (proh-**lack**-tih-**NOH**-mah), is a benign tumor of the pituitary gland that causes it to produce too much prolactin. In females this causes infertility and changes in menstruation. In males it causes impotence.

Diabetes Insipidus

Diabetes insipidus (dye-ah-**BEE**-teez in-**SIP**-ih-dus) is caused by insufficient production of the antidiuretic hormone (ADH) or by the inability of the kidneys to respond to ADH. This allows too much fluid to be excreted. This produces extreme polydipsia and polyuria.

- **Polydipsia** (**pol**-ee-**DIP**-see-ah) is excessive thirst (**poly** means many and **dipsia** means thirst).
- **Polyuria** (**pol**-ee-**YOU**-ree-ah) is excessive urination (**poly** means many and **uria** means urination).
- Diabetes insipidus is *not* similar to diabetes mellitus.

Treatment Procedures of the Pituitary Gland

- A **hypophysectomy** (high-**pof**-ih-**SECK**-toh-mee) is use of radiation or surgery to remove all or part of the pituitary gland.
- **Human growth hormone therapy** (GH), also known as recombinant GH, is a synthetic version of naturally occurring growth hormone. It is administered to stimulate growth when the natural supply of growth hormone is insufficient for normal development.

The Thyroid Gland

The butterfly-shaped **thyroid gland** lies on either side of the larynx, just below the thyroid cartilage (see Figure 13.1).

- The secretion of the thyroid hormones (T_4 and T_3) is controlled by the thyroid-stimulating hormone (TSH) secreted by the anterior lobe of the pituitary gland.
- The body's ability to secrete thyroid hormones depends on the uptake of iodine from food and water.

Functions of the Thyroid Gland

The primary function of the thyroid gland is to regulate the body's metabolism. **Metabolism** (meh-**TAB**-oh-**lizm**) is the rate at which the body uses energy and the speed at which body functions work.

- The thyroid secretions also influence growth and the functioning of the nervous system.

Secretions of the Thyroid Gland

- The primary thyroid hormones are **thyroxine** (T_4) (thigh-**ROCK**-sin) and **triiodothyronine** (T_3) (try-**eye**-oh-doh-**THIGH**-roh-neen).
- **Calcitonin** (**kal**-sih-**TOH**-nin), also known as **thyrocalcitonin**, works with the parathyroid hormone (PTH) to regulate calcium levels in the blood and tissues. Calcitonin decreases blood levels by moving calcium into storage in the bones and teeth. Compare with PTH.

Pathology of the Thyroid Gland

- **Thyroid cancer** is commonly first indicated by an enlargement of the thyroid gland. With early detection and treatment the survival rate is high. Without treatment the cancer will spread to other parts of the body.

Insufficient Thyroid Secretion

- **Hypothyroidism** (high-poh-**THIGH**-roid-izm), also known as an **underactive thyroid**, is a deficiency of

thyroid secretion (**hypo** means deficient, **thyroid** means thyroid, and **ism** means condition). Symptoms include fatigue, depression, sensitivity to cold, and a decreased metabolic rate.

- **Cretinism** (**CREE**-tin-izm) is a congenital lack of thyroid secretion. If treatment is not started soon after birth, it causes arrested physical and mental development.
- **Myxedema** (**mick**-seh-**DEE**-mah) is a severe form of adult hypothyroidism. Symptoms include an enlarged tongue and puffiness of the hands and face.
- **Hashimoto's thyroiditis** (hah-shee-**MOH**-tohz **thigh**-roi-**DYE**-tis) is an autoimmune disorder in which the immune system mistakenly attacks thyroid tissue, setting up an inflammatory process that may progressively destroy the gland. This may cause goiter or hypothyroidism.

Excessive Thyroid Secretion

- **Hyperthyroidism** (high-per-**THIGH**-roid-izm) is a condition of excessive thyroid hormones in the blood (**hyper** means excessive, **thyroid** means thyroid, and **ism** means condition). Symptoms include an increased metabolic rate, increased sweating, nervousness, and weight loss.
- **Graves' disease** (**GRAYVZ** dih-**ZEEZ**) is an autoimmune disorder characterized by hyperthyroidism, goiter, and exophthalmos.
- **Goiter** (**GOI**-ter), also known as **thyromegaly** (**thigh**-roh-**MEG**-ah-lee), is an abnormal enlargement of the thyroid gland that produces a swelling in the front part of the neck.
- **Exophthalmos** (**eck**-sof-**THAL**-mos) is an abnormal protrusion of the eyes.
- **Thyrotoxicosis** (**thy**-roh-**tock**-sih-**KOH**-sis), also known as **thyroid storm**, is a life-threatening condition resulting from the release of excessive quantities of the thyroid hormones into the bloodstream.

Diagnostic and Treatment Procedures Related to the Thyroid Gland

- A **thyroid scan** is one means to measure thyroid function (see Chapter 15).
- An **antithyroid drug** is a medication administered to slow the ability of the thyroid gland to produce thyroid hormones.
- A **chemical thyroidectomy** (**thigh**-roi-**DECK**-toh-mee), also known as **radioactive iodine therapy**, is the administration of radioactive iodine to destroy thyroid cells. This is used to treat hyperthyroid disorders such as Graves' disease.
- A **lobectomy** (loh-**BECK**-toh-mee) is the removal of one lobe of the thyroid gland. This term is also used to describe the removal of a lobe of the liver, brain, or lung.
- A **thyroid-stimulating hormone assay** is a diagnostic test to measure circulating blood levels of TSH. This

test is used to detect abnormal thyroid activity resulting from excessive pituitary stimulation.

The Parathyroid Glands

The four **parathyroid glands**, each of which is about the size of a grain of rice, are located within the thyroid gland (see Figure 13.1).

Functions of the Parathyroid Glands

The primary function of the parathyroid glands is to regulate calcium levels throughout the body. These calcium levels are important to the smooth functioning of the muscular and nervous systems.

Secretions of the Parathyroid Glands

Parathyroid hormone, also known as **PTH** or **parathormone**, works with calcitonin to regulate calcium levels in the blood and tissues. PTH increases calcium levels in the blood by mobilizing the release of calcium from storage in the bones and teeth. Compare with calcitonin.

Pathology of the Parathyroid Glands

Insufficient Parathyroid Secretion

- **Hypoparathyroidism** (**high**-poh-**par**-ah-**THIGH**-roid-izm) is a condition caused by an insufficient or absent secretion of the parathyroid glands. This is usually accompanied by hypocalcemia and in severe cases this leads to tetany.
- **Hypocalcemia** (**high**-poh-kal-**SEE**-mee-ah) is characterized by abnormally low levels of calcium in the blood (**hypo** means deficient, **calc** means calcium, and **emia** means blood condition.)
- **Tetany** (**TET**-ah-nee) is an abnormal condition characterized by periodic painful muscle spasms (cramps) and tremors.

Excessive Parathyroid Secretion

- **Hyperparathyroidism** (**high**-per-**par**-ah-**THIGH**-roid-izm), also known as **HP**, is the overproduction of PTH.

This causes hypercalcemia and may lead to weakened bones and the formation of kidney stones.

- **Hypercalcemia** (**high**-per-kal-**SEE**-mee-ah) is characterized by abnormally high concentrations of calcium circulating in the blood instead of being stored in the bones (**hyper** means excessive, **calc** means calcium, and **emia** means blood condition).
- **Primary HP** is caused by a diseased parathyroid gland. **Secondary HP** is caused by a problem elsewhere in the body. As an example, kidney failure makes the body resistant to the action of the PTH.

Treatment Procedure of the Parathyroid Glands

- A **parathyroidectomy** (**par**-ah-**thigh**-roi-**DECK**-toh-mee), which is the surgical removal of one or more of the parathyroid glands, is performed to control hyperparathyroidism.

The Adrenal Glands

The **adrenal glands**, also referred to as the **adrenals**, are located one on top of each kidney. Each adrenal gland consists of two parts: the **adrenal cortex** that is the outer portion and the **adrenal medulla** that is the inner portion (Figure 13.3).

Functions of the Adrenal Glands

One of the primary functions of the adrenals is to control electrolyte levels within the body. **Electrolytes** (ee-**LECK**-troh-lytes) are mineral substances, such as sodium and potassium, found in the blood.

- Other important functions include helping to regulate metabolism and interacting with the sympathetic nervous system in response to stress.

Secretions of the Adrenal Cortex

- A **corticosteroid** (**kor**-tih-koh-**STEHR**-oid) is the name given to any of the steroid hormones produced by the adrenal cortex or their synthetic equivalents. These are

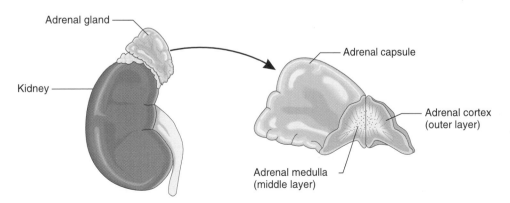

FIGURE 13.3 One adrenal gland is located on top of each kidney.

described in three groups: mineralocorticoids, gluco-corticoids, and gonadocorticoids.

- **Mineralocorticoids** regulate the mineral salts in the body. The primary mineralocorticoid is **aldosterone** (al-**DOSS**-ter-ohn) that regulates the salt and water levels in the body by increasing sodium reabsorption in the kidneys. (**Reabsorption** means that instead of excreting the sodium, the kidneys return it to the bloodstream.)

- **Glucocorticoids** regulate the metabolism of carbohydrates, fats, and proteins in the body. They also influence blood pressure and have an anti-inflammatory effect. The primary glucocorticoid is **cortisol** (**KOR**-tih-sol), which is also known as **hydrocortisone**.

- **Gonadocorticoids**, also known as **androgens** (**AN**-droh-jenz), are hormones that influence sex-related characteristics. Normally in adults production here is minimal and these hormones are produced in the male and female gonads.

Secretions of the Adrenal Medulla

- **Epinephrine** (**ep**-ih-**NEF**-rin), also called **adrenaline** (ah-**DREN**-uh-lin), and **norepinephrine** (**nor**-ep-ih-**NEF**-rin) stimulate the sympathetic nervous system. This stimulation causes an increase in the heart rate and increased blood pressure as well as the other symptoms associated with severe stress.

Pathology of the Adrenal Glands

- **Adrenalitis** (ah-**dree**-nal-**EYE**-tis) is an inflammation of the adrenal glands (adrenal means adrenal glands and itis means inflammation).

Insufficient Adrenal Secretions

- **Addison's disease** (**AD**-ih-sonz) is a progressive disease that occurs when adrenal glands do not produce enough cortisol. This may be due to a disorder of the adrenal glands or to inadequate secretion of ACTH by the pituitary gland. If untreated it can produce a life-threatening addisonian crisis.

Excessive Adrenal Secretions

- **Aldosteronism** (al-**DOSS**-teh-roh-**niz**-em *or* al-doh-**STER**-ohn-izm) is an abnormality of electrolyte balance caused by excessive secretion of aldosterone.

- **Primary aldosteronism**, also known as **Conn's syndrome**, is aldosteronism due to disorders of the adrenal gland.

- **Secondary aldosteronism** is *not* caused by a disorder of the adrenal gland. It results from a disorder elsewhere in the body, such as a nephrotic syndrome (see Chapter 9).

- A **pheochromocytoma** (fee-oh-**kroh**-moh-sigh-**TOH**-mah) is a benign tumor of the adrenal medulla that causes the gland to produce excess epinephrine.

Cushing's Syndrome

- **Cushing's syndrome** (**KUSH**-ingz **SIN**-drohm), also known as **CS** or **hypercortisolism**, is caused by prolonged exposure to high levels of cortisol. The symptoms include a rounded or moon face (Figure 13.4).

- CS may be caused by overproduction of cortisol by the body or by taking glucocorticoid hormone medications to treat inflammatory diseases such as asthma and rheumatoid arthritis.

FIGURE 13.4 Cushing's syndrome causes a characteristic round moon face. (*Courtesy of Matthew C. Leinung, M.D., Albany Medical College, Albany, NY*)

Treatment Procedures of the Adrenal Glands

- A **laparoscopic adrenalectomy** (ah-**dree**-nal-**ECK**-toh-mee) is a minimally invasive surgical procedure to remove one or both adrenal glands (adrenal means adrenal gland and ectomy means surgical removal).

- **Cortisone** (**KOR**-tih-sohn), also known as **hydrocortisone**, is the synthetic equivalent of corticosteroids produced by the body. Cortisone is administered to suppress inflammation and in transplant recipients it is administered as an immunosuppressant to prevent organ rejection by the body.

- **Epinephrine** is a synthetic pharmaceutical used as a vasoconstrictor to treat conditions such as heart dysrhythmias and asthma attacks. (A **vasoconstrictor** causes the blood vessels to contract.)

The Pancreatic Islets

The **pancreas** (**PAN**-kree-as) is a feather-shaped organ located posterior to (behind) the stomach (see Figure

13.1). Its primary functions are part of the digestive system and these are discussed in Chapter 8.

- The **pancreatic islets** (**pan**-kree-**AT**-ick **EYE**-lets), also known as the **islets of Langerhans** (**EYE**-lets of **LAHNG**-er-hahnz) or simply as **islets**, are cells within the pancreas that have an endocrine function.

Functions of the Pancreatic Islets

The functions of the islets are to control blood sugar levels and glucose metabolism throughout the body.

Secretions of the Pancreatic Islets

- **Glucagon** (**GLOO**-kah-gon), which is produced by the **alpha cells** of the islets, is secreted in response to low blood sugar. Glucagon increases the amount of glucose (sugar) in the bloodstream by stimulating the liver to convert glycogen into glucose.

- **Insulin** (**IN**-suh-lin), also known as **In**, is secreted by the **beta cells** of the islets in response to high blood sugar. It functions in two ways. First insulin allows glucose to enter the cells for use as energy. When additional glucose is *not* needed, insulin stimulates the liver to convert glucose into glycogen for storage (Figure 13.5).

Pathology of the Pancreas

- **Hyperglycemia** (**high**-per-glye-**SEE**-mee-ah) is an abnormally high concentration of glucose in the blood

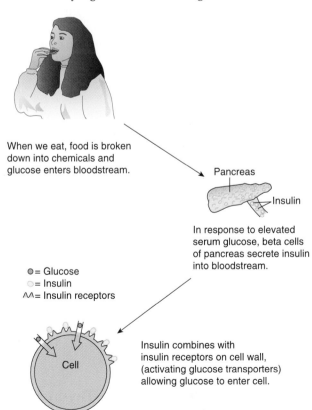

When we eat, food is broken down into chemicals and glucose enters bloodstream.

Pancreas

Insulin

In response to elevated serum glucose, beta cells of pancreas secrete insulin into bloodstream.

● = Glucose
○ = Insulin
∧∧ = Insulin receptors

Cell

Insulin combines with insulin receptors on cell wall, (activating glucose transporters) allowing glucose to enter cell.

FIGURE 13.5 How insulin works.

(**hyper** means excessive, **glyc** means sugar, and **emia** means blood condition). Symptoms of hyperglycemia include polyuria and polydipsia.

- **Hyperinsulinism** (**high**-per-**IN**-suh-lin-izm) is a condition marked by excessive secretion of insulin that produces hypoglycemia (**hyper** means excessive, **insulin** means insulin, and **ism** means condition).

- **Hypoglycemia** (**high**-poh-glye-**SEE**-mee-ah) is an abnormally low concentration of glucose (sugar) in the blood (**hypo** means deficient, **glyc** means sugar, and **emia** means blood condition).

- An **insulinoma** (in-suh-lin-**OH**-mah) is a benign tumor of the pancreas that causes hypoglycemia (**insulin** means insulin and **oma** means tumor).

- **Pancreatalgia** (**pan**-kree-ah-**TAL**-jee-ah) means pain in the pancreas (**pancreat** means pancreas and **algia** means pain).

- **Pancreatitis** (**pan**-kree-ah-**TYE**-tis) is an inflammation of the pancreas (**pancreat** means pancreas and **itis** means inflammation).

Diabetes Mellitus

- **Diabetes mellitus** (**dye**-ah-**BEE**-teez mel-**EYE**-tus *or* **MEL**-ih-tus) is a group of metabolic diseases characterized by hyperglycemia resulting from defects in insulin secretion, insulin action, or both.

- Although these are described as distinct types, many patients do not fit into a single category and the treatment goal is to most effectively control the blood sugar levels and prevent diabetic complications.

Type 1 Diabetes

Type 1 diabetes, also known as **insulin-dependent diabetes mellitus** (IDDM) or **juvenile diabetes**, is an autoimmune insulin deficiency disorder (*Note:* type 1 and type 2 diabetes are spelled with a small *t*).

- Due to the destruction of pancreatic islet beta cells the body does not secrete enough insulin. Type 1 diabetes is treated with carefully regulated insulin replacement therapy.

- Symptoms include increased urination, constant thirst and hunger, weight loss, blurred vision, extreme fatigue, and slow healing. Only 1 in 10 individuals with diabetes has this form of the disease.

Type 2 Diabetes

Type 2 diabetes, also known as **non–insulin-dependent diabetes mellitus** (NIDDM) or **adult-onset diabetes**, is an insulin resistance disorder. Although insulin is being produced, the body does not use it effectively. In an attempt to compensate the body secretes more insulin.

- Type 2 diabetes may have no symptoms for years. When symptoms do occur they include those of type 1 diabetes, plus recurring infections, irritability, and a tingling sensation in the hands or feet.

- Type 2 diabetes is treated with diet, exercise, and medications. Sulfonylureas are medications that lower blood sugar by causing the body to release more insulin. Other types of medications, such as Glucophage (metformin hydrochloride), work within the cells to help insulin let blood sugar in.

Gestational Diabetes Mellitus

Gestational diabetes mellitus (jes-TAY-shun-al dye-ah-BEE-teez mel-EYE-tus *or* MEL-ih-tus), also known as GDM, is the form of diabetes that occurs during some pregnancies. GDM usually disappears after delivery; however, many of these women later develop type 2 diabetes.

Diabetes Mellitus Diagnostic Procedures

- A **fasting blood sugar**, also known as **FBS**, measures the glucose (blood sugar) levels after the patient has not eaten for 8 to 12 hours. This test is used to screen for and to monitor treatment of diabetes mellitus.

- A **glucose tolerance test** (GLOO-kohs), also known as **GTT**, is used to confirm diabetes mellitus and to aid in diagnosing hypoglycemia (low blood sugar).

- A finger stick **blood sugar monitoring test** is performed at least once daily to determine how much insulin or other medications are required.

- **Hemoglobin** A_{1C} **testing**, also known as the **HgA$_{1c}$** or **glycohemoglobin test**, use blood tests that measures the average blood glucose level over the previous 3 to 4 months. This test monitors how well blood sugar levels have been controlled during this time period. **Glycohemoglobin** (glye-koh-**hee**-moh-GLOH-bin), also known as GHb, forms when glucose in the blood attaches to the hemoglobin.

- The **fructosamine test** (fruck-TOHS-ah-meen) measures average glucose levels over the past 3 weeks and is used to detect changes more rapidly.

Diabetic Emergencies

- **Hypoglycemia**, which is very low blood sugar, is caused by failing to eat at the proper time or not adjusting medications properly. Treatment is to raise blood sugar rapidly with glucose tablets or another form of readily absorbed sugar.

- **Hyperglycemia**, which is very high blood sugar, is also known as **diabetic ketoacidosis** (kee-toh-**ass**-ih-**DOH**-sis) or **DKA**. This acute, life-threatening complication is caused by a severe insulin deficiency. If untreated it may lead to a **diabetic coma** and possibly death.

Diabetic Complications

- Most diabetic complications result from the damage to blood vessels, particularly capillaries, caused by long-term high blood sugar. This affects the capillary beds in many organs such as the eyes and kidneys.

- **Heart disease** occurs because excess blood sugar makes the walls of the blood vessels sticky. This encourages atherosclerosis (plaque buildup) within these vessels that slows or blocks the normal flow of blood.

- **Kidney disease** may lead to renal failure due to blood vessel damage that reduces blood flow through the kidneys.

- **Peripheral neuropathy** (new-ROP-ah-thee) is damage to the nerves of the hands and feet. This can cause either extreme sensitivity or numbness.

- **Diabetic retinopathy**, also known as **DR**, is a complication of diabetics that causes damage to the retina of the eye. **Retinopathy** (ret-ih-NOP-ah-thee) means any disease of the retina (**retino** means retina and **pathy** means disease).

- One form of DR is **macular edema** in which fluids from blood vessels leaking into the eye cause the macula to swell. Another form is **proliferative retinopathy**. Here fragile new blood vessels form and break, clouding vision and damaging the retina.

Treatment Procedure of the Pancreas

- A **pancreatectomy** (pan-kree-ah-TECK-toh-mee) is the surgical removal of the pancreas (**pancreat** means pancreas and **ectomy** means surgical removal).

The Thymus

The **thymus** (THIGH-mus) is located near the midline in the anterior portion of the thoracic cavity. It is posterior to (behind) the sternum and slightly superior to (above) the heart. *Note:* The word part **thym/o** means thymus; however, it also means relationship to the soul or emotions.

Functions of the Thymus

The thymus plays an important role in the immune system and these functions are discussed in Chapter 6.

Secretions of the Thymus

- **Thymosin** (THIGH-moh-sin) stimulates the maturation of lymphocytes into T cells of the immune system.

Pathology of the Thymus

- **Thymitis** (thigh-MY-tis) is an inflammation of the thymus gland (**thym** means thymus and **itis** means inflammation).

- A **thymoma** (thigh-MOH-mah) is a usually benign tumor derived from the tissue of the thymus (**thym** means thymus and **oma** means tumor).

Treatment Procedure of the Thymus

- A **thymectomy** (thigh-MECK-toh-mee) is the surgical removal of the thymus gland (**thym** means thymus and **ectomy** means surgical removal).

The Pineal Gland

The **pineal gland** (**PIN**-ee-al) is located in the central portion of the brain.

Functions of the Pineal Gland

- The function of the pineal gland is not clearly understood; however, it is known to influence the sleep–wakefulness cycle.

Secretion of the Pineal Gland

- **Melatonin** (**mel**-ah-**TOH**-nin) influences the sleep and wakefulness portions of the circadian cycle. The term **circadian cycle** refers to the biologic functions that occur within a 24-hour period.

Pathology of the Pineal Gland

- **Pinealopathy** (**pin**-ee-ah-**LOP**-ah-thee) is any disorder of the pineal gland (**pinealo** means pineal gland and **pathy** means disease).

Treatment Procedures of the Pineal Gland

- A **pinealectomy** (**pin**-ee-al-**ECK**-toh-mee) is the surgical removal of the pineal body (**pineal** means pineal gland and **ectomy** means surgical removal).

The Gonads

The **gonads** (**GOH**-nadz), which are ovaries in females and testicles in males, are the gamete-producing glands. A **gamete** (**GAM**-eet) is a reproductive cell. This is the sperm in the male and ova (eggs) in the female.

- A **gonadotropic hormone** (**gon**-ah-doh-**TROHP**-ick), also known as **gonadotropin**, is any hormone that stimulates the gonads.

Functions of the Gonads

- The gonads secrete the hormones that are responsible for the development and maintenance of secondary sex characteristics.
- The additional functions of the glands are discussed in Chapter 14.

Secretions of the Testicles

- **Testosterone** (tes-**TOS**-teh-rohn), which is secreted by the testicles, stimulates the development of male secondary sex characteristics (Figure 13.6).

Secretions of the Ovaries

- **Estrogen** (**ES**-troh-jen) is important in the development and maintenance of the female secondary sex characteristics and regulation of the menstrual cycle (Figure 13.7).

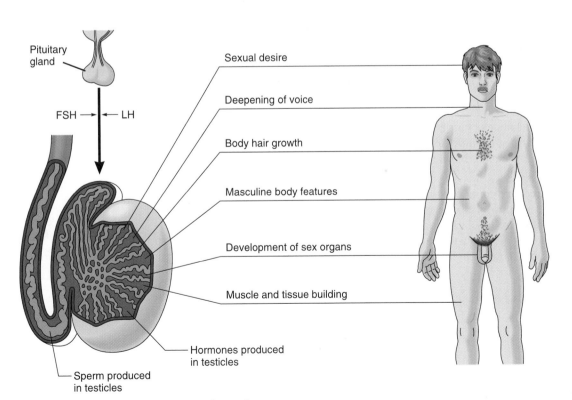

FIGURE 13.6 Secondary sex characteristics in the male.

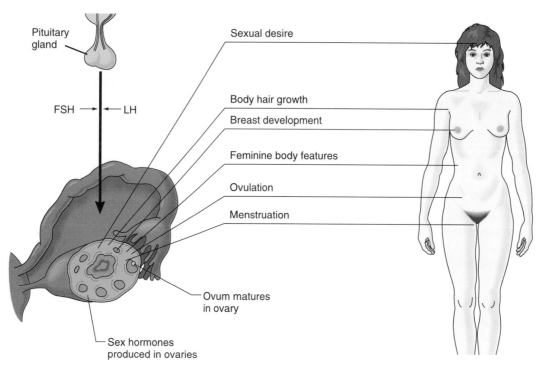

FIGURE 13.7 Secondary sex characteristics in the female.

- **Progesterone** (proh-JES-ter-ohn) is the hormone released during the second half of the menstrual cycle by the corpus luteum in the ovary. Its function is to complete the preparations for pregnancy.

- If pregnancy occurs, the placenta takes over the production of progesterone.

- If pregnancy does not occur, secretion of the hormone stops and is followed by the menstrual period.

The Placenta

- The **placenta** is an organ formed during pregnancy that allows the exchange of nutrients, oxygen, and waste products between the mother and child during pregnancy. After the child is born, the placenta is expelled as the afterbirth.

- **Human chorionic gonadotropin** (kor-ee-ON-ick gon-ah-doh-TROH-pin), also known as **HCG**, is the hormone secreted by the placenta during pregnancy. HCG stimulates the corpus luteum to continue producing the hormones required to maintain the pregnancy.

- It also stimulates the hormones required to stimulate lactation after childbirth.

Pathology of the Gonads

- **Hypergonadism** (**high**-per-**GOH**-nad-izm) is the condition of excessive secretion of hormones by the sex glands (**hyper** means excessive, **gonad** means sex gland, and **ism** means condition).

- **Hypogonadism** (**high**-poh-**GOH**-nad-izm) is the condition of deficient secretion of hormones by the sex glands (**hypo** means deficient, **gonad** means sex gland, and **ism** means condition).

- **Gynecomastia** (**guy**-neh-koh-**MAS**-tee-ah) is the condition of excessive mammary development in the male (**gyneco** means female, **mast** means breast, and **ia** means abnormal condition).

Treatment Procedures of the Gonads

- These procedures are discussed in Chapter 14.

Learning Exercises

● Matching Word Parts—1

Write the letter of the correct answer on the line provided in the left column.

13.1. _____ acr/o   A. adrenal glands

13.2. _____ adren/o   B. extremities

13.3. _____ crin/o   C. ovaries or testicles

13.4. _____ -dipsia   D. to secrete

13.5. _____ gonad/o   E. thirst

● Matching Word Parts—2

Write the letter of the correct answer on the line provided in the left column.

13.6. _____ -ism   A. pituitary

13.7. _____ pancreat/o   B. pineal gland

13.8. _____ parathyroid/o   C. pancreas

13.9. _____ pineal/o   D. parathyroid

13.10. _____ pituit/o   E. condition

● Matching Word Parts—3

Write the letter of the correct answer on the line provided in the left column.

13.11. _____ poly-   A. to stimulate

13.12. _____ somat/o   B. thyroid gland

13.13. _____ thym/o   C. soul, emotions

13.14. _____ thyr/o,   D. many
          thyroid/o

13.15. _____ -tropin   E. body

● Definitions

Circle the letter next to the correct answer.

13.16. Which hormone stimulates ovulation?

 a. estrogen

 b. follicle-stimulating hormone (FSH)

 c. luteinizing hormone (LH)

 d. progesterone

13.17. Which endocrine gland is known as the master gland?

 a. adrenal

 b. hypothalamus

 c. pituitary

 d. thymus

13.18. Which hormone stimulates the growth and secretion of the adrenal cortex?

 a. adrenocorticotropic hormone (ACTH)

 b. growth hormone (GH)

 c. melanocyte-stimulating hormone (MSH)

 d. thyroid-stimulating hormone (TSH)

13.19. Which endocrine gland(s) play(s) an important role in immune reactions?

 a. adrenal glands

 b. parathyroids

 c. pineal gland

 d. thymus

13.20. Which hormone works with the parathyroid hormone to regulate calcium levels in the blood and tissues?

 a. aldosterone

 b. calcitonin

 c. glucagon

 d. luteotropin

13.21. Which endocrine gland secretes cortisol?

    a. adrenal cortex

    b. pituitary gland (posterior lobe)

    c. thymus

    d. thyroid

13.22. Which hormone increases the amount of glucose in the bloodstream?

    a. adrenaline

    b. glucagon

    c. hydrocortisone

    d. insulin

13.23. Which endocrine glands secrete norepinephrine?

    a. adrenal medulla

    b. pancreatic islets

    c. ovaries

    d. testicles

13.24. Which hormone stimulates uterine contractions during childbirth?

    a. estrogen

    b. lactogenic hormone (LTH)

    c. oxytocin (OXT)

    d. thymosin

13.25. Which hormone stimulates the development of the male secondary sex characteristics?

    a. aldosterone

    b. parathyroid

    c. progesterone

    d. testosterone

● Matching Structures

Write the letter of the correct answer on the line provided in the left column.

13.26. _____ adrenal glands   A. control blood sugar levels

13.27. _____ pancreatic islets   B. influences the sleep–wakefulness cycle

13.28. _____ pineal gland   C. regulate electrolyte levels

13.29. _____ pituitary gland   D. stimulates metabolism

13.30. _____ thyroid gland   E. the master gland

● Which Word?

Circle the correct term in each sentence.

13.31. Insufficient secretion of the parathyroid glands causes *hyperparathyroidism* / *hypoparathyroidism.*

13.32. The growth hormone is also known as *somatotropin* / *thyrotropin.*

13.33. The hormones that influence sex-related characteristics are known as *glucocorticoids* / *gonadocorticoids.*

13.34. Insulin replacement therapy is always used in *type 1* / *type 2* diabetes mellitus.

13.35. An insufficient production of ADH causes *diabetes insipidus* / *diabetes mellitus.*

● Spelling Counts

Find the misspelled word in each sentence. Then write that word, spelled correctly, on the line provided.

13.36. Metebolism is the rate at which the body uses energy and the speed at which body functions work. _____

13.37. Diabetes melletus is a group of diseases characterized by defects in insulin production, use, or both. _____

13.38. Hydrocortizone has an anti-inflammatory effect. _____

13.39. The hormone progestarone is released during the second half of the menstrual cycle. _____

13.40. Thymosin is secreted by the thymas gland. _____

● Matching Abbreviations

Write the letter of the correct answer on the line provided in the left column.

13.41. _____ ACTH   A. luteinizing hormone

13.42. _____ GDM   B. glucose tolerance test

13.43. _____ GTT   C. lactogenic hormone

13.44. _____ LH   D. adrenocorticotropic hormone

13.45. _____ LTH   E. gestational diabetes mellitus

● Term Selection

Circle the letter next to the correct answer.

13.46. Which term means a condition caused by excessive secretion of any gland, especially an endocrine gland.

    a. endocrinopathy

    b. goiter

    c. hypercrinism

    d. hypocrinism

13.47. Which life-threatening condition can result from the presence of excessive quantities of the thyroid hormones?

    a. aldosteronism

    b. Cushing's syndrome

    c. goiter

    d. thyrotoxicosis

13.48. Which endocrine gland is located behind the sternum?

    a. pancreas

    b. parathyroid

    c. pineal

    d. thymus

13.49. Polydipsia and polyuria are symptoms of which condition?

    a. Cushing's syndrome

    b. diabetes insipidus

    c. pituitary adenoma

    d. prolactinoma

13.50. Which blood test measures the average blood sugar over the past 3 months?

    a. blood sugar monitoring

    b. fructosamine test

    c. glucose tolerance test

    d. hemoglobin A_{1C} testing

● Sentence Completion

Write the correct term on the line.

13.51. Substances, such as sodium and potassium, that are found in the blood are known as _____ .

13.52. Calcitonin and thyroxine are secreted by the _____ gland.

13.53. Damage to the retina of the eye caused by diabetes mellitus is known as diabetes _____ .

13.54. The medical term that describes a severe form of adult hypothyroidism with symptoms that include an enlarged tongue and puffiness of the hands and face is _____ .

13.55. Abnormal protrusion of the eyes associated with Graves' disease is known as _____ .

● True/False

If the statement is true, write T on the line. If the statement is false, write F on the line.

13.56. _____ Pancreatalgia is an inflammation of the pancreas.

13.57. _____ Polyuria means excessive urination.

13.58. _____ Secondary aldosteronism is due to a disorder of the adrenal gland.

13.59. _____ Hypoglycemia is an abnormally decreased concentration of glucose in the blood.

13.60. _____ Gynecomastia is the condition of excessive mammary development in the male.

13.61. _____ The alpha cells of the pancreatic islets secrete insulin.

13.62. _____ Type 1 and adult-onset describe the same form of diabetes mellitus.

13.63. _____ Human chorionic gonadotropin is secreted by the adrenal cortex.

13.64. _____ The growth hormone (GH) is secreted by the pineal gland.

13.65. _____ A chemical thyroidectomy is used to treat disorders such as Graves' disease.

● Clinical Conditions

Write the correct answer on the line.

13.66. Grace McClelland was treated for a tumor derived from the tissue of the thymus. The medical term for this condition is a/an

_____ _____ .

13.67. Joseph Butler complains of being thirsty all the time. His doctor listed this excessive thirst on his chart as _____ .

13.68. During her pregnancy, Carmella DeFillipo was treated for _____ diabetes.

13.69. Linda Thomas has a progressive disease that occurs when adrenal glands do not produce enough cortisol. This condition is known as _____ disease.

13.70. Patty Edward requires daily insulin injections to control her _____ -dependent (type 1) diabetes mellitus.

13.71. When "the champ" was training for the Olympics, he was tempted to use _____ steroids to increase his strength and muscle mass.

13.72. Leigh Franklin developed a condition that is characterized by extremely large hands and feet. The medical term for this condition is

_____ .

13.73. As a result of a congenital lack of thyroid secretion, the Vaugh-Eames child suffers from arrested physical and mental development. The medical term for this condition is

_____ .

13.74. Raymond Grovenor is excessively tall and large. This condition, which was caused by excessive functioning of the pituitary gland before puberty is known as

_____ .

13.75. Rose Liu required the surgical removal of her pancreas. The medical term for this procedure is a/an _____ .

● Which is the correct medical term?

Circle the letter next to the correct answer.

13.76. Which condition is also known as Conn's syndrome?

    a. hypercortisolism

    b. hypothyroidism

    c. primary aldosteronism

    d. secondary aldosteronism

13.77. Which term means a benign tumor of the pituitary gland that causes the excess secretion of ACTH?

    a. hyperpituitarism

    b. hypopituitarism

    c. pituitary adenoma

    d. prolactinoma

13.78. Which condition is an autoimmune disorder in which thyroid tissue is gradually destroyed?

    a. Graves' disease

    b. hypothyroidism

    c. Hashimoto's thyroiditis

    d. thyrotoxicosis

13.79. Which condition may progress to diabetic ketoacidosis?

    a. diabetic neuropathy

    b. diabetic retinopathy

    c. hyperglycemia

    d. hypoglycemia

13.80. Which hormone plays an important role in the immune system?

    a. glucagon

    b. melatonin

    c. parathyroid hormone

    d. thymosin

● Challenge Word Building

These terms are *not* found in this chapter; however, they are made up of these familiar word parts. You may want to look in the glossary or use a medical dictionary to check your answers!

endo-	insulin/o	-emia
	adren/o	-itis
	crin/o	-megaly
	pancreat/o	-ology
	thyroid/o	-oma
	thym/o	-otomy
	pineal/o	-pathy

13.81. The medical term meaning a surgical incision into the thyroid gland is a/an

_____ .

13.82. The study of the endocrine glands and their secretions is known as _____ .

13.83. The medical term meaning enlargement of the adrenal glands is _____ .

13.84. The medical term meaning any disease of the thymus gland is _____ .

13.85. The medical term meaning an inflammation of the thyroid gland is _____ .

13.86. The medical term meaning a surgical incision into the pancreas is a/an

_____ .

13.87. The medical term meaning any disease of the adrenal glands is _____ .

13.88. The medical term meaning a tumor of the pineal gland is a/an _____ .

13.89. The medical term meaning abnormally high levels of insulin in the blood is

_____ .

13.90. The medical term meaning an inflammation of the adrenal glands is _____ .

● **Labeling Exercises**

Identify the numbered items on this diagram.

13.91. _____ gland

13.92. _____ glands

13.93. _____ gland

13.94. _____ of the female

13.95. _____ gland

13.96. _____ lobe

13.97. _____ gland

13.98. _____ gland

13.99. _____ islets

13.100. _____ of the male

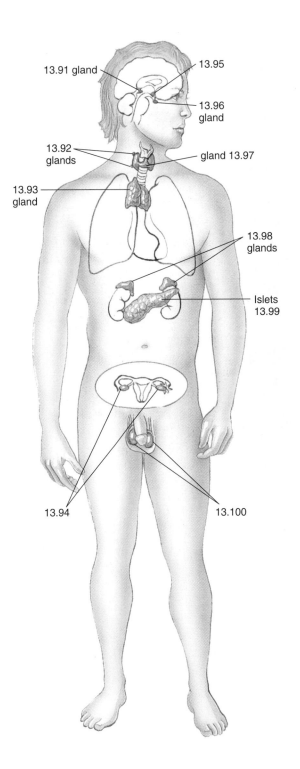

The Human Touch: Critical Thinking Exercise

The following story and questions are designed to stimulate critical thinking through class discussion or as a brief essay response. There are no easy or right-wrong answers to these questions.

By the time 14-year-old Jacob Tuls got home, he was sick enough for his mom to notice. His seemed shaky and confused and was sweaty even though the fall weather was cool. "Jake, let's get you a glass of juice right away," his mother said as calmly as she could. She was all too familiar with the symptoms of hypoglycemia brought on by Jake's type I diabetes. Ever since he was diagnosed at age 6, she had carefully monitored his insulin, eating, and exercise. But now that he was in middle school, the ball was in his court — and it really worried her that he often seemed to mess up.

"Yeah, I know I shouldn't have gone so long without eating," Jake muttered once he was feeling better. "But you don't understand — I don't want to be different from the other kids." Before he could finish, his mom was on the telephone to the school nurse's office.

Jacob needed to inject himself with insulin three times a day. He knew what happened when his blood sugar got too high, or if he didn't eat on schedule and it got too low. But when he was with his friends, he hated to go up to the chaperone on a field trip and say that he needed to eat something right away. And he hated it when some kid walked in while he was injecting. His mom made arrangements with the school nurse for him to go to her office to get some privacy — but whenever he didn't show up between 4th and 5th period, she'd come into the classroom to get him like he was some kind of sick "dweeb."

He was tired of having this disease, sick of shots, and mad that he couldn't sleep late and skip meals like other kids. He made a face at his mother as she talked on the telephone to the nurse, and slammed the back door on his way out to find his friend Joe.

Suggested Discussion Topics:

1. What could Jacob's parents do to help him get through this rough time of his life?

2. Why is it more difficult for Jacob to maintain his injection routine in middle school than it was in elementary school?

3. Knowing that missing an insulin injection could cause a diabetic coma and death, why wouldn't Jacob be more conscientious?

4. Do you think Jacob's schoolmates talk about him — or is it just his perception? Discuss both options.

5. People with juvenile diabetes can live close to a normal life span if they follow a healthy routine. Discuss stages in their lives where they might have the most difficulties with this disease.

14

The Reproductive Systems

● Overview of Structures, Word Parts, and Functions of the Reproductive Systems

MAJOR STRUCTURES	RELATED WORD ROOTS	PRIMARY FUNCTIONS
Male:		
Testicles, testes	orch/o, orchid/o, test/i, test/o, testicul/o	Produce sperm and the male hormone testosterone.
Female:		
Ovaries	oophor/o, ovari/o	Produce ova (eggs) and female hormones.
Fallopian tubes	salping/o	Catch mature ova, provide the site for fertilization, transport ova to uterus.
Uterus	hyster/o, metr/o, metri/o, uter/o	Protects and supports the developing child.
Placenta	placent/o	Exchanges nutrients and waste between the mother and fetus during pregnancy.

VOCABULARY Related to the Reproductive Systems

Check the box as you master each word part or term. Terms marked with the ❖ symbol are pronounced on the optional student audiotape.

Key Word Parts

- ☐ cervic/o
- ☐ colp/o
- ☐ episi/o
- ☐ -gravida
- ☐ gynec/o
- ☐ mamm/o
- ☐ men/o
- ☐ metr/o
- ☐ nulli-
- ☐ oophor/o
- ☐ orchid/o
- ☐ ov/o
- ☐ -pexy
- ☐ prostat/o
- ☐ salping/o

Key Medical Terms

- ☐ **ablation** (ab-LAY-shun) ❖
- ☐ **abruptio placentae** (ab-RUP-shee-oh plah-SEN-tee) ❖
- ☐ **amenorrhea** (ah-**men**-oh-REE-ah *or* ay-**men**-oh-REE-ah) ❖
- ☐ **anorchism** (an-OR-kizm) ❖
- ☐ **azoospermia** (ay-**zoh**-oh-SPER-mee-ah) ❖
- ☐ **benign prostatic hypertrophy** ❖
- ☐ **cervical dysplasia** (dis-PLAY-see-ah) ❖
- ☐ **cervicitis** (ser-vih-SIGH-tis)
- ☐ **cesarean section** (seh-ZEHR-ee-un SECK-shun)
- ☐ **chlamydia** (klah-MID-ee-ah)
- ☐ **circumcision** (ser-kum-SIZH-un)
- ☐ **colposcopy** (kol-POS-koh-pee)
- ☐ **curettage** (kyou-reh-TAHZH) ❖
- ☐ **dilation** (dye-LAY-shun) ❖
- ☐ **dysmenorrhea** (dis-men-oh-REE-ah) ❖
- ☐ **eclampsia** (eh-KLAMP-see-ah) ❖
- ☐ **ectopic pregnancy** (eck-TOP-ick) ❖
- ☐ **endocervicitis** (en-doh-ser-vih-SIGH-tis) ❖
- ☐ **endometriosis** (en-doh-mee-tree-OH-sis) ❖
- ☐ **epididymitis** (ep-ih-did-ih-MY-tis)
- ☐ **episiorrhaphy** (eh-piz-ee-OR-ah-fee) ❖
- ☐ **episiotomy** (eh-piz-ee-OT-oh-mee) ❖
- ☐ **fibrocystic breast disease** (figh-broh-SIS-tick) ❖
- ☐ **gonorrhea** (gon-oh-REE-ah) ❖
- ☐ **gynecologist** (guy-neh-KOL-oh-jist) ❖
- ☐ **human papilloma virus** (pap-ih-LOH-mah) ❖
- ☐ **hypomenorrhea** (high-poh-men-oh-REE-ah) ❖
- ☐ **hysterectomy** (hiss-teh-RECK-toh-mee) ❖
- ☐ **hysteropexy** (HISS-ter-oh-peck-see) ❖
- ☐ **hysterosalpingography** (hiss-ter-oh-sal-pin-GOG-rah-fee) ❖

- ☐ **hysterosalpingo-oophorectomy** (hiss-ter-oh-sal-ping-goh oh-ahf-oh-RECK-toh-mee) ❖
- ☐ **hysteroscopy** (hiss-ter-OSS-koh-pee) ❖
- ☐ **leiomyoma** (lye-oh-my-OH-mah) ❖
- ☐ **leukorrhea** (loo-koh-REE-ah) ❖
- ☐ **mammography** (mam-OG-rah-fee) ❖
- ☐ **mammoplasty** (MAM-oh-plas-tee) ❖
- ☐ **menarche** (meh-NAR-kee)
- ☐ **menometrorrhagia** (men-oh-met-roh-RAY-jee-ah) ❖
- ☐ **menopause** (MEN-oh-pawz)
- ☐ **menstruation** (men-stroo-AY-shun) ❖
- ☐ **metrorrhea** (mee-troh-REE-ah) ❖
- ☐ **metrorrhexis** (mee-troh-RECK-sis) ❖
- ☐ **mittelschmerz** (MIT-uhl-schmehrts) ❖
- ☐ **multiparous** (mul-TIP-ah-rus) ❖
- ☐ **neonate** (NEE-oh-nayt) ❖
- ☐ **nulligravida** (null-ih-GRAV-ih-dah) ❖
- ☐ **nullipara** (nuh-LIP-ah-rah) ❖
- ☐ **obstetrician** (ob-steh-TRISH-un) ❖
- ☐ **oligomenorrhea** (ol-ih-goh-men-oh-REE-ah) ❖
- ☐ **oligospermia** (ol-ih-goh-SPER-mee-ah) ❖
- ☐ **oophorectomy** (oh-ahf-oh-RECK-toh-mee) ❖
- ☐ **oophoritis** (oh-ahf-oh-RYE-tis) ❖
- ☐ **orchidectomy** (or-kih-DECK-toh-mee) ❖
- ☐ **orchitis** (or-KYE-tis) ❖
- ☐ **ovariectomy** (oh-vay-ree-ECK-toh-me) ❖
- ☐ **ovariorrhexis** (oh-vay-ree-oh-RECK-sis) ❖
- ☐ **Papanicolaou test** (pap-ah-nick-oh-LAY-ooh) ❖
- ☐ **perimenopause** (pehr-ih-MEN-oh-pawz) ❖
- ☐ **perineum** (pehr-ih-NEE-um)
- ☐ **placenta previa** (plah-SEN-tah PREE-vee-ah) ❖
- ☐ **preeclampsia** (pree-ee-KLAMP-see-ah) ❖
- ☐ **primigravida** (prye-mih-GRAV-ih-dah)
- ☐ **primipara** (prye-MIP-ah-rah)
- ☐ **prostatectomy** (pros-tah-TECK-toh-mee)
- ☐ **prostatitis** (pros-tah-TYE-tis)
- ☐ **pruritus vulvae** (proo-RYE-tus VUL-vee)
- ☐ **salpingo-oophorectomy** (sal-ping-goh oh-ahf-oh-RECK-toh-mee) ❖
- ☐ **syphilis** (SIF-ih-lis)
- ☐ **trichomonas** (trick-oh-MOH-nas) ❖
- ☐ **vaginal candidiasis** (kan-dih-DYE-ah-sis) ❖
- ☐ **vaginoplasty** (vah-JIGH-noh-plas-tee) ❖
- ☐ **varicocele** (VAR-ih-koh-seel) ❖
- ☐ **varicocelectomy** (var-ih-koh-sih-LECK-toh-mee) ❖
- ☐ **vasectomy** (vah-SECK-toh-mee) ❖
- ☐ **vasovasostomy** (vas-oh-vah-ZOS-toh-mee *or* vay-zoh-vay-ZOS-toh-mee) ❖

1 Identify and describe the major functions and structures of the male reproductive system.

2 Recognize, define, spell, and pronounce the terms related to the pathology and diagnostic and treatment procedures of the male reproductive system.

3 Name at least six sexually transmitted diseases.

4 Identify and describe the major functions and structures of the female reproductive system.

5 Recognize, define, spell, and pronounce the terms related to the pathology and diagnostic and treatment procedures of the female reproductive system.

6 Recognize, define, spell, and pronounce the terms related to the pathology and diagnostic and treatment procedures of the female during pregnancy, childbirth, and the postpartum period.

Functions of the Male Reproductive System

The primary function of the male reproductive system is to produce millions of sperm and deliver them to unite with a single ovum (egg) to create a new life.

Structures of the Male Reproductive System

Some of the structures of the male reproductive system also function as part of the urinary system. Urinary functions are discussed in Chapter 9.

External Male Genitalia

The term **genitalia** (jen-ih-TAY-lee-ah) means reproductive organs. The external genitalia are those reproductive organs located outside of the body cavity.

- Major external male organs include the penis, scrotum, and two testicles each with an attached epididymis (Figure 14.1).

Scrotum

The **scrotum** (SKROH-tum), also known as the **scrotal sac**, encloses, protects, and supports the testicles. It is suspended from the pubic arch behind the penis and lies between the thighs.

- In the male, the **perineum** (pehr-ih-NEE-um) is the region between the scrotum and the anus.

Testicles

The **testicles**, also known as **testes**, are the two small egg-shaped glands that produce the spermatozoa (Figure 14.2). (Singular, **testis**.)

- The testicles develop within the abdomen of the male fetus and normally descend into the scrotum before birth or soon after birth.

- The **epididymis** (ep-ih-DID-ih-mis) is a tube at the upper part of each testicle. It runs down the length of the testicle, then turns upward into the body where it becomes a narrower tube called the vas deferens.

The Penis

The **penis** (PEE-nis) is the male sex organ that transports the sperm into the female vagina. The penis is composed of erectile tissue that, during sexual stimulation, fills with blood (under high pressure) causing an erection.

- The **glans penis** (glanz PEE-nis) is a soft sensitive region located at the tip of the penis.

- The **prepuce** (PREE-pyous), also known as the **foreskin**, covers and protects the glans penis.

Internal Male Genitalia

Vas Deferens

The **vas deferens** (vas DEF-er-enz) leads from the epididymis to the ejaculatory duct in the prostate.

Seminal Vesicles

The **seminal vesicles** (SEM-ih-nal) are glands located at the base of the urinary bladder. These open into the vas deferens as it joins the urethra.

- These glands secrete a thick, yellow substance that nourishes the sperm cells and forms much of the volume of ejaculated semen.

- The **ejaculatory duct** is one of the two final portions of the seminal vesicles. This duct, which is formed by the union of the ductus deferens and the duct from the seminal vesicle, passes through the prostate gland and enters the urethra.

The Prostate Gland

The **prostate gland** (PROS-tayt) lies under the bladder and surrounds the upper end of the urethra in the region where the vas deferens enters the urethra.

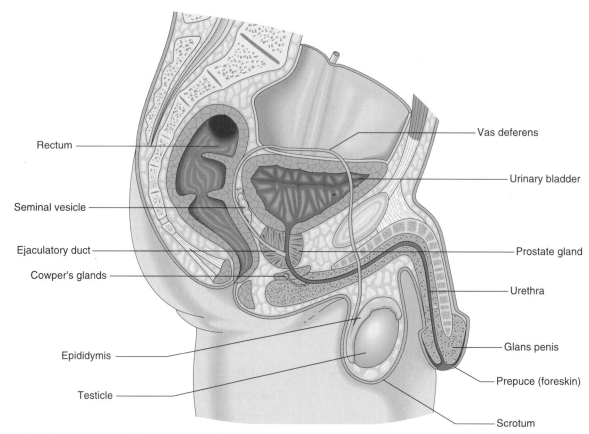

FIGURE 14.1 Cross section of the male reproductive organs.

Rectum
Seminal vesicle
Ejaculatory duct
Cowper's glands
Epididymis
Testicle

Vas deferens
Urinary bladder
Prostate gland
Urethra
Glans penis
Prepuce (foreskin)
Scrotum

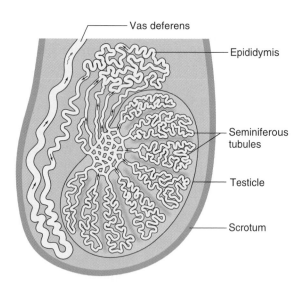

Vas deferens
Epididymis
Seminiferous tubules
Testicle
Scrotum

FIGURE 14.2 Cross section of structures contained within the scrotum. The flow through these structures is indicated by arrows.

- The prostate gland secretes a thick fluid that, as part of the semen, aids the motility of the sperm.

Cowper's Glands

Cowper's glands, also known as **bulbourethral glands** (**bul**-boh-you-**REE**-thral), are located on either side of the urethra just below the prostate gland, and their ducts open into the urethra.

- These glands secrete thick mucus that acts as a lubricant that tends to flow early during sexual excitement.

The Urethra

The **urethra** passes through the penis to the outside of the body. In the male it serves both the reproductive and urinary systems.

Sperm and Semen Formation

- The **sperm** are the male gametes. A **gamete** (**GAM**-eet) is a reproductive cell. Also known as **spermatozoa** (**sper**-mah-toh-**ZOH**-ah), sperm are formed in the seminiferous tubules of the testicles (singular, **spermatozoon**).
- After sperm are formed, they move into the epididymis where they become motile and are temporarily stored. (**Motile** means capable of spontaneous motion.)
- From the epididymis the sperm travel upward into the body and enter the vas deferens. Here the seminal vesicles and prostate gland add their secretions to form **semen** (**SEE**-men).
- At the peak of male sexual excitement, semen is ejaculated through the urethra.

Medical Specialties Related to the Male Reproductive System

- A **urologist** (you-**ROL**-oh-jist) specializes in diagnosing and treating diseases and disorders of the urinary system of females and the genitourinary system of males (**ur** means urine and **ologist** means specialist).

Pathology of the Male Reproductive System

The Penis

- **Balanitis** (**bal**-ah-**NIGH**-tis) is an inflammation of the glans penis and is often associated with phimosis (**balan** means glans penis and **itis** means inflammation).

- **Impotence** (**IM**-poh-tens), also known as **erectile dysfunction**, is the inability of the male to achieve or maintain a penile erection.
- **Phimosis** (figh-**MOH**-sis) is a narrowing of the opening of the foreskin so it cannot be retracted (pulled back) to expose the glans penis.

Testicles and Related Structures

- **Anorchism** (an-**OR**-kizm) is the congenital absence of one or both testicles (**an** means without, **orch** means testicle, and **ism** means abnormal condition) (Figure 14.3A).
- **Cryptorchidism** (krip-**TOR**-kih-dizm), also known as an **undescended testis**, is a developmental defect in which one testicle fails to descend into the scrotum (**crypto** means hidden, **orchid** means testicle, and **ism** means abnormal condition).

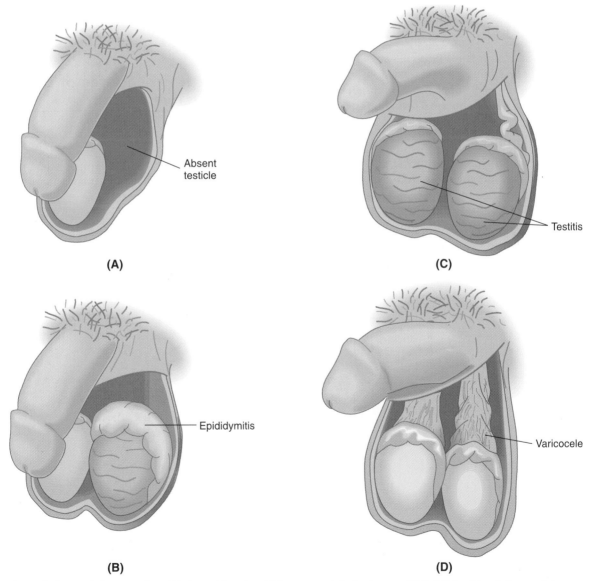

(A)   (B)   (C)   (D)

FIGURE 14.3 Pathology of the testicles. (A) Anorchism in which one testicle is absent. (B) Epididymitis of the testicle on the right. (C) Orchitis (inflammation) of both testicles. (D) Varicocele (varicose veins) of the testicles.

- **Epididymitis** (ep-ih-did-ih-**MY**-tis) is inflammation of the epididymis (**epididym** means epididymis and **itis** means inflammation) (Figure 14.3B).
- A **hydrocele** (**HIGH**-droh-seel) is a hernia filled with fluid in the testicles or the tubes leading from the testicles (**hydro** means relating to water and **cele** means hernia).
- **Testitis** (test-**TYE**-tis), also known as **orchitis** (or-**KYE**-tis), is inflammation of one or both testicles (**test** means testicle and **itis** means inflammation) (Figure 14.3C).
- **Varicocele** (**VAR**-ih-koh-seel), which is a varicose vein (abnormal enlargement of the vein) of the testicles that may cause male infertility (**varico** means varicose veins and **cele** means swelling) (Figure 14.3D).

Sperm Count

- **Azoospermia** (ay-**zoh**-oh-**SPER**-mee-ah) is the absence of sperm in the semen (**a** means without, **zoo** means life, **sperm** means sperm, and **ia** means abnormal condition).
- **Oligospermia** (**ol**-ih-goh-**SPER**-mee-ah), also known as a **low sperm count**, is an abnormally low number of sperm in the ejaculate (**oligo** means few, **sperm** means sperm, and **ia** means abnormal condition).

Prostate Gland

- **Benign prostatic hypertrophy** (BPH), also known as **prostatomegaly** (pros-tah-toh-**MEG**-ah-lee) or an **enlarged prostate**, is an abnormal enlargement of the prostate gland (Figure 14.4).
- **Prostate cancer** is one of the most common cancers among men. The disease may grow slowly with no symptoms, or it may grow aggressively and spread throughout the body.

- **Prostatitis** (pros-tah-**TYE**-tis) is an inflammation of the prostate gland (**prostat** means prostate gland and **itis** means inflammation).
- **Prostatorrhea** (pros-tah-toh-**REE**-ah) is an abnormal flow of prostatic fluid discharged through the urethra (**prostato** means prostate gland and **rrhea** means abnormal discharge).

Diagnostic Procedures of the Male Reproductive System

- **Prostate-specific antigen**, also known as **PSA**, is a blood test to screen for prostate cancer. Values greater than 10 are significant indicators for malignancy.
- **Sperm analysis**, also known as **SA** or a **sperm count**, is the testing of freshly ejaculated semen to determine the volume plus the sperm count, shape, size, and motility (ability to move).
- **Testicular self-examination**, also known as **TSE**, is an important self-help step in early detection of testicular cancer.

Treatment Procedures of the Male Reproductive System

General

- **Circumcision** (ser-kum-**SIZH**-un) is the surgical removal of the foreskin of the penis and is usually performed a few days after birth.
- An **orchidectomy** (or-kih-**DECK**-toh-mee) is the surgical removal of one or both testicles (**orchid** means testicle and **ectomy** means surgical removal). This procedure is also known as an **orchectomy**, **orchiectomy** (or-kee-**ECK**-toh-mee), or **testectomy**.

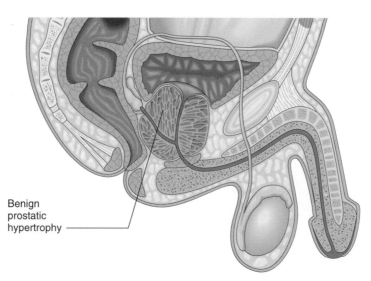

Benign prostatic hypertrophy

Figure 14.4 Benign prostatic hypertrophy. this enlarged prostate impinges on the bladder and slows the flow of urine through the urethra.

- A **varicocelectomy** (**var**-ih-koh-sih-**LECK**-toh-mee) is the removal of a portion of an enlarged vein to relieve a varicocele (**varico** means varicose vein, **cele** means swelling, and **ectomy** means surgical removal).

Male Sterilization

- **Castration** (kas-**TRAY**-shun), also known as **bilateral orchidectomy**, is the surgical removal or destruction of both testicles. (In the female this term describes the removal or destruction of the ovaries.)
- **Sterilization** is any procedure rendering an individual (male or female) incapable of reproduction.
- A **vasectomy** (vah-**SECK**-toh-mee) is the male sterilization procedure in which a portion of the vas deferens is surgically removed (**vas** means vas deferens and **ectomy** means surgical removal). This prevents sperm from entering the ejaculate but does not change the volume of semen (Figure 14.5).
- A **vasovasostomy** (vas-oh-vah-**ZOS**-toh-mee *or* vay-zoh-vay-**ZOS**-toh-mee) is a procedure to restore fertility to a vasectomized male.

Prostate Cancer Treatment

- The term **ablation** (ab-**LAY**-shun) means the removal or destruction of the function of a body part. This technique, which is used to treat conditions such as prostate cancer, may involve surgery, chemical destruction, electrocautery, extreme cold, or radiation.

FIGURE 14.5 In a vasectomy a portion of the vas deferens is removed to prevent sperm from becoming part of the semen.

- A **prostatectomy** (pros-tah-**TECK**-toh-mee) is the surgical removal of all or part of the prostate gland (**prostat** means prostate and **ectomy** means surgical removal).
- A **radical prostatectomy** is the surgical removal of the entire prostate gland, the seminal vesicles, and some surrounding tissue.
- A **transurethral prostatectomy** (**trans**-you-**REE**-thral **pros**-tah-**TECK**-toh-mee), also known as a **transurethral resection of the prostate** or **TURP**, is the removal of all or part of the prostate through the urethra (Figure 14.6).
- **Radiation therapy** (RT) and **hormone therapy** (HT) are additional treatments used to control prostate cancer.

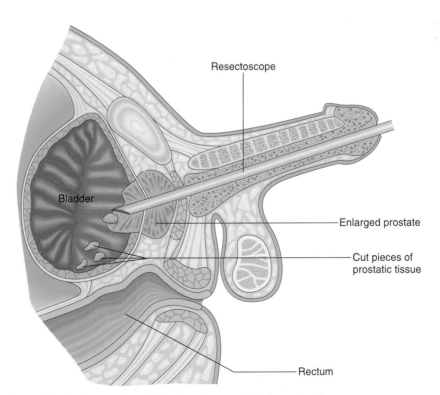

FIGURE 14.6 Transurethral resection being performed for benign prostatic hypertrophy.

Sexually Transmitted Diseases

Sexually transmitted diseases (STDs), also known as **venereal diseases** (VDs), are transmitted through sexual intercourse or other genital contact. **Venereal** (veh-**NEER**-ee-ahl) means pertaining to, relating to, or transmitted by sexual contact.

- **Bacterial vaginosis** (vaj-ih-**NOH**-sis), also known as **BV**, is a sexually transmitted bacterial infection of the vagina (**vagin** means vagina and **osis** means abnormal condition). BV may cause complications during pregnancy and an increased risk of HIV.

- **Chlamydia** (klah-**MID**-ee-ah), which is caused by the bacteria *Chlamydia trachomatis*, is highly contagious. Unless there is early treatment with antibiotics, it may cause sterility in both males and females.

- **Genital herpes** (**HER**-peez), also known as **HSV-2**, is caused by the herpes simplex virus and is highly contagious. Symptoms include itching or burning before the appearance of lesions (sores). Antiviral drugs ease symptoms; however, currently there is no cure and lesions may recur at anytime.

- **Gonorrhea** (gon-oh-**REE**-ah), which is caused by the bacteria *Neisseria gonorrhoeae* is highly contagious. It is characterized by painful urination and an abnormal discharge, and may affect other body structures including the eyes. This disease may be transmitted to the child during birth. To prevent possible gonorrhea infection of the eyes, all newborns receive one drop of silver nitrate or penicillin in each eye immediately after birth.

- **Human immunodeficiency virus** (HIV), which affects the immune system (see Chapter 6), is transmitted through exposure to infected body fluids particularly through sexual intercourse with an infected partner.

- The **human papilloma virus** (pap-ih-**LOH**-mah), also known as **HPV** or **genital warts**, is caused by the *human papillomavirus*. It is highly contagious, and increases the risk of genital and cervical cancer.

- **Syphilis** (**SIF**-ih-lis) is highly contagious and is caused by the spirochete *Treponema pallidum*. Before symptoms appear syphilis can be detected through the VDRL (Venereal Disease Research Laboratory) blood test.

- **Trichomonas** (trick-oh-**MOH**-nas), also known as **trich**, is a vaginal inflammation caused by the protozoan parasite *Trichomonas vaginalis*. It may cause complications during pregnancy and increases the risk of HIV infection.

Functions of the Female Reproductive System

The primary functions of the female reproductive system are the creation and support of new life.

- The ovaries produce eggs to be fertilized by the sperm.
- The uterus provides the environment and support for the developing child.
- After birth, the breasts produce milk to feed the child.

Structures of the Female Reproductive System

External Female Genitalia

- The external female genitalia are located below the mons pubis. The **mons pubis** (monz **PYOU**-bis) is a rounded fleshy prominence over the pubic symphysis (Figures 14.7 and 14.8).

- The female external genitalia are also known collectively as the **vulva** (**VUL**-vah) or the **pudendum** (pyou-**DEN**-dum) (plural, **pudenda**).

Labia

The **labia majora** and **labia minora** are the vaginal lips that protect the external genitalia and the urethral meatus. The **urethral meatus** is the external opening of the urethra (see Chapter 9).

Clitoris

The **clitoris** (**KLIT**-oh-ris) is an organ of sensitive, erectile tissue located anterior to (in front of) the vaginal opening and the urethral meatus.

Bartholin's Glands

Bartholin's glands are two small, rounded glands on either side of the vaginal opening that produce a mucus secretion to lubricate the vagina.

Perineum

In the female, the **perineum** (pehr-ih-**NEE**-um) is the region between the vaginal orifice and the anus.

Mammary Glands

The **mammary glands**, also known as **breasts**, are milk-producing glands that develop during puberty (Figure 14.9). Each breast is fixed to the overlying skin and the underlying pectoral muscles by suspensory ligaments (see also Figure 6.12).

- The **areola** (ah-**REE**-oh-lah) is the dark-pigmented area that surrounds the **nipple**.

- The **mammary glands**, also known as **lactiferous glands** of the breast, produce milk after childbirth.

- The **lactiferous duct** (lack-**TIF**-er-us) carries milk from the mammary glands to the nipple.

Internal Female Genitalia

The major female reproductive organs are located in the pelvic cavity and are protected by the bony pelvis (Figure 14.10, also see Figure 14.7). They include two ovaries, two fallopian tubes, one uterus, and the vagina.

Ovaries

The **ovaries** (**OH**-vah-rees) are a pair of small almond-shaped organs located in the lower abdomen, one on either side of the uterus.

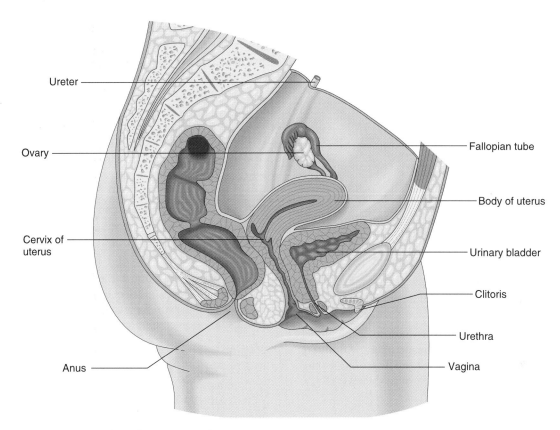

FIGURE 14.7 Cross section of the female reproductive organs.

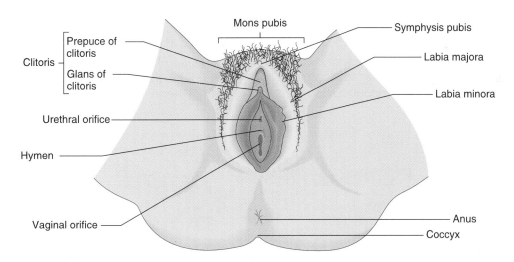

FIGURE 14.8 External genitalia of the female.

- A **follicle** (**FOL**-lick-kul) is a fluid-filled sac containing a single ovum (egg). There are thousands of these sacs on the surface of the ovaries.

- The **ova** (**OH**-vah), also known as eggs, are the female gametes (singular, **ovum**). Normally each month one ovum matures and is released.

Fallopian Tubes

The two **fallopian tubes**, also known as **uterine tubes**, carry the ovum downward from the ovary to the uterus. These tubes also carry sperm upward from the vagina and uterus.

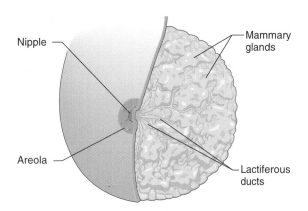

FIGURE 14.9 Structures of the breast.

- Each **fallopian tube** (fal-**LOH**-pee-an) extends from the upper end of the uterus to a point near but not attached to an ovary.
- The **infundibulum** (in-fun-**DIB**-you-lum) is the funnel-shaped opening into each fallopian tube. The **fimbriae** (**FIM**-bree-ee), which are the fringed finger-like extensions of this opening, catch the ovum when it leaves the ovary (singular, **fimbria**).

Uterus

The **uterus** (**YOU**-ter-us) is a pear-shaped organ with muscular walls and a mucous membrane lining filled with a rich supply of blood vessels.

- The uterus is situated between the urinary bladder and the rectum and midway between the sacrum and the pubic bone.

Parts of the Uterus

The uterus consists of three major anatomic areas.

- **Fundus** (**FUN**-dus) is the bulging rounded part above the entrance of the fallopian tubes (see Figure 14.10).
- **Corpus** (**KOR**-pus), also known as the **body**, is the middle portion.
- **Cervix** (**SER**-vicks), also known as the **cervix uteri**, is the lower narrow portion that extends into the vagina.

Tissues of the uterus

The uterus is composed of three major layers of tissue.

- **Perimetrium** (pehr-ih-**MEE**-tree-um) is the tough membrane outer layer (**peri** means surrounding, **metri** means uterus, and **um** is a singular noun ending).
- **Myometrium** (my-oh-**MEE**-tree-um) is the muscular middle layer (**myo** means muscle, **metri** means uterus, and **um** is a singular noun ending).
- **Endometrium** (en-doh-**MEE**-tree-um) is the inner layer that consists of specialized epithelial mucosa (**endo** means within, **metri** means uterus, and **um** is a singular noun ending).

Vagina

The **vagina** (vah-**JIGH**-nah) is a muscular tube lined with mucosa that extends from the cervix to the outside of the body (the word parts **colp/o** and **vagin/o** both mean vagina).

- The **hymen** (**HIGH**-men) is a membranous fold of tissue that partly or completely covers the external vaginal orifice. (An **orifice** is an entrance into, or an outlet from, a body cavity or canal.)

Menstruation

Menstruation (**men**-stroo-**AY**-shun), also known as **menses** (**MEN**-seez), is the normal periodic discharge of a bloody fluid from the nonpregnant uterus.

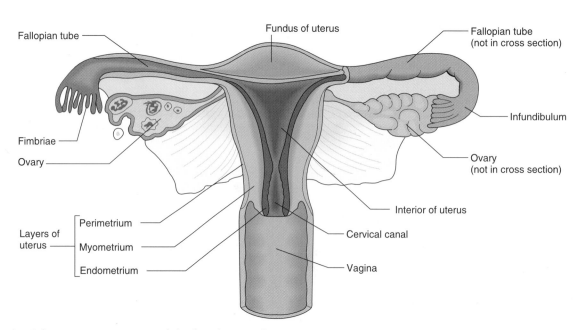

FIGURE 14.10 Schematic anterior view of the female reproductive organs.

- **Menarche** (meh-**NAR**-kee) is the beginning of the menstrual function that begins at puberty (**men** means menstruation and **arche** means beginning).
- The average **menstrual cycle** consists of 28 days. These are grouped into four phases and are summarized in Table 14.1.
- **Menopause** (**MEN**-oh-pawz) is the normal stopping of the monthly menstrual periods (**meno** means menstruation and **pause** means stopping). Menopause, which officially begins 12 months after a woman's final menstrual period, occurs at the average age of 52.
- **Perimenopause** (pehr-ih-**MEN**-oh-pawz) is the term used to designate the transition phase between regular menstrual periods and no periods at all (**peri** means surrounding, **meno** means menstruation, and **pause** means stopping). During this phase, which can last as long as 10 years, changes in hormone production may cause symptoms including hot flashes, mood swings, and disturbed sleep.

Medical Specialties Related to the Female Reproductive System

- A **gynecologist** (guy-neh-**KOL**-oh-jist) specializes in diagnosing and treating diseases and disorders of the female reproductive system (**gynec** means female and **ologist** means specialist).
- An **obstetrician** (ob-steh-**TRISH**-un) specializes in providing medical care to women during pregnancy, childbirth, and immediately thereafter. This specialty is referred to as **obstetrics** (ob-**STET**-ricks).
- A **neonatologist** (nee-oh-nay-**TOL**-oh-jist) specializes in diagnosing and treating disorders of the newborn (**neo** means new, **nat** means born, and **ologist** means specialist).
- A **pediatrician** (pee-dee-ah-**TRISH**-un) specializes in diagnosing, treating, and preventing disorders and diseases of children. This specialty is known as **pediatrics** (**ped** means child and **iatrics** means the medical practice of).

Pathology of the Female Reproductive System

Ovaries and Fallopian Tubes

- **Anovulation** (an-ov-you-**LAY**-shun) is the failure to ovulate. Menstruation may continue although ovulation does not occur.
- **Oophoritis** (oh-ahf-oh-**RYE**-tis) is an inflammation of an ovary (**oophor** means ovary and **itis** means inflammation).
- **Ovarian cancer** is the third most common cancer of the female reproductive system; however, more women die of it than from other forms.

Table 14.1
PHASES OF THE MENSTRUAL CYCLE

Days 1–5	**Menstrual Phase.** These are the days when the endometrial lining of the uterus is sloughed off and discharged through the vagina as the menstrual flow.
Days 6–12	**Postmenstrual Phase.** After the menstrual period, estrogen secreted by the ovary stimulates the lining of the uterus to prepare itself to receive a zygote (fertilized egg). The pituitary gland secretes follicle-stimulating hormone (FSH) causing an ovum to mature.
Days 13–14	**Ovulatory Phase.** On about the 13th or 14th day of the cycle, a mature ovum is released. When ovulation occurs, the egg leaves the ovary to travel slowly down the fallopian tube. During this time, the female is fertile and can become pregnant.
Days 15–28	**Premenstrual Phase.** If fertilization does not occur, hormone levels change to cause the breakdown of the uterine endometrium and the beginning of a new menstrual cycle.

- **Ovariorrhexis** (oh-vay-ree-oh-**RECK**-sis) is the rupture of an ovary (**ovario** means ovary and **rrhexis** means to rupture).
- **Pelvic inflammatory disease**, also known as **PID**, is any inflammation of the female reproductive organs not associated with surgery or pregnancy. PID frequently occurs as a complication of STDs and can lead to infertility, tubal pregnancy, and other serious disorders.
- The **polycystic ovary syndrome**, also known as **PCOS** or **Stein-Leventhal syndrome**, is characterized by enlargement of the ovaries caused by the presence of many cysts. This condition, which is due to a hormonal imbalance, may cause infertility, menstrual abnormalities, and the development of secondary male characteristics such as hair growth.
- **Pyosalpinx** (pye-oh-**SAL**-pinks) is an accumulation of pus in the fallopian tube (**pyo** means pus and **salpinx** means fallopian tube).
- **Salpingitis** (sal-pin-**JIGH**-tis) is an inflammation of a fallopian tube (**salping** means fallopian or eustachian tube and **itis** means inflammation). ■ **Caution:** This term also means inflammation of the eustachian tube of the middle ear.

The Uterus

- **Endometriosis** (**en**-doh-**mee**-tree-**OH**-sis) is a condition in which endometrial tissue escapes the uterus and grows outside the uterus on other structures in the pelvic cavity (**endo** means within, **metri** means uterus, and **osis** means abnormal condition).

- A **fibroid**, also known as a **leiomyoma** (**lye**-oh-my-**OH**-mah), is a benign tumor composed of muscle and fibrous tissue that occurs in the wall of the uterus.

- **Metrorrhea** (**mee**-troh-**REE**-ah) is an abnormal uterine discharge (**metro** means uterus and **rrhea** means abnormal flow).

- **Metrorrhexis** (**mee**-troh-**RECK**-sis) means rupture of the uterus (**metro** means uterus and **rrhexis** means to rupture).

- **Pyometritis** (**pye**-oh-meh-**TRY**-tis) is a purulent (pus-containing) inflammation of the uterus (**pyo** means pus, **metr** means uterus, and **itis** means inflammation).

- **Uterine cancer** occurs most commonly after menopause and one of the earliest symptoms is abnormal bleeding from the uterus.

Abnormal Uterine Positions

- **Anteflexion** (**an**-tee-**FLECK**-shun), as shown in Figure 14.7, is the normal position of the uterus. In this position it is bent forward (**ante** means forward, **flex** means bend, and **ion** means condition).

- **Anteversion** (**an**-tee-**VER**-zhun), as shown in Figure 14.11, is abnormal tipping, tilting, or turning forward of the entire uterus, including the cervix (**ante** means forward and **version** means to turn).

- **Prolapse of uterus**, as shown in Figure 14.11, is a falling or sinking down of the uterus until it protrudes through the vaginal opening. **Prolapse** (proh-**LAPS**) means downward placement.

- **Retroflexion** (**ret**-roh-**FLECK**-shun), as shown in Figure 14.11, is abnormal tipping with the body of the uterus bent forming an angle with the cervix (**retro** means backward, **flex** means to bend, and **ion** means condition).

- **Retroversion** (**ret**-roh-**VER**-zhun), as shown in Figure 14.11, is abnormal tipping of the entire uterus backward with the cervix pointing toward the pubic symphysis (**retro** means backward and **version** means to turn).

The Cervix

- **Cervical cancer** is the second most common cancer in women and usually affects women between the ages of 35 and 55. It can be detected early through routine Pap tests.

- **Cervical dysplasia**, also known as **precancerous lesions**, is the abnormal growth of cells of the cervix that may be detected on a Pap smear. If not treated, these cells may become malignant. **Dysplasia** (dis-**PLAY**-see-ah) means the abnormal growth of cells (**dys** means bad and **plasia** means formation).

- **Cervicitis** (**ser**-vih-**SIGH**-tis) is an inflammation of the cervix (**cervic** means cervix and **itis** means inflammation).

- **Endocervicitis** (**en**-doh-**ser**-vih-**SIGH**-tis) is an inflammation of the mucous membrane lining of the cervix (**endo** means within, **cervic** means cervix, and **itis** means inflammation).

The Vagina

- **Colporrhexis** (**kol**-poh-**RECK**-sis) means laceration of the vagina (**colpo** means vagina and **rrhexis** means to rupture).

- **Leukorrhea** (**loo**-koh-**REE**-ah) is a profuse white mucus discharge from the uterus and vagina (**leuko** means white and **rrhea** means abnormal flow).

- **Pruritus vulvae** (proo-**RYE**-tus **VUL**-vee) is a condition of severe itching of the external female genitalia. **Pruritus** means itching.

- **Vaginal candidiasis** (**kan**-dih-**DYE**-ah-sis), which is caused by the yeast *Candida albicans*, is the most commonly occurring vaginal yeast infection. Symptoms include itching, burning, and irritation.

- **Vaginitis** (**vaj**-ih-**NIGH**-tis), also known as **colpitis** (kol-**PYE**-tis), is an inflammation of the lining of the vagina (**vagin** means vagina and **itis** means inflammation).

External Genitalia

- **Vulvodynia** (**vul**-voh-**DIN**-ee-ah) is a nonspecific syndrome of unknown cause characterized by chronic burning, pain during sexual intercourse, itching, or stinging irritation of the vulva (**vulv** means vulva and **dynia** means pain).

Anteversion Marked retroversion Retroflexion Prolapse

FIGURE 14.11 Abnormal positions of the uterus.

- **Vulvitis** (vul-**VYE**-tis) is an inflammation of the vulva (**vulv** means vulva and **itis** means inflammation).

Breasts

- **Breast cancer** and its treatment are discussed in Chapter 6.
- **Fibrocystic breast disease** (**figh**-broh-**SIS**-tick) is the presence of single or multiple cysts in the breasts. These cysts are usually benign but may become malignant.
- A **galactocele** (gah-**LACK**-toh-seel), also known as a **galactoma** (**gal**-ack-**TOH**-mah), is a cystic enlargement of the mammary gland containing milk (**galacto** means milk and **cele** means hernia).
- **Mastitis** (mas-**TYE**-tis) is an inflammation of the breast usually associated with lactation but may occur for other reasons (**mast** means breast and **itis** means inflammation).

Menstrual Disorders

- **Amenorrhea** (ah-**men**-oh-**REE**-ah *or* ay-**men**-oh-**REE**-ah) is an absence of menstrual periods (**a** means without, **meno** means menstruation, and **rrhea** means abnormal flow). This condition is normal only before puberty, during pregnancy, while breast-feeding, and after menopause.
- **Dysmenorrhea** (dis-**men**-oh-**REE**-ah) is abdominal pain caused by uterine cramps during a menstrual period (**dys** means bad, **meno** means menstruation, and **rrhea** means abnormal flow).
- **Hypomenorrhea** (**high**-poh-men-oh-**REE**-ah) is a small amount of menstrual flow during a shortened regular menstrual period (**hypo** means deficient, **meno** means menstruation, and **rrhea** means abnormal flow).
- **Menorrhagia** (**men**-oh-**RAY**-jee-ah) is an excessive amount of menstrual flow over a longer duration than of a normal period (**meno** means menstruation and **rrhagia** means abnormal bleeding).
- **Menometrorrhagia** (**men**-oh-**met**-roh-**RAY**-jee-ah) is excessive uterine bleeding occurring both during the menses and at irregular intervals (**meno** means menstruation, **metro** means uterus, and **rrhagia** means abnormal bleeding).
- **Mittelschmerz** (**MIT**-uhl-schmehrts) means pain between menstrual periods (from the German, meaning middle pain). This usually occurs at the time of ovulation.
- **Oligomenorrhea** (ol-ih-goh-**men**-oh-**REE**-ah) means a markedly reduced menstrual flow and also abnormally infrequent menstruation or relative amenorrhea (**oligo** means scanty, **meno** means menstruation, and **rrhea** means abnormal flow).
- **Polymenorrhea** (**pol**-ee-**men**-oh-**REE**-ah) means abnormally frequent menstruation (**poly** means many, **meno** means menstruation, and **rrhea** means abnormal flow).
- **Premenstrual syndrome**, also known as **PMS**, includes symptoms occurring within the 2-week period before menstruation such as bloating, edema, headaches, mood swings, and breast discomfort.

Diagnostic Procedures of the Female Reproductive System

- **Breast self-examination**, also known as **BSE**, is an important self-care procedure for the early detection of breast cancer.
- **Colposcopy** (kol-**POS**-koh-pee) is the direct visual examination of the tissues of the cervix and vagina using a **colposcope** (**colpo** means vagina and **scopy** means visual examination).
- **Endovaginal ultrasound** (en-doh-**VAJ**-ih-nal) is a diagnostic test to determine the cause of abnormal vaginal bleeding. In this procedure an ultrasound transducer placed in the vagina uses sound waves to create images of the uterus and ovaries.
- **Hysterosalpingography** (hiss-ter-oh-**sal**-pin-**GOG**-rah-fee) is a radiographic examination of the uterus and fallopian tubes after the injection of radiopaque material (**hystero** means uterus, **salpingo** means tube, and **graphy** means process of recording).
- **Hysteroscopy** (hiss-ter-**OSS**-koh-pee) is the direct visual examination of the interior of the uterus using the magnification of a **hysteroscope** (**HISS**-ter-oh-skope) (see Figure 15.18).
- **Mammography** (mam-**OG**-rah-fee) is a radiographic examination of the breast (Figures 14.12 and 14.13). The resulting record is called a **mammogram**.

FIGURE 14.12 In mammography, the breast is gently flattened and then radiographed from above.

(A)

(B)

Figure 14.13 Mammograms. (A) A normal film. (B) A large mass is visible.

- A **Papanicolaou test** (**pap**-ah-**nick**-oh-**LAY**-ooh), also known as a **Pap smear,** is an exfoliative biopsy for the detection and diagnosis of conditions of the cervix and surrounding tissues (Figure 14.14). As used here, **exfoliative** (ecks-**FOH**-lee-ay-tiv) means that cells are scraped from the tissue and examined under a microscope.

Treatment Procedures of the Female Reproductive System

Medications

- **Birth control pills** are a form of hormones taken daily as a contraceptive to prevent pregnancy. A **contraceptive** is the measure taken or device used to lessen the likelihood of conception and pregnancy.

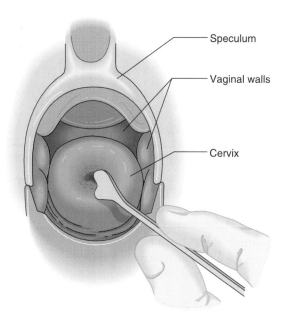

Figure 14.14 Performing a pap smear. A speculum is used to spread the vaginal walls. A disposable Ayer blade, similar to a tongue depressor, is used to scrape away a few cells. These are fixed on a glass slide and sent to the laboratory for examination.

- **Hormone replacement therapy** (HRT) is used to replace the estrogen and progesterone that are no longer produced during perimenopause and after menopause.

Ovaries and Fallopian Tubes

- An **oophorectomy** (oh-ahf-oh-**RECK**-toh-mee), also known as **ovariectomy** (oh-vay-ree-**ECK**-toh-me), is the surgical removal of an ovary (**oopho** means ovary and **ectomy** means surgical removal).
- A **salpingectomy** (sal-pin-**JECK**-toh-mee) is the surgical removal of a fallopian tube (**salping** means tube and **ectomy** means surgical removal).
- **Tubal ligation** is a surgical procedure performed for purpose of female sterilization. Each fallopian tube is ligated and a section is removed to prevent the ovum from reaching the uterus. **Ligate** means to bind or tie (Figure 14.15).

Uterus, Cervix, and Vagina

- A **cervicectomy** (ser-vih-**SECK**-toh-mee) is surgical removal of the cervix (**cervico** means cervix and **ectomy** means surgical removal).
- A **colpopexy** (**KOL**-poh-**peck**-see) is the surgical fixation of the vagina to a surrounding structure (**colpo** means vagina and **pexy** means surgical fixation in place).
- **Conization** (kon-ih-**ZAY**-shun *or* koh-nih-**ZAY**-shun), also known as a **cone biopsy,** is the surgical removal of a cone-shaped section of tissue from the cervix. This

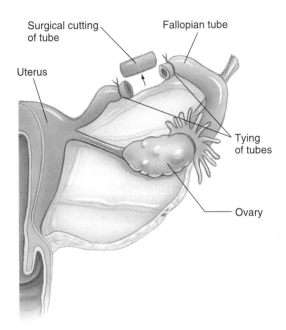

Surgical cutting of tube

Fallopian tube

Uterus

Tying of tubes

Ovary

FIGURE 14.15 Tubal ligation is performed as a form of female sterilization.

may be performed as a diagnostic procedure or to remove an abnormal area.

- **Colporrhaphy** (kol-**POR**-ah-fee) means suturing the vagina (**colpo** means vagina and **rrhaphy** means to suture).

- **Dilation and curettage** (D & C) is the dilation of the cervix and curettage of the uterus. **Dilation** (dye-**LAY**-shun) is the expansion of an opening and **curettage** (**kyou**-reh-**TAHZH**) is the removal of material from the surface. This may be by scraping with a **curette** or with the use of suction. This may be performed as a diagnostic or treatment procedure (Figure 14.16).

- A **hysteropexy** (**HISS**-ter-oh-**peck**-see) is the surgical fixation of a misplaced or abnormally movable uterus (**hystero** means uterus and **pexy** means surgical fixation).

- **Vaginoplasty** (vah-**JIGH**-noh-**plas**-tee) is the surgical repair of the vagina (**vagino** means vagina and **plasty** means surgical repair).

Hysterectomies

- A **hysterectomy** (**hiss**-teh-**RECK**-toh-mee) is the surgical removal of the uterus and may or may not include the cervix (**hyster** means uterus and **ectomy** means surgical removal) (Figure 14.17).

- A **vaginal hysterectomy**, also known as a **VH**, is performed through the vagina (Figure 14.17A).

- A **total abdominal hysterectomy** is performed through an incision in the abdomen. Because this procedure includes the removal of the uterus, cervix, fallopian tubes, and ovaries its full name is a **total hysterectomy, plus bilateral salpingo-oophorectomy**.

- A **bilateral salpingo-oophorectomy** (sal-**ping**-goh oh-**ahf**-oh-**RECK**-toh-mee), also known as **SO**, is the surgical removal of both fallopian tubes and ovaries (**salpingo** means tube, **oophor** means ovary, and **ectomy** means surgical removal).

- A **bilateral hysterosalpingo-oophorectomy** (**hiss**-ter-oh-sal-**ping**-goh oh-**ahf**-oh-**RECK**-toh-mee) is the surgical removal of the uterus and cervix, plus both ovaries and fallopian tubes (**hystero** means uterus, **salpingo** means tube, **oophor** means ovary, and **ectomy** means surgical removal) (Figure 14.17B).

- A **radical hysterectomy** includes the surgical removal of the uterus, tubes, ovaries, adjacent lymph nodes, and part of the vagina. This surgery is performed as part of the treatment of cancer in any of these organs.

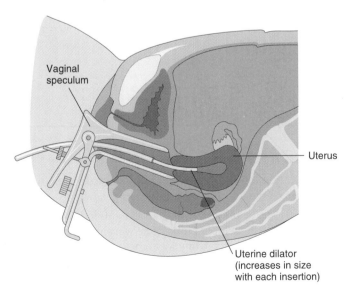

Vaginal speculum

Uterus

Uterine dilator (increases in size with each insertion)

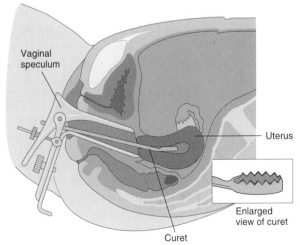

Vaginal speculum

Uterus

Enlarged view of curet

Curet

FIGURE 14.16 Dilation and curettage. (A) Dilation is the expansion of the cervical opening. (B) Curettage is the removal of material from the surface of the uterus.

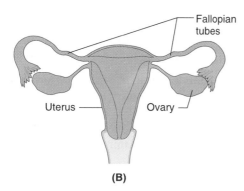

FIGURE 14.17 Types of hysterectomies. (A) In a vaginal hysterectomy, only the uterus and cervix are removed. (B) In a total hysterectomy, the cervix, uterus, tubes, and ovaries are removed.

Breasts

- **Mastectomy** as treatment of breast cancer is discussed in Chapter 6.
- **Mammoplasty** (**MAM**-oh-**plas**-tee), which is also spelled **mammaplasty**, is the surgical repair or restructuring of the breast (**mammo** means breast and **plasty** means surgical repair).
- **Breast augmentation** is mammoplasty to increase breast size.
- **Mastopexy** (**MAS**-toh-**peck**-see) is surgery to affix sagging breasts in a more elevated position (**masto** means breast and **pexy** means surgical fixation).

Assisted Reproduction

Infertility is the inability of a couple to achieve pregnancy after 1 year of regular, unprotected intercourse or the inability of a woman to carry a pregnancy to a live birth.

- An infertile couple may seek the help of an **infertility specialist**, also known as a **fertility specialist**, who diagnoses and treats problems associated with conception and maintaining pregnancy.

Table 14.2 summarizes the abbreviation and terms commonly associated with assisted reproduction.

Table 14.2

ABBREVIATIONS AND TERMS RELATED TO ASSISTED FERTILIZATION	
AMA	**Advanced maternal age** decreases the possibility of pregnancy. This term is applied to women in their late thirties to middle forties.
ART	**Assisted reproductive technology** is the term used to describe techniques used to aid an infertile couple in achieving a viable pregnancy.
GIFT	**Gamete intrafallopian transfer** is a procedure in which ovum and sperm are mixed outside of the body then transferred by laparoscopic surgery into the fallopian tube where hopefully fertilization will occur.
ICSI	**Intracytoplasmic sperm injection**, which is pronounced *icksy*, is a procedure outside of the body in which one sperm is placed into one egg thereby fertilizing it. This procedure is used in the case of severe male factor infertility.
IVF	**In vitro fertilization** is a procedure in which mature ova are removed from the mother and fertilized outside of the body. The resulting embryos are transferred into the uterus with the hope that they will implant and continue to develop as in a normal pregnancy.
ZIFT	**Zygote intrafallopian transfer** is a laparoscopic procedure in which a zygote is placed in the fallopian tube allowing it to travel down the tube to the uterus where it implants.

Pregnancy and Childbirth

Ovulation

Ovulation (**ov**-you-**LAY**-shun) is the release of a mature egg from the follicle on the surface of the ovary.

- After the ovum is released, it is caught up by the fimbriae of the fallopian tube. Here wavelike peristaltic actions move the ovum down the fallopian tube toward the uterus.
- It usually takes an ovum about 5 days to pass through the fallopian tube. If sperm are present, fertilization occurs within the fallopian tube.

- After the ovum has been released, the ruptured follicle enlarges, takes on a yellow fatty substance, and becomes the corpus luteum.
- The **corpus luteum** (**KOR**-pus **LOO**-tee-um) secretes the hormone progesterone during the second half of the menstrual cycle. This maintains the growth of the uterine lining in preparation for the fertilized egg.
- If the ovum is not fertilized the corpus luteum dies and the endometrium sloughs off as the menstrual flow.

Fertilization

- During **coitus** (**KOH**-ih-tus), also known as **copulation** (**kop**-you-**LAY**-shun) or **sexual intercourse**, the male **ejaculates** approximately 100 million sperm cells into the female's vagina. The sperm travel upward through the vagina, into the uterus, and on into the fallopian tube.
- When a sperm penetrates the descending ovum, **fertilization**, also known as **conception**, occurs and a new life begins.
- After fertilization occurs in the fallopian tube the fertilized egg, which is now called a **zygote** (**ZYE**-goht), travels to the uterus.
- **Implantation** is the embedding of the zygote into the endothelial lining of the uterus.
- From implantation through the eighth week of pregnancy the developing child is known as an **embryo** (**EM**-bree-oh).
- A **fetus** (**FEE**-tus) is the developing child from the ninth week of pregnancy to the time of birth (see Figure 14.20).

Multiple Births

- If more than one egg is passing down the fallopian tube when sperm are present the fertilization of more than one egg is possible.
- **Fraternal twins** result from the fertilization of separate ova by separate sperm cells. These develop into two separate embryos.
- **Identical twins** are formed from the fertilization of a single egg cell by a single sperm. As the fertilized egg cell divides, it separates into two parts and each part forms a separate embryo.

The Chorion and Placenta

- The **chorion** (**KOR**-ee-on) is the outer membrane that encloses the fetus. It contributes to the formation of the placenta (Figure 14.18).
- The **placenta** (plah-**SEN**-tah) is a temporary organ that forms with the uterus to allow the exchange of nutrients, oxygen, and waste products between the mother and child without allowing maternal blood and fetal blood to mix. The placenta also produces hormones necessary to maintain the pregnancy (Figure 14.19).
- At delivery the placenta is expelled as the **afterbirth**.

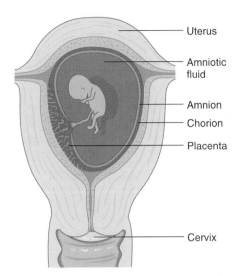

FIGURE 14.18 Structures related to the developing fetus.

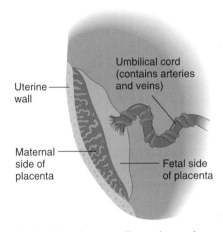

FIGURE 14.19 The placenta allows the exchange of nutrients and waste materials between mother and child without intermingling blood.

Amnion

The **amnion** (**AM**-nee-on), also known as the **amniotic sac**, is the innermost of the membranes that surround the embryo in the uterus and forms the **amniotic cavity** (am-nee-**OT**-ick).

- **Amnionic fluid** (am-nee-**ON**-ick), also known as **amniotic fluid**, is the liquid in which the fetus floats and is protected (see Figure 14.18).

The Umbilical Cord

The **umbilical cord** (um-**BILL**-ih-kal) is the structure that connects the fetus to the placenta.

- After birth the **navel**, also known as the **belly button**, is formed where the umbilical cord was attached to the fetus.

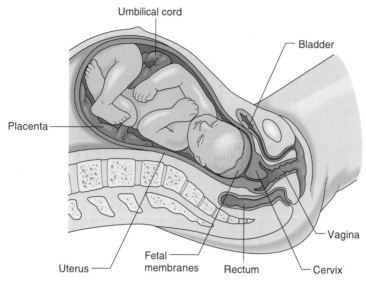

Figure 14.20 The fetus in position at term.

Gestation

Gestation (jes-**TAY**-shun), which lasts approximately 280 days, is the period of development of the child in the mother's uterus.

- The term **pregnancy**, which is often used interchangeably with gestation, means the condition of having a developing child in the uterus.

- Pregnancy is described in terms of the number of weeks of gestation (40 total) or it may be divided into three **trimesters** of 3 months each (Figure 14.20).

- The **due date**, or **estimated date of confinement** or **EDC**, is calculated from the first day of the **last menstrual period** (LMP).

- **Quickening** is the first movement of the fetus felt in the uterus. This usually occurs during the 16th to 20th week of pregnancy.

- The fetus is **viable** when it is capable of living outside the mother. Viability depends on the developmental age, birth weight of the fetus, and developmental stage of the lungs.

The Mother

- A **nulligravida** (null-ih-**GRAV**-ih-dah) is a woman who has never been pregnant (**nulli** means none and **gravida** means pregnant).

- A **nullipara** (nuh-**LIP**-ah-rah) is a woman who has never borne a viable child (**nulli** means none and **para** means to bring forth).

- A **primigravida** (prye-mih-**GRAV**-ih-dah) is a woman during her first pregnancy (**primi** means first and **gravida** means pregnant).

- A **primipara** (prye-**MIP**-ah-rah) is a woman who has borne one child (**primi** means first and **para** means to bring forth).

- **Multiparous** (mul-**TIP**-ah-rus) means a woman who has given birth two or more times (**multi** means many and **parous** means having borne one or more children).

Childbirth

Parturition (par-tyou-**RISH**-un), also known as **labor** and **childbirth**, is the act of giving birth to an offspring. The term **antepartum** means before the onset of labor with reference to the mother.

- **Labor and delivery** (L & D) occur in three stages. The first stage begins with contractions of the uterus and gradual **dilatation** (enlargement) of the cervix. During this stage **effacement** (eh-**FAYSS**-ment) is the thinning and shortening of the cervix during labor.

- The second stage is the delivery of the infant. The **amniotic sac**, also known as the **bag of waters**, ruptures. Then the uterine contractions become stronger and more frequent until the child is expelled.

- **Presentation** is the term used to describe the portion of the fetus that can be touched by the examining finger during labor.

- Normally the head presents first, and the stage at which the head can be seen at the vaginal orifice is called **crowning** (Figure 14.21).

- The third stage is the expulsion of the placenta as the **afterbirth**. The term **delivery** means the expulsion of the infant and afterbirth.

Postpartum

The term **postpartum** (pohst-**PAR**-tum) means after childbirth.

The Mother

- For the mother, **puerperium** (pyou-er-**PEE**-ree-um) is the period of 3 to 6 weeks after childbirth until the uterus returns to its normal size.

Figure 14.21 In a normal delivery, the baby's head emerges first.

- **Colostrum** (kuh-**LOS**-trum) is the fluid secreted by the breasts during the first days postpartum. This fluid is rich in antibodies and confers passive immunity to the newborn.
- **Lactation** (lack-**TAY**-shun) is the process of forming and secreting milk from the breasts as nourishment for the infant.
- **Lochia** (**LOH**-kee-ah) is the vaginal discharge during the first week or two after childbirth. It consists of blood, tissue, and mucus.
- **Uterine involution** is the return of the uterus to its normal size and former condition.

The Baby

- The newborn infant is known as a **neonate** (**NEE**-oh-nayt) during the first 4 weeks after birth.
- **Meconium** (meh-**KOH**-nee-um) is a greenish material that collects in the intestine of a fetus and forms the first stools of a newborn.

Pathology of Pregnancy and Childbirth

Pregnancy

- An **abortion** (ah-**BOR**-shun) (AB) is the interruption or termination of pregnancy before the fetus is viable. A **spontaneous abortion**, also known as **SAB** or a **miscarriage**, occurs without outside action. An **induced abortion**, also known as a **therapeutic abortion** (TAB), is deliberately caused by human action for medical purposes.
- An **ectopic pregnancy** (eck-**TOP**-ick), also known as an **extrauterine pregnancy**, is a pregnancy in which the fertilized egg is implanted and begins to develop outside of the uterus. (**Ectopic** means out of place.)
- A **tubal pregnancy** is an ectopic pregnancy implanted within the fallopian tube rather than the uterus (Figure 14.22).

- **Preeclampsia** (pree-ee-**KLAMP**-see-ah), also known as **toxemia of pregnancy**, is a complication of pregnancy characterized by hypertension (high blood pressure), edema (swelling), and proteinuria. **Proteinuria** (proh-tee-in-**YOU**-ree-ah) is an abnormally high level of protein in the urine.
- **Eclampsia** (eh-**KLAMP**-see-ah), a more serious form of preeclampsia, is characterized by convulsions and sometimes coma.

Ectopic (tubal) pregnancy

Figure 14.22 A tubal pregnancy may occur anywhere along the fallopian tube.

The Rh Factor

- When the mother's blood is **Rh-negative** (lacking the Rh factor) and the father's is **Rh-positive** (containing the Rh factor), the baby may inherit the Rh-positive factor from the father.
- During labor or a miscarriage, some of the baby's blood may enter the mother's circulation. This sensitizes her to the Rh-positive factor and causes her body to develop Rh-positive antibodies. These antibodies will cause a problem during her *next* pregnancy.
- Blood tests of the parents can identify this potential problem and, if it exists, the mother is vaccinated with Rh immune globulin to prevent the development of these antibodies (Figure 14.23).

Childbirth

- **Abruptio placentae** (ab-**RUP**-shee-oh plah-**SEN**-tee) is an abnormal condition in which the placenta separates from the uterine wall prematurely before the birth of the fetus.
- **Breech presentation** is when the buttocks or feet of the fetus are presented first.
- **Placenta previa** (plah-**SEN**-tah **PREE**-vee-ah) is the abnormal implantation of the placenta in the lower portion of the uterus. Symptoms include painless sudden onset bleeding during the third trimester. Treatment ranges from bedrest to immediate delivery by cesarean section (Figure 14.24).

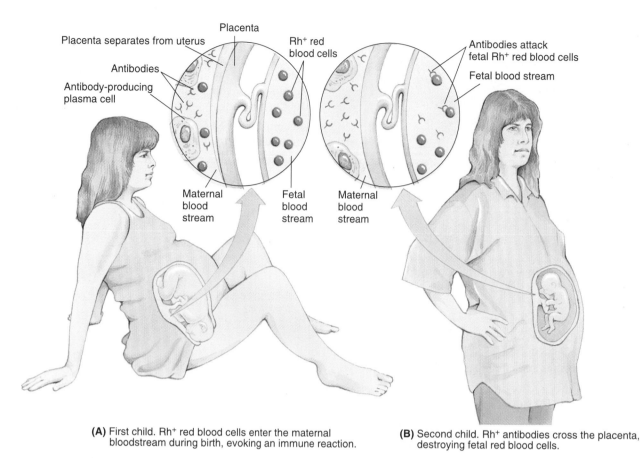

(A) First child. Rh⁺ red blood cells enter the maternal bloodstream during birth, evoking an immune reaction.

(B) Second child. Rh⁺ antibodies cross the placenta, destroying fetal red blood cells.

FIGURE 14.23 Rh incompatibility can cause problems for the fetus during a second pregnancy.

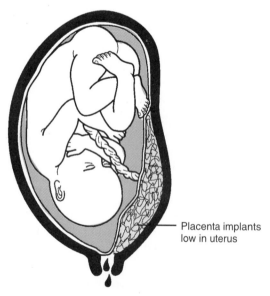

Placenta implants low in uterus

FIGURE 14.24 In placenta previa the placenta has attached abnormally low in the uterus.

- A **premature infant**, also known as a **preemie**, is any neonate born before the 37th week of gestation.
- **Stillbirth** is the birth of a fetus that died before or during delivery.

Diagnostic Procedures Related to Pregnancy

- **Amniocentesis** (**am-nee-oh-sen-TEE**-sis) is a surgical procedure in which a needle is passed through the abdominal and uterine walls to obtain a specimen of amniotic fluid (**amnio** means amnion and fetal membrane and **centesis** means a surgical puncture to remove fluid). This specimen, which is performed after the 16ᵗʰ week of pregnancy, is used to evaluate fetal health and diagnose certain congenital disorders (Figure 14.25).
- **Chorionic villus sampling** (CVS) is retrieval of chorionic cells from the placenta between the 8th to 10th week of pregnancy. These cells are evaluated to test for genetic abnormalities in the developing child.
- An **electronic fetal monitor** is a device that allows observation of the fetal heart rate and the maternal uterine contractions during labor (see Figure 1.6).

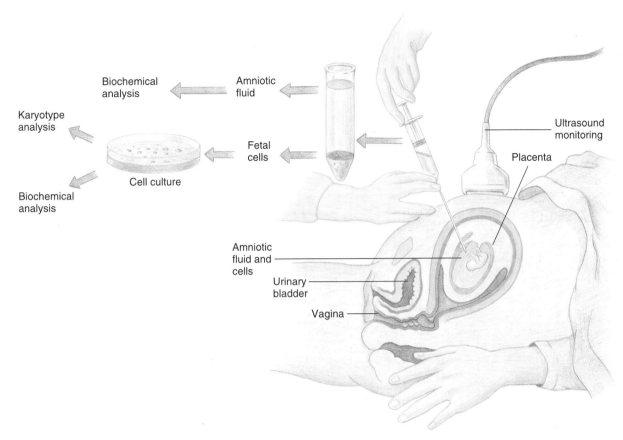

Biochemical analysis ← Amniotic fluid

Karyotype analysis

Ultrasound monitoring

Placenta

Fetal cells

Cell culture

Biochemical analysis

Amniotic fluid and cells

Urinary bladder

Vagina

Figure 14.25 Amniocentesis is performed to obtain a specimen of amniotic fluid for analysis.

- **Fetal ultrasound** is a noninvasive procedure used to evaluate fetal development (see Chapter 15 and Figure 15.28).

- **Pelvimetry** (pel-**VIM**-eh-tree) is the measurement of the dimensions of the pelvis to determine its capacity to allow passage of the fetus through the birth canal.

- A **pregnancy test** is performed on either a blood or urine specimen to determine human chorionic gonadotropin (HCG) levels. An unusually high level usually indicates pregnancy.

Treatment Procedures Related to Pregnancy and Childbirth

- An **Apgar score** is an evaluation of a newborn infant's physical status by assigning numerical values (0 to 2) to each of five criteria: (1) heart rate, (2) respiratory effort, (3) muscle tone, (4) response stimulation, and (5) skin color. The newborn is evaluated at 1 and 5 minutes after birth, and a total score of 8 to 10 indicates the best possible condition.

- A **cesarean delivery**, also known as a **cesarean section** (seh-**ZEHR**-ee-un **SECK**-shun) or **C-section**, is the delivery of the child through an incision in the maternal abdominal and uterine wall.

- The vaginal delivery of a subsequent child after a cesarean birth is referred to as a **VBAC** (vaginal birth after cesarean).

- An **episiotomy** (eh-**piz**-ee-**OT**-oh-mee) is a surgical incision of the perineum and vagina to facilitate delivery and prevent laceration of the tissues (episi means vulva and otomy means a surgical incision). A **laceration** (**lass**-er-**AY**-shun) is a jagged tear of the tissue.

- An **episiorrhaphy** (eh-**piz**-ee-**OR**-ah-fee) is a sutured repair of an episiotomy (episio means vulva and rrhaphy means to suture).

14 ● Learning Exercises

● Matching Word Parts—1

Write the letter of the correct answer on the line provided in the left column.

14.1. _____ cervic/o   A. menstruation

14.2. _____ colp/o   B. pregnant

14.3. _____ gynec/o   C. female

14.4. _____ men/o   D. vagina

14.5. _____ -gravida   E. cervix

● Matching Word Parts—2

Write the letter of the correct answer on the line provided in the left column.

14.6. _____ metr/o   A. egg

14.7. _____ ov/o   B. ovary

14.8. _____ oophor/o   C. prostate

14.9. _____ orchid/o   D. testicle

14.10. _____ prostat/o   E. uterus

● Matching Word Parts—3

Write the letter of the correct answer on the line provided in the left column.

14.11. _____ nulli-   A. vulva

14.12. _____ mamm/o   B. surgical fixation

14.13. _____ salping/o   C. tube

14.14. _____ -pexy   D. breast

14.15. _____ episi/o   E. none

● Definitions

Circle the letter next to the correct answer.

14.16. Which term describes the inner layer of the uterus?

a. corpus

b. endometrium

c. myometrium

d. perimetrium

14.17. Which term is used to describe the fertilized egg immediately after conception?

a. embryo

b. fetus

c. gamete

d. zygote

14.18. Which term describes the glands on either side of the vaginal opening that produce mucus to lubricate the vagina?

a. Bartholin's glands

b. bulbourethral glands

c. Cowper's glands

d. follicles

14.19. Which term describes the finger-like structures of the fallopian tube that catch the ovum as it is released by the ovary?

a. fimbriae

b. fundus

c. infundibulum

d. oviduct

14.20. Which phase of the menstrual cycle occurs approximately between days 15 and 28?

    a. menstrual

    b. ovulatory

    c. postmenstrual

    d. premenstrual

14.21. Which term describes the normal position of the uterus?

    a. anteflexion

    b. anteversion

    c. retroflexion

    d. retroversion

14.22. Which term means the beginning of the menstrual function that begins at puberty?

    a. menarche

    b. menopause

    c. menses

    d. menstruation

14.23. Which structure runs down the length of the testicle, then turns upward into the body where it becomes a narrower tube called the vas deferens?

    a. ejaculatory duct

    b. epididymis

    c. seminal vesicles

    d. urethra

14.24. Which term describes the region between the vaginal orifice and the anus?

    a. clitoris

    b. mons pubis

    c. perineum

    d. vulva

14.25. Which term describes the release of a mature egg by the ovary?

    a. coitus

    b. fertilization

    c. implantation

    d. ovulation

● Matching Structures

Write the letter of the correct answer on the line provided in the left column.

14.26. _____ clitoris   A. carries milk from the mammary glands

14.27. _____ lactiferous duct   B. encloses the testicles

14.28. _____ prepuce   C. external female genitalia

14.29. _____ scrotum   D. protects the tip of the penis

14.30. _____ vulva   E. sensitive tissue near vaginal opening

● Which Word?

Circle the correct term in each sentence.

14.31. The term used to describe a woman during her first pregnancy is *primigravida* / *primipara*.

14.32. The fluid secreted by the breasts during the first days after giving birth is *colostrum* / *meconium*.

14.33. The term meaning inflammation of the vulva is *vulvodynia* / *vulvitis*.

14.34. The total absence of sperm in the semen is known as *azoospermia* / *oligospermia*.

14.35. The term used to describe a woman who has never borne a viable child is *nulligravida* / *nullipara*.

● Spelling Counts

Find the misspelled word in each sentence. Then write that word, spelled correctly, on the line provided.

14.36. The prostrate gland secretes a thick fluid that aids the motility of the sperm. _____

14.37. Menstration is the normal periodic discharge from the uterus. _____

14.38. The plasenta is also known as the afterbirth. _____

14.39. A Papanicola test is an exfoliative biopsy for the detection and diagnosis of conditions of the cervix and surrounding tissues. _____

14.40. Cercumsion is the surgical removal of the foreskin of the penis and is usually performed a few days after birth. _____

● Matching Veneral Diseases

Write the letter of the correct answer on the line provided in the left column.

14.41._____ genital herpes   A. Characterized by painful urination and an abnormal discharge

14.42. _____ gonorrhea   B. Caused by the spirochete *Treponema pallidum*

14.43. _____ human papilloma virus   C. Antiviral drugs ease symptoms but do not cure.

14.44. _____ syphilis   D. Also known as genital warts

14.45. _____ trichomonas   E. A vaginal inflammation caused by a protozoan parasite

● Term Selection

Circle the letter next to the correct answer.

14.46. Which term describes an accumulation of pus in the fallopian tube?

   a. leiomyoma

   b. pelvic inflammatory disease

   c. pyosalpinx

   d. salpingitis

14.47. Which term describes a varicose vein of the testicles?

   a. cryptorchidism

   b. hydrocele

   c. phimosis

   d. varicocele

14.48. Which term describes abnormal tipping with the body of the uterus bent forming an angle with the cervix?

   a. anteflexion

   b. anteversion

   c. retroflexion

   d. retroversion

14.49. Which term means a markedly reduced menstrual flow and abnormally infrequent menstruation?

   a. amenorrhea

   b. hypomenorrhea

   c. oligomenorrhea

   d. polymenorrhea

14.50. Which term describes the surgical removal of the uterus, tubes, ovaries, adjacent lymph nodes, and part of the vagina?

   a. bilateral hysterosalpingo-oophorectomy

   b. bilateral salpingo-oophorectomy

   c. radical hysterectomy

   d. total abdominal hysterectomy

● Sentence Completion

Write the correct term on the line.

14.51. The dark area surrounding the nipple is known as the _____ .

14.52. During delivery when the buttocks or feet are presented first this is known as a/an _____ birth.

14.53. The most serious form of toxemia of pregnancy is known as _____ .

14.54. The term meaning suturing the vagina is _____ .

14.55. The structure that connects the fetus to the placenta is known as the _____ cord.

● True/False

If the statement is true, write T on the line. If the statement is false, write F on the line.

14.56. _____ When the mother's blood is Rh-negative, and the father's is Rh-positive, the baby may inherit the Rh-positive factor from the father.

14.57. _____ Meconium is the vaginal discharge that occurs during the first week or two after childbirth.

14.58. _____ A hysteroscope is an endoscope used in the direct visual examination of the interior of the uterus.

14.59. _____ The chorion is also known as the bag of waters.

14.60. _____ Dilation is the expansion of an opening.

14.61. _____ Mittelschmerz means pain between menstrual periods and usually occurs at the time of ovulation.

14.62. _____ A PSA test is used to determine the number of sperm in a semen specimen.

14.63. _____ An Apgar score is an evaluation of a newborn infant's physical status.

14.64. _____ Hysterosalpingography is the use of ultrasound to image the uterus and fallopian tubes.

14.65. _____ An ectopic pregnancy may occur in a fallopian tube.

● Clinical Conditions

Write the correct answer on the line.

14.66. Mr. Romer was treated for prostatomegaly. This condition is also known as benign _____ _____ .

14.67. Mary Smith required the delivery of her baby through an incision in the maternal abdominal and uterine wall. The full medical term for this procedure is a/an _____ section.

14.68. Daniel Grossman was treated for a urethral discharge coming from the prostate gland. The medical term for this condition is _____ .

14.69. Rita Liu, who is 25, is concerned because her menstrual periods have stopped and she knows that she is not pregnant. Her doctor described this condition as _____ .

14.70. To prevent laceration of the tissues during the delivery Barbara Klein's doctor performed a/an _____ .

14.71. Early in her pregnancy Mary Jimenez suffered a miscarriage. The medical term for this condition is a spontaneous _____ .

14.72. Harriet Ingram was diagnosed as having a leiomyoma, which is a benign tumor derived from the smooth muscle of the uterus. This condition is also known as a/an _____ .

14.73. Harry Belcher's doctor removed a portion of both vas deferens. The medical term for this sterilization procedure is a/an _____ .

14.74. There were complications in Jane Marsall's pregnancy caused by the abnormal implantation of the placenta in the lower portion of the uterus. The medical term for this condition is placenta _____ .

14.75. Immediately after birth the Reicher baby was described as being a newborn or a/an _____ .

● Which is the correct medical term?

Circle the letter next to the correct answer.

14.76. Which device allows observation of the fetal heart rate and the maternal uterine contractions during labor?

  a. electronic fetal monitor

  b. endovaginal ultrasound

  c. fetal ultrasound

  d. pelvimetry

14.77. Which term describes a condition of excessive uterine bleeding that occurs during both the menses and at irregular intervals?

  a. menorrhagia

  b. menometrorrhagia

  c. mittelschmerz

  d. polymenorrhea

14.78. Which term describes an inflammation of the glans penis?

    a. anorchism

    b. balanitis

    c. epididymitis

    d. orchitis

14.79. Which term describes precancerous lesions of the cervix?

    a. cervical dysplasia

    b. cervicitis

    c. colporrhexis

    d. vaginitis

14.80. Which term means a profuse white mucus discharge from the uterus and vagina?

    a. endocervicitis

    b. leukorrhea

    c. pruritus vulvae

    d. vaginitis

14.81. The medical term meaning a hernia protruding into the vagina is _____ .

14.82. The medical term meaning pain in the breast is _____ .

14.83. The medical term meaning an inflammation of the endometrium is _____ .

14.84. The medical term meaning the surgical repair of an ovary is a/an _____ .

14.85. The medical term meaning pain in the vagina is _____ .

11.86. The medical term meaning to suture the uterus is _____ .

14.87. The medical term meaning a hernia of the uterus, particularly during pregnancy, is a/an _____ .

14.88. The medical term meaning the surgical fixation of a displaced ovary is _____ .

14.89. The medical term meaning the rupture of the uterus, particularly during pregnancy, is _____ .

14.90 The medical term meaning an inflammation of the vulva and the vagina is _____ .

● **Challenge Word Building**

These terms are *not* found in this chapter; however, they are made up of these familiar word parts. You may want to look in the glossary or use a medical dictionary to check your answers!

endo-	hyster/o	-cele
	mast/o	-dynia
	metr/i	-itis
	oophor/o	-plasty
	vagin/o	-pexy
	vulv/o	-rrhaphy
		-rrhexis

● **Labeling Exercises**

Identify the numbered items on these diagrams.

14.91. _____ bladder

14.92. _____ gland

14.93. _____

14.94. _____

14.95. _____

14.96. _____ tube

14.97. _____

14.98. _____ bladder

14.99. _____

14.100. _____

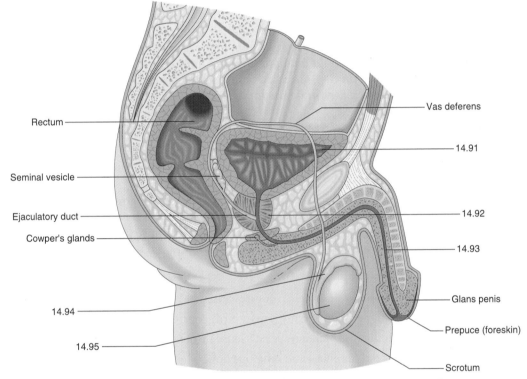

Rectum

Seminal vesicle

Ejaculatory duct

Cowper's glands

14.94

14.95

Vas deferens

14.91

14.92

14.93

Glans penis

Prepuce (foreskin)

Scrotum

Ureter

Ovary

Cervix of uterus

Anus

14.96

14.97

14.98

Clitoris

14.99

14.100

The Human Touch: Critical Thinking Exercise

The following story and questions are designed to stimulate critical thinking through class discussion or as a brief essay response. There are no easy or right-wrong answers to these questions.

"But Sam, you promised!" Jamie Chu began.

"Please do not get so upset," her husband interrupted. "I know I agreed to a vasectomy, but Grandmother may have a point. I do not have a son. Our family name has to be considered. I just feel that we should think about this."

"But Sam, we already discussed it. You're scheduled for the procedure." It seemed to Jamie that they had already spent plenty of time considering the number of children they wanted, and talking about various contraceptive methods. Jamie had problems taking the pill, and Sam didn't like using a condom. A tubal ligation could have been the answer, but Jamie had a fear of not waking up from the anesthesia. Besides, she had been the one to go through two pregnancies and childbirths. Sam had reluctantly agreed that it was his turn to take responsibility for family planning.

Their two daughters, 2-year-old Nanyn and her big sister Nadya, made the perfect size family, Jamie thought. She had grown up in a large family. A lot of her childhood was spent taking care of her brothers and sisters, and she rarely had her mother's undivided attention. She didn't want that for her children.

Sam's story was different. Before his parents immigrated to America they had had four daughters. His father was so proud when he was born, a son to carry on the family tradition.

It had taken quite a long time to convince Sam that a family of only daughters could be considered complete. And now Grandmother was questioning that decision . . .

Suggested Discussion Topics:

1. Which partner is responsible for birth control and why?
2. If a couple cannot agree about family size or birth control methods, what should they do?
3. Compare large families to small families. Discuss the good and bad points of each.
4. Discuss how cultural differences and religious beliefs influence choices like family size and birth control.
5. Why do some cultures value male children over female children?

CHAPTER

Diagnostic Procedures and Pharmacology

● **Overview of Diagnostic Procedures and Pharmacology**

Basic Diagnostic Procedures	Vital signs
	Auscultation
	Palpation and percussion
	Basic examination instruments
	Basic examination positions
Laboratory Tests	Blood tests
	Urinalysis
Endoscopy	Visual examination
	Endoscopic surgery
Imaging Techniques	Radiography (x-ray)
	Computed tomography (CT)
	Magnetic resonance imaging (MRI)
	Fluoroscopy
	Diagnostic ultrasound
Nuclear Medicine	Nuclear medicine
Radiographic Projections and Positioning	Projections
	Positioning
	Basic radiographic projections
Pharmacology	Terms Related to Pharmacology
	Routes of Administration

VOCABULARY   Related to Diagnostic Procedures and Pharmacology

Check the box as you master each word part or term. Terms marked with the ❖ symbol are pronounced on the optional student audiotape.

Key Word Parts

- [ ] albumin/o
- [ ] calc/i
- [ ] cin/e
- [ ] fluor/o
- [ ] glycos/o
- [ ] -graph
- [ ] -graphy
- [ ] hemat/o
- [ ] -ous
- [ ] per-
- [ ] phleb/o
- [ ] radi/o
- [ ] -scope
- [ ] -scopy
- [ ] -uria

Key Medical Terms

- [ ] abdominocentesis (ab-**dom**-ih-noh-sen-**TEE**-sis) ❖
- [ ] addiction
- [ ] adverse drug reaction
- [ ] agglutination (ah-**gloo**-tih-**NAY**-shun) ❖
- [ ] albuminuria (al-byou-mih-**NEW**-ree-ah) ❖
- [ ] assay (**ASS**-ay) ❖
- [ ] assessment
- [ ] auscultation (aws-kul-**TAY**-shun) ❖
- [ ] bacteriuria (back-**tee**-ree-**YOU**-ree-ah) ❖
- [ ] blood urea nitrogen (you-**REE**-ah)
- [ ] bruit (**BREW**-ee *or* **BROOT**) ❖
- [ ] calciuria (kal-sih-**YOU**-ree-ah) ❖
- [ ] cardiocentesis (**kar**-dee-oh-sen-**TEE**-sis) ❖
- [ ] centesis (sen-**TEE**-sis) ❖
- [ ] cineradiography (**sin**-eh-ray-dee-**OG**-rah-fee) ❖
- [ ] compliance
- [ ] computed tomography (toh-**MOG**-rah-fee) ❖
- [ ] contraindication
- [ ] creatinuria (kree-**at**-ih-**NEW**-ree-ah) ❖
- [ ] decubitus (dee-**KYOU**-bih-tus) ❖
- [ ] endoscopy (en-**DOS**-koh-pee) ❖
- [ ] extraoral radiography
- [ ] fluoroscopy (floo-or-**OS**-koh-pee) ❖
- [ ] glycosuria (glye-koh-**SOO**-ree-ah) ❖
- [ ] hematocrit (hee-**MAT**-oh-krit) ❖
- [ ] hematuria (hee-mah-**TOO**-ree-ah *or* hem-ah-**TOO**-ree-ah) ❖
- [ ] hypodermic (**high**-poh-**DER**-mick) ❖
- [ ] idiosyncratic (**id**-ee-oh-sin-**KRAT**-ick) ❖
- [ ] immunofluorescence (**im**-you-noh-**floo**-oh-**RES**-ens) ❖

- [ ] intradermal injection
- [ ] intramuscular injection
- [ ] intraoral radiography
- [ ] intravenous injection
- [ ] ketonuria (kee-toh-**NEW**-ree-ah) ❖
- [ ] lithotomy (lih-**THOT**-oh-mee)
- [ ] lymphangiography (lim-**fan**-jee-**OG**-rah-fee) ❖
- [ ] magnetic resonance imaging ❖
- [ ] ophthalmoscope (ahf-**THAL**-moh-skope) ❖
- [ ] otoscope (**OH**-toh-skope) ❖
- [ ] palliative (**PAL**-ee-**ay**-tiv *or* **PAL**-ee-ah-tiv) ❖
- [ ] palpation (pal-**PAY**-shun) ❖
- [ ] parenteral (pah-**REN**-ter-al) ❖
- [ ] percussion (per-**KUSH**-un) ❖
- [ ] percutaneous (**per**-kyou-**TAY**-nee-us) ❖
- [ ] perfusion (per-**FYOU**-zuhn)
- [ ] pericardiocentesis (**pehr**-ih-**kar**-dee-oh-sen-**TEE**-sis) ❖
- [ ] phlebotomist (fleh-**BOT**-oh-mist) ❖
- [ ] phlebotomy (fleh-**BOT**-oh-mee) ❖
- [ ] placebo (plah-**SEE**-boh) ❖
- [ ] positron emission tomography ❖
- [ ] potentiation (poh-**ten**-shee-**AY**-shun) ❖
- [ ] proteinuria (**proh**-tee-in-**YOU**-ree-ah) ❖
- [ ] prothrombin (proh-**THROM**-bin) ❖
- [ ] pyuria (pye-**YOU**-ree-ah) ❖
- [ ] radioimmunoassay (**ray**-dee-oh-**im**-you-noh-**ASS**-ay) ❖
- [ ] radiologist (ray-dee-**OL**-oh-jist) ❖
- [ ] radiolucent (ray-dee-oh-**LOO**-sent) ❖
- [ ] radionuclide imaging (ray-dee-oh-**NEW**-klyd) ❖
- [ ] radiopaque (ray-dee-oh-**PAYK**) ❖
- [ ] radiopharmaceuticals
- [ ] rale (**RAHL**) ❖
- [ ] recumbent (ree-**KUM**-bent) ❖
- [ ] regimen (**REJ**-ih-men) ❖
- [ ] rhonchus (**RONG**-kus) ❖
- [ ] single photon emission computed tomography ❖
- [ ] speculum (**SPECK**-you-lum) ❖
- [ ] sphygmomanometer (**sfig**-moh-mah-**NOM**-eh-ter) ❖
- [ ] stethoscope (**STETH**-oh-skope) ❖
- [ ] stridor (**STRYE**-dor) ❖
- [ ] subcutaneous injection
- [ ] supine (**SUE**-pine) ❖
- [ ] thoracentesis (thoh-rah-sen-**TEE**-sis) ❖
- [ ] ultrasonography (ul-trah-son-**OG**-rah-fee) ❖
- [ ] urinalysis (you-rih-**NAL**-ih-sis) ❖
- [ ] venipuncture (**VEN**-ih-**punk**-tyour) ❖

● OBJECTIVES

On completion of this chapter, you should be able to:

1 Describe the four vital signs recorded for most patients.

2 Recognize, define, spell, and pronounce the terms associated with basic examination procedures.

3 Identify and describe the basic examination positions.

4 Recognize, define, spell, and pronounce terms associated with frequently performed blood and urinalysis laboratory tests.

5 Recognize, define, spell, and pronounce terms associated with radiography and other imaging techniques.

6 Differentiate between projection and position and describe basic radiographic projections.

7 Recognize, define, spell, and pronounce the pharmacology terms introduced in this chapter.

Basic Examination Procedures

Basic examination procedures are performed during the assessment of the patient's condition. As used in medicine, **assessment** means the evaluation or appraisal of a condition. This information is used in reaching a diagnosis and in formulating a patient care plan.

Vital Signs

Four vital signs are recorded for most patients. These are temperature, pulse, respiration, and blood pressure.

- **Temperature** (T). An average normal temperature is 98.6°F (Fahrenheit) or 37.0°C (Celsius) (Figure 15.1).

- **Pulse** (P). The pulse rate is the number of times the heart beats per minute. The pulse may be measured at different points on the body (Figure 15.2). A normal adult pulse ranges from 50 to 80 beats per minute (bpm).

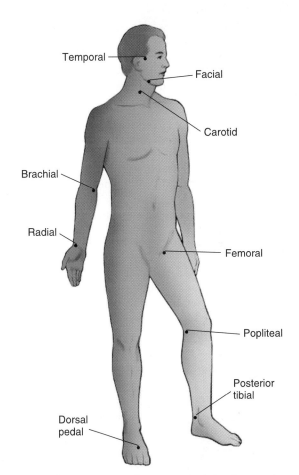

FIGURE 15.2 Major sites where an arterial pulse can be detected.

Celsius	Fahrenheit
42	107.6
41	105.8
40	104.0
39	102.2
38	100.4
37	98.6
36	96.8
35	95.0
34	93.2

FIGURE 15.1 The average normal temperature is 98.6°F (Fahrenheit) or 37.0°C (Celsius).

- **Respiration rate** (RR). The rate is recorded as the number of respirations per minute. (A single respiration is one inhalation and one exhalation.) The average respiratory rate for an adult ranges from 10 to 20 breaths per minute.

FIGURE 15.3 A sphygmomanometer and stethoscope are being used to measure blood pressure.

- **Blood pressure** (BP). A **sphygmomanometer** (sfig-moh-mah-**NOM**-eh-ter) is an instrument used to measure blood pressure. A **stethoscope** (**STETH**-oh-skope) is used to listen to sounds within the body and during the measurement of blood pressure (Figure 15.3). Blood pressure is discussed in Chapter 5.

Auscultation Sounds

Auscultation (**aws**-kul-**TAY**-shun) is listening through a stethoscope for sounds within the body to determine the condition of the lungs, pleura, heart, and abdomen (Figure 15.4). Table 15.1 contains tips for remembering some of the auscultation sounds.

Table 15.1

AN AID TO REMEMBERING AUSCULTATION SOUNDS

To remember the meaning of these terms, say each out loud so it resembles the sound heard from the body.

- A **bruit** sounds "murmury."
- A **rale** sounds "rattley."
- **Rhonchus** sounds musical.
- **Stridor** sounds harsh.

- A **bruit** (BREW-ee *or* BROOT) is an abnormal sound or murmur heard in auscultation.
- A **rale** (RAHL) is an abnormal rattle or crackle-like respiratory sound heard during inspiration (breathing in).
- **Rhonchus** (RONG-kus), also known as **wheezing**, is an added sound with a musical pitch occurring during inspiration or expiration that results from a partially obstructed airway caused by inflammation, spasm of smooth muscles, or the presence of mucus in the airways (plural, **rhonchi**).
- **Stridor** (STRYE-dor) is an abnormal, high-pitched, harsh or crowing sound heard during inspiration that results from a partial blockage of the pharynx, larynx, and trachea.

Palpation and Percussion

- **Palpation** (pal-**PAY**-shun) is an examination technique in which the examiner's hands are used to feel the texture, size, consistency, and location of certain body parts (Figure 15.5).

FIGURE 15.4 Auscultation is listening through a stethoscope to sounds within the body.

FIGURE 15.5 Palpation is the use of the fingertips to detect tenderness and determine structure size.

- **Percussion** (per-KUSH-un) is a diagnostic procedure to determine the density of a body area by the sound produced by tapping the surface with the finger or instrument (Figure 15.6).

FIGURE 15.6 Percussion is the use of the fingers in a tapping motion to evaluate air content in the lungs and over the abdomen to detect air in the loops of intestine.

Additional Examination Procedures

- An **ophthalmoscope** (ahf-THAL-moh-skope) is used to examine the interior of the eye (**ophthalmo** means eye and **scope** means instrument for visual examination) (Figure 15.7).

- The abbreviation **PERRLA** means *pupils are equal, round, responsive to light and accommodation.* This is a diagnostic observation and any abnormality might indicate a head injury or damage to the brain.

- An **otoscope** (OH-toh-skope) is used to visually examine the external ear canal and tympanic membrane (**oto** means ear and **scope** means instrument for visual examination) (Figure 15.8).

FIGURE 15.7 An ophthalmoscope is used to examine the interior of the eye.

FIGURE 15.8 An otoscope is used to examine the ear canal and tympanic membrane.

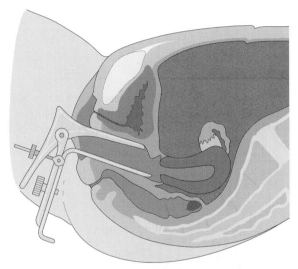

FIGURE 15.9 A speculum in place for inspection of the vagina.

- A **speculum** (SPECK-you-lum) is used to enlarge the opening of any canal or cavity to facilitate inspection of its interior (Figure 15.9).

Basic Examination Positions

Recumbent Position

The term **recumbent** (ree-KUM-bent) may be used to describe any position in which the patient is lying down either on the back, front, or side.

- The term **decubitus** (dee-KYOU-bih-tus) also means the act of lying down or the position assumed in lying down.

- In radiography, the term **decubitus** is used to describe the position of the patient when lying in a recumbent position. However, decubitus is most commonly used to describe a decubitus ulcer, which is also known as a bedsore (see Chapter 12).

Prone Position

In a **prone position**, the recumbent patient is lying on the belly *face down*. The arms may be placed under the head for comfort (Figure 15.10). This position is used for the examination and treatment of the back and buttocks.

FIGURE **15.10** The prone position.

Supine Position

In the **supine position** (SUE-pine), also known as the **horizontal recumbent position**, the patient is lying on the back with the *face up* (Figure 15.11). This position is used for examination and treatment of the anterior surface of the body and for x-rays.

FIGURE **15.11** The horizontal recumbent (supine) position.

Dorsal Recumbent Position

In the **dorsal recumbent position** the patient is supine (lying on the back) with the knees bent (Figure 15.12). This position is used for the examination and treatment of the abdominal area and for vaginal or rectal examinations.

Sims' Position

In the **Sims' position** the patient is lying on the left side with the right knee and thigh drawn up with the left arm placed along the back (Figure 15.13). This position is used in the examination and treatment of the rectal area.

FIGURE **15.12** The dorsal recumbent position.

FIGURE **15.13** The Sims' position.

Knee-Chest Position

In the **knee-chest position**, the patient is lying face down with the hips flexed (bent) so the knees and chest rest on the table (Figure 15.14). This position is used for rectal examinations.

Lithotomy Position

In the **lithotomy position** (lih-THOT-oh-mee) the patient is supine with the feet and legs raised and supported in stirrups (Figure 15.15). This position is used for vaginal and rectal examinations.

FIGURE **15.14** The knee-chest position.

FIGURE 15.15 The lithotomy position.

- Lithotomy also means a surgical incision for the removal of a stone, usually from the urinary bladder. This is discussed in Chapter 9.

Trendelenburg Position

In the **Trendelenburg position** the patient is lying on the back with the knees bent and the legs elevated slightly higher than the head (Figure 15.16). This position is used for some radiographic examinations and also for the treatment of shock.

FIGURE 15.16 The Trendelenburg position.

Laboratory Tests

- When used in regard to laboratory tests, the term **profile** means tests that are frequently performed as a group on automated multichannel laboratory testing equipment.
- When a laboratory test is ordered **stat** the results are needed immediately and the tests should have top priority in the laboratory. (Stat comes from the Latin word meaning immediately.)

Blood Tests

Obtaining Specimens

- **Phlebotomy** (fleh-**BOT**-oh-mee) is the puncture of a vein for the purpose of drawing blood (**phleb** means

vein and **otomy** means a surgical incision). This is also known as **venipuncture** (**VEN**-ih-**punk**-tyour).
- A **phlebotomist** (fleh-**BOT**-oh-mist) is an individual trained and skilled in phlebotomy.
- A **capillary puncture** is the technique used when only a small amount of blood is needed as a specimen for a blood test. Named for where it is performed it may be a finger stick, heel stick, or earlobe stick.

Complete Blood Cell Counts

A **complete blood cell count** (CBC) is a series of tests performed as a group to evaluate several blood conditions.

- **Erythrocyte sedimentation rate** (eh-**RITH**-roh-site) test, also known as **sed** or **ESR**, is based on the rate at which the red blood cells separate from the plasma and settle to the bottom of the container. An elevated count indicates the presence of inflammation in the body.
- **Hematocrit** (hee-**MAT**-oh-krit), also known as **Hct** or **HCT**, measures the percentage by volume of packed red blood cells in a whole blood sample (**hemato** means blood and **crit** means to separate). This test is used to diagnose abnormal states of hydration (fluid level in the body), polycythemia (excess red blood cells), and anemia (deficient red blood cells).
- A **platelet count** (PLC) measures the number of platelets in a specified amount of blood. This test is used to assess the effects of chemotherapy and radiation therapy and to aid in the diagnosis of thrombocytopenia (an abnormal decrease in the number of platelets).
- A **red blood cell** (RBC) **count** is a determination of the number of erythrocytes in the blood. A depressed count may indicate anemia or hemorrhage lasting more than 24 hours.
- **Total hemoglobin** (Hb) measures the amount of hemoglobin found in whole blood (**hemo** means blood and **globin** means protein). Test results measure the severity of anemia or polycythemia and monitor the response to therapy.
- A **white blood cell** (WBC) **count** is a determination of the number of leukocytes in the blood. An elevated count may be an indication of infection or inflammation.
- A **white blood cell differential** determines what percentage of the total WBC count is composed of each of the five types of leukocytes. This test provides information about the patient's immune system, detects certain types of leukemia, and determines the severity of infection.

Additional Blood Tests

- **Agglutination testing** (ah-**gloo**-tih-**NAY**-shun) includes a variety of tests that involve the clumping together of cells or particles when mixed with incompatible serum. These tests are performed to determine the patient's blood type and to check compatibility of donor and recipient blood before a transfusion.

- **Blood urea nitrogen** (you-REE-ah), also known as **BUN**, is the amount of urea present in the blood. Urea is the major end product of protein metabolism found in urine and blood and this test is a rough indicator of kidney function.

- **Lipid tests**, also known as a **lipid panel**, measure the amounts of cholesterol (high-density lipoprotein [HDL] and low-density lipoprotein [LDL]) and triglycerides in a blood sample.

- **Prothrombin time** (proh-THROM-bin), also known as **pro time**, is a test used to diagnose conditions associated with abnormal bleeding and to monitor anticoagulant therapy.

- **Serum enzyme tests** are used to measure the blood enzymes. These tests are useful as evidence of a myocardial infarction.

- The **serum bilirubin test** measures how well red blood cells are being broken down. Elevated levels of bilirubin, which causes jaundice, may indicate liver problems or gallstones.

- A **thyroid-stimulating hormone assay** measures circulating blood levels of thyroid-stimulating hormone (TSH) that may indicate abnormal thyroid activity.

Urinalysis

Urinalysis (you-rih-NAL-ih-sis) is the examination of the physical and chemical properties of urine to determine the presence of abnormal elements. Routine urinalysis is performed to screen for urinary and systemic disorders.

- For routine analysis a **dipstick** is used (Figure 15.17). Chemicals impregnated on this plastic strip react with substances in the urine and change color when abnormalities are present.

- More detailed testing requires **microscopic examination** of the specimen. As an example, casts are identified through microscopic examination. **Casts** are fibrous or protein materials, such as pus and fats, that are thrown off into the urine in kidney disease.

Figure 15.17 A dipstick is used for routine urinalysis.

- The average normal **pH** range of urine is from 4.5 to 8.0. A pH value *below* 7 indicates acid urine and is an indication of acidosis. A pH value *above* 7 indicates alkaline urine and may indicate conditions including a urinary tract infection. (The abbreviation pH describes the degree of acidity or alkalinity of a substance. A pH of 7 is neutral, that is, neither acid nor alkaline. Maximum acidity is 0 pH and maximum alkalinity is pH 14.)

- The **specific gravity** reflects the amount of wastes, minerals, and solids in the urine. Low specific gravity (dilute urine) is characteristic of diabetes insipidus. High specific gravity (concentrated urine) occurs in conditions such as dehydration, liver failure, and shock.

Conditions Identified through Urinalysis

- **Acetone** (ASS-eh-tohn), which has a sweet fruity odor, is found in small quantities in normal urine and in larger amount in diabetic urine.

- **Albuminuria** (al-byou-mih-NEW-ree-ah) is the presence of the serum protein albumin in the urine and is a sign of impaired kidney function (**albumin** means albumin or protein and **uria** means urine).

- **Bacteriuria** (back-tee-ree-YOU-ree-ah) is the presence of bacteria in the urine (**bacteri** means bacteria and **uria** means urine).

- **Calciuria** (kal-sih-YOU-ree-ah) is the presence of calcium in the urine (**calci** means calcium and **uria** means urine). Abnormally high levels may be diagnostic for hyperparathyroidism. Lower than normal levels may indicate osteomalacia.

- **Creatinuria** (kree-at-ih-NEW-ree-ah) is an increased concentration of creatine in the urine (**creatin** means creatinine and **uria** means urine). **Creatinine**, a waste product of muscle metabolism, is normally removed by the kidneys. Its presence in urine is an indication of increased muscle breakdown or a disruption of kidney function.

- **Glycosuria** (glye-koh-SOO-ree-ah) is the presence of glucose in the urine and is most commonly caused by diabetes (**glycos** means glucose and **uria** means urine).

- **Hematuria** (hee-mah-TOO-ree-ah *or* hem-ah-TOO-ree-ah) is the presence of blood in the urine (**hemat** means blood and **uria** means urine). This condition may be caused by kidney stones, infection, benign prostatic hyperplasia, damage to the kidney, or bladder cancer.

- In **gross hematuria** the urine may look pink, brown, or bright red and the presence of blood can be detected without magnification. In **microscopic hematuria** the urine is clear but blood cells can be seen under a microscope.

- **Ketonuria** (kee-toh-NEW-ree-ah) is the presence of ketones in the urine (**keton** means ketones and **uria** means urine). **Ketones** are formed when the body breaks down fat. Their presence in urine may indicate starvation or uncontrolled diabetes.

- **Proteinuria** (**proh**-tee-in-**YOU**-ree-ah) is an excess of serum protein in the urine and is usually a sign of kidney disease (**protein** means protein and **uria** means urine).
- **Pyuria** (pye-**YOU**-ree-ah) is the presence of pus in the urine (**py** means pus and **uria** means urine).
- **Urine culture and sensitivity** is an additional laboratory test to identify the cause of a urinary tract infection and to determine which antibiotic would be the most effective treatment.

Endoscopy

Endoscopy (en-**DOS**-koh-pee) is the visual examination of the interior of a body cavity (**endo** means within and **scopy** means visual examination). The fiber optic instrument used in this examination is an **endoscope**.

Endoscopic Surgery

The term endoscopy also describes surgical procedures requiring only very small incisions. Examples of these procedures include reconstructive knee surgery, laparoscopic cholecystectomy (gallbladder removal), bladder cancer treatment, hysterectomy, appendectomy, and lung biopsy.

The procedures and instruments are named for the body parts involved. As an example, Figure 15.18 shows an **arthroscope** being used to perform knee surgery.

Centesis

Centesis (sen-**TEE**-sis) is a surgical puncture to remove fluid for diagnostic purposes or to remove excess fluid.

- **Abdominocentesis** (ab-**dom**-ih-noh-sen-**TEE**-sis) is the surgical puncture of the abdominal cavity (**abdomino** means abdomen and **centesis** means a surgical puncture to remove fluid).
- **Amniocentesis** (am-nee-oh-sen-**TEE**-sis) is a diagnostic test to evaluate fetal health and is discussed in Chapter 14.
- **Cardiocentesis** (**kar**-dee-oh-sen-**TEE**-sis), also known as **cardiopuncture**, is the puncture of a chamber of the heart for diagnosis or therapy (**cardio** means heart and **centesis** means a surgical puncture to remove fluid).
- **Pericardiocentesis** (**pehr**-ih-**kar**-dee-oh-sen-**TEE**-sis) is the drawing of fluid from the pericardial sac (**peri** means surrounding, **cardio** means heart, and **centesis** means a surgical puncture to remove fluid).
- **Thoracentesis** (**thoh**-rah-sen-**TEE**-sis) is the puncture of the chest wall to obtain fluid for diagnostic purposes, to drain pleural effusions, or to reexpand a collapsed lung (**thora** means chest and **centesis** means a surgical puncture to remove fluid).

Imaging Techniques

Imaging techniques are used to visualize and examine internal body structures. The three most commonly used techniques are compared in Table 15.2 and Figure 15.19.

Two of these techniques involve the use of ionizing radiation, commonly known as **x-rays**, which is invisible, has no odor, and cannot be felt. This radiation is beneficial in producing images and in treating cancer; however, excessive exposure is dangerous and can cause death.

(A) Arthroscope in use

(B) Internal view of the knee during arthroscopy

FIGURE 15.18 Arthroscopic surgery. (A) The doctor views progress on a monitor. (B) Internal view as diseased tissue is removed during surgery.

FIGURE 15.19 Computed tomography provides cross-sectional images. Conventional x-rays superimpose anatomy and can capture images only in one plane.

Table 15.2

IMAGING SYSTEMS COMPARED

Method	How It Works
Conventional radiography (x-ray)	Uses radiation (x-rays) passing through the patient to expose a film that shows the body in profile. Hard tissues are light, soft tissues appear as shades of gray, and air is black.
Computed tomography (CT)	Uses radiation (x-rays) with computer assistance to produce multiple cross-sectional views of the body. Hard tissues are light and soft tissues appear as shades of gray.
Magnetic resonance imaging (MRI)	Uses a combination of radio waves and a strong magnetic field to produce images. Hard tissues are dark and soft tissues appear as shades of gray.

Contrast medium

A **radiographic contrast medium** is a substance used to make visible structures that are otherwise hard to see.

- A **radiopaque contrast medium** (ray-dee-oh-**PAYK**), such as barium sulfate, *does not* allow the x-rays to pass through and appears white or light gray on the resulting film.

- A **radiolucent contrast medium** (ray-dee-oh-**LOO**-sent), such as air or nitrogen gas, *does* allow the x-rays to pass through and appears black or dark gray on the resulting film.

Barium (Ba)

Barium is a radiopaque contrast medium used primarily to visualize the digestive system (Figure 15.20). It is administered orally as a barium swallow (upper gastrointestinal [GI] study) or rectally as a barium enema (lower GI study). X-rays and fluoroscopy are used to trace the barium flow through the digestive system.

Intravenous Contrast Medium

An **intravenous contrast medium** is injected into the vein to make visible the flow of blood through blood vessels and organs (see Figure 5.17). These techniques are usually named for the vessels or organs involved.

FIGURE 15.20 A radiograph after a barium swallow. The stomach and a portion of the small intestine are visible.

- For example, **lymphangiography** (lim-**fan**-jee-**OG**-rah-fee) is the radiographic examination of the lymphatic vessels following the injection of a contrast medium (**lymphangio** means lymph vessel and **graphy** means process of recording).

Radiology

- A **radiologist** (**ray**-dee-**OL**-oh-jist) is a physician who specializes in diagnosing and treating diseases and disorders with x-rays and other forms of radiant energy (**radi** means radiation and **ologist** means specialist).

- In conventional **radiology**, also known as **x-ray** or **radiography**, an image of hard tissue internal structures is created by the exposure of sensitized film to x-radiation (**radio** means radiation and **graphy** means the process of recording). The resulting film is known as an **x-ray** or **radiograph** (**radio** means radiation and **graph** means the resulting record).

- Radiographs are made up of shades of gray. Radiopaque hard tissues, such as bone and tooth enamel, do not permit x-rays to pass through and they appear white or light gray on the radiograph.

- Radiolucent air and soft tissues do permit x-rays to pass through and they appear as shades of gray to black on the radiograph (Figure 15.21).

Radiographic Projections and Positioning

Positioning

The term **positioning** describes the body placement and the part of the body closest to the film. For example, in a

FIGURE 15.21 A posteroanterior chest x-ray. Bones of the spine are white and soft tissues are shades of gray.

left lateral position, the left side of the body is placed nearest the film.

- The basic projections described in the next section may be used for most body parts (Figure 15.22). These projections may be exposed with the patient in a standing or recumbent position.

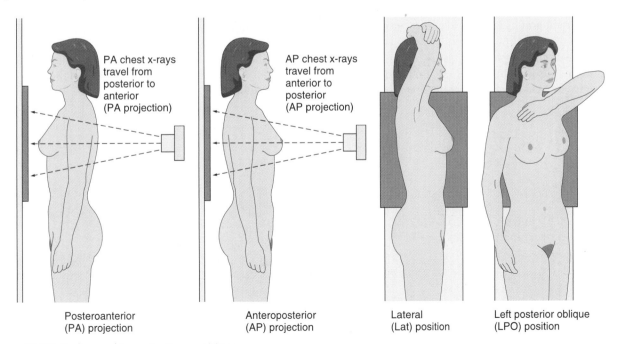

Posteroanterior (PA) projection

Anteroposterior (AP) projection

Lateral (Lat) position

Left posterior oblique (LPO) position

FIGURE 15.22 Radiographic projection positions.

Projections

The term **projection** describes the path that the x-ray beam follows through the body from entrance to exit.

- When the name of the projection combines two terms into a single word, the term listed first is the one that the x-ray penetrates first. As an example, in a posteroanterior projection the x-rays travel through the body from posterior (back) toward the anterior (front) to expose the film (see Figure 15.22).

Basic Radiographic Projections

- An **anteroposterior projection** (AP) has the patient positioned with the back parallel to the film. The x-ray beam travels from anterior (front) to posterior (back).

- A **posteroanterior projection** (PA) has the patient positioned facing the film and parallel to it. The x-ray beam travels through the body from posterior to anterior.

- A **lateral projection** (Lat), also known as a **side view**, has the patient positioned at right angles to the film. This view is named for the side of the body nearest the film.

- An **oblique projection** (Obli) has the patient positioned so the body is slanted sideways to the film. This is halfway between a parallel and a right angle position. This view is named for the side of the body nearest the film. **Oblique** means slanted sideways and these projections are named for the portion of the body nearest the film.

Dental Radiography

Specialized techniques and equipment are used in obtaining dental radiographs.

Extraoral Radiography

Extraoral radiography, as used in dentistry, means that the film is placed outside of the mouth. Figure 15.23 is a **panoramic radiograph**, which is also known as a **Panorex**.

Intraoral Radiography

Intraoral radiography, as used in dentistry, means that the film is placed within the mouth (Figure 15.24).

- **Periapical radiographs**, which show the entire tooth and some surrounding tissue, are used to detect abnormalities, such as an abscess, at the tip of the root.

FIGURE 15.23 A Panorex radiograph shows all of the teeth and surrounding structures of the upper and lower dental arches on a single film.

(A) **(B)**

FIGURE 15.24 Intraoral dental radiographs. (A) A periapical film shows the entire length of a tooth and some of the tissues surrounding the root. (B) A bitewing film shows the crowns of the upper and lower teeth in one area of the jaws. The white areas on these teeth are amalgam (silver) fillings.

- **Bitewing radiographs**, which show the crowns of teeth in both arches, are used primarily to detect decay (cavities) between the teeth.

Computed Tomography

Computed tomography (toh-**MOG**-rah-fee), also known as **CT** or **computed axial tomography** (CAT), uses a thin, fan-shaped x-ray beam that rotates around the patient to produce multiple cross-sectional views of the body (Figure 15.25).

Sagittal   Transverse   Coronal (frontal)

FIGURE 15.25 Computed tomography provides cross-sectional views of different body planes.

- Information gathered by radiation detectors is downloaded to a computer, analyzed, and converted into gray-scale images corresponding to anatomic slices of the body (Figure 15.26). These images are viewed on a monitor or printed as hard copy (films).

FIGURE **15.26** An abdominal CT scan in which the liver is predominant in the upper left and the stomach is visible in the upper right.

Magnetic Resonance Imaging

Magnetic resonance imaging, also known as **MRI**, uses a combination of radio waves and a strong magnetic field to create signals that are sent to a computer and converted into images of any plane through the body. In an MRI hard tissues appear dark and soft tissues are bright (Figure 15.27, see also Figure 10.12).

FIGURE **15.27** An MRI of the brain with a tumor visible in the upper left.

- In **closed architecture MRI**, also known as **high-field MRI**, patients may be uncomfortable because of the noise generated by the machine and feeling of being closed in. In **open architecture MRI** the design of the equipment is less confining and more comfortable for some patients.

- Because of the strong magnetic field, patients with pacemakers or other implanted electronic devices cannot be examined using this technique.

Fluoroscopy

Fluoroscopy (**floo**-or-**OS**-koh-pee) is used to visualize body parts in motion by projecting x-ray images on a luminous fluorescent screen (**fluoro** means glowing and **scopy** means visual examination).

- **Cineradiography** (**sin**-eh-**ray**-dee-**OG**-rah-fee) is the recording of images as they appear in motion on a fluorescent screen (**cine** means relationship to movement, **radio** means radiation, and **graphy** means process of recording).

- Fluoroscopy may also be used in conjunction with conventional x-ray techniques to capture a record of parts of the examination.

Diagnostic Ultrasound

Diagnostic ultrasound, also known as **ultrasonography** (**ul**-trah-son-**OG**-rah-fee), is imaging of deep body structures by recording the echoes of pulses of sound waves above the range of human hearing. The resulting record is called a **sonogram** (**SOH**-noh-gram).

- Ultrasound is most effective for viewing solid organs of the abdomen and soft tissues where the signal is not stopped by intervening bone or air. Ultrasound is used during pregnancy to evaluate fetal development (Figure 15.28).

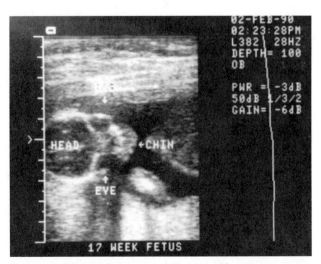

FIGURE **15.28** Fetal ultrasound (*Prepared by Lynne Schreiber, BS, RDMS, RT[R]*)

Nuclear Medicine

Nuclear medicine (NM), also known as **radionuclide imaging** (ray-dee-oh-NEW-klyd), is used for both diagnosis and treatment. Although other imaging techniques focus on the anatomic structures, NM looks at physiologic processes to determine how well body organs or systems are functioning.

- Nuclear medicine involves the use of **radiopharmaceuticals** that are injected or inhaled into the body and taken up (absorbed) by a particular organ.

- Each radiopharmaceutical contains a **radionuclide tracer**, also known as a **radioactive tracer**, that is specific to the body system being examined.

- A **gamma-ray camera** attached to a computer is used to generate an image showing the pattern of absorption. It is the pattern of absorption that indicates pathology.

Nuclear Scans

A **nuclear scan**, also known as a **scintigram** (SIN-tih-gram), uses this technology to gather information about the structure and function of organs or systems that cannot be seen on conventional x-rays.

Bone Scans

In a **bone scan** the radionuclide tracer is injected into the bloodstream and then the patient waits while the material travels through the body tissues. Only pathology in the bones absorbs the radionuclide and these are visible as dark areas on the scan (Figure 15.29).

Thyroid Scans

For a **thyroid scan** a radiopharmaceutical containing radioactive iodine is administered. The rate of iodine uptake by the thyroid is an indicator of thyroid function.

Single Photon Emission Computed Tomography

Single photon emission computed tomography, also known as **SPECT**, is a nuclear imaging technique in which

pictures are taken by one to three gamma cameras after a radionuclide tracer has been injected into the blood.

- In SPECT these **gamma cameras**, also known as **detectors**, rotate around the patient's body collecting data and producing images on a variety of planes.

- This technique is used to study myocardial perfusion. **Perfusion** (per-FYOU-zuhn) is the flow of blood through the vessels of an organ (see Chapter 5).

Positron Emission Tomography

Positron emission tomography, also known as **PET**, combines tomography with radionuclide tracers to produce enhanced images of selected body organs or areas. PET is used to determine cardiac or cerebral perfusion plus brain imaging for epilepsy, dementia, and recurrent brain tumors.

Radioimmunoassay

Radioimmunoassay (ray-dee-oh-**im**-you-noh-**ASS**-ay), also known as **radioassay**, is a laboratory technique in which a radioactively labeled substance is mixed with a blood specimen.

- **Assay** (**ASS**-ay) means to determine the amount of a particular substance in a mixture. These techniques can be used to evaluate function of the pituitary and thyroid glands.

- **Immunofluorescence** (**im**-you-noh-**floo**-oh-**RES**-ens) is a method of tagging antibodies with a fluorescent dye to detect or localize antigen-antibody combinations.

Pharmacology

Pharmacology is the study of the nature, uses, and effects of drugs for medical purposes. A **pharmacist** is a specialist who is licensed in formulating and dispensing medications.

Prescription and Over-the-Counter Drugs

- A **prescription** (Rx) is an order for medication, therapy, or a therapeutic device given (usually in writing) by an authorized person to a person properly authorized to dispense or perform the order.

- A **prescription drug** is a medication that may be dispensed only with a prescription from an appropriately licensed professional such as a physician or dentist. The abbreviations commonly used in relation to prescriptions and drug administration are shown in Table 15.3.

- An **over-the-counter drug** (OTC) is a medication that may be dispensed without a written prescription.

(A)   **(B)**

FIGURE 15.29 A bone scan of the head, shoulders, and upper spine (A) Anterior view. (B) Posterior view.

Table 15.3

FREQUENTLY USED DRUG ADMINISTRATION ABBREVIATIONS

Abbreviation	Meaning
a.c.	before meals
ad lib	as desired
b.i.d.	twice a day
c̄	with
NPO	nothing by mouth
p.c.	after meals
p.r.n.	as needed
p.o.	by mouth
qd	every day
q.h	every hour
q.i.d.	four times a day
t.i.d.	three times a day

Generic and Brand Name Drugs

- A **generic drug** is usually named for its chemical structure and not protected by a brand name or trademark. For example, diazepam is the generic name of a drug frequently used as a muscle relaxant.
- A **brand name** drug is sold under the name given the drug by the manufacturer. A brand name is always spelled with a capital letter. For example, Valium is the brand name for diazepam.

Terminology Related to Pharmacology

- **Addiction** is compulsive, uncontrollable dependence on a substance, habit, or practice to the degree that stopping causes severe emotional, mental, or physiologic reactions.
- An **adverse drug reaction** (ADR), also known as a **side effect** or an **adverse drug event** (ADE), is an undesirable drug response that accompanies the principal response for which the drug was taken.
- **Compliance** is the patient's consistency and accuracy in following the regimen prescribed by a physician or other health professional. As used here, **regimen** (REJ-ih-men) means directions or rules.
- A **contraindication** is a factor in the patient's condition that makes the use of a drug dangerous or ill advised.

- A **drug interaction** occurs when the effect of one drug is modified (changed) when it is administered at the same time as another drug.
- An **idiosyncratic reaction** (**id**-ee-oh-sin-**KRAT**-ick) is an unexpected reaction to a drug.
- A **palliative** (**PAL**-ee-**ay**-tiv *or* **PAL**-ee-ah-tiv) is a substance that eases the pain or severity of a disease but does not cure it.
- A **placebo** (plah-**SEE**-boh) is a substance containing no active ingredients that is given for its suggestive effects. In research, a placebo identical in appearance with the material being tested is administered to distinguish between drug action and suggestive effect of the material under study.
- **Potentiation** (poh-ten-shee-**AY**-shun), also known as **synergism** (**SIN**-er-jizm), is a drug interaction that occurs when the effect of one drug is potentiated (increased) by another drug.

Routes of Drug Administration

- **Inhalation administration** refers to vapor and gases taken in through the nose or mouth and absorbed into the bloodstream through the lungs. For example, the gases used for general anesthesia are administered by inhalation.
- **Oral administration** refers to drugs taken by mouth to be absorbed from the stomach or small intestine. These drugs may be in forms such as liquids, pills, or capsules. An **enteric coating** is applied to some tablets or capsules to prevent the release and absorption of their contents until they reach the small intestine.
- **Percutaneous treatment** (per-kyou-**TAY**-nee-us) means a procedure performed through the skin (**per** means through, **cutane** means skin, and **ous** means pertaining to). For example, a needle passed through the skin is used to aspirate fluid from a space below the skin.
- **Rectal administration** is the insertion of medication in the rectum by use of either **suppositories** or liquid solutions.
- With **sublingual administration** the medication is placed under the tongue and allowed to dissolve slowly. Once dissolved, the medication is quickly absorbed through the sublingual tissue directly into the bloodstream.
- **Topical administration** refers to the drugs, such as lotions, ointments, and eyedrops that are applied for local action.
- **Transdermal delivery** is a method of applying a drug to unbroken skin via a patch worn on the patient's skin. The drug is absorbed through the skin and into systemic circulation.

Parenteral Administration

- **Parenteral administration** (pah-**REN**-ter-al) is the administration of medication by injection through a

hypodermic syringe (**high**-poh-**DER**-mick) (Figure 15.30).

- An **intramuscular injection** (IM) is made directly into muscle tissue.

- A **subcutaneous injection** (SC) is made into the fatty layer just below the skin.

- An **intravenous injection** (IV) is made directly into a vein.

- An **intradermal injection** (ID) is made into the middle layers of the skin.

FIGURE 15.30 Types of injections.

Learning Exercises

Matching Word Parts—1

Write the letter of the correct answer on the line provided in the left column.

15.1. _____ albumin/o   A. relationship to motion

15.2. _____ calc/i   B. glowing

15.3. _____ cin/e   C. sugar

15.4. _____ fluor/o   D. albumin, protein

15.5. _____ glycos/o   E. calcium

Matching Word Parts—2

Write the letter of the correct answer on the line provided in the left column.

15.6. _____ -graph   A. blood

15.7. _____ -graphy   B. pertaining to

15.8. _____ hemat/o   C. the process of recording a picture or record

15.9. _____ -ous   D. the record or picture

15.10. _____ per-   E. through

Matching Word Parts—3

Write the letter of the correct answer on the line provided in the left column.

15.11. _____ phleb/o   A. instrument for visual examination

15.12. _____ radi/o   B. urine

15.13. _____ -scope   C. vein

15.14. _____ -scopy   D. visual examination

15.15. _____ -uria   E. radiation

Definitions

Circle the letter next to the correct answer.

15.16. Which projection has the patient positioned at right angles to the film?

a. anteroposterior

b. lateral

c. oblique

d. posteroanterior

15.17. Which instrument is used to examine the interior of the eye?

a. ophthalmoscope

b. otoscope

c. speculum

d. sphygmomanometer

15.18. Which imaging technique produces multiple cross-sectional images using x-radiation?

a. conventional x-ray

b. computed tomography

c. magnetic resonance imaging

d. ultrasound

15.19. Which blood test is used to indicate the presence of inflammation in the body?

a. agglutination

b. lipid tests

c. erythrocyte sedimentation rate

d. serum enzyme

15.20. Which technique uses the echoes of sound waves to image deep structures of the body?

a. cineradiography

b. fluoroscopy

c. magnetic resonance imaging

d. ultrasound

338 CHAPTER 15

15.21. Which term describes the presence of calcium in the urine?

   a. albuminuria

   b. calciuria

   c. creatinuria

   d. glycosuria

15.22. Which of these tests is used to monitor anti-coagulant therapy?

   a. agglutination

   b. lipid panel

   c. prothrombin time

   d. serum enzyme

15.23. Which test measures the percentage by volume of packed red blood cells in a whole blood sample?

   a. hematocrit

   b. hemoglobin

   c. red blood count

   d. white blood count

15.24. Which term describes an abnormal respiratory sound heard while listening to the chest while the patient is breathing in. This is a "rattley" sound.

   a. bruit

   b. rale

   c. rhonchus

   d. stridor

15.25. Which term describes the substance formed when the body breaks down fat and their presence in urine may indicate starvation or uncontrolled diabetes?

   a. albumin

   b. creatinine

   c. ketones

   d. urea

Matching Techniques

Write the letter of the correct answer on the line provided in the left column.

15.26. _____ centesis — A. uses powerful magnets

15.27. _____ computed tomography — B. uses a glowing screen

15.28. _____ conventional radiography — C. provides cross-sectional views

15.29. _____ fluoroscopy — D. removal of fluid for diagnostic purposes

15.30. _____ MRI — E. shows hard tissues as white

Which Word?

Circle the correct term in each sentence.

15.31. The term meaning an unexpected reaction to a drug is *idiosyncratic* / *palliative*.

15.32. The technology that combines tomography with radionuclide traces is called *positron emission tomography* / *radioimmunoassay*.

15.33. A substance that does not allow x-rays to pass through is called *radiolucent* / *radiopaque*.

15.34. A periapical film is an example of an *extraoral* / *intraoral* dental radiograph.

15.35. The name of a *brand name* / *generic* drug is always spelled with a capital letter.

Spelling Counts

Find the misspelled word in each sentence. Then write that word, spelled correctly, on the line provided.

15.36. Listening through a stethoscope for sounds within the body to determine the condition of the lungs, pleura, heart and abdomen is known as asultation _____

15.37. A sphygnomanometer is used to measure blood pressure. _____

15.38. The technique used to visualize body parts in motion is known as fluroscopy.
_____

15.39. The clumping together of cells or particles when mixed with incompatible blood is called agelutination. _____

15.40. A stethescope is used to listen for sounds within the body. _____

● Matching Abbreviations

Write the letter of the correct answer on the line provided in the left column.

15.41. _____ b.i.d.   A. as needed

15.42. _____ NPO   B. four times a day

15.43. _____ p.r.n.   C. nothing by mouth

15.44. _____ q.i.d.   D. three times a day

15.45. _____ t.i.d.   E. twice a day

● Term Selection

Circle the letter next to the correct answer.

15.46. Which term means the drawing of fluid from the sac surrounding the heart?

a. abdominocentesis

b. cardiocentesis

c. pericardiocentesis

d. thoracentesis

15.47. Which term means the abnormal presence of blood in the urine?

a. albuminuria

b. creatinuria

c. hematuria

d. ketonuria

15.48. Which term means a projection in which the patient is facing the film and parallel to it?

a. anteroposterior

b. lateral

c. oblique

d. posteroanterior

15.49. Which term describes a laboratory technique in which a radioactively labeled substance is mixed with a blood specimen?

a. nuclear scan

b. perfusion

c. radioactive tracer

d. radioimmunoassay

15.50. Which term means the administration of a medication by injection?

a. parenteral

b. percutaneous

c. transcutaneous

d. transdermal

● Sentence Completion

Write the correct term on the line.

15.51. The path that the x-ray beam follows through the body from entrance to exit is known as the _____ .

15.52. When a factor in the patient's condition makes the use of a drug dangerous or ill-advised this is known as a/an _____ .

15.53. A "murmury" sound heard in auscultation, especially an abnormal one, is known as a/an _____ .

15.54. The instrument used to visually examine the external ear and the eardrum is a/an _____ .

15.55. A compulsive, uncontrollable dependence on a substance or drug is known as a/an _____ .

● True/False

If the statement is true, write T on the line. If the statement is false, write F on the line.

15.56. _____ Excessive exposure to x-radiation is dangerous and may cause death.

15.57. _____ A barium enema makes the stomach visible in a GI series.

15.58. _____ Compliance means that the patient has accurately followed instructions.

15.59. _____ A contrast medium makes it possible to image internal structures that otherwise cannot be seen on x-ray films.

15.60. _____ Ultrasound is used to produce images of cross sections of the body.

15.61. _____ For an oblique projection, the patient is positioned so that his body is parallel to the film.

15.62. _____ Prothrombin time is the number of seconds required for thromboplastin to coagulate plasma.

15.63. _____ A placebo has the potential of curing a disease.

15.64. _____ An MRI can safely be recommended for a patient with a pacemaker.

15.65. _____ Nuclear medicine is used to construct a three-dimensional image of the body.

● **Clinical Conditions**

Write the correct answer on the line.

15.66. The urinalysis for Rosita LaPinta showed the presence of pus. The medical term for this condition is _____ .

15.67. For the rectal examination, Mr. Johnson was placed in the _____-_____ position with his face down, his hips flexed and his knees and chest resting on the table.

15.68. In preparation for Kelly Harrison's thyroid scan, radioactive _____ was administered.

15.69. During her examination of the patient, Dr. Wong used _____ to feel the texture, size, consistency and location of certain body parts.

15.70. Dr. McDowell ordered a blood _____ _____ (BUN) test for his patient because this is a rough indicator of kidney function.

15.71. In preparation for his upper GI series, Dwight Oshone swallowed a liquid containing the contrast medium _____ .

15.72. Maria Martinez underwent _____ to reexpand her collapsed lung.

15.73. For the examination, Scott Cunningham was placed lying on his belly with his face down. This is a/an _____ position.

15.74. The urinalysis for Kathleen McCaffee showed the presence of glucose in the urine. The medical term for this condition is _____ .

15.75. During the examination, Dr. Roberts used _____ . This involves tapping the surface of the body with a finger or instrument.

● **Which is the correct medical term?**

Circle the letter next to the correct answer.

15.76. Which term means an undesirable drug response?

    a. adverse drug response

    b. idiosyncratic reaction

    c. potentiation

    d. synergism

15.77. Which examination position is also used for the treatment of shock?

    a. lithotomy

    b. recumbent

    c. Sims'

    d. Trendelenburg

15.78. Which dental radiograph shows the entire tooth and some of the surrounding tissue?

    a. bitewing

    b. extraoral

    c. intraoral

    d. periapical

15.79. Which imaging technique uses one to three gamma cameras to capture images?

    a. MRI

    b. positron emission tomography

    c. radioimmunoassay

    d. single photon emission computed tomography

15.80. Which examination position has the patient in a supine position with the feet and legs supported in stirrups?

a. decubitus

b. dorsal recumbent

c. lithotomy

d. Sims'

● **Challenge Word Building**

These terms are *not* found in this chapter; however, they are made up of these familiar word parts. You may want to look in the glossary or use a medical dictionary to check your answers!

hyper-	albumin/o	-centesis
hypo-	arthr/o	-emia
	calc/i	-gram
	cyst/o	-ology
	py/o	-scope
	glycos/o	-scopy
	protein/o	-uria
	radi/o	

15.81. The medical term meaning the visual examination of the interior of a joint is

_____ .

15.82. The medical term meaning an abnormally high level of albumin in the blood is

_____ .

15.83. The medical term meaning the presence of excess sugar in the urine is

_____ .

15.84. The instrument used to visually examine the interior of the urinary bladder is a/an

_____ .

15.85. The term meaning the study of the use radiant energy and radioactive substances in medicine is _____ .

15.86. The term meaning a surgical puncture to remove fluid from the interior of a joint is

_____ .

15.87. The medical term meaning an abnormally low level of calcium in the circulating blood is

_____ .

15.88. The term meaning the record produced by a radiographic study of blood vessels is a/an

_____ .

15.89. The medical term meaning the presence of pus-forming organisms in the blood is

_____ .

15.90. The medical term meaning the presence of excess protein in the urine is

_____ .

● Labeling Exercises

Identify the numbered items on these diagrams.

15.91. This is the _____ position.

15.92. This is the _____ recumbent position.

15.93. This is the _____ position.

15.94. This is the _____ recumbent position.

15.95. This is the _____ position.

15.96. This is the _____ position.

15.97. This is a/an _____ injection.

15.98. This is a/an _____ injection.

15.99. This is a/an _____ injection.

15.100. This is a/an _____ injection.

15.91

15.92

15.93

15.94

15.95

15.96

15.97   15.98   15.99   15.100

Epidermis
Dermis
Subcutaneous tissue
Muscle

The Human Touch: Critical Thinking Exercise

The following story and questions are designed to stimulate critical thinking through class discussion or as a brief essay response. There are no easy or right-wrong answers to these questions.

Seth and Hiroshi grew up at the beach, surfing and playing the party scene. After high school Hiroshi studied law enforcement and joined the police department. Seth bummed around the world chasing waves for a few more years before going to computer school and getting a job at Sebring Software.

One night while they were watching the game at the Tradewinds Sports Bar, Seth said to his old friend, "You'll never guess what Sebring's security is doing now." Seth's employer was always worried about an employee stealing programming ideas and marketing them to the competition.

"Don't tell me," Hiroshi smirked. "A guard makes surprise raids on your home computer to see if you've downloaded any Sebring secrets."

"Not that," Seth spoke seriously, "but just as bad. They're going to do random drug testing. Whether a person does a little weed at night to relax is nobody else's business!"

"Our department does drug testing all the time." Hiroshi pointed out.

"Yeah, but you carry guns. I wouldn't want to be pulled over by some drugged-out cop waving a weapon. Someone could get hurt!"

Hiroshi thought a moment and finished his drink. "Seth, you design programs that operate traffic lights. What would happen if you messed up?"

Suggested Discussion Topics:

1. Drug testing by urine sample is a common practice at many places of employment. Discuss how you would feel if it were required of you.

2. Some drugs can be detected in urine 72 hours after they have been taken. Should an employer be able to reprimand employees for something they did on their own time? Why?

3. What types of jobs do you think should have mandatory drug testing? Why?

4. If someone were taking recreational drugs and wanted to hide that fact, is there any way he or she could avoid testing positive?

5. Do you think mandatory drug testing makes the workplace or job safer? If so, why?

Comprehensive Medical Terminology Review

● **Overview of Comprehensive Medical Terminology Review**

Study Tips	Hints to help you review more effectively.
Review Session	A 100-question practice session with an answer key to let you determine where you need more study emphasis.
Confirming Mastery	A 100-multiple choice question "mock" final test with an answer key to help evaluate your progress.

VOCABULARY Vocabulary Review List

These terms, which were selected from the first 15 chapters, are those that most students have difficulty remembering. Review these terms and word parts then add others that you need to work on. *Note:* These terms *are not* on your audiotape.

Key Word Parts

- [ ] brady-
- [ ] colp/o
- [ ] -desis
- [ ] -emia
- [ ] encepha/o
- [ ] -ic
- [ ] -lysis
- [ ] mening/o
- [ ] metr/o
- [ ] -osis
- [ ] -pexy
- [ ] -pnea
- [ ] -ptosis
- [ ] tachy-
- [ ] -uria

Key Medical Terms

- [ ] **abdominocentesis** (ab-**dom**-ih-noh-sen-**TEE**-sis)
- [ ] **abruptio placentae** (ab-**RUP**-shee-oh plah-**SEN**-tee)
- [ ] **Alzheimer's disease** (**ALTZ**-high-merz)
- [ ] **amyotrophic lateral sclerosis** (ah-**my**-oh-**TROH**-fick)
- [ ] **angina** (an-**JIGH**-nah *or* **AN**-jih-nuh)
- [ ] **anorexia** (an-oh-**RECK**-see-ah)
- [ ] **arteriosclerosis** (ar-**tee**-ree-oh-skleh-**ROH**-sis)
- [ ] **astigmatism** (ah-**STIG**-mah-tizm)
- [ ] **atherosclerosis** (**ath**-er-oh-skleh-**ROH**-sis)
- [ ] **auscultation** (aws-kul-**TAY**-shun)
- [ ] **bruit** (**BREW**-ee *or* **BROOT**)
- [ ] **bulimia** (byou-**LIM**-ee-ah *or* boo-**LEE**-mee-ah)
- [ ] **carcinoma** (**kar**-sih-**NOH**-mah)
- [ ] **cerebral palsy** (**SER**-eh-bral *or* she-**REE**-bral **PAWL**-zee)
- [ ] **cerebrovascular accident** (**ser**-eh-broh-**VAS**-kyou-lar)
- [ ] **cholecystitis** (koh-lee-sis-**TYE**-tis)
- [ ] **cirrhosis** (sih-**ROH**-sis)
- [ ] **cystic fibrosis** (**SIS**-tick figh-**BROH**-sis)
- [ ] **diabetes mellitus** (**dye**-ah-**BEE**-teez mel-**EYE**-tus *or* **MEL**-ih-tus)
- [ ] **embolism** (**EM**-boh-lizm)
- [ ] **embolus** (**EM**-boh-lus)
- [ ] **emphysema** (**em**-fih-**SEE**-mah)
- [ ] **encephalitis** (**en**-sef-ah-**LYE**-tis)
- [ ] **esophageal reflux** (eh-**sof**-ah-**JEE**-al **REE**-flucks)
- [ ] **esophageal varices** (eh-**sof**-ah-**JEE**-al **VAYR**-ih-seez)
- [ ] **Guillain-Barré syndrome** (gee-**YAHN**-bah-**RAY**)
- [ ] **hemangioma** (hee-**man**-jee-**OH**-mah *or* heh-**man**-jee-**OH**-mah)
- [ ] **hemodialysis** (hee-moh-dye-**AL**-ih-sis)

- [ ] **hysterosalpingo-oophorectomy** (**hiss**-ter-oh-sal-**ping**-goh-oh-**ahf**-oh-**RECK**-toh-mee)
- [ ] **intussusception** (**in**-tus-sus-**SEP**-shun)
- [ ] **ischemia** (iss-**KEE**-me-ah)
- [ ] **jaundice** (**JAWN**-dis)
- [ ] **laparoscopy** (**lap**-ah-**ROS**-koh-pee)
- [ ] **leukemia** (loo-**KEE**-me-ah)
- [ ] **lithotripsy** (**LITH**-oh-**trip**-see)
- [ ] **lymphoma** (lim-**FOH**-mah)
- [ ] **melanoma** (mel-ah-**NOH**-mah)
- [ ] **Menière's syndrome** (**men**-ee-**AYRZ** *or* men-**YEHRS**)
- [ ] **meningitis** (**men**-in-**JIGH**-tis)
- [ ] **metastasis** (meh-**TAS**-tah-sis)
- [ ] **metastasize** (meh-**TAS**-tah-sighz)
- [ ] **multiple sclerosis** (skleh-**ROH**-sis)
- [ ] **muscular dystrophy** (**DIS**-troh-fee)
- [ ] **myocardial infarction** (**my**-oh-**KAR**-dee-al in-**FARK**-shun)
- [ ] **myopia** (my-**OH**-pee-ah)
- [ ] **nephrolithiasis** (**nef**-roh-lih-**THIGH**-ah-sis)
- [ ] **osteomyelitis** (**oss**-tee-oh-**my**-eh-**LYE**-tis)
- [ ] **Papanicolaou test** (**pap**-ah-**nick**-oh-**LAY**-ooh)
- [ ] **perimenopause** (**pehr**-ih-**MEN**-oh-pawz)
- [ ] **peritoneal dialysis** (**pehr**-ih-toh-**NEE**-al dye-**AL**-ih-sis)
- [ ] **phlebitis** (fleh-**BYE**-tis)
- [ ] **placenta previa** (plah-**SEN**-tah **PREE**-vee-ah)
- [ ] **pleurisy** (**PLOOR**-ih-see)
- [ ] **pneumothorax** (new-moh-**THOR**-racks)
- [ ] **presbycusis** (**pres**-beh-**KOO**-sis)
- [ ] **presbyopia** (**pres**-bee-**OH**-pee-ah)
- [ ] **psoriasis** (soh-**RYE**-uh-sis)
- [ ] **rale** (**RAHL**)
- [ ] **Raynaud's** (ray-**NOHZ**)
- [ ] **rhonchus** (**RONG**-kus)
- [ ] **salpingo-oophorectomy** (sal-**ping**-goh-oh-**ahf**-oh-**RECK**-toh-mee)
- [ ] **sarcoma** (sar-**KOH**-mah)
- [ ] **scoliosis** (skoh-lee-**OH**-sis)
- [ ] **strabismus** (strah-**BIZ**-mus)
- [ ] **stridor** (**STRYE**-dor)
- [ ] **thrombosis** (throm-**BOH**-sis)
- [ ] **thrombus** (**THROM**-bus)
- [ ] **tracheostomy** (**tray**-kee-**OS**-toh-mee)
- [ ] **tracheotomy** (**tray**-kee-**OT**-oh-mee)
- [ ] **transient ischemic attack** (iss-**KEE**-mick)
- [ ] **trauma** (**TRAW**-mah)
- [ ] **triage** (tree-**AHZH**)
- [ ] **volvulus** (**VOL**-view-lus)
- [ ] **xeroderma** (zee-roh-**DER**-mah)
- [ ] **xerophthalmia** (**zeer**-ahf-**THAL**-mee-ah)

● OBJECTIVES

On completion of this chapter, you should be able to:

1. Recognize, define, spell, and pronounce the terms on the vocabulary lists for the first 15 chapters.

2. Recognize and define the word parts from the flash cards.

3. Recognize, define, spell, and pronounce the medical terms in Appendix C.

Study Tips

Use Your Vocabulary Lists

- After you have added any terms suggested by your instructor, photocopy the vocabulary list for each chapter. These sheets are easy to carry with you for additional review whenever you have a free minute.

- Review the terms on each list. When you have mastered a term, put a check in the box next to it. If you cannot spell and define a term, highlight it for further study.

- Look up the meanings of the highlighted terms in the text or glossary and work toward mastering them.

Use Your Flash Cards

- Use your flash cards from the back of the book.

- As you go through them, remove from the stack all those word parts you can define.

- Keep working until you've mastered all of these word parts.

Use Appendix C

- Appendix C contains all of the pathology and procedure terms from the textbook — plus those challenge word-building terms you encountered at the end of each chapter.

- Review the terms in this section. Put a check mark next to the terms you know. Highlight terms you have not mastered and next time through concentrate on these terms.

Make Your Own Study List

- By now you should have greatly reduced the number of terms still to be mastered. Make a list of these terms and word parts and concentrate on them.

Help Someone Else

- One of the greatest ways to really learn something is by teaching it! If a classmate is having trouble, tutoring that person will help both of you learn the material.

Review Session

Number a paper from RS.1 to RS.100 and write your answers on this sheet — then check them against the answer key. All answer choices are actual medical terms that you should be able to define. If you are not sure of a meaning, look the term up in the glossary or in your medical dictionary.

This section contains exercises that bring together information from *all* of the chapters. A wrong answer means you need more work on that area!

Review Questions

● Matching Word Parts—1

Write the letter of your answer on the answer sheet.

RS.1. _____ brady-   A. abnormal condition

RS.2. _____ colp/o   B. rapid

RS.3. _____ metr/o   C. slow

RS.4. _____ -osis   D. uterus

RS.5. _____ tachy-   E. vagina

● Matching Word Parts—2

Write the letter of the your answer on the answer sheet.

RS.6. _____ -desis   A. prolapse

RS.7. _____ -ic   B. setting free

RS.8. _____ -lysis   C. surgical fixation

RS.9. _____ -pexy   D. to bind together

RS.10. _____ -ptosis   E. pertaining to

● Matching Word Parts—3

Write the letter of the your answer on the answer sheet.

RS.11. _____ -emia   A. breathing

RS.12. _____ encephal/o   B. urine

RS.13. _____ mening/o   C. blood condition

RS.14. _____ -pnea   D. brain

RS.15. _____ -uria   E. brain covering

● Definitions

Write the letter of the your answer on the answer sheet.

RS.16. Which term means the surgical removal of a joint?

a. angiectomy

b. arteriectomy

c. atherectomy

d. arthrectomy

RS.17. Which term means the abnormal development or growth of cells?

a. dyscrasia

b. dyslexia

c. dysmenorrhea

d. dysplasia

RS.18. Which form of anemia is a genetic disorder?

a. aplastic anemia

b. hemolytic anemia

c. megaloblastic anemia

d. sickle cell anemia

RS.19. Which condition is characterized by rapidly worsening muscle weakness that may lead to temporary paralysis?

a. Becker's muscular dystrophy

b. Bell's palsy

c. Guillain-Barré syndrome

d. Raynaud's phenomenon

RS.20. Which term describes a benign tumor made up of newly formed blood vessels?

a. hemangioma

b. hematemesis

c. hematoma

d. hematuria

RS.21. Which term means slight paralysis of one side of the body?

a. hemiparesis

b. hemiplegia

c. myoparesis

d. quadriplegia

RS.22. Which term means the surgical removal of part of the stomach and upper portion of the small intestine?

a. esophagogastrectomy

b. esophagoplasty

c. gastroduodenostomy

d. gastrostomy

RS.23. Which term describes an added sound with a musical pitch during breathing that is also known as wheezing?

a. bruit

b. rale

c. rhonchus

d. stridor

RS.24. Which term means bleeding from the bladder?

a. cystoptosis

b. cystorrhagia

c. cystorrhaphy

d. cystorrhexis

RS.25. Which skin condition is caused by a staphylo-coccal infection and is commonly known as a boil?

a. abscess

b. carbuncle

c. furuncle

d. pustule

● Matching Genetic Disorders

Write the letter of the your answer on the answer sheet.

RS.26. _____ cystic fibrosis   A. Missing an essential digestive enzyme.

RS.27. _____ hemochroma-   B. Characterized by short-tosis   lived red blood cells.

RS.28. _____ phenylketo-   C. Causes abnormal nuria   hemoglobin.

RS.29. _____ sickle cell   D. Also known as iron anemia   overload disease.

RS.30. _____ thalassemia   E. Affects the lungs and digestive system

● Which Word?

Write the term you selected on the answer sheet.

RS.31. The term meaning the absence of normal sensitivity to pain is *anesthesia* / *anesthetic*.

RS.32. The term meaning any fungus infection of the nail is *onychocryptosis* / *onychomycosis*.

RS.33. The term meaning the ongoing presence of a disease within a population, group, or area is *endemic* / *pandemic*.

RS.34. The surgical stiffening of a joint or joining of spinal vertebrae is called *arthrodesis* / *arthrolysis*.

RS.35. The term meaning an accumulation of pus in the pleural cavity is *atelectasis* / *empyema*.

● Spelling Counts

Find the misspelled word in each sentence. Then write that word, spelled correctly, on your answer sheet.

RS.36. An opthalmologist specializes in diagnosing and treating diseases and disorders of the eye.

RS.37. The progressive loss of lung function due a decrease in the total number of alveoli is known as empysema.

RS.38. Altzheimer's disease is group of disorders associated with degenerative changes in the brain structure.

RS.39. The term blepharodema means swelling of the eyelid.

RS.40. The term oligospermism is also known as a low sperm count.

● Matching Bone Conditions

Write the letter of the your answer on the answer sheet.

RS.41. _____ osteomalacia   A. Abnormal hardening of bone.

RS.42. _____ osteonecrosis   B. Abnormal softening of bones.

RS.43. _____ osteoporosis   C. Death of bone tissue.

RS.44. _____ osteosarcoma   D. Loss of bone density.

RS.45. _____ osteosclerosis   E. Malignant bone tumor.

● Term Selection

Write the letter of the your answer on the answer sheet.

RS.46. Which condition is commonly known as a bruise?

  a. ecchymosis

  b. embolus

  c. emesis

  d. epistaxis

RS.47. Which respiratory condition in children and infants is characterized by obstruction of the larynx, hoarseness, and a barking cough?

  a. asthma

  b. croup

  c. diphtheria

  d. pneumonia

RS.48. Which term means a neoplasm composed of immature undifferentiated cells?

  a. adenocarcinoma

  b. blastoma

  c. malignant melanoma

  d. squamous cell carcinoma

RS.49. Which of these sexually transmitted diseases is caused by a spirochete?

  a. chlamydia

  b. gonorrhea

  c. syphilis

  d. trichomonas

RS.50. Which term describes a blood clot attached to the interior wall of a vein or artery?

    a. embolism

    b. embolus

    c. thrombosis

    d. thrombus

● Sentence Completion

Write the answer, spelled correctly, on your answer sheet.

RS.51. The term meaning abnormal enlargement of the liver is _____ .

RS.52. The term meaning a pounding or racing heart is _____ .

RS.53. The surgical removal of a portion of the tissue surrounding the heart is a/an

_____ .

RS.54. A surgical connection between two hollow or tubular structures is a/an

_____ .

RS.55. Medication administered to expand the opening of the passages into the lungs is a/an

_____ .

● True/False

Write the answer on your answer sheet. Use T if the statement is true. Use F if the answer is false.

RS.56. _____ Ileus is a temporary stoppage of intestinal peristalsis.

RS.57. _____ Hypothyroidism is a condition of excessive thyroid hormones in the blood.

RS.58. _____ Hysterorrhexis means to suture the uterus.

RS.59. _____ Nyctalopia is also known as night blindness.

RS.60. _____ Hypoglycemia is an abnormally low concentration of glucose in the blood.

RS.61. _____ Volvulus is the telescoping of one part of the intestine into the opening of an immediately adjacent part.

RS.62. _____ Nocturia is excessive urination during the night.

RS.63. _____ Myelography is a radiographic study of the bone marrow after the injection of a contrast medium.

RS.64. _____ Muscular dystrophy is a group of inherited muscle disorders that cause muscle weakness without affecting the nervous system.

RS.65. _____ Nephromalacia is abnormal hardening of the kidney.

● Clinical Conditions

Write the term, spelled correctly, on the answer sheet.

RS.66. Jewel Martin has a progressive autoimmune disorder characterized by scattered patches of demyelination of nerve fibers of the brain and spinal cord. The medical term for this condition is _____

_____ .

RS.67. Mr. Kuebler suffers from fine muscle tremors, has a masklike facial expression, and walks with a shuffling gait. The medical term for his progressive condition is _____

_____ .

RS.68. Jose Ramirez told his friends that he had a heart attack. The medical term for this is a/an

_____ _____ .

RS.69. Wayne Oliveri, who works all day at a keyboard, was diagnosed as having inflammation of the tendons passing through the carpal tunnel of the wrist. The condition is known as

_____ _____

syndrome.

RS.70. After the accident, Todd suffered from nerve pain caused by pressure on the spinal nerve roots in the neck region. The medical term for this condition is _____

_____ .

RS.71. Nurse Ortega observed his patient's pattern of alternating periods of rapid breathing, slow breathing, and the absence of breathing. He recorded this on the chart as

_____ _____

respiration.

RS.72. At age 45, George was diagnosed as having a hereditary disorder with symptoms that first appear in midlife and cause the irreversible and progressive loss of muscle control and mental ability. George has _____ disease.

RS.73. Megan Wilson's surgeon removed her gallbladder while working through very small openings in the abdominal wall. The medical term for this procedure is a/an _____

_____ .

RS.74. Carrie is abnormally afraid of being in narrow or enclosed spaces. This medical term for this condition is _____ .

RS.75. Brian was diagnosed as having peptic ulcers in the upper part of the small intestine. The medical term for this condition is

_____ _____ .

● Which is the correct medical term?

Write the letter of the your answer on the answer sheet.

RS.76. Which term means the removal or destruction of the function of a body part?

    a. ablation

    b. abrasion

    c. cryosurgery

    d. exfoliative cytology

RS.77. Which term means a woman who has delivered one child?

    a. nulligravida

    b. nullipara

    c. primigravida

    d. primipara

RS.78. Which term means inflammation of the pancreas?

    a. pancreatalgia

    b. pancreatectomy

    c. pancreatitis

    d. pancreatotomy

RS.79. Which term means an abnormally increased amount of cerebrospinal fluid within the brain?

    a. hydrocele

    b. hydrocephalus

    c. hydronephrosis

    d. hydroureter

RS.80. Which term means the surgical repair of the vagina?

    a. colpopexy

    b. colporrhaphy

    c. vaginoplasty

    d. valvoplasty

● Word Building With the "Double RR's"

Write the term, spelled correctly, on the answer sheet.

RS.81. The term meaning to suture torn fascia is

_____ .

RS.82. The term meaning an excessive flow of mucus from the nose is _____ .

RS.83. The term meaning rupture of the bladder is

_____ .

RS.84. The term meaning rupture of the stomach is

_____ .

RS.85. The term meaning bleeding from the spleen is

_____ .

RS.86. The term meaning to suture the ends of a severed nerve is _____ .

RS.87. The term meaning bleeding from the ureter is

_____ .

RS.88. The term meaning the rupture of a muscle is

_____ .

RS.89. The term meaning the excessive flow of gastric secretions is _____ .

RS.90. The term meaning to suture the tissue surrounding the heart is _____ .

● Medical Specialty Review

Write the term, spelled correctly, on the answer sheet.

RS.91. A specialist in diagnosing and treating diseases, disorders, and problems associated with aging is a/an _____ .

RS.92. A specialist, other than a physician, trained in administering anesthesia is a/an

_____ .

RS.93. A specialist in measuring the accuracy of vision to determine if corrective lenses or eyeglasses are needed is a/an _____ .

RS.94. A specialist in diagnosing and treating diseases and disorders of the female reproductive system is a/an _____ .

RS.95. A specialist in diagnosing, treating, and preventing disorders and diseases of children is a/an _____ .

RS.96. A specialist in manipulative treatment of disorders originating from misalignment of the spine is a/an _____ .

RS.97. A specialist in the prevention and treatment of disorders of the tissues surrounding the teeth is a/an _____ .

RS.98. A specialist diagnosing and treating diseases and disorders of the lungs and associated tissues is a/an _____ .

RS.99. A specialist diagnosing, treating and correcting disorders of the foot is a/an

_____ .

RS.100. A specialist in providing medical care to women during pregnancy, childbirth, and immediately thereafter is a/an

_____ .

● Review Session Answer Key

RS.1	C	RS.26	E	RS.51	hepatomegaly	RS.76	A
RS.2	E	RS.27	D	RS.52	palpitation	RS.77	D
RS.3	D	RS.28	A	RS.53	pericardiectomy	RS.78	C
RS.4	A	RS.29	C	RS.54	anastomosis	RS.79	B
RS.5	B	RS.30	B	RS.55	bronchodilator	RS.80	C
RS.6	D	RS.31	anesthesia	RS.56	T	RS.81	fasciorrhaphy
RS.7	E	RS.32	onychomycosis	RS.57	F	RS.82	rhinorrhea
RS.8	B	RS.33	endemic	RS.58	F	RS.83	cystorrhexis
RS.9	C	RS.34	arthrodesis	RS.59	T	RS.84	gastrorrhexis
RS.10	A	RS.35	empyema	RS.60	T	RS.85	splenorrhagia
RS.11	C	RS.36	ophthalmologist	RS.61	F	RS.86	neurorrhaphy
RS.12	D	RS.37	emphysema	RS.62	T	RS.87	ureterorrhagia
RS.13	E	RS.38	Alzheimer's	RS.63	F	RS.88	myorrhexis
RS.14	A	RS.39	blepharedema	RS.64	T	RS.89	gastrorrhea
RS.15	B	RS.40	oligospermia	RS.65	F	RS.90	pericardiorrhaphy
RS.16	D	RS.41	B	RS.66	multiple sclerosis	RS.91	gerontologist
RS.17	D	RS.42	C	RS.67	Parkinson's disease	RS.92	anesthetist
RS.18	D	RS.43	D	RS.68	myocardial infarction	RS.93	optometrist
RS.19	C	RS.44	E	RS.69	carpel tunnel	RS.94	gynecologist
RS.20	A	RS.45	A	RS.70	cervical radiculopathy	RS.95	pediatrician
RS.21	A	RS.46	A	RS.71	Cheyne-Stokes	RS.96	chiropractor
RS.22	C	RS.47	B	RS.72	Huntington's	RS.97	periodontist
RS.23	C	RS.48	B	RS.73	laparoscopic cholecystecomy	RS.98	pulmonologist
RS.24	B	RS.49	C	RS.74	claustrophobia	RS.99	podiatrist
RS.25	C	RS.50	D	RS.75	duodenal ulcers	RS.100	obstetrician

Confirming Mastery

Number a paper from FT.1 to FT.100 and write the letter of your answers on this sheet. When you have finished, check your answers against the answer key.

A wrong answer identifies an area where you need more work. All answer choices are actual medical terms that you should be able to define. If you are not sure of their meanings, look in the glossary or use your medical dictionary.

Because this is not actually the final test, you can go back and retake it as often as you want. Good Luck!

● Medical Terminology Final Examination

FT.1. Which medical term describes a torn or ragged wound?

a. fissure

b. fistula

c. laceration

d. lesion

FT.2. The term cystopexy means

a. drooping of the urinary bladder.

b. inflammation of the gallbladder.

c. laparoscopic examination of the gallbladder.

d. surgical fixation of the urinary bladder.

FT.3. Which medical term is commonly known as a heart attack?

a. arthrostenosis

b. myocardial infarction

c. transient ischemic attack

d. ventricular fibrillation

FT.4. Which term means inflammation of the connective tissues that enclose the spinal cord and brain?

a. encephalitis

b. encephalopathy

c. meningitis

d. myelopathy

FT.5. Which disease is also known as osteitis deformans?

a. Crone's disease

b. Ewing's sarcoma

c. Paget's disease

d. Raynaud's phenomenon

FT.6. The term myorrhexis means

a. bleeding from the spinal cord.

b. rupture of a muscle.

c. rupture of the spinal cord.

d. to suture a muscle.

FT.7. Which term means abnormal softening of the kidney?

a. nephromalacia

b. nephrosclerosis

c. neuromalacia

d. neurosclerosis

FT.8. A life-threatening complication of uncontrolled diabetes mellitus is

a. an embolism.

b. a thrombus.

c. convulsions.

d. diabetic ketoacidosis.

FT.9. A carotid endarterectomy is performed to

a. prevent a heart attack.

b. prevent a stroke.

c. relieve angina symptoms.

d. treat hypertension.

FT.10. Which medical term means the flow of pus from the ear?

a. otopyorrhea

b. otorrhagia

c. pyoderma

d. pyosalpinx

FT.11. Which term is commonly known as itching?

a. perfusion

b. pruritus

c. purpura

d. suppuration

FT.12. Which term means spasmodic choking pain due to interference with the oxygen supply to the heart muscle?

a. angina pectoris

b. claudication

c. cyanosis

d. myocardial infarction

FT.13. Which condition is also known as trigeminal neuralgia?

a. Hodgkin's disease

b. Lou Gehrig's disease

c. tic douloureux

d. torticollis

FT.14. Which term means an unexpected reaction to a drug?

a. adverse

b. idiosyncratic

c. placebo

d. palliative

FT.15. Which term means a prediction of the probable course and outcome of a disease or disorder?

a. differential diagnosis

b. diagnosis

c. prognosis

d. syndrome

FT.16. Which term means blue discoloration of the skin caused by a lack of adequate oxygen?

a. cyanosis

b. erythroderma

c. leukoplakia

d. melanosis

FT.17. A Colles' fracture is associated with which bone disease?

a. osteomalacia

b. osteomyelitis

c. osteoporosis

d. otosclerosis

FT.18. Which medical term is commonly known as bed-wetting?

a. nocturnal myoclonus

b. nocturnal enuresis

c. nocturia

d. urinary incontinence

FT.19. Which medical term describes any benign skin condition in which there is overgrowth and thickening of the epidermis?

a. epithelioma

b. keratosis

c. melanoma

d. papilloma

FT.20. Which term means inflammation of the lymph nodes?

a. adenoiditis

b. angiitis

c. lymphadenitis

d. lymphangioma

FT.21. Which term describes a sudden, involuntary contraction of a muscle?

a. adhesion

b. contracture

c. spasm

d. stricture

FT.22. Which respiratory disease is commonly known as whooping cough?

a. croup

b. diphtheria

c. emphysema

d. pertussis

FT.23. Which body system is affected by the autoimmune disorder known as Crohn's disease?

a. digestive

b. endocrine

c. nervous

d. reproductive

FT.24. Which condition is commonly known as low back pain?

a. kyphosis

b. lordosis

c. lumbago

d. scoliosis

FT.25. Which term means the surgical creation of an opening between the small intestine and the body surface?

a. colostomy

b. enteropexy

c. gastroptosis

d. ileostomy

FT.26. Which visualization technique is used to examine body parts in motion?

a. computed tomography

b. fluoroscopy

c. magnetic resonance imaging

d. radiography

FT.27. Which term means bleeding from the pharynx?

a. epistaxis

b. pharyngoplegia

c. pharyngorrhagia

d. pharyngorrhea

FT.28. Which autoimmune disease gradually destroys thyroid tissue?

a. Cushing's syndrome

b. goiter

c. Hashimoto's

d. Parkinson's disease

FT.29. Which term means a pus-producing inflammation of the uterus?

a. leukorrhea

b. metrorrhea

c. pyometritis

d. pyosalpinx

FT.30. Which term describes the syndrome characterized by sudden, severe, sharp headache usually present only on one side?

a. cephalagia

b. migraine headache

c. myxedema

d. tic douloureux

FT.31. Which term means vomiting blood?

a. epistaxis

b. hemarthrosis

c. hematemesis

d. hyperemesis

FT.32. Which term describes the condition commonly known as a bruise?

a. ecchymosis

b. exophthalmos

c. hematoma

d. hemangioma

FT.33. Which term means abnormally rapid, deep breathing resulting in decreased levels of carbon dioxide at the cellular level?

a. apnea

b. dyspnea

c. hyperventilation

d. hypoventilation

FT.34. Which medical term means difficult or painful urination?

a. dyskinesia

b. dyspepsia

c. dysphagia

d. dysuria

FT.35. Which terms means a false personal belief that is maintained despite obvious proof to the contrary?

a. delirium

b. delusion

c. dementia

d. hallucination

FT.36. Which type of abnormal heartbeat is known as tachycardia?

a. fast

b. fluttering

c. weak

d. slow

FT.37. Which eye condition is characterized by increased intraocular pressure?

a. cataracts

b. glaucoma

c. macular degeneration

d. monochromatism

FT.38. Which diagnostic tool is used to image the brain and spinal cord?

a. echoencephalography

b. electroencephalography

c. magnetic resonance imaging

d. ultrasound

FT.39. Which vision condition is commonly known as nearsightedness?

a. hyperopia

b. myopia

c. presbyopia

d. strabismus

FT.40. Which body cavity protects the brain?

a. anterior

b. cranial

c. superior

d. ventral

FT.41. Which term means a hernia of the bladder through the vaginal wall?

a. cystocele

b. cystopexy

c. vaginocele

d. vesicovaginal fissure

FT.42. Which term means a violent shaking up or jarring of the brain caused by a direct blow or explosion?

a. cerebral concussion

b. cerebral contusion

c. intracerebral hematoma

d. subdural hematoma

FT.43. Which term means a ringing sound in the ears?

a. presbycusis

b. syncope

c. tinnitus

d. vertigo

FT.44. Which term means a sudden and widespread outbreak of a disease within a population group or area?

a. endemic

b. epidemic

c. pandemic

d. syndrome

FT.45. Which term means an excessive flow of gastric secretions?

a. achlorhydria

b. aerophagia

c. gastrorrhea

d. gastrorrhexis

FT.46. Which term describes a small flat discolored lesion such as a freckle?

a. macule

b. papule

c. plaque

d. vesicle

FT.47. The Western blot blood test is used to

a. confirm an HIV infection.

b. detect hepatitis B.

c. diagnose Kaposi's sarcoma.

d. test for tuberculosis.

FT.48. Which term means excessive uterine bleeding occurring both during the menses and at irregular intervals?

a. dysmenorrhea

b. menometrorrhagia

c. menorrhagia

d. mittelschmerz

FT.49. Which term describes an injury that does not break the skin and is characterized by swelling, discoloration, and pain?

a. concussion

b. contusion

c. laceration

d. lesion

FT.50. Which term describes an abnormal rattle or crackle-like respiratory sound heard during inspiration?

a. bruit

b. rale

c. rhonchus

d. stridor

FT.51. Which medical term is commonly known as wear and tear arthritis?

a. gouty arthritis

b. osteoarthritis

c. rheumatoid arthritis

d. spondylosis

FT.52. Which term means to free a tendon from adhesions?

a. tenodesis

b. tenolysis

c. tenorrhaphy

d. tenotomy

FT.53. The term debilitated means

a. lacking adequate fluid.

b. mental impairment.

c. mentally confused due to a high fever.

d. weakened or having lost strength.

FT.54. Which term describes a progressive degenerative disease characterized by disturbance of structure and function of the liver?

a. cirrhosis

b. hepatitis A

c. hepatitis E

d. jaundice

FT.55. Which procedure removes waste products directly from the blood of patients whose kidneys no longer function?

a. diuresis

b. epispadias

c. hemodialysis

d. peritoneal dialysis

FT.56. Which medical condition is commonly known as fainting?

a. comatose

b. narcolepsy

c. stupor

d. syncope

FT.57. Which term means a deficiency of blood supply due to the constriction or obstruction of a blood vessel?

a. embolism

b. infarction

c. ischemia

d. thrombosis

FT.58. Which term means an accumulation of blood in the pleural cavity?

a. hemophilia

b. hemoptysis

c. hemostasis

d. hemothorax

FT.59. Which term means the return of swallowed food into the mouth?

a. emesis

b. nausea

c. reflux

d. regurgitation

FT.60. Which condition is caused by prolonged exposure to high levels of cortisol?

a. Addison's disease

b. Cushing's syndrome

c. Huntington's disease

d. Parkinson's disease

FT.61. Which term describes a yellow discoloration of the skin caused by abnormal amounts of bilirubin in the blood?

a. cyanosis

b. ileus

c. jaundice

d. volvulus

FT.62. Which term means excessive urination?

a. anuria

b. oliguria

c. polyuria

d. pyuria

FT.63. Which term means the surgical removal of the gallbladder?

a. cholecystectomy

b. cholecystostomy

c. cholecystotomy

d. choledocholithotomy

FT.64. Which blood test is used to detect the presence of inflammation in the body?

a. agglutination

b. a platelet count

c. complete blood cell count

d. erythrocyte sedimentation rate

FT.65. Which term means a closed sac or pouch containing fluid or semisolid material?

a. abscess

b. cyst

c. pustule

d. ulcer

FT.66. Which type of injection is administered within the substance of a muscle?

a. intradermal

b. intramuscular

c. intravenous

d. subcutaneous

FT.67. Which term means abnormal tipping forward of the uterus and cervix?

a. anteversion

b. prolapse

c. retroflexion

d. retroversion

FT.68. Which term means inflammation of the brain?

a. encephalitis

b. mastitis

c. meningitis

d. myelitis

FT.69. Which term means a spasm or twitching of a muscle or group of muscles?

a. contractures

b. myoclonus

c. seizures

d. tremors

FT.70. Which term describes the condition when the heart is unable to pump enough blood to meet the body's needs?

a. congestive heart failure

b. hypoperfusion

c. myocarditis

d. mitral valve prolapse

FT.71. Which term means a hospital-acquired infection?

a. functional disorder

b. iatrogenic illness

c. idiopathic disorder

d. nosocomial infection

FT.72. Which term means a malignant tumor that arises from connective tissue?

a. blastoma

b. carcinoma

c. malignant melanoma

d. sarcoma

FT.73. Which term describes the eye disorder that may develop as a complication of diabetes?

a. diabetic neuropathy

b. diabetic retinopathy

c. papilledema

d. retinal detachment

FT.74. Which term describes an eating disorder characterized by refusing to maintain a minimally normal body weight and an intense fear of gaining weight?

a. anorexia nervosa

b. bulimia nervosa

c. hypochondriasis

d. pica

FT.75. Which term means the presence of blood in the urine?

a. albuminuria

b. blood urea nitrogen

c. hematuria

d. proteinuria

FT.76. Which term describes the condition caused when a blood vessel in the brain leaks or ruptures?

a. cerebral hematoma

b. embolism

c. hemorrhagic stroke

d. ischemic stroke

FT.77. Which term describes the condition characterized by enlargement of the hands and feet caused by excessive secretion of the growth hormone *after* puberty?

a. acromegaly

b. acrophobia

c. cretinism

d. gigantism

FT.78. Which terms means an ingrown toenail?

a. cryptorchidism

b. onychocryptosis

c. onychophagia

d. oophoropexy

FT.79. An otoscope is used to examine the

a. adnexa of the eye.

b. auditory canal and tympanic membrane.

c. eustachian tube.

d. retina and optic nerve of the eye.

FT.80. Which term means protrusion of part of the stomach through the esophageal opening in the diaphragm.

a. esophageal hernia

b. esophageal varices

c. hiatal hernia

d. hiatal varices

FT.81. Which term means a surgical incision of the vulva to facilitate delivery of a baby?

a. episiorrhaphy

b. episiotomy

c. epispadias

d. epistaxis

FT.82. Which term describes a condition of severe itching of the external female genitalia?

a. colpitis

b. leukorrhea

c. pruritus vulvae

d. vaginal candidiasis

FT.83. Which term describes an infestation commonly known as head lice?

a. pediculosis capitis

b. pediculosis pubis

c. tinea capitis

d. tinea pedis

FT.84. Which instrument is used to enlarge the opening of a canal or body cavity to make it possible to inspect its interior?

a. endoscope

b. speculum

c. sphygmomanometer

d. stethoscope

FT.85. Cellulitis is a

a. diffuse infection of connective tissue.

b. dry patch made up of excess dead epidermal cells.

c. groove or crack-like sore.

d. localized collection of pus.

FT.86. Which term means a malignant tumor composed of cells derived from hemopoietic tissues of the bone marrow?

a. mycosis

b. myelitis

c. myeloma

d. myelosis

FT.87. Which term means an inflammation of the lungs in which the air sacs fill with pus and other liquid?

a. pneumoconiosis

b. pneumonia

c. pneumonitis

d. pneumothorax

FT.88. Which term means ankylosis of the bones of the middle ear resulting in a conductive hearing loss?

a. labyrinthitis

b. mastoiditis

c. osteosclerosis

d. otosclerosis

FT.89. Which term means to free a tendon from adhesions?

a. arthrodesis

b. arthrolysis

c. tenodesis

d. tenolysis

FT.90. Which term means to suture the vagina?

    a. colporrhaphy

    b. cystorrhaphy

    c. hepatorrhaphy

    d. hysterorrhaphy

FT.91. Which term means the surgical removal of plaque from the interior lining of an artery?

    a. angiectomy

    b. arteriectomy

    c. atherectomy

    d. arthrectomy

FT.92. Which term means abnormally increased motor function or activity?

    a. bradykinesia

    b. dyskinesia

    c. hyperkinesia

    d. hypokinesia

FT.93. Which term means difficulty in swallowing?

    a. dyspepsia

    b. dysphagia

    c. dysphonia

    d. dysplasia

FT.94. Which term means the process of recording electrical brain wave activity?

    a. echoencephalography

    b. electroencephalography

    c. electromyography

    d. electroneuromyography

FT.95. Which term means a woman who has never been pregnant?

    a. nulligravida

    b. nullipara

    c. primigravida

    d. primipara

FT.96. Which eye condition causes the loss of central vision but not total blindness?

    a. cataracts

    b. glaucoma

    c. macular degeneration

    d. presbyopia

FT.97. Which term means the surgical removal of excess skin for the elimination of wrinkles?

    a. blepharoplasty

    b. plication

    c. rhytidectomy

    d. sclerotherapy

FT.98. Which term means a group of inherited muscle disorders that cause muscle weakness without affecting the nervous system?

    a. multiple sclerosis

    b. muscular dystrophy

    c. myasthenia gravis

    d. Parkinson's disease

FT.99. Which term describes the process by which cancer spreads from one place to another?

    a. metabolism

    b. metastasis

    c. metastasize

    d. staging

FT.100. Which term means a collection of blood trapped within tissues?

    a. hemangioma

    b. hematemesis

    c. hematoma

    d. hematuria

● Final Test Answer Key

FT.1	C	FT.21	C	FT.41	A	FT.61	C	FT.81	B
FT.2	D	FT.22	D	FT.42	A	FT.62	C	FT.82	C
FT.3	B	FT.23	A	FT.43	C	FT.63	A	FT.83	A
FT.4	C	FT.24	C	FT.44	B	FT.64	D	FT.84	B
FT.5	C	FT.25	D	FT.45	C	FT.65	B	FT.85	A
FT.6	B	FT.26	B	FT.46	A	FT.66	B	FT.86	C
FT.7	A	FT.27	C	FT.47	A	FT.67	A	FT.87	B
FT.8	D	FT.28	C	FT.48	B	FT.68	A	FT.88	D
FT.9	B	FT.29	C	FT.49	B	FT.69	B	FT.89	D
FT.10	A	FT.30	B	FT.50	B	FT.70	A	FT.90	A
FT.11	B	FT.31	C	FT.51	B	FT.71	D	FT.91	C
FT.12	A	FT.32	A	FT.52	B	FT.72	D	FT.92	C
FT.13	C	FT.33	C	FT.53	D	FT.73	B	FT.93	B
FT.14	B	FT.34	D	FT.54	A	FT.74	A	FT.94	B
FT.15	C	FT.35	B	FT.55	C	FT.75	C	FT.95	A
FT.16	A	FT.36	A	FT.56	D	FT.76	C	FT.96	C
FT.17	C	FT.37	B	FT.57	C	FT.77	A	FT.97	C
FT.18	B	FT.38	C	FT.58	D	FT.78	B	FT.98	B
FT.19	B	FT.39	B	FT.59	D	FT.79	B	FT.99	C
FT.20	C	FT.40	B	FT.60	B	FT.80	C	FT.100	C

Appendix A:
Prefixes, Word Roots (Combining Forms), and Suffixes

Pertaining to

-ac	pertaining to
-al	pertaining to
-ar	pertaining to
-ary	pertaining to
-eal	pertaining to
-ical	pertaining to
-ial	pertaining to
-ic	pertaining to
-ine	pertaining to
-ior	pertaining to
-ory	pertaining to
-ous	pertaining to
-tic	pertaining to

Abnormal Conditions

-ago	abnormal condition, disease
-esis	abnormal condition, disease
-ia	abnormal condition, disease
-iasis	abnormal condition, disease
-ion	condition
-ism	condition, state of
-osis	abnormal condition, disease

Noun Endings

-a	noun ending
-e	noun ending
-um	singular noun ending
-us	singular noun ending
-y	noun ending

A

a-	no, not without, away from, negative
-a	noun ending
ab-	away from, negative absent
abdomin/o	abdomen
-able	capable of, able to
abort/o	premature expulsion of a nonviable fetus
abrad/o, abras/o	rub or scrape off
abrupt/o	broken away from
abs-	away from
abscess/o	going away, collection of pus
absorpt/o	suck up, suck in
-ac	pertaining to
acanth/o	spiny, thorny
acetabul/o	acetabulum (hip socket)
-acious	characterized by
acne/o	point or peak
acous/o, acoust/o	hearing, sound
acquir/o	get, obtain
acr/o	extremities (hands and feet), top, extreme point
acromi/o	acromion, point of shoulder blade
actin/o	light
acu/o	sharp, severe, sudden
acuit/o, acut/o	sharp, sharpness
acust/o, -acusia, -acusis	hearing, sense of hearing
ad-	toward, to, in direction of
aden/o	gland
adenoid/o	adenoids
adhes/o	stick to, cling to
adip/o	fat
adnex/o	bound to
adren/o, adrenal/o	adrenal glands
aer/o	air, gas
aesthet/o	sensation, sense of perception
af-	toward, to
affect/o	exert influence on
agglutin/o	clumping, stick together
aggress/o	attack, step forward
-ago	abnormal condition, disease
agor/a	marketplace
-agra	excessive pain, seizure, attack of severe pain
-aise	comfort, ease
-al	pertaining to
alb/i, alb/o, albin/o	white
albumin/o	albumin, protein
alg/e, algi/o, alg/o, algesi/o	relationship to pain
-algesia, -algesic	painful, pain sense
-algia	pain, painful condition
align/o	bring into line or correct position
aliment/o	to nourish
all/o, all-	other, different from normal, reversal
alopec/o	baldness, mangy

alveol/o	alveolus, air sac, small sac
ambi-	both sides, around or about, double
ambly/o	dull, dim
ambul/o, ambulat/o	walk
ametr/o	out of proportion
-amine	nitrogen compound
amni/o	amnion, fetal membrane
amph-	around, on both sides, doubly
amput/o, amputat/o	cut away, cut off a part of the body
amyl/o	starch
an-	no, not, without
an-, ana-	up, apart, backward, excessive
an/o	anus, ring
-an	characteristic of, pertaining to
-ancy	state of
andr/o	relationship to the male
aneurysm/o	aneurysm
angi/o	blood or lymph vessels
angin/o	angina, choking, strangling
anis/o	unequal
ankyl/o	crooked, bent, stiff
anomal/o	irregularity
ante-	before, in front of
anter/o	before, front
anthrac/o	coal, coal dust
anti-	against
anxi/o, anxiet/o	uneasy, anxious
aort/o	aorta
ap-	toward, to
-apheresis	removal
aphth/o	ulcer
apic/o	apex
aplast/o	defective development, lack of development
ap-, apo-	separation, away from, opposed, detached
aponeur/o	aponeurosis (type of tendon)
apoplect/o	a stroke
append/o, appendic/o	appendix
aqu/i, aqu/o, aque/o	water
-ar	pertaining to
arachn/o	spider web, spider
arc/o	bow, arc or arch
-arche	beginning
areat/o	occurring in patches or circumscribed areas
areol/o	little open space
-aria	connected with
arrect/o	upright, lifted up, raised
arter/o, arteri/o	artery
arthr/o	joint
articul/o	joint
-ary	pertaining to
as-	toward, to
-ase	enzyme

aspir/o, aspirat/o	to breathe in
asthen-, -asthenia	weakness, lack of strength
asthmat/o	gasping, choking
astr/o	star, star-shaped
at-	toward, to
atel/o	incomplete, imperfect
ather/o	plaque, fatty substance
athet/o	uncontrolled
atop/o	strange, out of place
atres/i	without an opening
atri/o	atrium
attenuat/o	diluted, weakened
aud-, audi/o, audit/o	ear, hearing, the sense of hearing
aur/i, aur/o	ear, hearing
auscult/o	listen
aut/o	self
-ax	a noun ending thorax
ax/o	axis, main stem
axill/o	armpit
azot/o	urea, nitrogen

B

bacill/o	rod-shaped bacterium (plural, bacteria)
bacteri/o	bacteria (singular, bacterium)
balan/o	glans penis
bar/o	pressure, weight
bartholin/o	Bartholin's gland
bas/o	base, opposite of acid
bi-, bis-	twice, double, two
bio-	life
bifid/o	split, divided into two parts
bifurcat/o	divide or fork into two branches
bil/i	bile, gall
bilirubin/o	bilirubin
bin-	two by two
-blast	embryonic, immature, formative element
blephar/o	eyelid
borborygm/o	rumbling sound
brachi/o	arm
brachy-	short
brady-	slow
brev/i, brev/o	short
bronch/i, bronchi/o, bronch/o	bronchial tube, bronchus
bronchiol/o	bronchiole, bronchiolus
brux/o	grind
bucc/o	cheek
burs/o	bursa, sac of fluid near joint
byssin/o	cotton dust

C

cadaver/o	dead body, corpse
calc/i	calcium, lime, the heel

calci-, calc/o	calcium
calcane/o	calcaneus, heel bone
calcul/o	stone, little stone
cali/o, calic/o	cup, calyx
call/i, callos/o	hard, hardened and thickened
calor/i	heat
canalicul/o	little canal or duct
canth/o	corner of the eye
capill/o	hair
capit/o	head
capn/o	carbon dioxide, sooty or smoky appearance
capsul/o	little box
carb/o	carbon
carbuncl/o	carbuncle
carcin/o	cancerous
cardi/o, card/o	heart
cari/o	rottenness, decay
carot/o	stupor, sleep
carp/o	wrist bones
cartilag/o	cartilage, gristle
caruncul/o	bit of flesh
cat-, cata-, cath-	down, lower, under, downward
catabol/o	a breaking down
cathart/o	cleansing, purging
cathet/o	insert, send down
caud/o	lower part of body, tail
caus/o, caust/o	burning, burn
cauter/o, caut/o	heat, burn
cav/i, cav/o	hollow, cave
cavern/o	containing hollow spaces
cec/o	cecum
-cele	hernia, tumor, swelling
celi/o, cel/o	abdomen, belly
cement/o	cementum, a rough stone
cent-	hundred
-centesis	surgical puncture to remove fluid
cephal/o, -ceps	head
cera-	wax
cerebell/o	cerebellum
cerebr/o	cerebrum, brain
cerumin/o	cerumen, earwax
cervic/o	neck, cervix (neck of uterus)
cheil/o	lip
cheir/o	hand
chem/i, chem/o, chemic/o	drug, chemical
chir/o	hand
chlor/o	green
chlorhydr/o	hydrochloric acid
chol/e	bile, gall
cholangi/o	bile duct
cholecyst/o	gallbladder
choledoch/o	common bile duct
cholesterol/o	cholesterol
chondr/o	cartilage
chord/o	spinal cord, cord
chore/o	dance
chori/o, chorion/o	chorion, membrane

choroid/o	choroid layer of eye	conjunctiv/o	conjunctiva, joined together, connected
chrom/o, chromat/o	color	consci/o	aware, awareness
chron/o	time	consolid/o	become firm or solid
chym/o	to pour, juice	constipat/o	pressed together, crowded together
cib/o	meal	constrict/o	draw tightly together
cicatric/o	scar	-constriction	narrowing
-cidal	pertaining to killing	contact/o	touched, infected
-cide	causing death	contagi/o	infection, unclean, touching of something
cili/o	eyelashes, microscopic hair-like projections	contaminat/o	render unclean by contact, pollute
cine-	relationship to movement	contine/o, continent/o	keep in, contain, hold back, restrain
circ/i	ring or circle		
circulat/o	circulate, go around in a circle	contra-	against, counter, opposite
circum-	around, about	contracept/o	prevention of conception
circumcis/o	cutting around	contus/o	bruise
circumscrib/o	confined, limited in space	convalesc/o	recover, become strong
cirrh/o	orange-yellow, tawny	convex/o	arched, vaulted
cis/o	cut	convolut/o	coiled, twisted
clasis, -clast	break down	convuls/o	pull together
claudicat/o	limping	copi/o	plentiful
claustr/o	barrier	copulat/o	joining together, linking
clav/i	key	cor/o	pupil
clavicul/o, cleid/o	clavicle, collar bone	cord/o	cord, spinal cord
climacter/o	crisis, rung of a ladder	cordi/o	heart
clitor/o	clitoris	core/o, cor/o	pupil
-clonus	violent action	cori/o	skin, leather
clus/o	shut or close	corne/o	cornea
-clysis	irrigation, washing	coron/o	coronary, crown
co-	together, with	corp/u, corpor/o	body
coagul/o, coagulat/o	clotting, coagulation	corpuscul/o	little body
		cort-	covering
coarct/o, coarctat/o	press together, narrow	cortic/o	cortex, outer region
cocc/i, cocc/o, -coccus	spherical bacteria	cost/o	rib
		cox/o	hip, hip joint
coccyg/o	coccyx, tailbone	crani/o	skull
cochle/o	spiral, snail, snail shell	-crasia	a mixture or blending
coher/o, cohes/o	cling, stick together	creatin/o	creatine
coit/o	a coming together	crepit/o, crepitat/o	crackling, rattling
col/o	colon, large intestine	crin/o, -crine	secrete
coll/a	glue	cris/o, critic/o	turning point
colon/o	colon, large intestine	-crit	to separate
colp/o	vagina	cry/o	cold
column/o	pillar	crypt/o	hidden
com-	together, with	cubit/o	elbow
comat/o	deep sleep	cuboid/o	cubelike
comminut/o	break into pieces	culd/o	cul-de-sac, blind pouch
communic/o	share, to make common	cult/o	cultivate
compatibil/o	sympathize with	-cusis	hearing
con-	together, with	cusp/i	point, pointed flap
concav/o	hollow	cutane/o	skin
concentr/o	condense, intensify, remove excess water	cyan/o	blue
		cycl/o	ciliary body of eye, cycle
concept/o	become pregnant	-cyesis	pregnancy
conch/o	shell	cyst-, -cyst	bladder, bag
concuss/o	shaken together, violently agitated	cyst/o	urinary bladder, cyst, sac of fluid
condyl/o	knuckle, knob	cyt/o, -cyte	cell
confus/o	confusion, disorder	-cytic	pertaining to a cell
coni/o	dust	- cytosis	condition of cells

D

dacry/o	tear, lacrimal duct (tear duct)
dacryocyst/o	lacrimal sac (tear sac)
dactyl/o	fingers, toes
de-	down, lack of, from, not, removal
debrid/e	open a wound
deca-, deci-	ten, tenth
decidu/o	shedding, falling off
decubit/o	lying down
defec/o, defecat/o	free from waste, clear
defer/o	carrying down or out
degenerat/o	gradual impairment, breakdown, diminished function
deglutit/o	swallow
dehisc/o	burst open, split
deliri/o	wandering in the mind
delt/o	Greek letter delta, triangular shape
delus/o	delude, mock, cheat
dem/o	people, population
-dema	swelling (fluid)
demi-	half
dendr/o	branching, resembling a tree
dent/i, dent/o	tooth, teeth
depilat/o	hair removal
depress/o	press down lower, pressed or sunk down
derma-, dermat/o, derm/o	skin
desic/o	drying
-desis	surgical fixation of bone or joint, to bind, tie together
deteriorat/o	worsening or gradual impairment
dextr/o	right side
di-	twice, twofold, double
dia-	through, between, apart, complete
diaphor/o	sweat
diaphragmat/o	diaphragm, wall across
diastol/o	standing apart, expansion
didym/o	testes, twins, double
diffus/o	pour out, spread apart
digest/o	divide, distribute
digit/o	finger or toe
dilat/o, dilatat/o	spread out, expand
-dilation	widening, stretching, expanding
dilut/o	dissolve, separate
diphther/o	membrane
dipl/o	double
dips/o, -dipsia	thirst
dis-	negative, apart, absence of
dislocat/o	displacement
dissect/o	cutting apart
disseminat/o	widely scattered
dist/o	far
distend/o, distent/o	stretch apart, expand
diur/o, diuret/o	tending to increase urine output
divert/i	turning aside
domin/o	controlling, ruling
don/o	give
dors/i, dors/o	back of body
-dote	what is given
-drome	to run, running
-duct	opening
duct/o	to lead, carry
duoden/i, duoden/o	duodenum
dural	pertaining to dura mater
-dynia	pain
dys-	bad, difficult, painful

E

e-	out of, from
-e	noun ending
-eal	pertaining to
ec-	out, outside
ecchym/o	pouring out of juice
ech/o	sound
eclamps/o, eclampt/o	flashing or shining forth
ectasia, -ectasis	stretching, dilation, enlargement
ecto-	out, outside
-ectomy	surgical removal, cutting out, excision
-ectopy	displacement
eczemat/o	eruption
-edema	swelling
edem-, edemat/o	swelling, fluid, tumor
edentul/o	without teeth
ef-	out
effect/o	bring about a response, activate
effus/o	pouring out
ejaculat/o	throw or hurl out
electr/o	electricity, electric
eliminat/o	expel from the body
em-	in
emaciat/o	wasted by disease
embol/o	something inserted or thrown in
embry/o	fertilized ovum, embryo
-emesis	vomiting
emet/o	vomit
-emia	blood, blood condition
emmetr/o	in proper measure
emolli/o	make soft, soften
en-	in, within, into
encephal/o	brain
end-, endo-	in, within, inside
endocrin/o	secrete within
enem/o	end in, inject
enter/o	small intestine
ento-	within
enzym/o	leaven
eosin/o	red, rosy
epi-	above, upon, on
epidemi/o	among the people, an epidemic
epididym/o	epididymis
epiglott/o	epiglottis
episi/o	vulva

epithel/i, epitheli/o	epithelium
equin/o	pertaining to a horse
-er	one who
erect/o	upright
erg/o, -ergy	work
erot/o	sexual love
eruct/o, eructat/o	belch forth
erupt/o	break out, burst forth
erythem/o, erythemat/o	flushed, redness
erythr/o	red
es-	out of, outside, away from
-esis	abnormal condition, disease
eso-	inward
esophag/o	esophagus
-esthesia, esthesi/o	sensation, feeling
esthet/o	feeling, nervous sensation, sense of perception
estr/o	female
ethm/o	sieve
eti/o	cause
eu-	good, normal, well, easy
-eurysm	widening
evacu/o, evacuat/o	empty out
ex-	out of, outside, away from
exacerbat/o	aggravate, irritate
exanthemat/o	rash
excis/o	cutting out
excori/o, excoriat/o	abrade or scratch
excret/o	separate, discharge
excruciat/o	intense pain, agony
exhal/o, exhalat/o	breathe out
exo-	out of, outside, away from
exocrin/o	secrete out of
expector/o	cough up
expir/o, expirat/o	breathe out
exstroph/o	turned or twisted out
extern/o	outside, outer
extra-	on the outside, beyond, outside
extrem/o, extremit/o	extremity, outermost
extrins/o	from the outside, contained outside
exud/o, exudat/o	to sweat out

F

faci/o	face, form
-facient	making, producing
fasci/o	fascia, fibrous band
fascicul/o	little bundle
fatal/o	pertaining to fate, death
fauc/i	narrow pass, throat
febr/i	fever
fec/i, fec/o	dregs, sediment, waste
femor/o	femur, thigh bone
fenestr/o	window
fer/o	bear, carry
-ferent	carrying
-ferous	bearing, carrying, producing

fertil/o	fertile, fruitful, productive
fet/i, fet/o	fetus, unborn child
fibr/o	fiber
fibrill/o	muscular twitching
fibrin/o	fibrin, fibers, threads of a clot
fibros/o	fibrous connective tissue
fibul/o	fibula
-fic, fic/o	making, producing, forming
-fication	process of making
-fida	split
filtr/o, filtrat/o	filter, to strain through
fimbri/o	fringe
fiss/o, fissur/o	crack, split, cleft
fistul/o	tube or pipe
flamme/o	flame colored
flat/o	flatus, breaking wind, rectal gas
flex/o	bend
flu/o	flow
fluor/o	luminous, glowing
foc/o	focus, point
foll/i	bag, sac
follicul/o	follicle, small sac
foramin/o	opening, foramen
fore-	before, in front of
-form, form/o	resembling, in the shape of
fornic/o	arch, vault, brothel
foss/o	ditch, shallow depression
fove/o	pit
fract/o	break, broken
fren/o	device that limits movement
frigid/o	cold
front/o	forehead, brow
-fuge	to drive away
funct/o, function/o	perform, function
fund/o	bottom, base, ground
fung/i	fungus
furc/o	forking, branching
furuncul/o	furunculus, a boil, an infection
-fusion	pour

G

galact/o	milk
gamet/o	wife or husband, sperm or egg
gangli/o, ganglion/o	ganglion
gangren/o	eating sore, gangrene
gastr/o	stomach, belly
gastrocnemi/o	gastrocnemius, calf muscle
gemin/o	twin, double
gen-, gen/o, -gen	producing, forming
-gene	production, origin, formation
-genic, -genesis	creation, reproduction
genit/o	produced by, birth, reproductive organs
-genous	producing
ger/i	old age
germin/o	bud, sprout, germ
geront/o	old age

gest/o, gestat/o	bear, carry young or offspring
gigant/o	giant, very large
gingiv/o	gingival tissue, gums
glauc/o	gray
glen/o	socket or pit
gli/o	neurologic tissue, supportive tissue of nervous system
globin/o, -globulin	protein
globul/o	little ball
glomerul/o	glomerulus
gloss/o	tongue
glott/i, glott/o	back of the tongue
gluc/o	glucose, sugar
glute/o	buttocks
glyc/o, glycos/o	glucose, sugar
glycer/o	sweet
glycogen/o	glycogen, animal starch
gnath/o	jaw
-gnosia	knowledge, to know,
-gog, -gogue	make flow
goitr/o	goiter, enlargement of the thyroid gland
gon/e, gon/o	seed
gonad/o	gonad, sex glands
goni/o	angle
gracil/o	slender
grad/i	move, go, step, walk
-grade	go
-gram	resulting record
granul/o	granule(s)
-graph	resulting record
-graphy	process of recording
gravid/o	pregnancy
-gravida	pregnant
gynec/o	woman, female
gyr/o	turning, folding

H

hal/o, halit/o	breath
halluc/o	great or large toe
hallucin/o	hallucination, to wander in the mind
hem/e	deep red iron-containing pigment
hem/o, hemat/o	blood, relating to the blood
hemangi/o	blood vessel
hemi-	half
hemoglobin/o	hemoglobin
hepat/o	liver
hered/o, heredit/o	inherited, inheritance
herni/o	hernia
herpet/o	creeping
heter/o	other, different
-hexia	habit
hiat/o	opening
hidr/o	sweat
hil/o	hilum, notch or opening from a body part
hirsut/o	hairy, rough
hist/o, histi/o	tissue

holo-	all
hom/o	same, like, alike
home/o	sameness, unchanging, constant
hormon/o	hormone
humer/o	humerus (upper arm bone)
hydr/o, hydra-	relating to water
hygien/o	healthful
hymen/o	hymen, a membrane
hyper-	excessive, increased
hyph-	under
hypn/o	sleep
hypo-	deficient, decreased
hyster/o	uterus

I

-ia	abnormal condition, disease, plural of -ium
-ial	pertaining to
-ian	specialist
-iasis	abnormal condition, disease
iatr/o	physician, treatment
-iatrics	field of medicine, healing
-iatrist	specialist
-iatry	field of medicine
-ible	capable of, able to
-ic	pertaining to
ichthy/o	dry, scaly
-ician	specialist
icter/o	jaundice
idi/o	peculiar to the individual or organ, one, distinct
-iferous	bearing, carrying, producing
-ific	making, producing
-iform	shaped or formed like, resembling
-igo	attack, diseased condition
-ile	capable of
ile/o	ileum, small intestine
ili/o	ilium, hip bone
illusi/o	deception
im-	not
immun/o	immune, protection, safe
impact/o	pushed against, wedged against, packed
impress/o	pressing into
impuls/o	pressure or pushing force, drive, urging on
in-	in, into, not, without
-ine	pertaining to
incis/o	cutting into
incubat/o	incubation, hatching
indurat/o	hardened
infarct/o	filled in, stuffed
infect/o	infected, tainted
infer/o	below, beneath
infest/o	attack, assail, molest
inflammat/o	flame within, set on fire
infra-	below, beneath, inferior to
infundibul/o	funnel

ingest/o	carry or pour in
inguin/o	groin
inhal/o, inhalat/o	breathe in
inject/o	to force or throw in
innominat/o	unnamed, nameless
inocul/o	implant, introduce
insipid/o	tasteless
inspir/o, inspirat/o	breathe in
insul/o	island
insulin/o	insulin
intact/o	untouched, whole
inter-	between, among
intermitt/o	not continuous
intern/o	within, inner
interstiti/o	the space between things
intestin/o	intestine
intim/o	innermost
intoxic/o	put poison in
intra-	within, inside
intrins/o	contained within
intro-	within, into, inside
introit/o	entrance or passage
intussuscept/o	take up or receive within
involut/o	rolled up, curled inward
iod/o	iodine
-ion	action, process, state or condition
ion/o	ion, to wander
-ior	pertaining to
ipsi-	same
ir-	in
ir/i, ir/o, irid/o, irit/o	iris, colored part of eye
is/o	same, equal
isch/o	to hold back
ischi/o	ischium
-is	noun ending
-ism	condition, state of
iso-	equal
-ist	a person who practices, specialist
-itis	inflammation
-ium	structure, tissue
-ize	to make, to treat

J

jejun/o	jejunum
jugul/o	throat
juxta-	beside, near, nearby

K

kal/i	potassium
kary/o	nucleus, nut
kata-, kath-	down
kel/o	growth, tumor
kera-	horn, hardness
kerat/o	horny, hard, cornea
ket/o, keton/o	ketones, acetones
kines/o, kinesi/o, -kinesia	movement

-kinesis	motion
klept/o	to steal
koil/o	hollow or concave
kraur/o	dry
kyph/o	bent, hump

L

labi/o	lip
labyrinth/o	maze, labyrinth, the inner ear
lacer/o, lacerat/o	torn, mangled
lacrim/o	tear, tear duct, lacrimal duct
lact/i, lact/o	milk
lactat/o	secrete milk
lamin/o	lamina
lapar/o	abdomen, abdominal wall
laps/o	slip, fall, slide
-lapse	to slide, fall, sag
laryng/o	larynx, throat
lat/i, lat/o	broad
later/o	side
lav/o, lavat/o	wash, bathe
lax/o, laxat/o	loosen, relax
leiomy/o	smooth (visceral) muscle
lemm/o	husk, peel, bark
-lemma	sheath, covering
lent/i	the lens of the eye
lenticul/o	shaped like a lens, pertaining to a lens
-lepsy	seizure
lept/o	thin, slender
-leptic	to seize, take hold of
lepto-	small, soft
letharg/o	drowsiness, oblivion
leuk/o	white
lev/o, levat/o	raise, lift up
lex/o, -lexia	word, phrase
libid/o, libidin/o	sexual drive, desire, passion
ligament/o	ligament
ligat/o	binding or tying off
lingu/o	tongue
lipid/o, lip/o	fat, lipid
-listhesis	slipping
lith/o, -lith	stone, calculus
lithiasis	presence of stones
lob/i, lob/o	lobe, well-defined part of an organ
loc/o	place
loch/i	childbirth, confinement
-logy	study of
longev/o	long-lived, long life
lord/o	curve, swayback bent
lumb/o	lower back, loin
lumin/o	light
lun/o, lunat/o	moon
lunul/o	crescent
lup/i, lup/o	wolf
lute/o	yellow
lux/o	to slide
lymph/o	lymph, lymphatic tissue

lymphaden/o	lymph gland
lymphangi/o	lymph vessel
-lysis	breakdown, separation, setting free, destruction, loosening
-lyst	agent that causes lysis or loosening
-lytic	to reduce, destroy

M

macro-	large, abnormal size or length, long
macul/o	spot
magn/o	great, large
major/o	larger
mal-	bad, poor, evil
-malacia	abnormal softening
malign/o	bad, evil
malle/o	malleus, hammer
malleol/o	malleolus, little hammer
mamm/o	breast
man/i	madness, rage
man/i, man/o	hand
mandibul/o	mandible, lower jaw
-mania	obsessive preoccupation
manipul/o	use of hands
manubri/o	handle
masset/o	chew
mast/o	breast
mastic/o, masticat/o	chew
mastoid/o	mastoid process
matern/o	maternal, of a mother
matur/o	ripe
maxill/o	maxilla (upper jaw)
maxim/o	largest, greatest
meat/o	opening or passageway
medi/o	middle
mediastin/o	mediastinum, middle
medic/o	medicine, physician, healing
medicat/o	medication, healing
medull/o	medulla (inner section), middle, soft, marrow
mega-	large, great
-megaly	enlargement
mei/o	less, meiosis
melan/o	black, dark
mellit/o	honey, honeyed
membran/o	membrane, thin skin
men/o	menstruation, menses
mening/o, meningi/o	membranes, meninges
menisc/o	meniscus, crescent
mens/o	menstruate, menstruation, menses
menstru/o, menstruat/o	occurring monthly
ment/o	mind, chin
mes-, meso-	middle
mesenter/o	mesentery
mesi/o	middle, median plane

meta-	change, beyond, subsequent to, behind, after or next
metabol/o	change
metacarp/o	metacarpals, bones of the hand
metatars/o	bones of the foot between the tarsus and toes
-meter	measure, instrument used to measure
metr/i, metr/o, metri/o	uterus
-metrist	one who measures
-metry	to measure
mio-	smaller, less
micr/o, micro-	small
mictur/o, micturit/o	urinate
mid-	middle
midsagitt/o	from front to back, at the middle
milli-	one-thousandth
-mimetic	mimic, copy
mineral/o	mineral
minim/o	smallest, least
minor/o	smaller
-mission	to send
mit/o	a thread
mitr/o	a miter having two points on top
mobil/o	capable of moving
mono-	one, single
monil/i	string of beads, genus of parasitic mold or fungi
morbid/o	disease, sickness
moribund/o	dying
morph/o	shape, form
mort/i, mort/o, mort/u	death, dead
mortal/i	pertaining to death, subject to death
mot/o, motil/o	motion, movement
mu/o	close, shut
muc/o, mucos/o	mucus
multi-	many, much
muscul/o	muscle
mut/a	genetic change
mut/o	unable to speak, inarticulate
mutagen/o	causing genetic change
my/o	muscle
myc/e, myc/o	fungus
mydri/o	wide
mydrias/i	dilation of the pupil
myel/o	spinal cord, bone marrow
myocardi/o	myocardium, heart muscle
myom/o	muscle tumor
myos/o	muscle
myring/o	tympanic membrane, eardrum
myx/o, myxa-	mucus

N

nar/i	nostril
narc/o	numbness, stupor

nas/i, nas/o	nose
nat/i	birth
natr/o	sodium
nause/o	nausea, seasickness
neo-	new, strange
necr/o	death
-necrosis	tissue death
nect/o	bind, tie, connect
nephr/o	kidney
nerv/o, neur/i, neur/o	nerve, nerve tissue
neutr/o	neither, neutral
nev/o	birthmark, mole
nid/o	next
niter-, nitro-	nitrogen
noct/i	night
nod/o	knot, swelling
nodul/o	little knot
nom/o	law, control
non-	no
nor-	chemical compound
norm/o	normal or usual
nuch/o	the nape
nucle/o	nucleus
nucleol/o	little nucleus, nucleolus
nulli-	none
numer/o	number, count
nunci/o	messenger
nutri/o, nutrit/o	nourishment, food, nourish, feed
nyct/o, nyctal/o	night

O

ob-	against
obes/o	obese, extremely fat
obliqu/o	slanted, sideways
oblongat/o	oblong, elongated
obstetr/i, obstetr/o	midwife, one who stands to receive
occipit/o	back of the skull, occiput
occlud/o, occlus/o	shut, close up
occult/o	hidden, concealed
ocul/o	eye
odont/o	tooth
-oid	like, resembling
-ole	little, small
olecran/o	elbow, olecranon
olfact/o	smell, sense of smell
olig/o	scanty, few
-ologist	specialist
-ology	the science or study of
-oma	tumor, neoplasm
om/o	shoulder
oment/o	omentum, fat
omphal/o	umbilical cord, the navel
onc/o	tumor
-one	hormone
onych/o	fingernail or toenail
o/o, oo/o	egg
oophor/o	ovary

-opaque	obscure
opac/o, opacit/o	shaded, dark, impenetrable to light
oper/o, operat/o	perform, operate, work
opercul/o	cover or lid
ophthalm/o	eye, vision
-opia	vision condition
opisth/o	backward
-opsia, -opsis, -opsy	vision, view of
opt/i, opt/o, optic/o	eye, vision
or/o	mouth, oral cavity
orbit/o	orbit, bony cavity or socket
orch/o, orchid/o, orchi/o	testicles, testis, testes
-orexia	appetite
organ/o	organ
orgasm/o	swell, be excited
orth/o	straight, normal, correct
-ory	pertaining to
os-	mouth, bone
-ose	full of, pertaining to, sugar
-osis	abnormal condition, disease
osm/o	pushing, thrusting
-osmia	smell, odor
oss/e, oss/i, oste/o, ost/o	bone
ossicul/o	ossicle (small bone)
-ostomy	surgically creating an opening
-ostosis	condition of bone
ot/o	ear, hearing
-otia	ear condition
-otomy	cutting, surgical incision
ov/i, ov/o	egg, ovum
ovari/o	ovary
ovul/o	egg
-oxia	oxygen condition
ox/i, ox/o, ox/y	oxygen
oxid/o	containing oxygen
oxy-	swift, sharp, acid,
oxysm/o	sudden

P

pachy-	heavy, thick
palat/o	palate, roof of mouth
pall/o, pallid/o	pale, lacking or drained of color
palliat/o	cloaked, hidden
palm/o	palm of the hand
palpat/o	touch, feel, stroke
palpebr/o	eyelid
palpit/o	throbbing, quivering
pan-	all, entire, every
pancreat/o	pancreas
papill/i, papill/o	nipple-like
papul/o	pimple
par-, para-	beside, near, beyond, abnormal, apart from opposite, along side of
par/o	to bear, bring forth, labor

-para	to give birth
paralys/o, paralyt/o	disable
parasit/o	parasite
parathyroid/o	parathyroid glands
pares/i	to disable
-paresi	partial or incomplete paralysis
paret/o	to disable
-pareunia	sexual intercourse
pariet/o	wall
parotid/o	parotid gland
-parous	having borne one or more children
paroxysm/o	sudden attack
-partum, parturit/o	childbirth, labor
patell/a, patell/o	patella, kneecap
path/o, -pathy	disease, suffering, feeling, emotion
paus/o	cessation, stopping
-pause	stopping
pector/o	chest
ped/o	child, foot
pedi/a	child
pedicul/o	louse (singular), lice (plural)
pelv/i, pelv/o	pelvic bone, pelvic cavity, hip
pen/i	penis
pendo	to hang
-penia	deficiency, lack, too few
peps/i, -pepsia, pept/o	digest, digestion
per-	excessive, through
percept/o	become aware, perceive
percuss/o	strike, tap, beat
peri-	surrounding, around
perine/o	perineum
peristals/o, peristalt/o	constrict around
peritone/o	peritoneum
perme/o	to pass or go through
pernici/o	destructive, harmful
perone/o	fibula
perspir/o	perspiration
pertuss/i	intensive cough
petechi/o	skin spot
-pexy	surgical fixation
phac/o	lens of eye
phag/o	eat, swallow
-phage	a cell that destroys, eat, swallow
-phagia	eating, swallowing
phak/o	lens of eye
phalang/o	phalanges, finger and toe
phall/o	penis
pharmac/o, pharmaceut/o	drug
pharyng/o	throat, pharynx
phas/o	speech
-phasia	speak or speech
phe/o	dusky
pher/o	to bear or carry
-pheresis	removal
phil/o, -phila, -philia	attraction to, like, love
phleb/o	vein
phlegm/o	thick mucus
phob/o, -phobia	abnormal fear
phon/o, -phonia	sound, voice
phor/o	carry, bear, movement
-phoresis	carrying, transmission
-phoria	to bear, carry, feeling, mental state
phot/o	light
phren/o	diaphragm, mind
-phthisis	wasting away
-phylactic	protective, preventive
-phylaxis	protection
physi/o, physic/o	nature
-physis	to grow
phyt/o, -phyte	plant
pigment/o	pigment, color
pil/i, pil/o	hair
pineal/o	pineal gland
pinn/i	external ear, auricle
pituit/o, pituitar/o	pituitary gland
plac/o	flat plate or patch
placent/o	placenta, round flat cake
plak/o, -plakia	plaque, plate, thin flat layer or scale
plan/o	flat
plant/i, plant/o	sole of foot
plas/i, plas/o	development, growth, formation
plas/o, -plasia	development, formation, growth
-plasm	formative material of cells
plasm/o	something molded or formed
plast/o	growth, development, mold
-plastic	pertaining to formation
-plasty	surgical repair
ple/o	more, many
-plegia	paralysis, stroke
-plegic	one affected with paralysis
pleur/o	pleura, side of the body
plex/o	plexus, network
plic/o	fold or ridge
-pnea	breathing
-pneic	pertaining to breathing
pne/o-	breath, breathing
pneum/o, pneumon/o	lung, air
pod/o	foot
-poiesis	formation, to make
poikil/o	varied, irregular
pol/o	extreme
poli/o	gray matter of brain and spinal cord
pollic/o	thumb
poly-	many
polyp/o	polyp, small growth
pont/o	pons (a part of the brain), bridge
poplit/o	back of the knee
por/o	pore, small opening
-porosis	lessening in density, porous condition
port/i	gate, door
post-	after, behind
poster/o	behind, toward the back

potent/o	powerful
pract/i, practic/o	practice, pursue an occupation
prandi/o, -prandial	meal
-praxia	action, condition concerning the performance of movements
-praxis	act, activity, practice use
pre-	before, in front of
precoc/i	early, premature
pregn/o	pregnant, full of
prematur/o	too early, untimely
preputi/o	foreskin, prepuce
presby/o	old age
press/o	press, draw
priap/o	penis
primi-	first
pro-	before, in behalf of
process/o	going forth
procident/o	fall down or forward
procreat/o	reproduce
proct/o	anus and rectum
prodrom/o	running ahead, precursor
product/o	lead forward, yield, produce
prolaps/o	fall downward, slide forward
prolifer/o	reproduce, bear offspring
pron/o, pronat/o	bent forward
pros-	before
prostat/o	prostate gland
prosth/o, prosthet/o	addition, appendage
prot/o, prote/o	first
protein/o	protein
proxim/o	near
prurit/o	itching
pseud/o	false
psor/i, psor/o	itch, itching
psych/o	mind
ptomat/o	a fall
-ptosis	droop, sag, prolapse, fall
-ptyal/o	saliva
-ptysis	spitting
pub/o	pubis, part of hip bone
pubert/o	ripe age, adult
pudend/o	pudendum
puerper/i	childbearing, labor
pulm/o, pulmon/o	lung
pulpos/o	fleshy, pulpy
puls/o	beat, beating, striking
punct/o	sting, prick, puncture
pupill/o	pupil
pur/o	pus
purpur/o	purple
purul/o	pus-filled
pustul/o	infected pimple
py/o	pus
pyel/o	renal pelvis, bowl of kidney
pylor/o	pylorus, pyloric sphincter
pyr/o, pyret/o	fever, fire
pyramid/o	pyramid shaped

Q

quadr/i, quadr/o	four

R

rabi/o	madness, rage
rachi/o	spinal column, vertebrae
radi/o	radiation, x-rays, radius (lateral lower arm bone)
radiat/o	giving off rays or radiant energy
radicul/o	nerve root
raph/o	seam, suture
re-	back, again
recept/o	receive, receiver
recipi/o	receive, take to oneself
rect/o	rectum, straight
recticul/o	network
recuperat/o	recover, regain health
reduct/o	bring back together
refract/o	bend back, turn aside
regurgit/o	flood or gush back
remiss/o	give up, let go, relax
ren/o	kidney
restor/o	rebuild, put back, restore
resuscit/o	revive
retent/o	hold back
reticul/o	network
retin/o	retina, net
retro-	behind, backward, back of
retract/o	draw back or in
rhabdomy/o	striated muscle
rheum/o, rheumat/o	watery flow, subject to flow
rhin/o	nose
rhiz/o	root
rhonc/o	snore, snoring
rhythm/o	rhythm
rhytid/o	wrinkle
rigid/o	stiff
ris/o	laugh
roentgen/o	x-ray
rotat/o	rotate, revolve
-rrhage, -rrhagia	bleeding, abnormal excessive fluid discharge
-rrhaphy	to suture
-rrhea	abnormal flow, discharge
-rrhexis	rupture
rube-	red
rug/o	wrinkle, fold

S

sacc/i, sacc/o	sac
acchar/o	sugar
sacr/o	sacrum
saliv/o	saliva
salping/o	uterine (fallopian) tube, auditory (eustachian) tube
-salpinx	uterine (fallopian) tube

san/o	sound, healthy, sane
sangu/i, sanguin/o	blood
sanit/o	soundness, health
saphen/o	clear, apparent, manifest
sapr/o	decaying, rotten
sarc/o	flesh, connective tissue
scalp/o	carve, scrape
scapul/o	scapula, shoulder blade
schiz/o	division, split
scintill/o	spark
scirrh/o	hard
scler/o	sclera, white of eye, hard
-sclerosis	abnormal hardening
scoli/o	curved, bent
-scope	instrument for visual examination
-scopic	pertaining to visual examination
-scopy	visual examination
scot/o	darkness
scrib/o, script/o	write
scrot/o	bag or pouch
seb/o	sebum
secret/o	produce, separate out
sect/o, secti/o	cut, cutting
segment/o	pieces
sell/o	saddle
semi-	half
semin/i	semen, seed, sperm
sen/i	old
senesc/o	grow old
senil/o	old age
sens/i	feeling, sensation
sensitiv/o	sensitive to, affected by
seps/o	infection
sept/o	infection, partition
ser/o	serum
seros/o	serous
sial/o	saliva
sialaden/o	salivary gland
sider/o	iron
sigm/o	Greek letter sigma
sigmoid/o	sigmoid colon
silic/o	glass
sin/o, sin/u	hollow, sinus
sinistr/o	left, left side
sinus/o	sinus
-sis	abnormal condition, disease
sit/u	place
skelet/o	skeleton
soci/o	companion, fellow being
-sol	solution
solut/o, solv/o	loosened, dissolved
soma-, somat/o	body
somn/i, somn/o	sleep
son/o	sound
sopor/o	sleep
spad/o	draw off, draw
-spasm, spasmod/o	sudden involuntary contraction, tightening or cramping
spec/i	look at, a kind or sort
specul/o	mirror
sperm/o, spermat/	sperm, spermatozoa, seed
sphen/o	sphenoid bone, wedge
spher/o	round, sphere, ball
sphincter/o	tight band
sphygm/o	pulse
spin/o	spine, backbone
spir/o	to breathe
spirill/o	little coil
spirochet/o	coiled microorganism
splen/o	spleen
spondyl/o	vertebrae, vertebral column, back bone
spontane/o	unexplained, of one's own accord
spor/o	seed, spore
sput/o	sputum, spit
squam/o	scale
-stalsis	contraction, constriction
staped/o, stapedi/o	stapes (middle ear bone)
staphyl/o	clusters, bunch of grapes
-stasis, -static	control, maintenance of a constant level
steat/o	fat, lipid, sebum
sten/o	narrowing, contracted
-stenosis	abnormal narrowing
ster/o	solid structure
stere/o	solid, three-dimensional
steril/i	sterile
stern/o	sternum, the breastbone
stert/o	snore, snoring
steth/o	chest
-sthenia	strength
stigmat/o	point, spot
stimul/o	goad, prick, incite
stol/o	send or place
stomat/o	mouth
-stomosis, -stomy	furnish with a mouth or outlet, new opening
strab/i	squint, squint-eyed
strat/i	layer
strept/o	twisted chain
striat/o	stripe, furrow, groove
stric-	narrowing
strict/o	draw tightly together, bind or tie
strid/o	harsh sound
stup/e	benumbed, stunned
styl/o	pen, pointed instrument
sub-	under, less, below
subluxat/o	partial dislocation
sucr/o	sugar
sudor/i	sweat
suffoc/o, suffocat/o	choke, strangle
sulc/o	furrow, groove
super-, super/o	above, excessive, higher than
superflu/o	overflowing, excessive
supin/o	lying on the back
supinat/o	bend backward, place on the back
suppress/o	press down

suppur/o, suppurat/o	to form pus
supra-	above, upper, excessive
supraren/o	above or on the kidney, suprarenal gland
sutur/o	stitch, seam
sym-	with, together, joined together
symptomat/o	falling together, symptom
syn-	together, with, union, association
synaps/o, synapt/o	point of contact
syncop/o	to cut short, cut off
-syndesis	surgical fixation of vertebrae
syndesm/o	ligament
syndrom/o	running together
synovi/o, synov/o	synovial membrane, synovial fluid
syphil/i, syphil/o	syphilis
syring/o	tube
system/o, systemat/o	body system
systol/o	contraction

T

-thorax	chest, pleural cavity
tachy-	fast, rapid
tact/i	touch
talip/o	foot and ankle deformity
tars/o	tarsus (ankle bone), instep, edge of the eyelid
tax/o	coordination, order
techn/o, techni/o	skill
tectori/o	covering, rooflike
tele/o	distant, far
tempor/o	temporal bone, temple
ten/o, tend/o	tendon, stretch out, extend, strain
tenac/i	holding fast, sticky
tendin/o	tendon
tens/o	stretch out, extend, strain
terat/o	malformed fetus
termin/o	end, limit
test/i, test/o, testicul/o	testis, testicle
tetan/o	rigid, tense
tetra-	four
thalam/o	thalamus, inner room
thalass/o	sea
thanas/o, thanat/o	death
the/o	put, place
thec/o	sheath
thel/o	nipple
therap/o, therapeut/o	treatment
therm/o	heat
thio-	sulfur
thora/o, thorac/o	chest
thromb/o	clot
thym/o	thymus gland, soul
-thymia	mind
-thymic	pertaining to the mind

thyr/o, thyroid/o	thyroid gland
tibi/o	tibia (shin bone)
-tic	pertaining to
tine/o	gnawing worm, ringworm
tinnit/o	ringing, buzzing, tinkling
-tion	process, state or quality of
toc/o, -tocia, -tocin	labor, birth
tom/o	cut, section, slice
-tome	instrument to cut
-tomy	process of cutting
ton/o	tension, tone, stretching
tone/o	to stretch
tonsill/o	tonsil, throat
top/o	place, position, location
tors/o	twist, rotate
tort/i	twisted
tox/o, toxic/o	poison, poisonous
trabecul/o	little beam marked with cross bars or beams
trache/i, trache/o	trachea, windpipe
trachel-	neck
tract/o	draw, pull, path, bundle of nerve fibers
tranquil/o	quiet, calm, tranquil
trans-	across, through
transfus/o	pour across, transfer
transit/o	changing
transvers/o	across, crosswise
traumat/o	injury
trem/o	shaking, trembling
tremul/o	fine tremor or shaking
treponem/o	coiled, turning microbe
-tresia	opening
tri-	three
trich/o	hair
trigon/o	trigone
-tripsy	to crush
-trite	instrument for crushing
trochle/o	pulley
trop/o, -tropia	turn, change
troph/o, -trophy	development, nourishment
-tropic	turning
-tropin	stimulate, act on
tub/i, tub/o	tube, pipe
tubercul/o	little knot, swelling
tunic/o	covering, cloak, sheath
turbinat/o	coiled, spiral shaped
tuss/i	cough
tympan/o	tympanic membrane, eardrum
-type	classification, picture

U

-ula	small, little
-ule	small one
ulcer/o	sore, ulcer
uln/o	ulna (medial lower arm bone)
ultra-	beyond, excess
-um	singular noun ending

umbilic/o	navel
un-	not
ungu/o	nail
uni-	one
ur/o	urine, urinary tract
-uresis	urination
ureter/o	ureter
urethr/o	urethra
urg/o	press, push
-uria	urination, urine
urin/o	urine or urinary organs
urtic/o	nettle, rash, hives
-us	thing, singular noun ending
uter/i, uter/o	uterus
uve/o	iris, choroid, ciliary body, uveal tract
uvul/o	uvula, little grape

V

vaccin/i, vaccin/o	vaccine
vacu/o	empty
vag/o	vagus nerve, wandering
vagin/o	vagina
valg/o	bent or twisted outward
valv/o, valvul/o	valve
var/o	bent or twisted inward
varic/o	varicose veins, swollen or dilated vein
vas/o	vas deferens, vessel
vascul/o	blood vessel, little vessel
vast/o	vast, great, extensive
vect/o	carry, convey
ven/o	vein
vener/o	sexual intercourse
venter-	abdomen
ventilat/o	expose to air, fan
ventr/o	in front, belly side of body
ventricul/o	ventricle of brain or heart, small chamber
venul/o	venule, small vein
verg/o	twist, incline

verm/i	worm
verruc/o	wart
-verse, -version	to turn
vers/o, vert/o	turn
vertebr/o	vertebra, backbone
vertig/o, vertigin/o	whirling round
vesic/o	urinary bladder
vesicul/o	seminal vesicle, blister, little bladder
vestibul/o	entrance, vestibule
vi/o	force
vill/i	shaggy hair, tuft of hair
vir/o	poison, virus
viril/o	masculine, manly
vis/o	seeing, sight
visc/o	sticky
viscer/o	viscera, internal organ
viscos/o	sticky
vit/a, vit/o	life
viti/o	blemish, defect
vitre/o	glassy, made of glass
voc/i	voice
vol/o	palm or sole
volv/o	roll, turn
vulgar/i	common
vulv/o	vulva, covering

X

xanth/o	yellow
xen/o	strange, foreign
xer/o	dry
xiph/i, xiph/o	sword

Y

-y	noun ending

Z

zo/o	animal life
zygomat/o	cheek bone, yoke
zygot/o	joined together

Appendix B:
Abbreviations and Meanings

A	

A2 or A$_2$	aortic valve closure
A	accommodation; age; anterior
AAA	abdominal aortic aneurysm
AAL	anterior axillary line
AAV	adeno-associated virus
Ab	antibody
AB, ab	abortion
AB	abnormal
A/B	acid–base ratio
ABC	aspiration; biopsy; cytology
abd	abdomen
ABE	acute bacterial endocarditis
ABG	arterial blood gases
ABP	arterial blood pressure
ABR	auditory brainstem response
AC	acromioclavicular; air conduction
ac	acute
AC, ac	before meals
Acc	accommodation
ACD	acid-citrate-dextrose; anterior chest diameter
ACG	angiocardiography; apex cardiogram
ACH	adrenocortical hormone
ACL	anterior cruciate ligament
ACLS	advanced cardiac life support
ACP	acid phosphatase
ACTH	adrenocorticotropic hormone
ACVD	acute cardiovascular disease
AD	abdominal diaphragmatic breathing; adenovirus; Alzheimer's disease; right ear
ADD	attention deficit disorder
ADE	adverse drug event
ADH	antidiuretic hormone

ADHD	attention deficit hyperactivity disorder
ADL	activities of daily living
ad lib	as desired
adm	admission
ADS	antibody deficiency syndrome
ADR	adverse drug reaction
ADT	admission; discharge; transfer
AE	above elbow
AED	automated external defibrillation
AF	acid-fast; atrial fibrillation
AFB	acid-fast bacilli
A fib	atrial fibrillation
AFP	alpha-fetoprotein
Ag	antigen
AG, A/G	albumin/globulin ratio
AH	abdominal hysterectomy
AHD	arteriosclerotic heart disease; autoimmune hemolytic disease
AHF	antihemophilic factor VIII
AHG	antihemophilic globulin factor VIII
AI	aortic insufficiency; atherogenic index
AID	acute infectious disease; artificial insemination donor
AIDS	acquired immune deficiency syndrome
AIH	artificial insemination homologous
AIHA	autoimmune hemolytic anemia
aj	ankle jerk
AK	above knee
AKA	above-knee amputation; also known as
alb	albumin
ALG	antilymphocytic globulin
alk	alkaline
alk phos	alkaline phosphatase
ALL	acute lymphoblastic leukemia; acute lymphocytic leukemia

ALP	alkaline phosphatase
ALS	aldolase; amyotrophic lateral sclerosis; antilymphocytic serum
ALT	alanine transaminase (liver and heart enzyme)
alt dieb	alternate days; every other day
alt hor	alternate hours
alt noct	alternate nights
AMA	advanced maternal age; against medical advice; American Medical Association
amb	ambulate; ambulatory
AMD	age-related macular degeneration
AMI	acute myocardial infarction
AML	acute myeloblastic leukemia; acute myelocytic leukemia
amp	ampule
AMS	amylase
amt	amount
AN	anesthesiology
ANA	antinuclear antibodies
ANF	antinuclear factor
ANLL	acute nonlymphocytic leukemia
ANS	autonomic nervous system
ant	anterior
AOD	adult-onset diabetes; arterial occlusive disease
AOM	acute otitis media
A & P	anterior and posterior; auscultation and percussion
AP	angina pectoris; anteroposterior; anterior-posterior
APLD	aspiration percutaneous lumbar diskectomy
aq	aqueous; water
ARD	acute respiratory disease
ARDS	adult respiratory distress syndrome
ARF	acute renal failure; acute respiratory failure
ARM	artificial rupture of membranes
ART	assisted reproductive technology
AS	ankylosing spondylitis; aortic stenosis; left ear
ASA	aspirin
ASAP	as soon as possible
ASCVD	arteriosclerotic cardiovascular disease
ASD	atrial septal defect
ASH	asymmetrical septal hypertrophy
ASHD	arteriosclerotic heart disease
ASIS	anterior superior iliac spine
ASO	arteriosclerosis obliterans
ASS	anterior superior spine
AST	aspartate aminotransferase
as tol	as tolerated
ATP	adenosine triphosphate
Au	gold
AU	aures unitas; both ears
AUL	acute undifferentiated leukemia
ausc	auscultation
A-V	aortic valve; artificial ventilation; atrioventricular; arteriovenous
AVM	arteriovenous malfunction

AVN	atrioventricular node
AVR	aortic valve replacement
Ax	axillary
AZT	Aschheim-Zondek test

B

B/A	backache
BA	bronchial asthma
Ba	barium
BAC	blood alcohol concentration
BaE	barium enema
BAO	basal acid output
bas	basophils
BBB	blood–brain barrier; bundle branch block
BBT	basal body temperature
BC	bone conduction
BCC	basal cell carcinoma
BE	barium enema; below elbow
BEAM	brain electrical activity map
BED	binge eating disorder
BFP	biologic false positive
BID, bid, b.i.d.	bis in die; twice a day
bil	bilateral
BIN, bin	twice a night
BK	below knee
BKA	below-knee amputation
Bld	blood
BJ	Bence Jones
BM	bone marrow; bowel movement
BMD	Becker's muscular dystrophy; bone mineral density
BMI	body mass index
BMR	basal metabolic rate
BMT	barium meal test; bone marrow transplant
BNO	bladder neck obstruction
BNR	bladder neck resection
BOM	bilateral otitis media
B/P, BP	blood pressure
BP&P	blood pressure and pulse
BPH	benign prostatic hyperplasia; benign prostatic hypertrophy
BPM, bpm	beats per minute; breaths per minute
BPPV	benign paroxysmal positional vertigo
BR	bedrest
BRBPR	bright red blood per rectum (hematochochezia)
Bronch	bronchoscopy
BRP	bathroom privileges
BS	blood sugar; bowel sounds; breath sounds
BSE	breast self-examination
BSO	bilateral salpingo-oophorectomy
BT	bleeding time
BUN	blood urea nitrogen
BV	bacterial vaginosis; blood volume
Bx, bx	biopsy

C

C_1 through C_7	cervical vertebrae
C	centigrade; Celsius
c	centimeter
c̄	with
c̲	without
Ca	calcium
CA, Ca	cancer; cardiac arrest; carcinoma; chronological age
CAB	coronary artery bypass
CABG	coronary artery bypass grafting
CAD	computer-assisted diagnosis; coronary artery disease
cal	calorie
cap, caps	capsule
CAPD	continuous ambulatory peritoneal dialysis
CAT	computerized axial tomography
cath	catheter; catheterize
CAVH	continuous arteriovenous hemofiltration
CBC, cbc	complete blood count
CBF	capillary blood flow; coronary blood flow
CBI	continuous bladder irrigation
CBR	complete bedrest
CBS	chronic brain syndrome
CC	chief complaint; colony count; cardiac cycle; creatinine clearance; cardiac catheterization
cc	cubic centimeter (1/1000 liter)
CCA	circumflex coronary artery
CCCR	closed chest cardiopulmonary resuscitation
CCPD	continuous cycle peritoneal dialysis
CCr	creatinine clearance
CCT	cranial computed tomography
CCU	coronary care unit
CDC	calculated date (day) of confinement; Centers for Disease Control and Prevention
CDE	common duct exploration
CDH	congenital dislocation of the hip
CDT	cumulative trauma disorders
CEA	carcinoembryonic antigen
CF	complete fixation; counting fingers; cystic fibrosis
CFS	chronic fatigue syndrome
C gl	with correction; with glasses
CGL	chronic granulomatous leukemia
Ch	cholesterol
CHB	complete heart block
CHD	congenital heart defects; coronary heart disease
CHF	congestive heart failure
CHO	carbohydrate
chol	cholesterol
chr	chronic
CI	coronary insufficiency
cib	food
CID	cytomegalic inclusion disease

CIE	counter-immunoelectrophoresis
CIN	cervical intraepithelial neoplasia
circ	circumcision
CIS	carcinoma in situ
CIT	conventional insulin treatment
CK	creatine kinase
ck	check
Cl, cl	clinic; chloride
CL	cholelithiasis; chronic leukemia; cirrhosis of the liver; cleft lip; corpus luteum
CLD	chronic liver disease
CLL	chronic lymphocytic leukemia
cl liq	clear liquid
cm	centimeter (1/100 meter)
cm^3	cubic centimeter
CME	cystoid macular edema
CMG	cystometrogram
CML	chronic myelocytic leukemia
CMM	cutaneous malignant melanoma
CMV	controlled mechanical ventilation; cystometrogram; cytomegalovirus
CNS	central nervous system; cutaneous nerve stimulation
c/o	complains of
Co	cobalt
CO	carbon monoxide; coronary occlusion; coronary output
CO_2	carbon dioxide
COH	carbohydrate
COLD	chronic obstructive lung disease
comp	compound
cond	condition
contra	against
COPD	chronic obstructive pulmonary disease
CP	cardiopulmonary; cerebral palsy
CPA	carotid phonoangiograph
CPAP	continuous positive airway pressure
CPC	clinicopathologic conference
CPD	cephalopelvic disproportion
CPE	cytopathic effect
CPK	creatine phosphokinase
CPN	chronic pyelonephritis
CPPB	continuous positive-pressure breathing
CPR	cardiopulmonary resuscitation
CPS	cycles per second
CRD	chronic respiratory disease
CRF	chronic renal failure
creat	creatinine
CR	conditioned reflex; complete response
CRF	chronic renal failure
CS	central supply; cesarean section; complete stroke; conditioned stimulus; Cushing's syndrome
C & S	culture and sensitivity
CSAP	cryosurgical ablation of the prostate
CSF	cerebrospinal fluid
CSR	central supply room; Cheyne-Stokes respiration
CT	computed tomography

CTCL	cutaneous T-cell lymphoma
CTS	carpal tunnel syndrome
CTT	computed transaxial tomography
CTZ	chemoreceptor trigger zone
cu	cubic
CUC	chronic ulcerative colitis
CUG	cystourethrogram
CV	cardiovascular
CVA	cardiovascular accident; cerebrovascular accident; costovertebral angle
CVD	cardiovascular disease
CVL	central venous line
CVP	central venous pressure; Cytoxan, vincristine, prednisone
CVS	chorionic villus sampling
CWP	childbirth without pain; coal workers' pneumoconiosis
Cx	cervix
CX, CXR	chest x-ray film
cysto	cystoscopic examination; cystoscopy

D

D	diopter (lens strength)
d	day
DAT	diet as tolerated
db	decibel
D & C	dilation and curettage
D/C, DC	discontinue
DCC	direct-current cardioversion
DCIS	ductal carcinoma in situ
DCR	direct cortical response
D & E	dilation and evacuation
del	delivery
DES	diethylstilbestrol
DGE	delayed gastric emptying
DEXA	dual energy x-ray absorptiometry
DHEA	dehydroepiandrosterone
DHFS	dengue hemorrhagic fever shock syndrome
DI	diabetes insipidus
diag	diagnosis
DIC	diffuse intravascular coagulation
diff	differential
DIP	distal interphalangeal
disch	discharge
DJD	degenerative joint disease
DKA	diabetic ketoacidosis
DL	danger list
DLE	discoid lupus erythematosus
DM	dermatomyositis; diabetes mellitus; diastolic murmur
DMD	Duchenne's muscular dystrophy
DNA	deoxyribonucleic acid
DNR	do not resuscitate
DNS	deviated nasal septum
DOA	dead on arrival
DOB	date of birth
DOE	dyspnea on exertion
DOMS	delayed-onset muscle soreness

DOT	directly observed therapy
DQ	developmental quotient
DPT	diphtheria-pertussis-tetanus
dr	dram; dressing
DR	diabetic retinopathy
DR	digital radiography; doctor
DRG	diagnosis-related group
D/S	dextrose in saline
DSA	digital subtraction angiography
DSD	dry sterile dressing
dsg	dressing
DT	diphtheria and tetanus toxoids
DTP	diphtheria, tetanus toxoids, and pertussis vaccine
DTs	delirium tremens
DTR	deep tendon reflex
DUB	dysfunctional uterine bleeding
DVA	distance visual acuity
DVI	digital vascular imaging
DW	distilled water
D/W	dextrose in water
Dx	diagnosis

E

E	enema
EBL	estimated blood loss
EBP	epidural blood patch
EBV	Epstein-Barr virus
ECC	endocervical curettage; extracorporeal circulation
ECCE	extracapsular lens extraction
ECG	electrocardiogram; electrocardiography
ECHO	echocardiogram; echocardiography
ECOM	extracorporeal membrane oxygenator
ECT	electroconvulsive therapy
ED	effective dose
EDC	estimated date (day) of confinement
EDD	end-diastolic dimension
EDG	electrodynogram
EDV	end-diastolic volume
EEG	electroencephalogram; electroencephalography
EENT	eye, ear, nose, and throat
EFM	electronic fetal monitor
EIA	enzyme immunoassay
EIB	exercise-induced bronchospasm
Ej	elbow jerk
EKG	electrocardiogram; electrocardiography
ELISA	enzyme-linked immunoassay; enzyme-linked immunosorbent assay
elix	elixir
EM	electron microscope; emmetropia
EMG	electromyogram; electromyography
EMR	educable mentally retarded; electronic medical record; eye movement record
EMS	early morning specimen; electromagnetic spectrum
ENG	electronystagmography

ENT	ear, nose, and throat
EOG	electro-oculogram
EOM	extraocular muscles; extraocular movement
Eos, eosins	eosinophils
EP	ectopic pregnancy; evoked potential
EPF	early pregnancy factor; exophthalmos-producing factor
EPO	erythropoietin
EPR	electron paramagnetic resonance; emergency physical restraint
EPS	extrapyramidal symptoms; exophthalmos-producing substance
ER	emergency room; epigastric region
ERCP	endoscopic retrograde cholangiopancreatography
ERG	electroretinogram
ERPF	effective renal plasma flow
ERT	estrogen replacement therapy; external radiation therapy
ERV	expiratory reserve volume
ESD	end-systolic dimension
ESPF	end-stage pulmonary fibrosis
ESR	erythrocyte sedimentation rate
ESRD	end-stage renal disease
ESWL	extracorporeal shock-wave lithotripsy
EST	electric shock therapy
ESV	end-systolic volume
ET	embryo transfer; enterically transmitted; esotropia
et	and
ETF	eustachian tube function
etiol	etiology
ETT	endotracheal tube; exercise tolerance test
EU	Ehrlich units; emergency unit; etiology unknown
EWB	estrogen withdrawal bleeding
ex	excision; exercise
exam	examination
exp	expiration
ext	extraction; external

F

F	Fahrenheit
FA	fluorescent antibody
FAS	fetal alcohol syndrome
FB	foreign body
FBS	fasting blood sugar
FCD	fibrocystic disease
FDP	fibrin-fibrinogen degradation products
Fe	iron
FECG	fetal electrocardiogram
FEF	forced expiratory flow
FEV	forced expiratory volume
FFA	free fatty acids
FH	family history
FHR	fetal heart rate
FHS	fetal heart sounds
FHT	fetal heart tones

FIA	fluorescent immunoassay; fluoroimmunoassay
FME	full mouth extractions
FMS	fibromyalgia syndrome
FOBT	fecal occult blood test
FPG	fasting plasma glucose
FR	fibrin-fibrinogen related
fr	French (catheter size)
FRC	functional residual capacity
FROM	full range of motion
FS	frozen section
FSH	follicle-stimulating hormone
FSP	fibrin-fibrinogen split products
FSS	functional endoscopic sinus surgery
FT	family therapy
FTA	fluorescent treponemal antibody
FTI	free thyroxine index
FTND	full-term normal delivery
FTT	failure to thrive
FU	follow-up; follow up
FUO	fever of unknown origin
FX, Fx	fracture

G

g	gram
g_1	gravida (pregnancy)
Ga	gallium
GA	gastric analysis; general anesthesia
GB	gallbladder
GBM	glomerular basement membrane
GBS	gallbladder series; Guillain-Barré syndrome
G-Cs	glucocorticoids
GC	gonorrhea
GDM	gestational diabetes mellitus
GER	gastroesophageal reflux
GERD	gastroesophageal reflux disease
GFR	glomerular filtration rate
GG	gamma globulin
GGT	gamma-glutamyl transferase
GH	growth hormone
GHb	glycohemoglobin
GIFT	gamete intrafallopian transfer
GIT	gastrointestinal tract
GLTT	glucose tolerance test
gm	gram
GMP	guanosine monophosphate
GOT	glutamic oxaloacetic transaminase
GP	general practice
gr	grain
grav I	pregnancy one; primigravida
GS	general surgery
GSW	gunshot wound
GT	glucose tolerance
GTP	guanosine triphosphate
GTT	glucose tolerance test
gtt	drops
GU	genitourinary
GVHD	graft-versus-host disease

GxT	graded exercise test
GYN, Gyn	gynecology

H

h	hour
H	hydrogen; hypodermic
H & H	hemoglobin and hematocrit
HAA	hepatitis associated antigen; hepatitis Australia antigen
HAI	hemagglutination-inhibition immunoassay
HASHD	hypertensive arteriosclerotic heart disease
HAV	hepatitis A virus
HB	heart block; hemoglobin
HBE	His bundle electrocardiogram
HbF	fetal hemoglobin
HBP	high blood pressure
HbS	sickle cell hemoglobin
HBV	hepatitis B virus
HC	Huntington's chorea
HCD	heavy-chain disease
HCFA	Health Care Financing Administration
HCG, hCG	human chorionic gonadotropin
HCl	hydrochloric acid
HCL	hairy cell leukemia
HCPCS	Health Care Financing Administration Common Procedure Coding System
HCT, hct	hematocrit
HCV	hepatitis C virus
HCVD	hypertensive cardiovascular disease
HD	hearing distance; heart disease; hemodialysis; hip disarticulation; Hodgkin's disease; Huntington's disease
HDL	high-density lipoprotein
He	helium
H & E	hematoxylin and eosin stain
HDN	hemolytic disease of the newborn
HDS	herniated disk syndrome
HE	hereditary elliptocytosis
HEENT	head, eyes, ears, nose, throat
HF	heart failure
Hg	mercury
HgA$_{1c}$	glycohemoglobin test
Hgb	hemoglobin
HGE	human granulocytic Ehrlichiosis
HI	hemagglutination-inhibition
HIE	hypoxic ischemic encephalopathy
HIV	human immunodeficiency virus
H & L	heart and lungs
HL	Hodgkin's lymphoma
HLA	human leukocyte antigen
HLR	heart-lung resuscitation
HM	hand motion
HMD	hyaline membrane disease
HMO	health maintenance organization
HNP	herniated nucleus pulposus
HO	hyperbaric oxygen
HOB	head of bed
H & P	history and physical

HP	hemipelvectomy; hyperparathyroidism
HPF	high-power field
HPL	human placental lactogen
HPN	hypertension
HPO	hypothalamic-pituitary-ovarian
HPS	hantavirus pulmonary syndrome
HPV	human papilloma virus
HR	heart rate
hr	hour
HRT	hormone replacement therapy
hs, h.s.	at bedtime; hour of sleep
HS	hereditary spherocytosis; herpes simplex
HSG	hysterosalpingogram
HSV	herpes simplex virus
ht	height; hematocrit; hormone therapy
HTO	high tibial osteotomy
HV	hospital visit
HVD	hypertensive vascular disease
Hx	history
hypo	hypodermic
HZ	herpes zoster

I

I	intensity of magnetism; iodine
IABP	intra-aortic balloon pump
IACP	intra-aortic counterpulsation
IADH	inappropriate antidiuretic hormone
IASD	interatrial septal defect
IBC	iron-binding capacity
IBD	inflammatory bowel disease
IBS	irritable bowel syndrome
IC	inspiratory capacity
ICCE	intracapsular lens extraction
ICCU	intensive coronary care unit
ICF	intracellular fluid
ICP	intracranial pressure
ICS	intercostal space
ICSI	intracytoplasmic sperm injection
ICT	indirect Coombs' test; insulin coma therapy
ict ind	icterus index
ICU	intensive care unit
I & D	incision and drainage
ID	infectious disease; intradermal
IDC	infiltrating ductal carcinoma; invasive ductal carcinoma
IDD	insulin-dependent diabetes
IDDM	insulin-dependent diabetes mellitus
IDK	internal derangement of the knee
IDS	immunity deficiency state
I/E	inspiratory-expiratory ratio
IEMG	integrated electromyogram
IFG	impaired fasting glucose
Ig	immunoglobulin
IgA	immunoglobulin A
IgD	immunoglobulin D
IgE	immunoglobulin E
IgG	immunoglobulin G
IgM	immunoglobulin M

IGT	impaired glucose tolerance
IH	infectious hepatitis
IHD	ischemic heart disease
IHSS	idiopathic hypertrophic subaortic stenosis
IL	interleukin
ILC	infiltrating lobar carcinoma; invasive lobular carcinoma
IM	infectious mononucleosis; intramuscular
IMAG	internal mammary artery graft
IMF	idiopathic myelofibrosis
IMV	intermittent mandatory ventilation
IN	insulin
inf	inferior; infusion
I & O	intake and output
IO	intraocular
IOD	iron-overload disease (hemochromatosis)
IOL	intraocular lens
IOP	intraocular pressure
IPF	idiopathic pulmonary fibrosis
IPG	impedance plethysmography
IPPB	intermittent positive-pressure breathing
IQ	intelligence quotient
irrig	irrigation
IS	intercostal space
ISG	immune serum globulin
isol	isolation
ITP	idiopathic thrombocytopenic purpura
IU	international unit
IUD	intrauterine device
IUP	intrauterine pressure
IV	intravenous; intravenously
IVC	inferior vena cava
IVCP	inferior vena cava pressure
IVD	intervertebral disk
IVDA	intravenous drug abuse
IVF	in vitro fertilization
IVFA	intravenous fluorescein angiography
IVP	intravenous pyelogram
IVSD	interventricular septal defect
IVU	intravenous urogram

J

jct	junctions
JOD	juvenile-onset diabetes
JRA	juvenile rheumatoid arthritis
Jt	joint
JVP	jugular venous pressure; jugular venous pulse

K

K	potassium
KB	ketone bodies
KCF	key clinical findings
KCl	potassium chloride
KD	knee disarticulation
KE	kinetic energy
kg	kilogram

kj	knee jerk
KO	keep open
KOH	potassium hydrochloride
KS	Kaposi's sarcoma
KUB	kidney, ureter, bladder
KVO	keep vein open

L

l, L	liter
L_1-L_5	lumbar vertebrae
L & A	light and accommodation
LA	left atrium
lab	laboratory
lac	laceration
LAD	left anterior descending
LAP	leucine aminopeptidase
lap	laparotomy
laser	light amplification by stimulated emission of radiation
LASIK	laser in situ keratomileusis
lat	lateral
LAVH	laparoscopically assisted vaginal hysterectomy
lb	pound
LB	large bowel; low back
LBBB	left bundle branch block
LBW	low birth weight
LBBX	left breast biopsy and examination
LBP	low back pain
LCIS	lobular carcinoma in situ
L & D	labor and delivery
LD	lactic dehydrogenase
LDD	light-dark discrimination
LDH	lactic dehydrogenase
LDL	low-density lipoprotein
LE	left eye; life expectancy; lower extremity; lupus erythematosus
LES	lower esophageal sphincter
lg	large
LH	luteinizing hormone
LHBD	left heart bypass device
LHF	left-sided heart failure
LHR	leukocyte histamine release test
lig	ligament
liq	liquid
L K & S	liver, kidney, and spleen
LLE	lower left extremity
LLL	left lower lobe
LLSB	left lower sternal border
LLQ	left lower quadrant
L/min	liters per minute
LMP	last menstrual period
LNMP	last normal menstrual period
LOC	level of consciousness; loss of consciousness
LOM	limitation of motion; loss of motion
LOS	length of stay
LP	light perception; lumbar puncture; lumboperitoneal

LPF	low-power field
LPS	lipase
LR	light reaction
LRDKT	living related donor kidney transplant
LSB	left sternal border
LSD	lysergic acid diethylamide
lt	left
LTB	laryngotracheobronchitis
LTC	long-term care
LTH	luteotropic hormone
LUE	left upper extremity
LUL	left upper lobe
LUQ	left upper quadrant
LV	left ventricle
LVH	left ventricle hypertrophy
lymphs	lymphocytes

M

M	meter; murmur
Mabs	monoclonal antibodies
MAO	maximal acid output; monoamine oxidase
MAR	multiple antibiotic resistant
MBC	maximal breathing capacity
MBD	minimal brain damage
mc	millicurie
mcg µg	microgram
MCH	mean corpuscular hemoglobin
MCHC	mean corpuscular hemoglobin concentration
MCT	mean circulation time
MCV	mean corpuscular volume
MD	macular degeneration; medical doctor; muscular dystrophy
MDR-TB	multidrug-resistant tuberculosis
MDS	myelodysplastic syndrome
ME	middle ear
MED	minimal effective dose; minimal erythema dose
mEq	milliequivalent
M & F	mother and father
MFT	muscle function test
mg	milligram
MG	myasthenia gravis
mgm	milligram
MH	malignant hyperpyrexia; malignant hyperthermia; marital history
MHA	microhemagglutination
MHC	major histocompatibility complex
MI	mitral insufficiency; myocardial infarction
MICU	medical intensive care unit; mobile intensive care unit
MID	multi-infarct dementia
MIDCAB	minimally invasive direct coronary artery bypass
MIP	maximal inspiratory pressure
ml, mL	milliliter
MLD	median lethal dose
mm	millimeter

mm Hg	millimeters of mercury
MM	multiple myeloma; malignant melanoma
MND	motor neuron disease
MNT	medical nutrition therapy
MODY	maturity-onset diabetes of the young
MOM	milk of magnesia
mono	monocytes
MP	metacarpal-phalangeal
MPD	myofacial pain dysfunction
MPJ	metacarpophalangeal joint
MR	mental retardation; metabolic rate; mitral regurgitation
MRD	medical record department
MRI	magnetic resonance imaging
MS	mitral stenosis; multiple sclerosis; musculoskeletal
MSH	melanocyte-stimulating hormone
MSL	midsternal line
MT	medical technician; medical technologist
MTD	right eardrum
MTS	left eardrum
MTX	methotrexate
MV	mitral valve
MVP	mitral valve prolapse
MVPS	Medicare volume performance standard
MY	myopia
myel	myelogram
myop	myopia

N

N/C	no complaints
NA	not applicable; numerical aperture
Na	sodium
NaCl	sodium chloride
NAD	no acute disease; no apparent distress
NB	newborn
NBT	nitroblue tetrazolium
NCV	nerve conduction velocity
NED	no evidence of disease
NEG	negative
neg	negative
neuro	neurology
NF	National Formulary; neurofibromatosis
N/G	nasogastric (tube)
ng	*Neisseria gonorrhoeae*
NGU	nongonococcal urethritis
NHL	non-Hodgkin's lymphoma
NICU	neurologic intensive care unit
NIDDM	non–insulin-dependent diabetes mellitus
NK	natural killer (cell)
NKA	no known allergies
NLP	neurolinguistic programming
NM	neuromuscular; nuclear medicine
N & M	nerves and muscles; night and morning
NMR	nuclear magnetic resonance
No.	number
noc, noct	night
NOFTT	nonorganic failure to thrive

NPC	no point of convergence
NPH	neutral protamine Hagedorn
NPN	nonprotein nitrogen
NPO	nothing by mouth
NR	no response
NREM	no rapid eye movements
N/S	normal saline
NS	nephrotic syndrome; normal saline; not stated; not sufficient
NSAID	nonsteroidal anti-inflammatory drug
NSR	normal sinus rhythm
NSU	nonspecific urethritis
Nt	neutralization
N & T	nose and throat
NTD	neural tube defect
NTG	nitroglycerin
N & V	nausea and vomiting
NVA	near visual acuity
NVD	nausea, vomiting, and diarrhea; neck vein distention
NVS	neural vital signs
NYD	not yet diagnosed

O

OA	osteoarthritis
OB	obstetrics
OB-GYN	obstetrics and gynecology
obl	oblique
OBS	organic brain syndrome
Obs	obstetrics
OC	office call; oral contraceptive
OCC	occasional
OCD	obsessive compulsive disorder; oral cholecystogram
OCT	oral contraceptive therapy
OD	overdose; right eye (oculus dexter)
od	once a day
OGN	obstetric-gynecologic-neonatal
OGTT	oral glucose tolerance test
oint	ointment
OJD	osteoarthritic joint disease
OM	otitis media
OME	otitis media with effusion
OMR	optic mark recognition
OOB	out of bed
O & P	ova and parasites
OP	outpatient
OPD	outpatient department
OPG	oculoplethysmography
Ophth	ophthalmic
OPT	outpatient
OPV	oral poliovirus vaccine
OR	operating room
ORIF	open reduction internal fixation
ORT	oral rehydration therapy
Orth	orthopedics
OS	left eye (oculus sinister)
os	mouth

OSA	obstructive sleep apnea
OT	occupational therapy; old tuberculin
OTC	over-the-counter
Oto	otology
OU	each eye (oculus unitas)
oz	ounce
OXT	oxytocin

P

P, p	after; phosphorus; pulse
P & A	percussion and auscultation
PA	pernicious anemia; physician's assistant; posteroanterior; posterior-anterior; pulmonary artery
PABA	para-aminobenzoic acid
PAC	premature atrial contraction
PACAB	port-access coronary artery bypass
PADP	pulmonary artery diastolic pressure
PAMP	pulmonary arterial mean pressure
Pap	Papanicolaou smear
PAR	perennial allergic rhinitis; postanesthetic recovery
PARA (P_1)	full-term infants delivered
paren	parenterally
PASP	pulmonary artery systolic pressure
PAT	paroxysmal atrial tachycardia
Path	pathology
PBC	primary biliary cirrhosis
PBI	protein-bound iodine
PBP	progressive bulbar palsy
PBT_4	protein-bound thyroxine
pc	after meals
PCO, PCOS	polycystic ovary syndrome
PCP	*Pneumocystis carinii* pneumonia
PCT	plasmacrit time
PCU	progressive care unit
PCV	packed cell volume
PD	interpupillary distance; Parkinson's disease; peritoneal dialysis
PDA	patent ductus arteriosus
PDD	pervasive developmental disorder
PDL	periodontal ligament
PE	physical examination
PEA	pulseless electrical activity
Peds	pediatrics
PEEP	positive end-expiratory pressure
PEF	peak expiratory flow rate
PEG	pneumoencephalogram; pneumoencephalography
PEL	permissible exposure limit
per	by; through
PERLA	pupils equally reactive to light and accommodation
PERRLA	pupils equal, round, react to light and accommodation
PET	positron emission tomography; preeclamptic toxemia
PFT	pulmonary function test

PG	pregnant; prostaglandin
PG, 2-h	post-load glucose (number indicates elapsed time)
PGH	pituitary growth hormone
PGL	persistent generalized lymphadenopathy
pH	acidity; hydrogen ion concentration
PH	past history; personal history; public health
PHN	postherpetic neuralgia
PI	present illness
PICU	pulmonary intensive care unit
PID	pelvic inflammatory disease
PIF	peak inspiratory flow
PIP	proximal interphalangeal
PK	pyruvate kinase; pyruvate kinase deficiency
PKR	partial knee replacement
PKU	phenylketonuria
PL	light perception
PLC	platelet count
PLMS	periodic limb movements in sleep
PLS	primary lateral sclerosis
PLTS	platelets
PM	evening or afternoon; physical medicine; polymyositis; postmortem
PMA	progressive muscular atrophy
PMH	past medical history
PMI	point of maximal impulse
PMN	polymorphonuclear neutrophils
PMP	past menstrual period; previous menstrual period
PMR	physical medicine and rehabilitation; polymyalgia rheumatica
PMS	premenstrual syndrome
PMT	premenstrual tension
PMVS	prolapsed mitral valve syndrome
PND	paroxysmal nocturnal dyspnea; postnasal drip
PNH	paroxysmal nocturnal hemoglobinuria
PNS	parasympathetic nervous system; peripheral nervous system
PO, p.o.	by mouth; orally; phone order; postoperative
POC	products of conception
polys	polymorphonuclear leukocytes
POMR	problem-oriented medical record
pos	positive
POS	polycystic ovary syndrome
post-op	postoperatively
PP	postpartum; postprandial (after meals); pulse pressure
PPA pos	phenylpyruvic acid positive
PPBS	postprandial blood sugar
PPD	purified protein derivative
PPLO	pleuropneumonia-like organisms
PPS	postperfusion syndrome; postpolio syndrome
PPV	positive-pressure ventilation
PR	peripheral resistance; pulse rate
Pr	presbyopia; prism
pr	by rectum

PRA	plasma renin activity
PRBC	packed red blood cells
PRC	packed red cells
PRE	progressive restrictive exercise
preg	pregnant
preop	preoperative
prep	prepare
PRK	photoreactive keratectomy
prn	as needed
proct	proctology
prog	prognosis
PROM	passive range of motion; premature rupture of membranes
pro time	prothrombin time
PRRE	pupils round, regular, and equal
PSA	prostate-specific antigen
PSP	phenolsulfonphthalein
PSS	progressive systemic sclerosis; physiologic saline solution
psych	psychiatry
PT	paroxysmal tachycardia; physical therapy; prothrombin time
pt	patient; pint
PTA	percutaneous transluminal angioplasty; plasma thromboplastin antecedent, factor XI
PPT	partial prothrombin time
PTB	patellar tendon bearing
PTC	percutaneous transhepatic cholangiography, plasma thromboplastic component, factor XI
PTCA	percutaneous transluminal coronary angioplasty
PTD	permanent and total disability
PTE	parathyroid extract
PTH	parathyroid hormone; parathormone
PTSD	posttraumatic stress disorder
PTT	partial thromboplastin time; prothrombin time
PU	peptic ulcer; pregnancy urine; prostatic urethra
PUD	peptic ulcer disease; pulmonary disease
pul	pulmonary
PV	peripheral vascular; plasma volume; polycythemia vera
P & V	pyloroplasty and vagotomy
PVC	premature ventricular contraction
PVD	peripheral vascular disease
PVE	prosthetic valve endocarditis
PVOD	peripheral vascular occlusive disease
PVS	persistent vegetative state
PVT	paroxysmal ventricular tachycardia
pvt	private
PWB	partial weight-bearing
PWP	pulmonary wedge pressure
Px	prognosis

Q

q	every
qd, q.d.	every day
qh, q.h.	every hour
q 2 h	every 2 hours
QID, qid, q.i.d.	four times a day
qm	every morning
qn	every night
qns	quantity not sufficient
qod	every other day
qoh	every other hour
QOL	quality of life
qs	quantity sufficient
qt	quart; quiet
q.q.	each
quad	quadrant

R

R	rectal; respiration; right
RA	refractory anemia; rheumatoid arthritis; right arm; right atrium
Ra	radium
rad	radiation absorbed dose
RAF	rheumatoid arthritis factor
RAI	radioactive iodine
RAIU	radioactive iodine uptake determination
RAS	reticular activating system
RAST	radioallergosorbent
RAT	radiation therapy
RBBB	right bundle branch block
RBC	red blood cell; red blood count
RBCV	red blood cell volume
RBE	relative biologic effects
RCA	right coronary artery
RD	respiratory distress; retinal detachment
RDA	recommended daily allowance
RDS	respiratory distress syndrome
reg	regular
rehab	rehabilitation
RE	right eye
rem	roentgen-equivalent-man
REM	rapid eye movement
RER	renal excretion rate
RES	reticuloendothelial system
RBRVS	resource-based relative value scale
resp	respirations
RF	renal failure; rheumatoid factor; rheumatic fever
RFS	renal function study
RH	right hand
Rh neg	Rhesus factor negative
Rh pos	Rhesus factor positive
RHD	rheumatic heart disease
RIA	radioimmunoassay
RICE	rest, ice, compression, elevate
RIF	right iliac fossa

RIST	radioimmunosorbent
RK	radial keratotomy
RL	right leg
RLC	residual lung capacity
RLD	related living donor
RLE	right lower extremity
RLL	right lower lobe
RLQ	right lower quadrant
RLS	restless legs syndrome
RM	respiratory movement
RML	right mediolateral
RMSF	Rocky Mountain spotted fever
RNA	ribonucleic acid
RND	radical neck dissection
R/O	rule out
ROA	right occipitis anterior
ROM	range of motion; rupture of membranes
ROP	right occipitis posterior
ROPS	roll over protection structures
ROS	review of systems
ROT	right occipitis transverse
RP	relapsing polychondritis; retrograde pyelogram
RPCF	Reiter protein complement fixation
RPF	renal plasma flow
RPG	retrograde pyelogram
rpm	revolutions per minute
RPO	right posterior oblique
RPR	rapid plasma reagin
RQ	respiratory quotient
R & R	rate and rhythm
RR	recovery room; respiratory rate
RSD	reflex sympathetic dystrophy
RSHF	right-sided heart failure
RSI	repetitive stress injuries
RSR	regular sinus rhythm
RSV	right subclavian vein
rt	right; routine
RT	radiation therapy; respiratory therapy
RTA	renal tubular acidosis
rt lat	right lateral
rtd	retarded
RUL	right upper lobe
RU	roentgen unit; routine urinalysis
RUE	right upper extremity
RUL	right upper lobe
RUQ	right upper quadrant
RV	residual volume; right ventricle
RVG	radionuclide ventriculogram
RVH	right ventricular hypertrophy
RVS	relative value schedule
RW	ragweed
Rx	prescription; take; therapy; treatment

S

s	without
S-A	sinoatrial node
S & A	sugar and acetone

SA	salicylic acid; sinoatrial; sperm analysis; surgeon's assistant
SAAT	serum aspartate aminotransferase
SAB	spontaneous abortion
SACH	solid ankle cushion heel
SACP	serum acid phosphatase
SAFP	serum alpha-fetoprotein
SALD	serum aldolase
SAL	sensorineural activity level; sterility assurance level; suction-assisted lipectomy
SALP	salpingectomy; salpingography; serum alkaline phosphatase
Salpx	salpingectomy
SAM	self-administered medication program
SAS	short arm splint; sleep apnea syndrome; social adjustment scale; subarachnoid space
SB	stillbirth
SBE	subacute bacterial endocarditis
SBO	small bowel obstruction
sc, SC	subcutaneous
SC	spinal cord
SCA	sickle cell anemia
SCC	squamous cell carcinoma
SCD	sudden cardiac death
SCI	spinal cord injury
schiz	schizophrenia
SCID	severe combined immune deficiency
SCPK	serum creatine phosphokinase
SCT	sickle cell trait
SD	septal defect; shoulder disarticulation; spontaneous delivery; sudden death
SDAT	senile dementia of Alzheimer's type
SDM	standard deviation of the mean
SDS	sudden death syndrome
sec, s	second
SED	suberythema dose
sed rate	sedimentation rate
seg	segmented neutrophils
SEM	scanning electron microscopy
semi	half
seq	sequela; sequestrum
SES	subcutaneous electric stimulation
sev	sever; severed
SF	scarlet fever; spinal fluid
SG	serum globulin; skin graft
SGA	small for gestational age
s gl	without correction; without glasses
SGGTP	serum gamma-glutamyl transpeptidase
SGOT	serum glutamic oxaloacetic transaminase
SGPT	serum glutamic pyruvic transaminase
SH	serum hepatitis; sex hormone; social history
sh	shoulder
SI	saturation index
SICU	surgical intensive care unit
SIDS	sudden infant death syndrome
SIRS	systemic inflammatory response syndrome
SIS	saline infusion sonohysterography
SISI	short increment sensitivity index

SLAP	serum leucine aminopeptidase
SLE	St. Louis encephalitis; systemic lupus erythematosus
SLPS	serum lipase
SM	simple mastectomy
sm	small
SMA	sequential multiple analysis
SMAC	sequential multiple analysis computer
SMG	senile macular degeneration
SMR	submucous resection
SMRR	submucous resection and rhinoplasty
SNR	signal-to-noise ratio
SNS	sympathetic nervous system; sensory nervous system
SO	salpingo-oophorectomy
SOAP	symptoms, observations, assessments, plan; subjective, objective, assessment, plan
SOB	shortness of breath
SOM	serous otitis media
SONO	sonography
SOP	standard operating procedure
sos	if necessary
SPBI	serum protein-bound iodine
SPE	serum protein electrophoresis
spec	specimen
SPECT	single photon emission computed tomography
SPF	skin protective factor
sp gr	specific gravity
SPHI	serum phosphohexoisomerase
SPK	serum pyruvate kinase
SPP	suprapubic prostatectomy
SPR	scanned projection radiography
SQ	subcutaneous
SR	sedimentation rate; stimulus response; system review
Sr	strontium
SRS	smoker's respiratory syndrome
ss	half
SS	signs and symptoms; Sjögren's syndrome; soap solution
SSE	soap suds enema
SSU	sterile supply unit
ST	esotropia
staph	staphylococcus
stat	immediately
STD	sexually transmitted disease; skin test dose
STH	somatotropic hormone
STK	streptokinase
strep	streptococcus
STS	serologic test for syphilis
STSG	split thickness skin graft
subcu	subcutaneous
sub-Q	subcutaneous
SUI	stress urinary incontinence
supp	suppository
surg	surgical; surgery
SVC	superior vena cava
SVD	spontaneous vaginal delivery

SVG	saphenous vein graft
SVN	small volume nebulizer
Sx	symptoms

T

T	temperature
T_1-T_{12}	thoracic vertebrae
TA	therapeutic abortion
T & A	tonsillectomy and adenoidectomy
TAB	therapeutic abortion
tab	tablet
TACT	target air-enema computed tomography
TAF	tumor angiogenesis factor
TAH	total abdominal hysterectomy
TAO	thromboangiitis obliterans
TB	tuberculosis
TBD	total body density
TBF	total body fat
TBG	thyroxine-binding globulin
TBI	thyroxine-binding index
TBW	total body weight
Tc	technetium
TCDB	turn, cough, deep breathe
TCP	time care profile
TD	total disability
TDM	therapeutic drug monitoring
TDT	tone decay test
TEE	transesophageal echocardiography
temp	temperature
TEN	toxic epidermal necrolysis
TENS	transcutaneous electrical nerve stimulation
TES	treadmill exercise score
TF	tactile fremitus
TFS	thyroid function studies
TGA	transposition of great arteries
THR	total hip replacement
TIA	transient ischemic attack
TIA-IR	transient ischemic attack incomplete recovery
TIBC	total iron-binding capacity
TID, tid, t.i.d.	times interval difference; three times a day
tinct	tincture
TKO	to keep open
TKR	total knee replacement
TLC	tender loving care; total lung capacity
TLE	temporal lobe epilepsy
TM	temporomandibular; tympanic membrane
TMD	temporomandibular disease; temporomandibular disorder
TMJ	temporomandibular joint
TMs	tympanic membranes
Tn	normal intraocular tension
TND	term normal delivery
TNF	tumor necrosis factor
TNI	total nodal irradiation
TNM	tumor, nodes, metastases
TO	telephone order
top	topically
TP	testosterone propionate; total protein
TPA	tissue plasminogen activator; *Treponema pallidum* agglutination
TPBF	total pulmonary blood flow
TPI	*Treponema pallidum* immobilization
TPN	total parenteral nutrition
TPR	temperature, pulse, respiration
TPUR	transperineal urethral resection
tr	tincture
TR	tuberculin residue
trach	tracheostomy
TRBF	total renal blood flow
TRH	thyrotropin-releasing hormone
TS	Tourette syndrome
TSD	Tay-Sachs disease
TSE	testicular self-examination
TSH	thyroid-stimulating hormone
TSP	total serum protein
TSS	toxic shock syndrome
TST	tuberculin skin test
TT	thrombin time
TTH	thyrotropic hormone
TULIP	transurethral ultrasound-guided laser-induced proctectomy
TUMT	transurethral microwave therapy
TUR	transurethral resection
TURP	transurethral resection of prostate; prostatectomy
TV	tidal volume; tricuspid valve
TVH	total vaginal hysterectomy
TW	tap water
TWE	tap water enema
Tx	traction; treatment

U

U	units
UA	urinalysis
UC	ulcerative colitis; urine culture; uterine contractions
UCD	usual childhood diseases
UCG	urinary chorionic gonadotropin; uterine chorionic gonadotropin
UCR	unconditioned reflex
UE	upper extremity
UFR	uroflowmeter; uroflowmetry
UG	upper gastrointestinal; urogenital
UGI	upper gastrointestinal
UK	unknown
UL	upper lobe
ULQ	upper left quadrant
umb	umbilicus
UN	urea nitrogen
ung	ointment
UOQ	upper outer quadrant
UP	uroporphyrin
UPP	urethral pressure profile
UR	upper respiratory

ur	urine
URD	upper respiratory disease
URI	upper respiratory infection
urol	urology
URQ	upper right quadrant
US	ultrasonic; ultrasonography
USP	United States Pharmacopeia
UTI	urinary tract infection
UV	ultraviolet
UVJ	ureterovesical junction

V

VA	vacuum aspiration; visual acuity
vag	vaginal
VB	viable birth
VBAC	vaginal birth after ceasarean
VBP	ventricular premature beat
VC	acuity of color vision; vena cava; vital capacity
VCG	vectorcardiogram
VCUG	voiding cystourethrogram
VD	venereal disease
VDG	venereal disease, gonorrhea
VDH	valvular disease of heart
VDRL	Venereal Disease Research Laboratory
VDS	venereal disease, syphilis
VE	visual efficiency
VEP	visual evoked potential
VER	visual evoked response
VF	visual field; vocal fremitus
V fib	ventricular fibrillation
VG	ventricular gallop
VH	vaginal hysterectomy
VHD	valvular heart disease, ventricular heart disease
VI	volume index
vit cap	vital capacity
VLDL	very-low-density lipoprotein
VP	venipuncture; venous pressure
V & P	vagotomy and pyloroplasty
VPC	ventricular premature contraction

VPRC	volume of packed red cells
VS, vs	vital signs
VSD	ventricular septal defect
VTAs	vascular targeting agents
VZV	varicella-zoster virus (chickenpox)

W

W	water
WA	while awake
WB	weight-bearing; whole blood
WBC	white blood cell; white blood count
W/C, w/c	wheelchair
wd	wound
WD	well-developed
w/d	well-developed
WDWN	well-developed; well-nourished
wf	white female
w/n	well-nourished
WNL	within normal limits
w/o	without
WR	Wassermann reaction
wt	weight
w/v	weight by volume

X

x	multiplied by; times
XDP	xeroderma pigmentosum
XM	cross-match
XR	x-ray
XT	exotropia
XU	excretory urogram

Y

y/o	year(s) old
YOB	year of birth
yr, y	year

Z

Z	atomic number; no effect; zero

Appendix C:
Glossary of Pathology and Procedures

A

abdominocentesis (ab-**dom**-ih-noh-sen-**TEE**-sis): Surgical puncture of the abdominal cavity to remove fluid for diagnostic purposes.

ablation (ab-**LAY**-shun): The removal or destruction of the function of a body part.

abortion (ah-**BOR**-shun): The interruption or termination of pregnancy before the fetus is viable.

abrasion (ah-**BRAY**-zhun): An injury in which superficial layers of skin are scraped or rubbed away; treatment involving scraping or rubbing away skin.

abruptio placentae (ab-**RUP**-shee-oh plah-**SEN**-tee): An abnormal condition in which the placenta separates from the uterine wall prematurely before the birth of the fetus.

abscess (**AB**-sess): A localized collection of pus within a circumscribed area that is associated with tissue destruction.

accommodation (ah-**kom**-oh-**DAY**-shun): The process whereby the eyes make adjustments for seeing objects at various distances.

ACE inhibitors (angiotensin-converting enzyme inhibitors): Medications administered to treat hypertension and congestive heart failure.

acetone (**ASS**-eh-tohn): a substance with a sweet fruity odor that is found in small quantities in normal urine and in larger amount in diabetic urine.

Achilles tendinitis (**ten**-dih-**NIGH**-tis): Inflammation of the Achilles tendon caused by excessive stress being placed on the tendon.

achlorhydria (ah-klor-**HIGH**-dree-ah): The absence of hydrochloric acid from gastric secretions.

acne vulgaris (**ACK**-nee vul-**GAY**-ris): A chronic inflammatory disease that is characterized by pustular eruptions of the skin in or near the sebaceous glands.

acquired immune deficiency syndrome: The advanced stage of HIV infection.

acromegaly (**ack**-roh-**MEG**-ah-lee): Enlargement of the extremities (hands and feet) caused by excessive secretion of the growth hormone *after* puberty.

acronym (**ACK**-roh-nim): A word formed from the initial letter or letters of the major parts of a compound term.

acrophobia (**ack**-roh-**FOH**-bee-ah): An excessive fear of being in high places.

actinic keratosis (ack-**TIN**-ick **kerr**-ah-**TOH**-sis): A precancerous skin lesion caused by excessive exposure to the sun.

acute nasopharyngitis (**nay**-zoh-**far**-in-**JIGH**-tis): Inflammation of the nose and throat; among the terms used to describe the common cold; also known as an upper respiratory infection.

acute respiratory distress syndrome: A type of lung failure resulting from many different disorders that cause pulmonary edema.

addiction: Compulsive, uncontrollable dependence on a substance, habit, or action to the degree that stopping causes severe emotional, mental, or physiologic reactions.

Addison's disease (**AD**-ih-sonz): A progressive disease in which the adrenal glands do not produce enough cortisol that if untreated can produce a life threatening addisonian crisis.

adenectomy (**ad**-eh-**NECK**-toh-mee): Surgical removal of a gland.

adenitis (**ad**-eh-**NIGH**-tis): Inflammation of a gland.

adenocarcinoma (ad-eh-noh-**kar**-sih-**NOH**-mah): Any one of a large group of carcinomas derived from glandular tissue.

adenoidectomy (ad-eh-noid-**ECK**-toh-mee *or* ad-eh-noy-**DECK**-toh-mee): Surgical removal of the adenoids.

adenoma (ad-eh-**NOH**-mah): A benign tumor in which the cells form recognizable glandular structures.

adenoma, pituitary (ad-eh-**NOH**-mah): A benign tumor of the pituitary gland that causes excess hormone secretion. An ACTH-secreting tumor stimulates the excess production of cortisol that causes most cases of Cushing's syndrome.

adenoma, prolactin-producing: A benign tumor of the pituitary gland that causes it to produce too much prolactin; also known as a prolactinoma.

adenomalacia (ad-eh-noh-mah-**LAY**-shee-ah): Abnormal softening of a gland.

adenosclerosis (ad-eh-noh-skleh-**ROH**-sis): Abnormal hardening of a gland.

adenosis (ad-eh-**NOH**-sis): Any disease condition of a gland.

adhesion (ad-**HEE**-zhun): A band of fibrous tissue that holds structures together abnormally.

adrenalitis (ah-**dree**-nal-**EYE**-tis): Inflammation of the adrenal glands.

adrenitis (ad-reh-**NIGH**-tis): Inflammation of the adrenal glands.

adrenomegaly (ah-**dree**-noh-**MEG**-ah-lee): Enlargement of the adrenal glands.

adrenopathy (**ad**-ren-**OP**-ah-thee): Any disease of the adrenal glands.

aerophagia (**ay**-er-oh-**FAY**-jee-ah): The spasmodic swallowing of air followed by eructations.

agglutination testing (ah-**gloo**-tih-**NAY**-shun): Laboratory tests that involve the clumping together of cells or particles when mixed with incompatible serum. These tests are performed to determine the patient's blood type and to check compatibility of donor and recipient blood before a transfusion.

agoraphobia (**ag**-oh-rah-**FOH**-bee-ah): An overwhelming and irrational fear of leaving the familiar setting of home or venturing into the open.

albinism (**AL**-bih-niz-um): An inherited deficiency or absence of pigment in the skin, hair, and eyes due to an abnormality in production of melanin.

albuminuria (**al**-byou-mih-**NEW**-ree-ah): The presence of the serum protein albumin in the urine.

alcoholism (**AL**-koh-hol-izm): Chronic dependence or abuse of alcohol with specific signs and symptoms of withdrawal.

aldosteronism (al-**DOSS**-teh-roh-**niz**-em *or* al-doh-**STER**-ohn-izm): An abnormality of electrolyte balance caused by excessive secretion of aldosterone.

allergen (**AL**-er-jen): An antigen that is capable of inducing an allergic response.

allergic rhinitis (rye-**NIGH**-tis), commonly referred to as an **allergy**, is an allergic reaction to airborne allergens that causes an increased flow of mucus.

allergist (**AL**-er-jist): A specialist in diagnosing and treating conditions of allergic reactions and altered immunologic reactivity.

allergy: An overreaction by the body to a particular antigen; also known as hypersensitivity.

allogenic (al-oh-**JEN**-ick): Originating within another.

alopecia (al-oh-**PEE**-shee-ah): The partial or complete loss of hair; also known as baldness.

alopecia areata: A disease of unknown cause in which there are well-defined bald areas, usually on the scalp and face.

alopecia capitis totalis: A condition characterized by the loss of all the hair on the scalp.

alopecia universalis: The total loss of hair on all parts of the body.

Alzheimer's disease (**ALTZ**-high-merz): A group of disorders associated with degenerative changes in the brain structure leading to characteristic symptoms including progressive memory loss, impaired cognition, and personality changes.

amblyopia (am-blee-**OH**-pee-ah): Dimness of vision or the partial loss of sight without detectable disease of the eye.

amebic dysentery (ah-**MEE**-bik **DIS**-en-ter-ee): An intestinal infection caused by *Entamoeba histolytica amoeba*.

amenorrhea (ah-men-oh-**REE**-ah *or* ay-**men**-oh-**REE**-ah): The absence of menstrual periods. This condition is normal only before puberty, during pregnancy, while breast-feeding, and after menopause.

ametropia (**am**-eh-**TROH**-pee-ah): An error of refraction in which only objects located a finite distance from the eye are focused on the retina.

amnesia (am-**NEE**-zee-ah): A disturbance in the memory marked by total or partial inability to recall past experiences.

amniocentesis (**am**-nee-oh-sen-**TEE**-sis): Surgical puncture to remove a specimen of amniotic fluid for diagnostic purposes

amobarbital (**am**-oh-**BAR**-bih-tal): A barbiturate used as a sedative and hypnotic.

amyotrophic lateral sclerosis (ah-**my**-oh-**TROH**-fick): A degenerative disease of the motor neurons in which patients become progressively weaker until they are completely paralyzed; also known as Lou Gehrig's disease.

analgesic (**an**-al-**JEE**-zick): A drug that relieves pain without affecting consciousness.

analgesic, narcotic: Medications, such as morphine and codeine, that are used to relieve severe pain but which may cause dependence or addiction.

analgesic, nonnarcotic: Medication, such as aspirin, that is used to relieve mild to moderate pain.

anaphylaxis (an-ah-fih-**LACK**-sis): A severe response to a foreign substance such as a drug, food, insect venom, or chemical.

anaplasia (an-ah-**PLAY**-zee-ah): Change in the structure of cells and in their orientation to each other.

anastomosis (ah-**nas**-toh-**MOH**-sis): A surgical connection between two hollow or tubular structures.

anemia (ah-**NEE**-mee-ah): A disorder characterized by lower than normal levels of red blood cells in the blood.

anemia, aplastic (ay-**PLAS**-tick ah-**NEE**-mee-ah): A marked absence of *all* formed blood elements.

anemia, Cooley's: A group of genetic disorders characterized by short-lived red blood cells that lack the normal ability to produce hemoglobin; also known as thalassemia.

anemia, hemolytic: A condition in which red blood cells are destroyed faster than the bone marrow can replace them.

anemia, megaloblastic (**MEG**-ah-loh-**blas**-tick ah-**NEE**-mee-ah): A form of anemia in which the bone marrow produces large abnormal red blood cells with a reduced capacity to carry oxygen.

anemia, pernicious: An autoimmune disorder results in the inability of the body to absorb vitamin B_{12} normally.

anemia, sickle cell: A genetic disorder that causes abnormal hemoglobin that results in the red blood cells assuming an abnormal sickle shape.

anesthesia (an-es-**THEE**-zee-ah): The absence of normal sensation, especially sensitivity to pain.

anesthesia, epidural (ep-ih-**DOO**-ral): Regional anesthesia produced by injecting a local anesthetic into the epidural space of the lumbar or sacral region of the spine.

anesthesia, general: The total loss of body sensation and consciousness as induced by various anesthetic agents, given primarily by inhalation or intravenous injection.

anesthesia, local: The loss of sensation in a limited area produced by injecting an anesthetic solution near that area.

anesthesia, regional: The temporary interruption of nerve conduction is produced by injecting an anesthetic solution near the nerves to be blocked.

anesthesia, spinal: Anesthesia produced by injecting an anesthetic into the subarachnoid space, which is located below the arachnoid membrane and above the pia mater that surrounds the spinal cord.

anesthesia, topical: An anesthetic that numbs only the tissue surface and is applied as a liquid, ointment, or spray.

anesthesiologist (an-es-**thee**-zee-**OL**-oh-jist): A physician who specializes in administering anesthetic agents before and during surgery.

anesthetic (an-es-**THET**-ick): The medication used to induce anesthesia. The anesthetic may be topical, local, regional, or general.

anesthetist (ah-**NES**-theh-tist): A specialist, other than a physician, trained in administering anesthesia.

aneurysm (**AN**-you-rizm): A localized weak spot or balloon-like enlargement of the wall of an artery.

aneurysmectomy (an-you-riz-**MECK**-toh-mee): Surgical removal of an aneurysm.

aneurysmorrhaphy (an-you-riz-**MOR**-ah-fee): To suture an aneurysm.

angiectomy (an-jee-**ECK**-toh-mee): Surgical removal of a blood vessel.

angiitis (an-je-**EYE**-tis): Inflammation of a blood or lymph vessel; also known as vasculitis.

angina pectoris (an-**JIGH**-nah *or* **AN**-jih-nuh **PECK**-toh-riss): Severe episodes of spasmodic choking or suffocating chest pain caused by an insufficient supply of oxygen to the heart muscle.

angiocardiography (an-jee-oh-**kar**-dee-**OG**-rah-fee): A radiographic study using x-rays and contrast medium to visualize the dimensions of the heart and large blood vessels.

angiogenesis (an-jee-oh-**JEN**-eh-sis): The ability of a tumor to support its growth by creating its own blood supply.

angiogram (**AN**-jee-oh-**gram**): The record produced by a radiographic study of blood vessels.

angiography (an-jee-**OG**-rah-fee): A radiographic study of blood vessels after the injection of a contrast medium.

angiomegaly (an-jee-oh-**MEG**-ah-lee): Abnormal enlargement of blood vessels.

angionecrosis (an-jee-oh-neh-**KROH**-sis): Death of the walls of blood vessels.

angiorrhaphy (an-jee-**OR**-ah-fee): A suture repair of any vessel, especially of a blood vessel.

angiosclerosis (an-jee-oh-skleh-**ROH**-sis): Abnormal hardening of the walls of blood vessels.

angiospasm (**AN**-jee-oh-**spazm**): Spasmodic contraction of the blood vessels.

angiostenosis (an-jee-oh-steh-**NOH**-sis): Abnormal narrowing of a blood vessel.

anhidrosis (an-high-**DROH**-sis): The condition of lacking or being without sweat.

anisocoria (an-ih-so-**KOH**-ree-ah): A condition in which the pupils are unequal in size.

ankylosing spondylitis (ang-kih-**LOH**-sing **spon**-dih-**LYE**-tis): Rheumatoid arthritis characterized by progressive stiffening of the spine caused by fusion of the vertebral bodies.

ankylosis (ang-kih-**LOH**-sis): Loss or absence of mobility in a joint due to disease, an injury, or a surgical procedure.

anomaly (ah-**NOM**-ah-lee): A deviation from what is regarded as normal.

anonychia (an-oh-**NICK**-ee-ah): Pertaining to the absence of fingernails or toenails.

anoplasty (**AY**-noh-**plas**-tee): Surgical repair of the anus.

anorchism (an-**OR**-kizm): The congenital absence of one or both testicles.

anorexia (an-oh-**RECK**-see-ah): The lack or loss of appetite for food.

anorexia nervosa: An eating disorder characterized by a refusal to maintain a minimally normal body weight and an intense fear of gaining weight.

anoscopy (ah-**NOS**-koh-pee): Visual examination of the anal canal and lower rectum using a short speculum called an anoscope).

anovulation (an-ov-you-**LAY**-shun): The failure to ovulate although menstruation may continue to occur.

anoxia (ah-**NOCK**-see-ah): The absence or almost complete absence of oxygen from inspired gases, arterial blood, or tissues.

anteflexion (an-tee-**FLECK**-shun): The normal position of the uterus.

anteversion (an-tee-**VER**-zhun): Abnormal tipping, tilting, or turning forward of the entire uterus, including the cervix.

anthracosis (an-thrah-**KOH**-sis): A form of pneumoconiosis caused by coal dust in the lungs; also known as black lung disease.

anti-angiogenesis: Treatment that cuts off the blood supply to the tumor.

antianxiety drugs: Medication administered to suppress anxiety and relax muscles; also known as tranquilizers.

antiarrhythmic (an-tih-ah-**RITH**-mick): Medication administered to control irregularities of the heartbeat.

antibiotic: A medication administered to combat bacterial infections.

anticoagulant (an-tih-koh-**AG**-you-lant): Medication administered to slow blood clotting and to prevent new clots from forming; also known as a thrombolytic.

anticonvulsant (an-tih-kon-**VUL**-sant): Medication that is administered to prevent seizures and convulsions.

antidepressant: Medication that is administered to prevent or relieve depression.

antiemetic (an-tih-ee-**MET**-ick): Medication administered to prevent or relieve nausea and vomiting.

antihypertensive (an-tih-**high**-per-**TEN**-siv): Medication administered to lower high blood pressure.

antineoplastic (an-tih-nee-oh-**PLAS**-tick): Medication that blocks the growth of neoplasms and is used to treat cancer.

antipsychotic (an-tih-sigh-**KOT**-ick): Medication that is administered to treat symptoms of severe psychiatric disorders.

antipyretic (an-tih-pye-**RET**-ick): Medication to reduce or relieve fever.

antisocial personality disorder: A pattern of disregard for, and violation of, the rights of others that brings the individual into continuous conflict with society.

antispasmodic: Medication that acts to control spasmodic activity of the smooth muscles such as those of the intestine.

antiviral (an-tih-**VYE**-ral): Medication used to treat viral infections or to provide temporary immunity.

anuresis (an-you-**REE**-sis): The complete suppression of urine formation by the kidneys; also known as anuria.

anuria (ah-**NEW**-ree-ah): See anuresis.

anxiety state: A feeling of apprehension, tension, or uneasiness that stems from the anticipation of danger, the source of which is largely unknown or unrecognized.

Apgar score: A system to evaluate a newborn infant's physical status.

aphakia (ah-**FAY**-kee-ah): The absence of the lens of an eye after cataract extraction.

aphasia (ah-**FAY**-zee-ah): A condition, often due to brain damage associated with a stroke, in which there is the loss of the ability to speak, write, or comprehend speech or the spoken word.

aphonia (ah-**FOH**-nee-ah): Loss of the ability to produce normal speech sounds.

aphthous ulcers (**AF**-thus): Recurrent blister-like sores that break and form lesions on the soft tissues lining the mouth; also known as canker sores.

aplasia (ah-**PLAY**-zee-ah): Lack of development of an organ or tissue.

apnea (**AP**-nee-ah *or* ap-**NEE**-ah): The absence of spontaneous respiration.

appendectomy (ap-en-**DECK**-toh-mee): The surgical removal of the appendix.

appendicitis (ah-**pen**-dih-**SIGH**-tis): Inflammation of the appendix.

arrhythmia, cardiac (ah-**RITH**-mee-ah): An irregularity or the loss of normal rhythm of the heartbeat; also known as dysrhythmia.

arteriectomy (ar-teh-ree-**ECK**-toh-mee): Surgical removal of part of an artery.

arteriogram (ar-**TEER**-ee-oh-gram): The record produced by arteriography.

arteriography (ar-tee-ree-**OG**-rah-fee): The process of recording a picture of an artery or arteries.

arteriomalacia (ar-**tee**-ree-oh-mah-**LAY**-shee-ah): Abnormal softening of the walls of an artery or arteries.

arterionecrosis (ar-tee-ree-oh-neh-**KROH**-sis): Tissue death of an artery or arteries.

arteriosclerosis (ar-tee-ree-oh-skleh-**ROH**-sis): Abnormal hardening of the walls of an artery or arteries.

arteriostenosis (ar-**tee**-ree-oh-steh-**NOH**-sis): Abnormal narrowing of an artery or arteries.

arteritis (ar-teh-**RYE**-tis): Inflammation of an artery.

arthralgia (ar-**THRAL**-jee-ah): Pain in a joint or joints.

arthrectomy (ar-**THRECK**-toh-mee): The surgical removal of a joint.

arthritis (ar-**THRIGH**-tis): Inflammation of one or more joints.

arthritis, gouty: Arthritis associated with the formation of uric acid crystals in the joint as the result of hyperuricemia.

arthritis, juvenile rheumatoid: Arthritis that affects children with pain and swelling in the joints, skin rash, fever, slowed growth, and fatigue.

arthritis, rheumatoid: Autoimmune disorder in which the synovial membranes are inflamed and thicken.

arthrocentesis (ar-throh-sen-**TEE**-sis): Surgical puncture of the joint space to remove synovial fluid for analysis.

arthrodesis (ar-throh-**DEE**-sis): Surgical stiffening of a joint or joining of spinal vertebrae; also known as fusion or surgical ankylosis.

arthrolysis (ar-**THROL**-ih-sis): Surgical loosening of an ankylosed joint.

arthroplasty (**AR**-throh-**plas**-tee): Surgical repair of a joint; also surgical replacement of a joint.

arthrosclerosis (**ar**-throh-skleh-**ROH**-sis): Stiffness of the joints, especially in the elderly.

arthroscopy (ar-**THROS**-koh-pee): Visual examination and treatment of the internal structure of a joint using an arthroscope.

arthrotomy (ar-**THROT**-oh-mee): A surgical incision into a joint.

asbestosis (**ass**-beh-**STOH**-sis): A form of pneumoconiosis caused by asbestos particles found in the lungs of workers from the ship building and construction trades.

asphyxia (ass-**FICK**-see-ah): Pathologic changes caused by a lack of oxygen in air that is inhaled.

asphyxiation (ass-**fick**-see-**AY**-shun): Any interruption of breathing that results in the loss of consciousness or death; also known as suffocation.

aspiration (ass-pih-**RAY**-shun): Inhaling or drawing a foreign substance into the upper respiratory tract; withdrawal by suction of fluids or gases from a body cavity.

assay (**ASS**-ay): To determine the amount of a particular substance in a mixture.

assessment: Evaluation or appraisal of a condition.

asthma (**AZ**-mah): A chronic allergic disorder characterized by episodes of severe breathing difficulty, coughing, and wheezing.

astigmatism (ah-**STIG**-mah-tizm): A condition in which the eye does not focus properly because of unequal curvatures of the cornea.

ataxia (ah-**TACK**-see-ah): Inability to coordinate the muscles in the execution of voluntary movement.

atelectasis (at-ee-**LEK**-tah-sis): A condition in which the lung fails to expand because air cannot pass beyond the bronchioles; also known as a collapsed lung.

atherectomy (**ath**-er-**ECK**-toh-mee): Surgical removal of plaque from the interior lining of an artery.

atheroma (**ath**-er-**OH**-mah): Fatty deposit within the wall of an artery.

atherosclerosis (**ath**-er-oh-skleh-**ROH**-sis): Hardening and narrowing of the arteries due to a buildup of cholesterol plaques.

atonic (ah-**TON**-ick): Lack of normal muscle tone.

atrophy (**AT**-roh-fee): Weakness and wasting away.

atropine (**AT**-roh-peen): Antispasmodic that may be administered preoperatively to relax smooth muscles.

attention deficit disorder: A condition in which a child has a short attention span and impulsiveness that are inappropriate for the child's developmental age.

attention deficit hyperactivity disorder: A pattern of inattention and hyperactivity that are inappropriate for the child's developmental age.

audiologist (aw-dee-**OL**-oh-jist): A specialist in the measurement of hearing function and the rehabilitation of persons with hearing impairments.

audiometer (aw-dee-**OM**-eh-ter): An electronic device that produces acoustic stimuli of a known frequency and intensity.

auscultation (aws-kul-**TAY**-shun): Listening through a stethoscope for sounds within the body to determine the condition of the lungs, pleura, heart, and abdomen.

autistic disorder (aw-**TISS**-tick): A disorder in which a young child cannot develop normal social relationships, behaves in compulsive and ritualistic ways, and frequently has poor communication skills; also known as an autism.

autism (**AW**-tizm): See autistic disorder.

autoimmune disorder (aw-toh-ih-**MYOUN**): A disorder of the immune system in which the body attacks itself.

autologous (aw-**TOL**-uh-guss): Originating within an individual.

autopsy (**AW**-top-see): A postmortem (after death) examination.

azoospermia (ay-**zoh**-oh-**SPER**-mee-ah): The absence of sperm in the semen.

B

bacilli (bah-**SILL**-eye): Rod-shaped spore-forming bacteria.

bacteria (back-**TEER**-ree-ah): A group of one-cell microscopic organisms some of which cause disease in humans.

bactericide (back-**TEER**-ih-sighd): A substance that causes the death of bacteria.

bacteriostatic (bac-**tee**-ree-oh-**STAT**-ick): An agent that inhibits, slows, or retards the growth of bacteria.

bacteriuria (back-**tee**-ree-**YOU**-ree-ah): The presence of bacteria in the urine.

balanitis (**bal**-ah-**NIGH**-tis): Inflammation of the glans penis, usually associated with phimosis.

balloon angioplasty: A procedure in which a small balloon on the end of a catheter is used to open a partially blocked coronary artery; also known as percutaneous transluminal coronary angioplasty.

barbiturate (bar-**BIT**-you-rayt): A class of drugs whose major action is a calming or depressed effect on the central nervous system.

barium: A radiopaque contrast medium used primarily to visualize the digestive system.

Becker's muscular dystrophy (**BECK**-urz): A less severe form of muscular dystrophy that does not appear until early adolescence or adulthood.

Bell's palsy: Paralysis of the facial nerve (seventh cranial) that causes drooping only on the affected side of the face.

benign prostatic hypertrophy: An abnormal enlargement of the prostate gland.

benign: Not recurring, nonmalignant, and with a favorable chance for recovery.

beta-blockers: Medications administered to slow the heartbeat.

bilateral hysterosalpingo-oophorectomy (**hiss**-ter-oh-sal-**ping**-goh-oh-**ahf**-oh-**RECK**-toh-mee): Surgical removal of the uterus and cervix, plus both ovaries and fallopian tubes.

bilateral salpingo-oophorectomy (sal-**ping**-goh-oh-**ahf**-oh-**RECK**-toh-mee): Surgical removal of both fallopian tubes and ovaries.

binaural (bye-**NAW**-rul *or* bin-**AW**-rahl): Involving both ears.

biopsy (**BYE**-op-see): The removal of a small piece of living tissue for examination to confirm or establish a diagnosis.

biopsy, excisional: The removal of an entire tumor or lesion plus a margin of surrounding healthy tissue.

biopsy, incisional: The removal of a piece, but not all, of the tumor or lesion.

biopsy, needle: The use of a hollow needle to remove a core of tissue for examination.

bipolar disorder: A clinical course characterized by the occurrence of manic episodes alternating with depressive episodes; also known as a manic-depressive episode.

birthmark: See hemangioma and port-wine stain.

blastoma (blas-**TOH**-mah): A neoplasm composed of immature undifferentiated cells.

blepharedema (blef-ahr-eh-**DEE**-mah): Swelling of the eyelid.

blepharitis (blef-ah-**RYE**-tis): Inflammation of the eyelid.

blepharoplasty (**BLEF**-ah-roh-**plas**-tee): Surgical reduction of the upper and lower eyelids; also known as a lid lift.

blepharoptosis (blef-ah-roh-**TOH**-sis *or* blef-ah-rop-**TOH**-sis): Drooping of the upper eyelid.

blindness: The inability to see.

blood urea nitrogen (you-**REE**-ah): A laboratory test to determine the amount of urea present in the blood.

bone density testing: Radiographic tests to determine bone density.

bone marrow transplant: A treatment for cancers such as leukemia and lymphomas that affect bone marrow.

botulism (**BOT**-you-lizm): Food poisoning that is characterized by paralysis and is often fatal, caused by *Clostridium botulinum.*

brachytherapy (brack-ee-**THER**-ah-pee): Radioactive materials in contact with or implanted into the tissues to be treated.

bradycardia (brad-ee-**KAR**-dee-ah): An abnormally slow heartbeat.

bradykinesia (brad-ee-kih-**NEE**-zee-ah *or* brad-ee-kih-**NEE**-zhuh): Extreme slowness in movement.

bradypnea (brad-ihp-**NEE**-ah *or* brad-ee-**NEE**-ah): An abnormally slow rate of respiration, usually less than 10 breaths per minute.

brain tumor: An abnormal growth within the brain that may be either benign or malignant.

breast augmentation: Mammoplasty to increase breast size.

breast self-examination: An important self-care procedure for the early detection of breast cancer.

breech presentation: An abnormal birth position in which the buttocks or feet of the fetus are presented first.

bronchiectasis (**brong**-kee-**ECK**-tah-sis): Chronic dilation of bronchi or bronchioles resulting from an earlier lung infection that was not cured.

bronchitis (brong-**KYE**-tis): Inflammation of the bronchial walls.

bronchoconstrictor (**brong**-koh-kon-**STRICK**-tor): Medication that narrows the opening of the passages into the lungs.

bronchodilator (**brong**-koh-dye-**LAY**-tor): Medication that expands the opening of the passages into the lungs.

bronchoplasty (**BRONG**-koh-**plas**-tee): Surgical repair of a bronchial defect.

bronchoplegia (**brong**-koh-**PLEE**-jee-ah): Paralysis of the walls of the bronchi.

bronchopneumonia (**brong**-koh-new-**MOH**-nee-ah): A form of pneumonia that begins in the bronchioles.

bronchorrhagia (**brong**-koh-**RAY**-jee-ah): Bleeding from the bronchi.

bronchorrhea (**brong**-koh-**REE**-ah): An excessive discharge of mucus from the bronchi.

bronchoscopy (brong-**KOS**-koh-pee): Visual examination of the bronchi using a bronchoscope.

bruit (**BREW**-ee *or* **BROOT**): An abnormal sound or murmur heard in auscultation.

bruxism (**BRUCK**-sizm): Involuntary grinding or clenching of the teeth that usually occurs during sleep and is associated with tension or stress.

bulimia (byou-**LIM**-ee-ah *or* boo-**LEE**-mee-ah): An eating disorder characterized by episodes of binge eating followed by self-induced vomiting or misuse of laxatives; also known as bulimia nervosa.

bulla (**BULL**-ah): A large blister that is *more than* 0.5 cm in diameter.

burn, first-degree: A burn that causes no blisters and only superficial damage to the epidermis; also known as a superficial burn.

burn, second-degree: A burn that causes blisters and superficial damage to the epidermis; also known as a partial thickness burn.

burn, third-degree: A burn that damages the epidermis, corium, and subcutaneous layers; also known as a full thickness burn.

burn: An injury to body tissues caused by heat, flame, electricity, sun, chemicals, or radiation.

bursectomy (ber-**SECK**-toh-mee): Surgical removal of a bursa.

bursitis (ber-**SIGH**-tis): Inflammation of a bursa.

byssinosis (biss-ih-**NOH**-sis): A form of pneumoconiosis caused by cotton, flax, or hemp dust in the lungs; also known as brown lung disease.

C

calcium channel blockers: Medications administered to treat hypertension, angina, and arrhythmia.

calciuria (kal-sih-**YOU**-ree-ah): The presence of calcium in the urine.

callus (**KAL**-us): A thickening of part of the skin on the hands or feet caused by repeated rubbing; the bulging deposit that forms around the area of the break in a fractured bone.

capillary puncture: The technique used to draw a small amount of blood for testing; also known as a finger stick.

carbuncle (**KAR**-bung-kul): A cluster of furuncles that result in extensive sloughing of skin and scar formation.

carcinoma (**kar**-sih-**NOH**-mah): A malignant tumor that occurs in epithelial tissue.

carcinoma, basal cell: A malignant tumor of the basal cell layer of the epidermis.

carcinoma in situ: A malignant tumor in its original position that has not yet disturbed or invaded the surrounding tissues.

cardiac catheterization (**KAR**-dee-ack **kath**-eh-ter-eye-**ZAY**-shun): Placement of a catheter through a vein or artery and into the heart.

cardiocentesis (**kar**-dee-oh-sen-**TEE**-sis): A puncture of a chamber of the heart to remove fluid for diagnosis or therapy.

cardiologist (**kar**-dee-**OL**-oh-jist): A specialist in diagnosing and treating abnormalities, diseases, and disorders of the heart.

cardiomegaly (**kar**-dee-oh-**MEG**-ah-lee): Abnormal enlargement of the heart.

cardioplegia (**kar**-dee-oh-**PLEE**-jee-ah): Paralysis of the muscles of the heart.

cardiorrhaphy (**kar**-dee-**OR**-ah-fee): To suture the wall of the heart.

cardiorrhexis (**kar**-dee-oh-**RECK**-sis): Rupture of the heart.

cardiotomy (**kar**-dee-**OT**-oh-mee): A surgical incision into the heart.

cardioversion (**kar**-dee-oh-**VER**-zhun): The use of electrical shock to restore the heart's normal rhythm; also known as defibrillation.

carditis (**kar**-**DYE**-tis): Inflammation of the heart.

carpal tunnel syndrome (**KAR**-pul): Inflammation of the tendons passing through the carpal tunnel of the wrist.

castration (**kas**-**TRAY**-shun): Surgical removal or destruction of both testicles.

cataract (**KAT**-ah-rakt): Loss of transparency of the lens of the eye.

catatonic (**kat**-ah-**TON**-ick): Behavior marked by a lack of responsiveness, stupor, and a tendency to remain in a fixed posture.

catheterization (**kath**-eh-ter-eye-**ZAY**-shun): Insertion of a sterile catheter through the urethra and into the urinary bladder.

causalgia (**kaw**-**ZAL**-jee-ah): Intense burning pain after an injury to a sensory nerve.

cauterization (**kaw**-ter-eye-**ZAY**-zhun): The destruction of tissue by burning for therapeutic purposes.

cellulitis (**sell**-you-**LYE**-tis): A diffuse infection of connective tissue with severe inflammation within the layers of the skin.

centesis (**sen**-**TEE**-sis): A surgical puncture to remove fluid for diagnostic purposes or to remove excess fluid.

cephalalgia (**sef**-ah-**LAL**-jee-ah): Pain in the head; also known as a headache or cephalodynia.

cephalodynia: See cephalalgia.

cerebral palsy (**SER**-eh-bral *or* seh-**REE**-bral **PAWL**-zee): A condition caused by a brain injury that occurs during pregnancy, birth, or soon after birth that is characterized by poor muscle control and other neurologic deficiencies

cerebrovascular accident (**ser**-eh-broh-**VAS**-kyou-lar): Damage to the brain when the blood flow to the brain is disrupted because a blood vessel supplying it is blocked; also known as a stroke.

cervical radiculopathy (rah-**dick**-you-**LOP**-ah-thee): Nerve pain caused by pressure on the spinal nerve roots in the neck region.

cervicectomy (**ser**-vih-**SECK**-toh-mee): Surgical removal of the cervix.

cervicitis (**ser**-vih-**SIGH**-tis): Inflammation of the cervix.

cesarean delivery (seh-**ZEHR**-ee-un): The delivery of the child through an incision in the maternal abdominal and uterine wall; also known as a cesarean section or a C-section.

chalazion (kah-**LAY**-zee-on): A localized swelling of the eyelid resulting from obstruction of one of the oil-producing glands of the eyelid.

chemabrasion (keem-ah-**BRAY**-shun): The use of chemicals to remove the outer layers of skin to treat acne scaring, fine wrinkling, and general keratoses; also known as a chemical peel.

chemotherapy: The use of chemical agents and drugs to destroy malignant cells and tissues.

Cheyne-Stokes respiration (**CHAYN**-**STOHKS**): A pattern of alternating periods of hyperpnea (rapid breathing), hypopnea (slow breathing), and apnea (the absence of breathing).

chickenpox: An acute highly contagious viral disease caused by the herpes virus *Varicella zoster*.

chiropractor (**KYE**-roh-**prack**-tor): A specialist in manipulative treatment of disorders originating from misalignment of the spine.

chlamydia (klah-**MID**-ee-ah): A highly contagious sexually transmitted disease caused by the bacteria *Chlamydia trachomatis*.

chloasma (kloh-**AZ**-mah): A pigmentation disorder characterized by brownish colored spots on the face; also known as melasma or the mask of pregnancy.

cholecystalgia (**koh**-lee-sis-**TAL**-jee-ah): Pain in the gallbladder.

cholecystectomy (**koh**-lee-sis-**TECK**-toh-mee): Surgical removal of the gallbladder.

cholecystitis (**koh**-lee-sis-**TYE**-tis): Inflammation of the gallbladder.

choledocholithotomy (koh-**led**-oh-koh-lih-**THOT**-oh-mee): An incision in the common bile duct for the removal of gallstones.

cholelithiasis (**koh**-lee-lih-**THIGH**-ah-sis): The presence of gallstones in the gallbladder or bile ducts.

cholera (**KOL**-er-ah): An intestinal infection caused by *Vibrio cholerae*.

cholesterol (koh-**LES**-ter-ol): Lipids that travel in the blood in packages called lipoproteins.

chondritis (kon-**DRY**-tis): Inflammation of cartilage.

chondroma (kon-**DROH**-mah): Benign tumor derived from cartilage cells.

chondromalacia (**kon**-droh-mah-**LAY**-shee-ah): Abnormal softening of the cartilage.

chondropathy (kon-**DROP**-ah-thee): A disease of the cartilage.

chondroplasty (**KON**-droh-**plas**-tee): Surgical repair of cartilage.

chorionic villus sampling: A diagnostic procedure using chorionic cells from the fetus to test for genetic abnormalities in the developing child.

chronic obstructive pulmonary disease: A general term used to describe a group of respiratory conditions characterized by chronic airflow limitations.

cicatrix (sick-**AY**-tricks): A "normal" scar resulting from the healing of a wound.

cineradiography (**sin**-eh-**ray**-dee-**OG**-rah-fee): The recording of images as they appear in motion on a fluorescent screen.

circumcision (**ser**-kum-**SIZH**-un): Surgical removal of the foreskin of the penis.

circumscribed (**SER**-kum-skryebd): Contained within a limited area.

cirrhosis (sih-**ROH**-sis): A progressive degenerative disease of the liver characterized by disturbance of structure and function of the liver.

claustrophobia (**klaws**-troh-**FOH**-bee-ah): An abnormal fear of being in narrow or enclosed spaces.

cleft lip: A congenital defect resulting in a deep fissure of the lip running upward to the nose; also known as a hare lip.

cleft palate: A congenital fissure of the palate that involves the upper lip, hard palate, and/or soft palate.

clubbing: Abnormal curving and shine on the nails that is often accompanied by enlargement of the fingertips. This condition can be hereditary or caused by changes associated with oxygen deficiencies related to coronary or pulmonary disease.

cognition (kog-**NISH**-un): The mental activities associated with thinking, learning, and memory.

colectomy (koh-**LECK**-toh-mee): Surgical removal of all or part of the colon.

colitis (koh-**LYE**-tis): Inflammation of the colon.

colonoscopy (**koh**-lun-**OSS**-koh-pee): Visual examination of the inner surface of the colon, from the rectum to the cecum.

colostomy (koh-**LAHS**-toh-mee): Surgical creation of an opening between the colon and the body surface.

colostrum (kuh-**LOS**-trum): The fluid secreted by the breasts during the first days postpartum.

colotomy (koh-**LOT**-oh-mee): A surgical incision into the colon.

colpitis (kol-**PYE**-tis): Inflammation of the lining of the vagina; also known as vaginitis.

colpopexy (**KOL**-poh-**peck**-see): Surgical fixation of the vagina to a surrounding structure.

colporrhaphy (kol-**POR**-ah-fee): Suturing the vagina.

colporrhexis (**kol**-poh-**RECK**-sis): Laceration of the vagina.

colposcopy (kol-**POS**-koh-pee): The direct visual examination of the tissues of the cervix and vagina using a colposcope.

coma (**KOH**-mah): A profound state of unconsciousness marked by the absence of spontaneous eye movements, no response to painful stimuli, and no vocalization.

comatose (**KOH**-mah-tohs): The condition of being in a coma.

comedo (**KOM**-eh-doh): A lesion formed by the buildup of sebum and keratin in a hair follicle.

communicable (kuh-**MEW**-nih-kuh-bul): Any disease transmitted from one person to another either by direct or indirect contact.

complete blood cell count: A series of tests performed as a group to evaluate several blood conditions.

compliance: The patient's consistency and accuracy in following the regimen prescribed by a physician or other health professional.

compulsions: Repetitive behaviors the goal of which is to prevent or reduce anxiety or stress.

computed tomography (toh-**MOG**-rah-fee): An imaging technique that uses a thin, fan-shaped x-ray beam that rotates around the patient to produce multiple cross-sectional views of the body.

concussion (kon-**KUSH**-un): A violent shaking up or jarring of the brain.

congenital disorder (kon-**JEN**-ih-tahl): An abnormal condition that exists at the time of birth and may be caused by a developmental disorder before birth, prenatal influences, premature birth, or injuries during birth.

congestive heart failure: A syndrome in which the heart is unable to pump enough blood to meet the body's needs for oxygen and nutrients.

conization (**kon**-ih-**ZAY**-shun *or* **koh**-nih-**ZAY**-shun): Surgical removal of a cone-shaped section of tissue from the cervix; also known as a cone biopsy.

conjunctivitis (kon-**junk**-tih-**VYE**-tis): Inflammation of the conjunctiva; also known as pinkeye.

conjunctivoplasty (**kon**-junk-**TYE**-voh-**plas**-tee): Surgical repair of the conjunctiva.

conscious: State of being awake, aware, and responding appropriately.

constipation: A decrease in frequency in the passage of stools, or difficulty in passing hard, dry stools.

contraceptive: A measure taken or device used to lessen the likelihood of conception and pregnancy.

contracture (kon-**TRACK**-chur): Abnormal shortening of muscle tissues making the muscle resistant to stretching.

contraindication: A factor in the patient's condition that makes the use of a drug dangerous or ill advised.

contrast medium: A substance used in radiography to make visible structures that are otherwise hard to see.

contrast medium, radiolucent: A substance such as air that *does* allow x-rays to pass through and appears black or dark gray on the resulting film.

contrast medium, radiopaque: A substance that *does not* allow x-rays to pass through and appears white or light gray on the resulting film.

contusion (kon-**TOO**-zhun): An injury that does not break the skin and is characterized by swelling, discoloration, and pain.

contusion, cerebral: Bruising of brain tissue as a result of a head injury.

convergence (kon-**VER**-jens): The simultaneous inward movement of both eyes in an effort to maintain single binocular vision as an object comes nearer.

conversion disorder: A change in function, such as the paralysis of an arm, that suggests a physical disorder but has no physical cause.

convulsion: A sudden, violent, involuntary contraction of a group of muscles caused by a disturbance in brain function; also known as a seizure.

convulsion, clonic: A state marked by alternate contraction and relaxation of muscles resulting in jerking movements of the face, trunk, or extremities.

convulsion, tonic: A state of continuous muscular contraction that results in rigidity and violent spasms.

corneal abrasion: An injury, such as a scratch or irritation, to the outer layers of the cornea.

corneal transplant: The replacement of a scarred or diseased cornea with clear corneal tissue from a donor; also known as keratoplasty.

corneal ulcer: Pitting of the cornea caused by an infection or injury.

coronary artery bypass graft: A surgical procedure to replace a blocked coronary artery with a piece of vein from the leg; also known as bypass surgery.

coronary artery disease: Atherosclerosis of the coronary arteries that may cause angina pectoris, myocardial infarction, and sudden death

coronary thrombosis (KOR-uh-**nerr**-ee throm-**BOH**-sis): Damage to the heart caused by a thrombus blocking a coronary artery.

corticosteroid: A hormone-like preparation used primarily as an anti-inflammatory and as an immunosuppressant.

cortisone (**KOR**-tih-sohn): The synthetic equivalent of corticosteroids produced by the body that is administered to suppress inflammation and as an immunosuppressant to prevent organ rejection by the body.

costectomy (kos-**TECK**-toh-mee): The surgical removal of a rib or ribs.

costotomy (kos-**TOT**-oh-mee): Surgical incision or division of a rib or ribs.

craniectomy (**kray**-nee-**EK**-toh-mee): Surgical removal of a portion of the skull.

craniocele (**KRAY**-nee-oh-**seel**): A congenital gap in the skull with herniation of brain substance; also known as an encephalocele.

craniomalacia (**kray**-nee-oh-mah-**LAY**-shee-ah): Abnormal softening of the skull.

cranioplasty (**KRAY**-nee-oh-**plas**-tee): Surgical repair of the skull.

craniotomy (**kray**-nee-**OT**-oh-mee): Surgical incision or opening into the skull that is performed to gain access to part of the brain; also known as a bone flap.

creatinuria (kree-**at**-ih-**NEW**-ree-ah): An increased concentration of creatine in the urine.

crepitation (**krep**-ih-**TAY**-shun): Crackling sensation that is felt and heard when the ends of a broken bone move together; also know as crepitus.

crepitus (**KREP**-ih-tus): See crepitation.

cretinism (**CREE**-tin-izm): A congenital lack of thyroid secretion.

Crohn's disease: A chronic autoimmune disorder involving any part of the gastrointestinal tract but most commonly resulting in scarring and thickening of the walls of the ileum, the colon or both.

croup (**KROOP**): An acute respiratory syndrome in children and infants characterized by obstruction of the larynx, hoarseness, and a barking cough.

crust: A collection of dried serum and cellular debris on the skin.

cryosurgery: The elimination of abnormal tissue cells through the application of extreme cold.

cryptorchidism (krip-**TOR**-kih-dizm): A developmental defect in which one testis fails to descend into the scrotum; also known as an undescended testis.

curettage (**kyou**-reh-**TAHZH**): The removal of material from the surface by scraping or with the use of suction.

Cushing's syndrome (**KUSH**-ingz **SIN**-drohm): A condition caused by prolonged exposure to high levels of cortisol produced by the body or taken as medication.

cyanosis (**sigh**-ah-**NOH**-sis): Blue discoloration of the skin caused by a lack of adequate oxygen.

cyst: A closed sac or pouch containing fluid or semisolid material.

cystalgia (sis-**TAL**-jee-ah): Pain in the urinary bladder.

cystectomy (sis-**TECK**-toh-mee): Surgical removal of all or part of the urinary bladder.

cystic fibrosis (**SIS**-tick figh-**BROH**-sis): A genetic disorder in which the lungs are clogged with large quantities of abnormally thick mucus and the digestive system is impaired by thick gluelike mucus that interferes with digestive juices.

cystitis (sis-**TYE**-tis): Inflammation of the bladder.

cystocele (**SIS**-toh-seel): A hernia of the bladder through the vaginal wall.

cystodynia (**sis**-toh-**DIN**-ee-ah): Pain in the urinary bladder.

cystography (sis-**TOG**-rah-fee): A radiographic examination of the bladder after instillation of a contrast medium via a urethral catheter.

cystolith (SIS-toh-lith): Presence of stones in the urinary bladder.

cystopexy (sis-toh-**peck**-see): Surgical fixation of the bladder to the abdominal wall.

cystoplasty (SIS-toh-**plas**-tee): Surgical repair of the bladder.

cystoptosis (**sis**-top-**TOH**-sis *or* **sis**-toh-**TOH**-sis): Prolapse of the bladder into the urethra.

cystorrhagia (**sis**-toh-**RAY**-jee-ah): Bleeding from the bladder.

cystorrhaphy (sis-**TOR**-ah-fee): To suture the bladder.

cystorrhexis (**sis**-toh-**RECK**-sis): Rupture of the bladder.

cystoscopy (sis-**TOS**-koh-pee): Visual examination of the urinary bladder using a cystoscope.

cystostomy (sis-**TOS**-toh-mee): Creation of an artifical opening between the urinary bladder and the exterior of the body.

cytomegalovirus (**sigh**-toh-**meg**-ah-loh-**VYE**-rus): An infection caused by a group of large herpes-type viruses with a wide variety of disease effects.

cytotoxic drug (**sigh**-toh-**TOK**-sick): Medication that kills or damages cells and is used as an immunosuppressant or an antineoplastic.

D

dacryocystitis (**dack**-ree-oh-sis-**TYE**-tis): An inflammation of the lacrimal sac that is associated with faulty tear drainage.

deafness: The complete or partial loss of the ability to hear.

debridement (day-breed-**MON**): The removal of dirt, foreign objects, damaged tissue, and cellular debris from a wound to prevent infection and to promote healing.

decubitus (dee-**KYOU**-bih-tus): The act of lying down or the position assumed in lying down.

defibrillation (dee-**fib**-rih-**LAY**-shun): The use of electrical shock to restore the heart's normal rhythm; also known as cardioversion.

dehydration: A condition in which fluid loss exceeds fluid intake and disrupts the body's normal electrolyte balance.

delirium (dee-**LIR**-ee-um): A potentially reversible condition often associated with a high fever that comes on suddenly in which the patient is confused, disoriented, and unable to think clearly.

delirium tremens (dee-**LIR**-ee-um **TREE**-mens): A form of acute organic brain syndrome due to alcohol withdrawal that is characterized by sweating, tremor, restlessness, anxiety, mental confusion, and hallucinations.

delusion (dee-**LOO**-zhun): A false personal belief that is maintained despite obvious proof or evidence to the contrary.

dementia (dee-**MEN**-shee-ah): A slowly progressive decline in mental abilities including impaired memory, thinking, and judgment.

dental calculus (**KAL**-kyou-luhs): Hardened dental plaque on the teeth that irritates the surrounding tissues.

dental caries (**KAYR**-eez): An infectious disease that destroys the enamel and dentin of the tooth; also known as tooth decay or a cavity.

dental plaque (**PLACK**): A soft deposit consisting of bacteria and bacterial by-products that builds up on the teeth and is a major cause of dental caries and periodontal disease.

dentist: A specialist in diagnosing and treating diseases and disorders of teeth and tissues of the oral cavity.

dermabrasion (**der**-mah-**BRAY**-zhun): A form of abrasion involving the use of revolving wire brushes or sandpaper.

dermatitis (**der**-mah-**TYE**-tis): Inflammation of the upper layers of skin.

dermatitis, contact: A localized allergic response caused by contact with an irritant or allergen that causes redness, itching, and rash.

dermatologist (**der**-mah-**TOL**-oh-jist): A specialist in diagnosing and treating disorders of the skin.

dermatomycosis (**der**-mah-toh-my-**KOH**-sis): A fungal infection that causes white to light brown areas on the skin; also known as tinea versicolor.

dermatopathy (**der**-mah-**TOP**-ah-thee): Any disease of the skin.

dermatoplasty (**DER**-mah-toh-**plas**-tee): The replacement of damaged skin with tissue taken from a donor site on the patient's body; also known as a skin graft.

dermatosis (**der**-mah-**TOH**-sis): A general term used to denote any skin lesion or group of lesions, or eruptions of any type that is *not* associated with inflammation.

detached retina: The retina is pulled away from its normal position of being attached to the choroid in the back of the eye.

developmental disorder: An anomaly or malformation that is present at birth.

diabetes insipidus (**dye**-ah-**BEE**-teez in-**SIP**-ih-dus): A condition caused by insufficient production of the antidiuretic hormone (ADH) or by the inability of the kidneys to respond to ADH that allows too much fluid to be excreted.

diabetes mellitus (**dye**-ah-**BEE**-teez mel-**EYE**-tus *or* MEL-ih-tus): A group of metabolic diseases characterized by hyperglycemia resulting from defects in insulin secretion, insulin action, or both.

diabetes mellitus, gestational: A form of diabetes that may occur during pregnancies and usually disappears after delivery.

diabetes mellitus, type 1: An insulin deficiency disorder; also known as insulin-dependent diabetes mellitus.

diabetes mellitus, type 2: An insulin resistance disorder; also known as non–insulin-dependent diabetes mellitus.

diabetic ketoacidosis (**kee**-toh-**ass**-ih-**DOH**-sis): An acute, life-threatening complication is caused by a severe insulin deficiency.

diabetic nephropathy: Disease of the kidney caused by long-term diabetes mellitus.

dialysis (dye-**AL**-ih-sis): A procedure to remove waste products from the blood of patients whose kidneys no longer function.

diaphoresis (**dye**-ah-foh-**REE**-sis): Profuse sweating.

diarrhea (**dye**-ah-**REE**-ah): Abnormal frequency of loose or watery stools.

diffuse: Widespread.

digitalis (**dij**-ih-**TAL**-is): Medication administered to slow and strengthen the heart muscle contractions; also known as digoxin.

dilation (dye-**LAY**-shun): The expansion of an opening.

dilation and curettage: The dilation of the cervix and curettage of the uterus; also known as a D & C.

diopter (dye-**AHP**-tur): A unit of measurement of lens refractive power.

diphtheria (dif-**THEE**-ree-ah): An acute infectious disease of the throat and upper respiratory tract caused by the presence of diphtheria bacteria.

diplopia (dih-**PLOH**-pee-ah): The perception of two images of a single object; also known as double vision.

diskectomy (dis-**KECK**-toh-mee): Surgical removal of an intervertebral disk.

diuresis (**dye**-you-**REE**-sis): Increased excretion of urine.

diuretics (**dye**-you-**RET**-icks): Mediation administered to increase urine secretion to rid the body of excess sodium and water.

diverticulectomy (**dye**-ver-**tick**-you-**LECK**-toh-mee): Surgical removal of a diverticulum.

diverticulitis (**dye**-ver-tick-you-**LYE**-tis): Inflammation of one or more diverticulum.

dorsal recumbent position: Lying on the back with the knees bent.

Down syndrome: A genetic syndrome characterized by varying degrees of mental retardation and multiple physical abnormalities; also known as trisomy 21.

drug, adverse reaction: An undesirable drug response that accompanies the principal response for which the drug was taken.

drug, brand name: Medication sold under the name given by the manufacturer. A brand name is always spelled with a capital letter.

drug, generic: Medication named for its chemical structure and not protected by a brand name or trademark.

drug, interaction: A reaction that occurs when the effect of one drug is changed if it is administered at the same time as another drug.

drug, over-the-counter: A medication that may be dispensed without a written prescription.

drug, prescription: A medication that may be dispensed only with a prescription from an appropriately licensed professional.

dual x-ray absorptiometry (ab-**sorp**-shee-**OM**-eh-tree): Low exposure radiographic measurement used to detect early signs of osteoposoris; also known as DXA.

Duchenne's muscular dystrophy (doo-**SHENZ**): A severe form of muscular dystrophy that appears between 2 to 6 years of age.

ductal carcinoma in situ: Breast cancer at its earliest stage before the cancer has broken through the wall of the duct.

duodenal ulcers (dew-oh-**DEE**-nal *or* dew-**ODD**-eh-nal **UL**-serz): Peptic ulcers occurring in the upper part of the small intestine.

dyschromia (dis-**KROH**-mee-ah): Any disorder of the pigmentation of the skin or hair.

dyscrasia (dis-**KRAY**-zee-ah): Any abnormal or pathologic condition of the blood.

dyskinesia (**dis**-kih-**NEE**-zee-ah): Distortion or impairment of voluntary movement as in a tic or spasm.

dyslexia (dis-**LECK**-see-ah): A learning disability characterized by reading achievement that falls substantially below that expected given the individual's chronological age, measured intelligence, and age-appropriate education.

dysmenorrhea (**dis**-men-oh-**REE**-ah): Abdominal pain caused by uterine cramps during a menstrual period.

dyspepsia (dis-**PEP**-see-ah): An impairment of digestion; also known as indigestion.

dysphagia (dis-**FAY**-jee-ah): Difficulty in swallowing.

dysphonia (dis-**FOH**-nee-ah): Any voice impairment including hoarseness, weakness, or loss of voice.

dysplasia (dis-**PLAY**-see-ah): Abnormal development or growth of cells.

dysplasia, cervical: The abnormal growth of cells of the cervix; also known as precancerous lesions.

dyspnea (**DISP**-nee-ah): Difficult or labored breathing; also known as shortness of breath.

dysrhythmia (dis-**RITH**-mee-ah): An irregularity or the loss of normal rhythm of the heartbeat; also known as cardiac arrhythmia.

dystaxia (dis-**TACK**-see-ah): Difficulty in controlling voluntary movement; also known as partial ataxia.

dystonia (dis-**TOH**-nee-ah): Condition of abnormal muscle tone.

dysuria (dis-**YOU**-ree-ah): Difficult or painful urination.

E

E. coli: An intestinal infection caused by *Escherichia coli*.

ecchymosis (**eck**-ih-**MOH**-sis): A purplish area caused by bleeding within the skin; also known as a bruise.

echocardiography (**eck**-oh-**kar**-dee-**OG**-rah-fee): An ultrasonic diagnostic procedure used to evaluate the structures and motion of the heart.

echoencephalography (**eck**-oh-en-**sef**-ah-**LOG**-rah-fee): The use of ultrasound imaging to diagnose a shift in the midline structures of the brain.

eclampsia (eh-**KLAMP**-see-ah): A more serious form of preeclampsia characterized by convulsions and sometimes coma.

ectopic pregnancy (eck-**TOP**-ick): A pregnancy in which the fertilized egg is implanted and begins to develop outside of the uterus; also known as an extrauterine pregnancy.

ectropion (eck-**TROH**-pee-on): The turning outward of the edge of the eyelid.

eczema (**ECK**-zeh-mah): An acute or chronic skin inflammation characterized by erythema, papules, vesicles, pustules, scales, crusts, scabs, and possibly itching.

edema (eh-**DEE**-mah): Excess fluid in body tissues, causing swelling.

effusion (eh-**FEW**-zhun): The escape of fluid from blood or lymphatic vessels into the tissues or a cavity.

effusion, pleural: Abnormal escape of fluid into the pleural cavity that prevents the lung from fully expanding.

electrocardiogram (ee-**leck**-troh-**KAR**-dee-oh-**gram**): A record of the electrical activity of the myocardium.

electroconvulsive therapy (ee-**leck**-troh-kon-**VUL**-siv): A controlled convulsion produced by the passage of an electric current through the brain to treat depression and mental disorders; also known as electroshock therapy.

electroencephalography (ee-**leck**-troh-en-**sef**-ah-**LOG**-rah-fee): The process of recording electrical brain-wave activity.

electromyography (ee-**leck**-troh-my-**OG**-rah-fee): Diagnostic test that records the strength of muscle contractions as the result of electrical stimulation.

electroneuromyography (ee-**leck**-troh-**new**-roh-my-**OG**-rah-fee): Recording neuromuscular activity by the electric stimulation of nerve trunk carrying fibers to and from the muscle; also known as nerve conduction studies.

electronic fetal monitor: A device used during labor to monitor the fetal heart rate and the maternal uterine contractions.

emaciated (ee-**MAY**-shee-ayt-ed): Abnormally thin.

embolism (**EM**-boh-lizm): Blockage of a vessel by an embolus.

embolus (**EM**-boh-lus): A foreign object, such as a blood clot, quantity of air or gas, or a bit of tissue or tumor that is circulating in the blood.

embryo (**EM**-bree-oh): The developing child from implantation through the eighth week of pregnancy.

emesis (**EM**-eh-sis): To expel the contents of the stomach through the esophagus and out of the mouth; also known as vomiting.

emetic (eh-**MET**-ick): Medication administered to produce vomiting.

emmetropia (em-eh-**TROH**-pee-ah): The normal relationship between the refractive power of the eye and the shape of the eye that enables light rays to focus correctly on the retina.

empathy (**EM**-pah-thee): The ability to understand another person's mental and emotional state without becoming personally involved.

emphysema (em-fih-**SEE**-mah): The progressive loss of lung function due a decrease in the total number of alveoli, the enlargement of the remaining alveoli, and then the progressive destruction of their walls.

empyema (em-pye-**EE**-mah): An accumulation of pus in the pleural cavity; also known as pyothorax.

encephalitis (en-sef-ah-**LYE**-tis): Inflammation of the brain.

encephalocele (en-**SEF**-ah-loh-**seel**): A congenital gap in the skull with herniation of brain substance; also known as a craniocele.

encephalography (en-**sef**-ah-**LOG**-rah-fee): A radiographic study demonstrating the intracranial fluid-containing spaces of the brain.

encephalomalacia (en-**sef**-ah-loh-mah-**LAY**-shee-ah): Abnormal softening of the brain.

encephalopathy (en-**sef**-ah-**LOP**-ah-thee): Any degenerative disease of the brain.

endarterectomy (**end**-ar-ter-**ECK**-toh-mee): Surgical removal of the lining of an artery that is clogged with plaque.

endemic (en-**DEM**-ick): Ongoing presence of a disease within a population, group, or area.

endocarditis (**en**-doh-kar-**DYE**-tis): Inflammation of the inner layer of the heart.

endocarditis, bacterial: Inflammation of the inner lining or valves of the heart caused by bacteria.

endocervicitis (**en**-doh-ser-vih-**SIGH**-tis): Inflammation of the mucous membrane lining of the cervix.

endocrinologist (en-doh-krih-**NOL**-oh-jist): A specialist in diagnosing and treating diseases and malfunctions of the glands of internal secretion.

endocrinology (en-doh-krih-**NOL**-oh-jee): Study of the endocrine glands and their secretions.

endocrinopathy (en-doh-krih-**NOP**-ah-thee): Any disease due to a disorder of the endocrine system.

endometriosis (en-doh-**mee**-tree-**OH**-sis): A condition in which endometrial tissue escapes the uterus and grows on other structures in the pelvic cavity.

endometritis (en-doh-mee-**TRY**-tis): Inflammation of the endometrium.

endoscopy (en-**DOS**-koh-pee): The visual examination of the interior of a body cavity with the use of an endoscope.

endotracheal intubation (en-doh-**TRAY**-kee-al **in**-too-**BAY**-shun): The passage of a tube through the nose or mouth into the trachea to establish an airway.

endovaginal ultrasound (en-doh-**VAJ**-ih-nal): An ultrasonic diagnostic test to determine the cause of abnormal vaginal bleeding.

enteritis (en-ter-**EYE**-tis): Inflammation of the small intestines.

entropion (en-**TROH**-pee-on): The turning inward of the edge of the eyelid.

enuresis (en-you-**REE**-sis): The involuntary discharge of urine.

enzyme-linked immunosorbent assay: A blood test to screen for the presence of HIV antibodies; also known as ELISA.

epicondylitis (ep-ih-**kon**-dih-**LYE**-tis): Inflammation of the tissues surrounding the elbow.

epidemic (**ep**-ih-**DEM**-ick): Sudden and widespread outbreak of a disease within a population group or area.

epidemiologist (**ep**-ih-**dee**-mee-**OL**-oh-jist): A specialist in the study of outbreaks of disease within a population group.

epididymitis (**ep**-ih-did-ih-**MY**-tis): Inflammation of the epididymis.

epiglottitis (**ep**-ih-glot-**TYE**-tis): Inflammation of the epiglottis.

epilepsy (**EP**-ih-**lep**-see) is a group of neurologic disorders characterized by recurrent episodes of seizures.

epilepsy, grand mal (**GRAN MAHL EP**-ih-**lep**-see): The more severe form of epilepsy that is characterized by generalized tonic-clonic seizures.

epilepsy, petit mal (peh-**TEE MAHL EP**-ih-**lep**-see): The milder form of epilepsy in which there is a sudden, temporary loss of consciousness, lasting only a few seconds; also known as absence epilepsy.

epinephrine: A medication used as a vasoconstrictor to treat conditions such as heart dysrhythmias and asthma attacks.

episiorrhaphy (eh-**piz**-ee-**OR**-ah-fee): A sutured repair of an episiotomy.

episiotomy (eh-**piz**-ee-**OT**-oh-mee): A surgical incision of the perineum and vagina to facilitate delivery and prevent laceration of the tissues.

epispadias (ep-ih-**SPAY**-dee-as): In the male, a congenital abnormality in which the urethral opening is located on the upper surface of the penis. In the female with epispadias, the urethral opening is in the region of the clitoris.

epistaxis (ep-ih-**STACK**-sis): Bleeding from the nose; also known as a nosebleed.

epithelioma (ep-ih-thee-lee-**OH**-mah): A benign or malignant tumor originating in the epidermis that may occur on the skin or mucous membranes.

ergonomics (er-goh-**NOM**-icks): Study of human factors that affect the design and operation of tools and the work environment.

eructation (eh-ruk-**TAY**-shun): The act of belching or raising gas orally from the stomach.

erythema (**er**-ih-**THEE**-mah): Any redness of the skin such as a nervous blush, an inflammation, or a mild sunburn.

erythrocytosis (eh-**rith**-roh-sigh-**TOH**-sis): An abnormal increase in the number of circulating red blood cells.

esophagalgia (eh-sof-ah-**GAL**-jee-ah): Pain in the esophagus.

esophageal reflux (eh-**sof**-ah-**JEE**-al **REE**-flucks): The upward flow of stomach acid into the esophagus; also known as gastroesophageal reflux disease.

esophageal varices (eh-**sof**-ah-**JEE**-al **VAYR**-ih-seez): Enlarged and swollen veins at the lower end of the esophagus.

esophagogastrectomy (eh-**sof**-ah-goh-gas-**TRECK**-toh-mee): Surgical removal of all or part of the esophagus and stomach.

esophagoplasty (eh-**SOF**-ah-go-**plas**-tee): Surgical repair of the esophagus.

esotropia (**es**-oh-**TROH**-pee-ah): Strabismus characterized by an inward deviation of one eye in relation to the other; also known as cross-eyes.

etiology (**ee**-tee-**OL**-oh-jee): Study of the causes of diseases.

eupnea (youp-**NEE**-ah): Easy or normal breathing.

eustachitis (**you**-stay-**KYE**-tis): Inflammation of the eustachian tube.

Ewing's sarcoma (**YOU**-ingz sar-**KOH**-mah): Cancer usually occurring in the diaphyses of long bones in the arms and legs of children or adolescents.

excision (eck-**SIH**-zhun): The complete removal of a lesion or organ.

exfoliative cytology (ecks-**FOH**-lee-**ay**-tiv sigh-**TOL**-oh-jee): A biopsy in which cells are scraped from the tissue and examined under a microscope.

exophthalmos (**eck**-sof-**THAL**-mos): Abnormal protrusion of the eyes.

exostosis (**eck**-sos-**TOH**-sis): Benign growth on the surface of a bone.

exotropia (**eck**-soh-**TROH**-pee-ah): Strabismus characterized by the outward deviation of one eye relative to the other; also known as wall-eye.

extracapsular cataract extraction: The removal of a cloudy lens that leaves the posterior lens capsule intact.

extracorporeal shock-wave lithotripsy (**LITH**-oh-**trip**-see): Destruction of a kidney stone with the use of ultrasonic waves traveling through water; also known as lithotripsy.

exudate (**ECKS**-you-dayt): Accumulated fluid in a cavity that has penetrated through vessel walls into the adjoining tissue.

F

fasciectomy (**fas**-ee-**ECK**-toh-mee): Surgical removal of fascia.

fasciitis (**fas**-ee-**EYE**-tis): Inflammation of a fascia.

fasciodesis (**fash**-ee-**ODD**-eh-sis): Binding fascia to a skeletal attachment.

fascioplasty (**FASH**-ee-oh-**plas**-tee): Surgical repair of a fascia.

fasciorrhaphy (**fash**-ee-**OR**-ah-fee): To suture torn fascia.

fasciotomy (**fash**-ee-**OT**-oh-mee): Surgical incision of fascia.

fasting blood sugar: A blood test used to screen for and to monitor treatment of diabetes mellitus.

fenestration (**fen**-es-**TRAY**-shun): A surgical procedure in which a new opening is made in the labyrinth of the inner ear to restore hearing.

fetus (**FEE**-tus): The developing child from the ninth week of pregnancy to the time of birth.

fibrillation (**fih**-brih-**LAY**-shun): Rapid, random, and ineffective contractions of the heart.

fibrillation, atrial: Condition in which the atria beat faster than the ventricles.

fibrillation, ventricular: The result of irregular contractions of the ventricles that is fatal unless reversed by electric defibrillation.

fibrocystic breast disease (figh-broh-**SIS**-tick): The presence of single or multiple cysts in the breasts.

fibroid: A benign tumor composed of muscle and fibrous tissue that occurs in the wall of the uterus; also known as a leiomyoma.

fibromyalgia syndrome (**figh**-broh-my-**AL**-jee-ah): A chronic disorder of unknown cause characterized by widespread aching pain, tender points, and fatigue.

fibrosis (figh-**BROH**-sis): The abnormal formation of fibrous tissue.

fissure: A groove or cracklike sore of the skin; normal folds in the contours of the brain.

fluorescein staining (flew-oh-**RES**-ee-in): A dye used to visualize a corneal abrasion.

fluoroscopy (floo-or-**OS**-koh-pee): An imaging technique used to visualize body parts in motion by projecting x-ray images on a luminous fluorescent screen.

flutter: A cardiac arrhythmia in which the atrial contractions are rapid but regular.

fructosamine test (fruck-**TOHS**-ah-meen): A blood test that measures average blood sugar levels over the previous 3 weeks.

functional: A disorder in which there are no detectable physical changes to explain the symptoms being experienced by the patient.

fungus (**FUNG**-gus): A simple parasitic plant some of which are pathogenic to humans.

furuncles (**FYOU**-rung-kuls): Large tender, swollen, areas caused by staphylococcal infection around hair follicles; also known as boils.

G

galactocele (gah-**LACK**-toh-seel): A cystic enlargement of the mammary gland containing milk; also known as a galactoma.

galactoma (**gal**-ack-**TOH**-mah): See galactocele.

gallstone: A hard deposit that forms in the gallbladder and bile ducts; also known as biliary calculus.

gangrene (**GANG**-green): Tissue death usually associated with a loss of circulation.

gastralgia (gas-**TRAL**-jee-ah): Pain in the stomach.

gastrectomy (gas-**TRECK**-toh-mee): Surgical removal of all or a part of the stomach.

gastritis (gas-**TRY**-tis): Inflammation of the stomach.

gastroduodenostomy (gas-troh-**dew**-oh-deh-**NOS**-toh-mee): Removal of the pylorus of the stomach and the establishment of an anastomosis between the upper portion of the stomach and the duodenum.

gastrodynia (**gas**-troh-**DIN**-ee-ah): Pain in the stomach.

gastroenteritis (gas-troh-en-ter-**EYE**-tis): Inflammation of the stomach and small intestine.

gastroenterocolitis (gas-troh-**en**-ter-oh-koh-**LYE**-tis): Inflammation of the stomach, small intestine, and large intestine.

gastroenterologist (gas-troh-**en**-ter-**OL**-oh-jist): A specialist in diagnosing and treating diseases and disorders of the stomach and intestines.

gastroesophageal reflux disease: The upward flow of stomach acid into the esophagus; also known as esophageal reflux.

gastrointestinal endoscopy: Endoscopic examination of the interior of the esophagus, stomach, and duodenum.

gastropexy (**GAS**-troh-**peck**-see): Surgical fixation of the stomach to correct displacement.

gastrorrhagia (**gas**-troh-**RAY**-jee-ah): Bleeding from the stomach.

gastrorrhaphy (gas-**TROR**-ah-fee): To suture the stomach.

gastrorrhea (**gas**-troh-**REE**-ah): Excessive flow of gastric secretions.

gastrorrhexis (**gas**-troh-**RECK**-sis): Rupture of the stomach.

gastrosis (gas-**TROH**-sis): Any abnormal condition of the stomach.

gastrostomy (gas-**TROS**-toh-mee): Surgical creation of an artificial opening into the stomach.

gastrotomy (gas-**TROT**-oh-mee): A surgical incision into the stomach.

geneticist (jeh-**NET**-ih-sist): A specialist in the field of genetics.

genital herpes (**HER**-peez): A highly contagious sexually transmitted disease caused by the herpes simplex virus.

genital warts: A highly contagious sexually transmitted disease caused by the *human papillomavirus*.

gerontologist (**jer**-on-**TOL**-oh-jist): A specialist in diagnosing and treating diseases, disorders, and problems associated with aging.

GI series, lower: A radiographic study of the lower portion of the digestive system using barium as a contrast medium; also known as a barium enema.

GI series, upper: A radiographic study of the upper portion of the digestive system using barium as a contrast medium; also known as a barium swallow.

gigantism (jigh-**GAN**-tiz-em *or* **JIGH**-en-tiz-em): Abnormal overgrowth of the body caused by excessive secretion of the growth hormone *before* puberty.

gingivectomy (**jin**-jih-**VECK**-toh-mee): Surgical removal of diseased gingival tissue.

gingivitis (**jin**-jih-**VYE**-tis): Inflammation of the gums that is the earliest stage of periodontal disease.

glaucoma (glaw-**KOH**-mah): Increased intraocular pressure that damages the optic nerve and may cause the loss of peripheral vision and eventually blindness.

glomerulonephritis (gloh-**mer**-you-loh-neh-**FRY**-tis): Inflammation of the kidney involving primarily the glomeruli.

glucose tolerance test (**GLOO**-kohs): A blood test used to confirm diabetes mellitus and to aid in diagnosing hypoglycemia.

glycohemoglobin (**glye**-koh-**hee**-moh-**GLOH**-bin): The substance that forms when glucose in the blood attaches to the hemoglobin.

glycosuria (glye-koh-**SOO**-ree-ah): The presence of glucose in the urine that is commonly caused by diabetes.

goiter (**GOI**-ter): An abnormal enlargement of the thyroid gland that produces a swelling in the front part of the neck; also known as thyromegaly.

gonorrhea (gon-oh-**REE**-ah): A highly contagious sexually transmitted disease caused by the bacteria *Neisseria gonorrhoeae*.

granulation tissue: Tissue that forms during the healing of a wound to create what will become scar tissue.

granuloma (gran-you-**LOH**-mah): A general term used to describe small knotlike swellings of granulation tissue.

Graves' disease (**GRAYVZ**-dih-**ZEEZ**): An autoimmune disorder characterized by hyperthyroidism, goiter, and exophthalmos.

Guillain-Barré syndrome (gee-**YAHN**-bah-**RAY**): A condition characterized by rapidly worsening muscle weakness that may lead to temporary paralysis.

gynecologist (guy-neh-**KOL**-oh-jist): A specialist in diagnosing and treating diseases and disorders of the female reproductive system.

gynecomastia (guy-neh-koh-**MAS**-tee-ah): The condition of excessive mammary development in the male.

H

halitosis (hal-ih-**TOH**-sis): An unpleasant breath odor that may be caused by dental diseases, respiratory, or gastric disorders; also known as bad breath.

hallucination (hah-**loo**-sih-**NAY**-shun): A sense perception that has no basis in external stimulation.

hallux valgus (**HAL**-ucks **VAL**-guss): Abnormal enlargement of the joint at the base of the great toe; also known as a bunion.

hamstring injury: Strain or tear of the posterior femoral muscles.

Hashimoto's thyroiditis (hah-shee-**MOH**-tohz **thigh**-roi-**DYE**-tis): An autoimmune disorder in which the immune system mistakenly attacks thyroid tissue, setting up an inflammatory process that may progressively destroy the gland.

hearing loss, conductive: A hearing loss in which the outer or middle ear does not conduct sound vibrations to the inner ear normally.

hearing loss, noise-induced: Damage to sensitive hairlike cells of the inner ear caused by repeated exposure to very intense noise such as aircraft engines, noisy equipment, and loud music.

hearing loss, sensorineural: A hearing loss caused by problems affecting the inner ear; also known as nerve deafness.

hemangioma (hee-**man**-jee-**OH**-mah): A benign tumor made up of newly formed blood vessels.

hemangioma, strawberry: This dark reddish purple growth is a benign tumor made up of newly formed blood vessels that is usually present at birth; also known as a birthmark.

hematemesis (**hee**-mah-**TEM**-eh-sis *or* **hem**-ah-**TEM**-eh-sis): Vomiting blood.

hematocrit (hee-**MAT**-oh-krit): A laboratory test that measures the percentage by volume of packed red blood cells in a whole blood sample.

hematologist (hee-mah-**TOL**-oh-jist *or* **hem**-ah-**TOL**-oh-jist): A specialist in diagnosing and treating diseases and disorders of the blood and blood-forming tissues.

hematoma (hee-mah-**TOH**-mah): A collection of blood trapped within tissues.

hematoma, cranial: A collection of blood trapped in the tissues of the brain.

hematoma, subungual: A collection of blood trapped in the tissues under a nail.

hematopoietic (**hee**-mah-toh-poi-**ET**-ick *or* **hem**-ah-toh-poi-**ET**-ick): Pertaining to the formation of blood.

hematuria (hee-mah-**TOO**-ree-ah *or* **hem**-ah-**TOO**-ree-ah): The presence of blood in the urine.

hematuria, gross: The presence of blood in urine that can be detected without magnification.

hematuria, microscopic: The presence of blood in urine that can be seen only under a microscope.

hemianopia (hem-ee-ah-**NOH**-pee-ah): Blindness in one half of the visual field.

hemiparesis (hem-ee-pah-**REE**-sis): Slight paralysis of one side of the body.

hemiplegia (hem-ee-**PLEE**-jee-ah): Paralysis of one side of the body.

hemoccult (**HEE**-moh-kult): A laboratory test for hidden blood in the stools; also known as the fecal occult blood test.

hemochromatosis (hee-moh-**kroh**-mah-**TOH**-sis): A genetic disorder in which the intestines absorb too much iron and the excess accumulates in organs; also known as iron-overload disease.

hemodialysis (hee-moh-dye-**AL**-ih-sis): Removal of waste products by filtering the patient's blood.

hemoglobin A_{1C} testing: A blood test that measures the average blood glucose level over the previous 3 to 4 months.

hemophilia (hee-moh-**FILL**-ee-ah): A group of hereditary bleeding disorders in which one of the factors needed to clot the blood is missing.

hemoptysis (hee-**MOP**-tih-sis): Spitting of blood or blood-stained sputum derived from the lungs or bronchial tubes as the result of a pulmonary or bronchial hemorrhage.

hemorrhage (**HEM**-or-idj): The loss of a large amount of blood in a short time.

hemorrhoidectomy (hem-oh-roid-**ECK**-toh-mee): Surgical removal of hemorrhoids.

hemorrhoids (**HEM**-oh-roids): Enlarged veins in or near the anus that may cause pain and bleeding; also known as piles.

hemostasis (hee-moh-**STAY**-sis): To control bleeding.

hemothorax (hee-moh-**THOH**-racks): An accumulation of blood in the pleural cavity.

hepatectomy (hep-ah-**TECK**-toh-mee): Surgical removal of all or part of the liver.

hepatitis (**hep**-ah-**TYE**-tis): Inflammation of the liver.

hepatoenteric (**hep**-ah-toh-en-**TER**-ick): Referring to the liver and intestines.

hepatomegaly (**hep**-ah-toh-**MEG**-ah-lee): Abnormal enlargement of the liver.

hepatorrhaphy (**hep**-ah-**TOR**-ah-fee): To suture the liver.

hepatorrhexis (**hep**-ah-toh-**RECK**-sis): Rupture of the liver.

hepatotomy (**hep**-ah-**TOT**-oh-mee): A surgical incision into the liver.

hereditary disorders: Diseases or conditions caused by a defective gene.

hernia (**HER**-nee-ah): Protrusion of a part or structure through the tissues normally containing it.

hernia, hiatal: Protrusion of part of the stomach through the esophageal sphincter in the diaphragm.

hernia, inguinal: Protrusion of a small loop of bowel through a weak place in the lower abdominal wall or groin.

herniated disk (**HER**-nee-**ayt**-ed): Rupture of the intervertebral disk resulting in pressure on spinal nerve roots; also known as a ruptured disk.

herniorrhaphy (**her**-nee-**OR**-ah-fee): To suture a defect in a muscular wall to repair a hernia.

herpes labialis (**HER**-peez lay-bee-**AL**-iss): Blister-like sores caused by the herpes simplex virus that occur on the lips and adjacent tissue; also known as cold sores or fever blisters.

herpes zoster (**HER**-peez **ZOS**-ter): An acute viral infection characterized by painful skin eruptions that follow the underlying route of the inflamed nerve; also known as shingles.

hirsutism (**HER**-soot-izm): Abnormal hairiness; the appearance of male body or facial hair patterns in the female.

Hodgkin's lymphoma (**HODJ**-kinz): A form of lymphoma distinguished by the presence of *Reed-Sternberg cells.*

homocysteine (**hoh**-moh-**SIS**-teen): An amino acid normally found in the blood and used by the body to build and maintain tissues.

hordeolum (hor-**DEE**-oh-lum): An infection of one or more glands at the border of the eyelid; also known as a stye.

hormone replacement therapy: Administration of artificially produced hormones to replace the estrogen and progesterone no longer produced during perimenopause and after menopause.

human growth hormone therapy (hGH): A synthetic version of naturally occurring growth hormone that is administered to stimulate growth when the supply of growth hormone is insufficient for normal development.

human immunodeficiency virus: A bloodborne pathogen that invades and then progressively impairs or kills cells of the immune system; also known as HIV.

human papilloma virus (pap-ih-**LOH**-mah): A highly contagious sexually transmitted disease caused by the *human papillomavirus*; also known as genital warts.

Huntington's disease: A hereditary disorder with symptoms that first appear in midlife and cause the irreversible and progressive loss of muscle control and mental ability; also known as Huntington's chorea.

hydrocele (**HIGH**-droh-seel): A hernia filled with fluid in the testicles or the tubes leading from the testicles.

hydrocephalus (high-droh-**SEF**-ah-lus): An abnormally increased amount of cerebrospinal fluid within the brain.

hydronephrosis (high-droh-neh-**FROH**-sis): Dilation of the renal pelvis of one or both kidneys.

hydroureter (**high**-droh-you-**REE**-ter): Distention of the ureter with urine that cannot flow because the ureter is blocked.

hyperalbuminemia (**high**-per-al-**byou**-mih-**NEE**-mee-ah): Abnormally high level of albumin in the blood.

hypercalcemia (**high**-per-kal-**SEE**-mee-ah): A condition characterized by abnormally high concentrations of calcium circulating in the blood instead of being stored in the bones.

hypercrinism (**high**-per-**KRY**-nism): A condition caused by excessive secretion of any gland, especially an endocrine gland.

hyperemesis (**high**-per-**EM**-eh-sis): Excessive vomiting.

hyperesthesia (**high**-per-es-**THEE**-zee-ah): A condition of excessive sensitivity to stimuli.

hyperglycemia (**high**-per-glye-**SEE**-mee-ah): An abnormally high concentration of glucose in the blood.

hyperglycosuria (**high**-per-**glye**-koh-**SOO**-ree-ah): Presence of excess sugar in the urine.

hypergonadism (**high**-per-**GOH**-nad-izm): The condition of excessive secretion of hormones by the sex glands.

hyperhidrosis (**high**-per-high-**DROH**-sis): The condition of excessive sweating.

hyperinsulinism (**high**-per-**IN**-suh-lin-izm): A condition marked by excessive secretion of insulin that produces hypoglycemia.

hyperkinesia (**high**-per-kye-**NEE**-zee-ah): Abnormally increased motor function or activity; also known as hyperactivity.

hyperlipemia (**high**-per-lye-**PEE**-mee-ah). A general term for elevated plasma concentrations of cholesterol, triglycerides, and lipoproteins; also known as hyperlipidemia.

hyperlipidemia (**high**-per-**lip**-ih-**DEE**-mee-ah): See hyperlipemia.

hyperopia (**high**-per-**OH**-pee-ah): A defect in which light rays focus beyond the retina; also known as farsightedness.

hyperparathyroidism (**high**-per-**par**-ah-**THIGH**-roid-izm): Overproduction of parathyroid hormone that causes hypercalcemia and may lead to weakened bones and the formation of kidney stones.

hyperpituitarism (**high**-per-pih-**TOO**-ih-tah-rizm): Pathology that results in the excessive secretion by the anterior lobe of the pituitary gland.

hyperplasia (**high**-per-**PLAY**-zee-ah): An abnormal increase in the number of normal cells in normal arrangement in a tissue.

hyperpnea (**high**-perp-**NEE**-ah): An abnormal increase in the depth and rate of the respiratory movements.

hyperproteinuria (**high**-per-**proh**-tee-in-**YOU**-ree-ah): Presence of excess of protein in the urine.

hypertension: Consistent abnormally elevated blood pressure levels.

hyperthyroidism (**high**-per-**THIGH**-roid-izm): A condition of excessive thyroid hormones in the blood.

hypertonia (**high**-per-**TOH**-nee-ah): Condition of excessive tone of the skeletal muscles with increased resistance of muscle to passive stretching.

hyperventilation (**high**-per-ven-tih-**LAY**-shun): Abnormally rapid deep breathing, resulting in decreased levels of carbon dioxide at the cellular level.

hypnotic: Medication that depresses the central nervous system and usually produces sleep.

hypocalcemia (**high**-poh-kal-**SEE**-mee-ah): A condition characterized by abnormally low levels of calcium in the blood.

hypochondriasis (**high**-poh-kon-**DRY**-ah-sis): A preoccupation with fears of having, or the idea that one has, a serious disease based on misinterpretation of one or more bodily signs or symptoms.

hypocrinism (**high**-poh-**KRY**-nism): A condition caused by deficient secretion of any gland, especially an endocrine gland.

hypoglycemia (**high**-poh-glye-**SEE**-mee-ah): An abnormally low concentration of glucose in the blood.

hypogonadism (**high**-poh-**GOH**-nad-izm): The condition of deficient secretion of hormones by the sex glands.

hypohidrosis (**high**-poh-high-**DROH**-sis): Abnormal condition resulting in the diminished flow of perspiration.

hypokinesia (**high**-poh-kye-**NEE**-zee-ah): Abnormally decreased motor function or activity.

hypomenorrhea (**high**-poh-men-oh-**REE**-ah): A small amount of menstrual flow during a shortened regular menstrual period.

hypoparathyroidism (**high**-poh-**par**-ah-**THIGH**-roid-izm): A condition caused by an insufficient or absent secretion of the parathyroid glands.

hypoperfusion (**high**-poh-per-**FYOU**-zhun): A deficiency of blood passing through an organ or body part.

hypophysectomy (**high**-pof-ih-**SECK**-toh-mee): Removal of all or part of the pituitary gland by the use of radiation or surgery.

hypopituitarism (**high**-poh-pih-**TOO**-ih-tah-**rizm**): A condition of reduced secretion due to the partial or complete loss of the function of the anterior lobe of the pituitary gland.

hypoplasia (**high**-poh-**PLAY**-zee-ah): Incomplete development of an organ or tissue, but less severe in degree than aplasia.

hypopnea (**high**-poh-**NEE**-ah): Shallow or slow respiration.

hypospadias (**high**-poh-**SPAY**-dee-as): In the male, a congenital abnormality in which the urethral opening is on the undersurface of the penis. In the female with hypospadias the urethral opening is into the vagina.

hypotension (**high**-poh-**TEN**-shun): Lower than normal blood pressure.

hypothyroidism (**high**-poh-**THIGH**-roid-izm): A deficiency of thyroid secretion; also known as an underactive thyroid.

hypotonia (**high**-poh-**TOH**-nee-ah): Condition of diminished tone of the skeletal muscles with decreased resistance of muscle to passive stretching.

hypoxia (**high**-**POCK**-see-ah): Subnormal oxygen levels in the cells that is less severe than anoxia.

hysterectomy (**hiss**-teh-**RECK**-toh-mee): The surgical removal of the uterus that may or may not include the cervix.

hysterectomy, radical: Surgical removal of the uterus, tubes, ovaries, adjacent lymph nodes, and part of the vagina.

hysterectomy, total abdominal: A hysterectomy performed through an incision in the abdomen that includes the removal of the uterus, cervix, fallopian tubes, and ovaries.

hysterectomy, vaginal: A hysterectomy performed through the vagina.

hysterocele (**HISS**-ter-oh-seel): Hernia of the uterus, particularly during pregnancy.

hysteropexy (**HISS**-ter-oh-**peck**-see): Surgical fixation of a misplaced or abnormally movable uterus.

hysterorrhaphy (**hiss**-ter-**OR**-ah-fee): To suture the uterus.

hysterorrhexis (**hiss**-ter-oh-**RECK**-sis): Rupture of the uterus, particularly during pregnancy.

hysterosalpingography (**hiss**-ter-oh-**sal**-pin-**GOG**-rah-fee): A radiographic examination of the uterus and fallopian tubes after the injection of radiopaque material.

hysteroscopy (**hiss**-ter-**OSS**-koh-pee): The direct visual examination of the interior of the uterus using the magnification of a hysteroscope.

I

iatrogenic (eye-**at**-roh-**JEN**-ick): An unfavorable response to medical treatment for a different disorder.

icterus (**ICK**-ter-us): Yellow discoloration of the skin and other tissues caused by greater than normal amounts of bilirubin in the blood; also known as jaundice.

idiopathic (**id**-ee-oh-**PATH**-ick): An illness without known cause.

idiosyncratic reaction (**id**-ee-oh-sin-**KRAT**-ick): An unexpected reaction to a drug.

ileectomy (**ill**-ee-**ECK**-toh-mee): Surgical removal of the ileum.

ileitis (**ill**-ee-**EYE**-tis): Inflammation of the ileum.

ileostomy (**ill**-ee-**OS**-toh-mee): Surgical creation of an opening between the ileum, at the end of the small intestine, and the abdominal wall.

ileus (**ILL**-ee-us): A temporary stoppage of intestinal peristalsis.

immunodeficiency (**im**-you-noh-deh-**FISH**-en-see): A condition that occurs when one or more parts of the immune system are deficient or missing.

immunofluorescence (**im**-you-noh-**floo**-oh-**RES**-ens): A method of tagging antibodies with a fluorescent dye to detect or localize antigen-antibody combinations.

immunoglobulin (**im**-you-noh-**GLOB**-you-lin): A type of antibody produced naturally by the body; synthetic immunoglobulins are administered as a postexposure preventive measure against certain viruses such as rabies and some types of hepatitis.

immunologist (**im**-you-**NOL**-oh-jist): A specialist in the study, diagnosis, and treatment of disorders of the immune system.

immunology (**im**-you-**NOL**-oh-jee): Study of the immune system.

immunosuppressant (**im**-you-noh-soo-**PRES**-ant): Medication that prevents or reduces the body's normal reactions to invasion by disease or by foreign tissues.

immunosuppression (**im**-you-noh-sup-**PRESH**-un): Treatment used to interfere with the ability of the immune system to respond to antigen stimulation.

immunotherapy (ih-**myou**-noh-**THER**-ah-pee): Treatment of disease either by enhancing or repressing the immune response.

impacted cerumen: An accumulation of ear wax that forms a solid mass adhering to the walls of the external auditory canal.

impetigo (**im**-peh-**TYE**-goh): A highly contagious bacterial skin infection characterized by isolated pustules that become crusted and rupture.

impingement syndrome (im-**PINJ**-ment): Inflammation of tendons that get caught in the narrow space between the bones within the shoulder joint.

impotence (**IM**-poh-tens): The inability of the male to achieve or maintain a penile erection; also known as erectile dysfunction.

incision and drainage: Cutting open a lesion such as an abscess and draining the contents.

incontinence (in-**KON**-tih-nents): The inability to control excretory functions.

incontinence, bowel: The inability to control the excretion of feces.

incontinence, urinary: The inability to control the voiding of urine.

infarct (**IN**-farkt): Localized area of necrosis (tissue death) caused by an interruption of the blood supply.

infectious (in-**FECK**-shus) Illness caused by a pathogenic organism.

infectious mononucleosis (**mon**-oh-**new**-klee-**OH**-sis): An infection caused by the Epstein-Barr virus (one of the herpes viruses) that is characterized by fever, a sore throat, and enlarged lymph nodes.

infertility: The inability of a couple to achieve pregnancy after 1 year of regular, unprotected intercourse or the inability of a woman to carry a pregnancy to a live birth.

infestation: The dwelling of a parasite on external surface tissue.

inflammation (in-flah-**MAY**-shun): A localized response to injury or destruction of tissues.

influenza (in-flew-**EN**-zah): An acute, highly contagious viral respiratory infection, that is spread by respiratory droplets and occurs most commonly during the colder months.

injection, intradermal: An injection made into the middle layers of the skin.

injection, intramuscular: An injection made directly into muscle tissue.

injection, intravenous: An injection made directly into a vein.

injection, subcutaneous: An injection made into the fatty layer just below the skin.

insomnia: The prolonged or abnormal inability to sleep.

insulinemia (in-suh-lih-**NEE**-mee-ah): Abnormally high levels of insulin in the blood.

insulinoma (in-suh-lin-**OH**-mah): A benign tumor of the pancreas that causes hypoglycemia.

intermittent claudication (klaw-dih-**KAY**-shun): A complex of symptoms including cramplike pain of the leg muscles caused by poor circulation.

internist: A specialist in diagnosing and treating diseases and disorders of the internal organs.

interstitial cystitis (in-ter-**STISH**-al sis-**TYE**-tis): Inflammation within the wall of the bladder.

intestinal adhesions (ad-**HEE**-zhunz): Abnormally hold together parts of the intestine where they normally should be separate.

intestinal obstruction: A complete stoppage or serious impairment to the passage of the intestinal contents.

intracapsular cataract extraction: The removal of a cloudy lens including the surrounding capsule.

intraocular lens: A plastic lens surgically implanted to replace the natural lens.

intravenous fluorescein angiography (**flew**-oh-**RES**-ee-in an-jee-**OG**-rah-fee): A diagnostic test in which a dye is injected into the arm and pictures are taken as the dye passes through the blood vessels in the retina.

intravenous pyelogram (**PYE**-eh-loh-**gram**): A radiographic examination of the kidneys and ureters using a contrast medium.

intravenous urography (you-**ROG**-rah-fee): A radiographic examination of the urinary tract with the use of a contrast medium.

intubation (in-too-**BAY**-shun): Insertion of a tube, usually for the passage of air or fluids.

intussusception (in-tus-sus-**SEP**-shun): Telescoping of one part of the intestine into the opening of an immediately adjacent part.

invasive ductal carcinoma: A form of breast cancer that starts in the milk duct, breaks through the wall of that duct, and invades fatty breast tissue; also known as infiltrating ductal carcinoma.

invasive lobular carcinoma: Breast cancer that starts in the milk glands, breaks through the wall of the gland and invades the fatty tissue of the breast; also known as infiltrating lobular carcinoma.

iridalgia (ir-ih-**DAL**-jee-ah): Pain felt in the iris.

iridectomy (ir-ih-**DECK**-toh-mee): Surgical removal of a portion of the iris tissue.

iridopathy (ir-ih-**DOP**-ah-thee): Any disease of the iris.

iridotomy (ir-ih-**DOT**-oh-mee): Incision into the iris.

iritis (eye-**RYE**-tis): Inflammation of the iris.

irritable bowel syndrome: A disorder of the motility of the entire gastrointestinal tract characterized by abdominal pain, nausea, gas, constipation, and/or diarrhea; also known as spastic colon.

ischemia (iss-**KEE**-mee-ah): Deficiency in blood supply due to either the constriction or the obstruction of a blood vessel.

ischemic heart disease (iss-**KEE**-mick): A group of cardiac disabilities resulting from an insufficient supply of oxygenated blood to the heart

J

jaundice (**JAWN**-dis): Yellow discoloration of the skin and other tissues caused by greater than normal amounts of bilirubin in the blood; also known as icterus.

K

Kaposi's sarcoma (**KAP**-oh-seez sar-**KOH**-mah): A form of sarcoma that is frequently associated with HIV and may affect the skin, mucous membranes, lymph nodes and internal organs.

keloid (**KEE**-loid): An abnormally raised or thickened scar that is usually smooth and shiny.

keratitis (ker-ah-**TYE**-tis): Inflammation of the cornea of the eye.

keratoplasty (**KER**-ah-toh-**plas**-tee): The replacement of a scarred or diseased cornea with clear corneal tissue from a donor; also known as a corneal transplant.

keratosis (kerr-ah-**TOH**-sis): Any skin condition in which there is overgrowth and thickening of the skin.

ketonuria (kee-toh-**NEW**-ree-ah): The presence of ketones in the urine.

kidney transplant: The grafting of a donor kidney into the body to replace the recipient's failed kidneys; also known as a renal transplantation.

kleptomania (klep-toh-**MAY**-nee-ah): A personality disorder characterized by a recurrent failure to resist impulses to steal objects not for immediate use or their monetary value.

knee-chest position: Lying face down with the hips bent so the knees and chest rest on the table.

koilonychia (koy-loh-**NICK**-ee-ah): A malformation of the nails that is often indicative of iron-deficiency anemia in which the outer surface is scooped out; also known as spoon nail.

kyphosis (kye-**FOH**-sis): Abnormal increase in the outward curvature of the thoracic spine as viewed from the side; also known as humpback or dowager's hump.

L

labyrinthectomy (lab-ih-rin-**THECK**-toh-mee): Surgical removal of the labyrinth of the inner ear.

labyrinthitis (lab-ih-rin-**THIGH**-tis): Inflammation of the labyrinth resulting in vertigo.

labyrinthotomy (lab-ih-rin-**THOT**-oh-mee): A surgical incision into the labyrinth of the inner ear.

laceration (lass-er-**AY**-shun): A torn, ragged wound.

lacrimotomy (lack-rih-**MOT**-oh-mee): Surgical incision into the lacrimal duct.

lactation (lack-**TAY**-shun): The process of forming and secreting milk from the breasts as nourishment for the infant.

laminectomy (lam-ih-**NECK**-toh-mee): Surgical removal of a lamina from a vertebra.

laparoscopic adrenalectomy (ah-**dree**-nal-**ECK**-toh-mee): A minimally invasive surgical procedure to remove one or both adrenal glands.

laparoscopic cholecystectomy (**koh**-lee-sis-**TECK**-toh-mee): Surgical removal of the gallbladder using a laparoscope and other instruments while working through very small openings in the abdominal wall.

laparoscopy (lap-ah-**ROS**-koh-pee): Visual examination of the interior of the abdomen with the use of a laparoscope.

laryngectomy (lar-in-**JECK**-toh-mee): Surgical removal of the larynx.

laryngitis (lar-in-**JIGH**-tis): Inflammation of the larynx.

laryngologist (lar-in-**GOL**-oh-jist): A specialist in the study of the larynx.

laryngoplasty (lah-**RING**-goh-**plas**-tee): Surgical repair of the larynx.

laryngoplegia (lar-ing-goh-**PLEE**-jee-ah): Paralysis of the larynx.

laryngorrhagia (lar-ing-goh-**RAY**-jee-ah): Bleeding from the larynx.

laryngoscopy (lar-ing-**GOS**-koh-pee): Visual examination of the larynx using a laryngoscope.

laryngospasm (lah-**RING**-goh-spazm): A sudden spasmodic closure of the larynx.

laser iridotomy (ir-ih-**DOT**-oh-mee): Laser treatment of closed-angle glaucoma.

laser trabeculoplasty (trah-**BECK**-you-loh-**plas**-tee): Laser treatment of open-angle glaucoma.

laser: The acronym for **l**ight **a**mplification by **s**timulated **e**mission of **r**adiation. Lasers are used to treat skin, eye, and many other conditions.

leiomyoma (lye-oh-my-**OH**-mah): A benign tumor composed of muscle and fibrous tissue that occurs in the wall of the uterus; also known as a fibroid.

lensectomy (len-**SECK**-toh-mee): The surgical removal of a cataract-clouded lens.

lesion (**LEE**-zhun): A pathologic change of the tissues due to disease or injury.

lethargy (**LETH**-ar-jee): A lowered level of consciousness marked by listlessness, drowsiness, and apathy.

leukemia (loo-**KEE**-mee-ah): A malignancy characterized by a progressive increase of abnormal leukocytes.

leukopenia (loo-koh-**PEE**-nee-ah): An abnormal decrease in the number of white blood cells.

leukorrhea (loo-koh-**REE**-ah): A profuse white mucus discharge from the uterus and vagina.

ligation (lye-**GAY**-shun): Binding or tying off blood vessels or ducts.

lipectomy (lih-**PECK**-toh-mee): Surgical removal of fat beneath the skin.

lipedema (lip-eh-**DEE**-mah): An abnormal swelling due to the collection of fat and fluid under the skin, usually between the calf and ankle.

lipid tests: Laboratory tests to measure the amounts of cholesterol and triglycerides in a blood sample; also known as a lipid panel.

lipoma (lih-**POH**-mah): A benign fatty deposit under the skin, causing a bump.

liposuction (**LIP**-oh-**suck**-shun *or* **LYE**-poh-**suck**-shun): Surgical removal of fat beneath the skin with the aid of suction; also known as suction-assisted lipectomy.

lithotomy (lih-**THOT**-oh-mee): Surgical incision for the removal of a stone; an examination position.

lithotomy position (lih-**THOT**-oh-mee): Lying on the back with the feet and legs raised and supported in stirrups.

lithotripsy (**LITH**-oh-**trip**-see): Destruction of a kidney stone with the use of ultrasonic waves traveling through water; also known as extracorporeal shock-wave lithotripsy.

lobectomy (loh-**BECK**-toh-mee): Surgical removal of a lobe of the brain, liver, lung, or thyroid gland.

lochia (**LOH**-kee-ah): The vaginal discharge during the first week or two after childbirth.

lordosis (lor-**DOH**-sis): Abnormal increase in the forward curvature of the lower or lumbar spine; also known as swayback.

Lou Gehrig's disease: A degenerative disease of the motor neurons in which patients become progressively weaker until they are completely paralyzed; also known as amyotrophic lateral sclerosis.

lumbago (lum-**BAY**-goh): Pain of the lumbar region; also known as low back pain.

lumpectomy: Surgical removal of only the cancerous tissue and a margin of normal tissue.

lupus erythematosus (**LOO**-pus er-ih-**thee**-mah-**TOH**-sus): An autoimmune disorder characterized by a red, scaly rash on the face and upper trunk.

luxation (luck-**SAY**-shun): Dislocation or displacement of a bone from its joint.

lymphadenectomy (**lim**-fad-eh-**NECK**-toh-mee): Surgical removal of a lymph node.

lymphadenitis (lim-**fad**-eh-**NIGH**-tis): Inflammation of the lymph nodes; also known as swollen glands.

lymphadenopathy (lim-**fad**-eh-**NOP**-ah-thee): Any disease process usually involving enlargement of the lymph nodes.

lymphadenopathy, persistent generalized: The continued presence of enlarged lymph nodes that is often an indication of the presence of a malignancy or deficiency in immune system function.

lymphangiogram (lim-**FAN**-jee-oh-**gram**): A radiographic study of the lymphatic vessels and nodes with the use of a contrast medium to make these structures visible.

lymphangiography (lim-**fan**-jee-**OG**-rah-fee): A radiographic examination of the lymphatic vessels following the injection of a contrast medium.

lymphangioma (lim-**fan**-jee-**OH**-mah): A benign abnormal collection of lymphatic vessels forming a mass.

lymphangitis (lim-fan-**JIGH**-tis): Inflammation of the lymph vessel.

lymphedema (**lim**-feh-**DEE**-mah): An abnormal accumulation of fluid primarily in the legs and ankles that occurs when veins or lymph vessels do not drain properly.

lymphoma (lim-**FOH**-mah): A general term applied to malignancies that develop in the lymphatic system.

M

macular degeneration (**MACK**-you-lar): A gradually progressive condition that results in the loss of central vision but not in total blindness.

macule (**MACK**-youl): A discolored, flat spot such as a freckle or *flat* mole that is *less than* 1 cm in diameter.

magnetic resonance imaging: The use of a combination of radio waves and a strong magnetic field to produce images of the structures of the body.

major depressive episode: A prolonged period during which there is either a depressed mood or the loss of interest or pleasure in nearly all activities.

malaria (mah-**LAY**-ree-ah): A disease caused by a parasite that lives within certain mosquitoes and is transferred to humans by the bite of the mosquito.

malignant: Harmful, tending to spread, becoming progressively worse, and life-threatening.

malingering (mah-**LING**-ger-ing): The intentional creation of false or grossly exaggerated physical or psychological symptoms, motivated by external incentives such as avoiding work.

malnutrition: Lack of proper food or nutrients in the body, either due to a shortage of food or the improper absorption or distribution of nutrients.

mammography (mam-**OG**-rah-fee): A radiographic study of the breasts. The resulting record is called a mammogram.

mammoplasty (**MAM**-oh-**plas**-tee): Surgical repair or restructuring of the breasts.

manic episode: A distinct period during which there is an abnormally, and persistently elevated, expansive, and irritable mood.

mastitis (mas-**TYE**-tis): Inflammation of the breast usually associated with lactation but which may occur for other reasons.

mastodynia (**mas**-toh-**DIN**-ee-ah): Pain in the breast.

mastoidectomy (**mas**-toy-**DECK**-toh-mee): Surgical removal of mastoid cells.

mastoiditis (**mas**-toy-**DYE**-tis): Inflammation of any part of the mastoid process.

mastopexy (**MAS**-toh-**peck**-see): Surgery to affix sagging breasts in a more elevated position.

maxillofacial surgery (mack-**sill**-oh-**FAY**-shul): Specialized surgery of the face and jaws to correct deformities, treat diseases, and repair injuries.

measles: An acute, highly contagious viral disease transmitted by respiratory droplets that is characterized by Koplik's spots and a spreading skin rash.

meatotomy (**mee**-ah-**TOT**-oh-mee): An incision of the urinary meatus to enlarge the opening.

meconium (meh-**KOH**-nee-um): A greenish material that collects in the intestine of a fetus and forms the first stools of a newborn.

melanodermatitis (mel-ah-noh-**der**-mah-**TYE**-tis): Excess melanin present in an area of skin inflammation.

melanoma, malignant: Skin cancer derived from cells capable of forming melanin.

melanosis (mel-ah-**NOH**-sis): Any condition of unusual deposits of black pigment in different parts of the body.

melasma: A pigmentation disorder characterized by brownish colored spots on the face; also known as chloasma or the mask of pregnancy.

melena (meh-**LEE**-nah *or* **MEL**-eh-nah): The passage of black stools containing digested blood.

Menière's syndrome (**men**-ee-**AYRZ** *or* men-**YEHRS**): A chronic disease of the inner ear characterized by three main symptoms: attacks of dizziness, a fluctuating hearing loss, and tinnitus.

meningitis (men-in-**JIGH**-tis): An inflammation of the meninges of the brain or spinal cord.

meningocele (meh-**NING**-goh-**seel**): The protrusion of the membranes of the brain or spinal cord through a defect in the skull or spinal column.

meningoencephalitis (meh-**ning**-goh-en-**sef**-ah-**LYE**-tis): Inflammation of the meninges and brain.

meningoencephalomyelitis (meh-**ning**-goh-en-**sef**-ah-loh-**my**-eh-**LYE**-tis): Inflammation of the meninges, brain, and spinal cord.

meningomalacia (meh-**ning**-goh-mah-**LAY**-shee-ah): Abnormal softening of the meninges.

menometrorrhagia (**men**-oh-**met**-roh-**RAY**-jee-ah): Excessive uterine bleeding occurring both during the menses and at irregular intervals.

menorrhagia (**men**-oh-**RAY**-jee-ah): An excessive amount of menstrual flow over a longer duration than a normal period.

mental retardation: Significantly below average general intellectual functioning that is accompanied by significant limitation in adaptive functioning.

metabolism (meh-**TAB**-oh-**lizm**): The rate at which the body uses energy and the speed at which body functions work.

metastasis (meh-**TAS**-tah-sis): The new cancer site that results from the spreading process.

metastasize (meh-**TAS**-tah-sighz): The process by which cancer spreads from one place to another.

metrorrhea (**mee**-troh-**REE**-ah): An abnormal uterine discharge.

metrorrhexis (**mee**-troh-**RECK**-sis): Rupture of the uterus.

migraine headache (**MY**-grayn): A syndrome characterized by sudden, severe, sharp headache usually present only on one side.

miliaria (mill-ee-**AYR**-ee-ah): Trapped sweat that produces a skin rash and itching; also known as heat rash or prickly heat.

mitral stenosis (steh-**NOH**-sis): Abnormal narrowing of the opening of the mitral valve.

mitral valve prolapse: Abnormal protrusion of the mitral value that results in the incomplete closure of the valve.

mittelschmerz (**MIT**-uhl-schmehrts): Pain between menstrual periods.

modified radical mastectomy: Surgical removal of the entire breast and lymph nodes under the arm.

Mohs' chemosurgery: A technique using a zinc chloride paste to remove recurrent tumors and scarlike basal cell carcinomas with a minimum of normal tissue loss but complete removal of the tumor.

monaural (mon-**AW**-rahl): Involving one ear.

monochromatism (mon-oh-**KROH**-mah-tizm): The lack of the ability to distinguish colors; also known as color blindness.

mucous (**MYOU**-kus): Specialized membranes that line the body cavities.

mucus (**MYOU**-kus): The substance secreted by the mucous membranes.

multiparous (mul-**TIP**-ah-rus): A woman who has given birth two or more times.

multiple sclerosis (skleh-**ROH**-sis): A progressive autoimmune disorder characterized by scattered patches of demyelination of nerve fibers of the brain and spinal cord.

mumps: An acute viral disease characterized by swelling of the parotid glands. (The parotid glands are salivary glands located on the face just in front of the ears.)

Munchausen syndrome (**MUHN**-chow-zen): A condition in which the "patient" repeatedly makes up clinically convincing simulations of disease for the purpose of gaining medical attention.

Munchausen syndrome by proxy: A form of child abuse in which the abusive parent will falsify an illness in a child by making up or creating symptoms and then seeking medical treatment.

muscle relaxant: Medication that acts on the central nervous system to relax muscle tone and relieve spasms.

muscular dystrophy (**DIS**-troh-fee): A group of inherited muscle disorders that cause muscle weakness without affecting the nervous system.

myalgia (my-**AL**-jee-ah): Muscle tenderness or pain.

myasthenia (**my**-as-**THEE**-nee-ah): Muscle weakness from any cause.

myasthenia gravis (**my**-as-**THEE**-nee-ah **GRAH**-vis): An autoimmune disease in which there is an abnormality in the neuromuscular function causing episodes of muscle weakness.

mycoplasma pneumonia (**my**-koh-**PLAZ**-mah new-**MOH**-nee-ah): A milder but longer lasting form of the pneumonia caused by the fungi *Mycoplasma pneumoniae*; also known as walking pneumonia.

mycosis (my-**KOH**-sis): Any disease caused by a fungus.

mydriatic drops (**mid**-ree-**AT**-ick): Medication placed in the eye to produce temporary paralysis that forces the pupils to remain wide open even in the presence of bright light.

myectomy (my-**ECK**-toh-mee): Surgical removal of a portion of a muscle.

myelitis (my-eh-**LYE**-tis): Inflammation of the spinal cord; also inflammation of bone marrow.

myelography (my-eh-**LOG**-rah-fee): A radiographic study of the spinal cord after the injection of a contrast medium.

myeloma (my-eh-**LOH**-mah): A malignant tumor composed of cells derived from hemopoietic tissues of the bone marrow.

myelopathy (my-eh-**LOP**-ah-thee): Any pathologic condition of the spinal cord.

myelosis (my-eh-**LOH**-sis): A tumor of the spinal cord; also an abnormal proliferation of bone marrow tissue.

myocardial infarction (my-oh-**KAR**-dee-al in-**FARK**-shun): Occlusion of a coronary artery resulting in an infarct of the affected myocardium; also known as a heart attack.

myocarditis (my-oh-kar-**DYE**-tis): Inflammation of the myocardium.

myocele (**MY**-oh-seel): Protrusion of a muscle through its ruptured sheath or fascia.

myoclonus (my-oh-**KLOH**-nus *or* my-**OCK**-loh-nus): Spasm or twitching of a muscle or group of muscles.

myofascial damage (my-oh-**FASH**-ee-ahl): Tenderness and swelling of the muscles and their surrounding tissues that is caused by overworking the muscles.

myolysis (my-**OL**-ih-sis): Degeneration of muscle tissue.

myoma (my-**OH**-mah): A benign neoplasm made up of muscle tissue.

myomalacia (my-oh-mah-**LAY**-shee-ah): Abnormal softening of muscle tissue.

myonecrosis (my-oh-neh-**KROH**-sis): Death of individual muscle fibers.

myoparesis (my-oh-**PAR**-eh-sis): Weakness or slight paralysis of a muscle.

myopathy (my-**OP**-ah-thee): Any pathologic change or disease of muscle tissue.

myopia (my-**OH**-pee-ah): A defect in which light rays focus in front of the retina; also known as nearsightedness.

myoplasty (**MY**-oh-**plas**-tee): Surgical repair of a muscle.

myorrhaphy (my-**OR**-ah-fee): To suture a muscle wound.

myorrhexis (my-oh-**RECK**-sis): Rupture of a muscle.

myosarcoma (my-oh-sahr-**KOH**-mah): A malignant tumor derived from muscle tissue.

myosclerosis (my-oh-skleh-**ROH**-sis): Abnormal hardening of muscle tissue.

myositis (my-oh-**SIGH**-tis): Inflammation of skeletal muscle tissue.

myotomy (my-**OT**-oh-mee): Surgical incision into, or division of, a muscle.

myotonia (my-oh-**TOH**-nee-ah): Delayed relaxation of a muscle after a strong contraction.

myringectomy (mir-in-**JECK**-toh-mee): Surgical removal of all or part of the tympanic membrane; also known as a tympanectomy.

myringitis (mir-in-**JIGH**-tis): Inflammation of the tympanic membrane.

myringotomy (mir-in-**GOT**-oh-mee): A surgical incision of the eardrum to create an opening for the placement of tympanostomy tubes.

myxedema (mick-seh-**DEE**-mah): A severe form of hypothyroidism in adults.

N

narcissistic personality disorder (nahr-sih-**SIS**-tick): A pattern of an exaggerated need for admiration and complete lack of empathy.

narcolepsy (**NAR**-koh-**lep**-see): A syndrome characterized by recurrent uncontrollable seizures of drowsiness and sleep.

nasogastric intubation (nay-zoh-**GAS**-trick in-too-**BAY**-shun): Placement of a tube through the nose and into the stomach.

natal (**NAY**-tal): Pertaining to birth.

nausea (**NAW**-see-ah): The sensation that leads to the urge to vomit.

neonate (**NEE**-oh-nayt): An infant during the first 4 weeks after birth.

neonatologist (nee-oh-nay-**TOL**-oh-jist): A specialist in diagnosing and treating disorders of the newborn.

neonatology (nee-oh-nay-**TOL**-oh-jee) Study of disorders of the newborn.

neoplasm (**NEE**-oh-plazm): A new and abnormal tissue formation that may be benign or malignant; also known as a tumor.

nephrectasis (neh-**FRECK**-tah-sis): Distention of a kidney.

nephrectomy (neh-**FRECK**-toh-mee): Surgical removal of a kidney.

nephritis (neh-**FRY**-tis): Inflammation of the kidney.

nephrolith (**NEF**-roh-lith): Presence of stones in the kidney; also known as renal calculus or a kidney stone.

nephrolithiasis (nef-roh-lih-**THIGH**-ah-sis): A disorder characterized by the presence of stones in the kidney.

nephrolithotomy (nef-roh-lih-**THOT**-oh-mee): Surgical removal of a kidney stone through an incision in the kidney.

nephrologist (neh-**FROL**-oh-jist): A specialist in diagnosing and treating diseases and disorders of the kidneys.

nephrolysis (neh-**FROL**-ih-sis): Freeing of a kidney from adhesions.

nephromalacia (nef-roh-mah-**LAY**-shee-ah): Abnormal softening of the kidney.

nephropathy (neh-**FROP**-ah-thee): Disease of the kidney.

nephropexy (**NEF**-roh-**peck**-see): Surgical fixation of a floating kidney.

nephroptosis (nef-rop-**TOH**-sis): The downward displacement of the kidney; also known as a floating kidney.

nephropyosis (nef-roh-pye-**OH**-sis): Formation or discharge of pus from the kidney.

nephrosclerosis (nef-roh-skleh-**ROH**-sis): Abnormal hardening of the kidney.

nephrosis (neh-**FROH**-sis): Any abnormal condition of the kidney.

nephrostomy (neh-**FROS**-toh-mee): Surgical establishment of an opening between the pelvis of the kidney through its cortex to the exterior of the body.

nephrotic syndrome (neh-**FROT**-ick): A group of kidney diseases characterized by edema, hyperproteinuria, hypoproteinemia, and hyperlipidemia.

nephrotomy (neh-**FROT**-oh-mee): Surgical incision into the kidney.

neuralgia (new-**RAL**-jee-ah): Pain in a nerve or nerves.

neurectomy (new-**RECK**-toh-mee): The surgical removal of a nerve.

neuritis (new-**RYE**-tis): Inflammation of a nerve or **nerves**.

neuroblastoma (**new**-roh-blas-**TOH**-mah): A sarcoma of nervous system origin.

neurologist (new-**ROL**-oh-jist): A specialist in diagnosing and treating disorders of the central nervous system.

neuroma (new-**ROH**-mah): A benign tumor made up nerve tissue.

neuromalacia (**new**-roh-mah-**LAY**-shee-ah): Abnormal softening of a nerve or nerves.

neuroplasty (**NEW**-roh-**plas**-tee): Surgical repair of a nerve or nerves.

neurorrhaphy (new-**ROR**-ah-fee): To suture the ends of a severed nerve.

neurosurgeon: A physician who specializes in surgery of the nervous system.

neurotomy (new-**ROT**-oh-mee): A surgical incision or the dissection of a nerve.

nevi (**NEE**-vye): Small dark skin growths that develop from melanocytes in the skin; also known as moles.

nevi, dysplastic: Atypical moles that may develop into skin cancer.

nitroglycerin: A vasodilator used to relieve the pain of angina.

nocturia (nock-**TOO**-ree-ah): Excessive urination during the night.

nocturnal enuresis: The involuntary discharge of urine during sleep; also known as bed-wetting.

nocturnal myoclonus (nock-**TER**-nal **my**-oh-**KLOH**-nus *or* my-**OCK**-loh-nus): Jerking of the limbs that may occur normally as a person is falling asleep.

nodule (**NOD**-youl): A small *solid* bump that may be felt within the skin or may be raised as if it had formed below the surface of the skin and pushed upward.

non-Hodgkin's lymphomas: The term used to describe all lymphomas *other than* Hodgkin's lymphoma.

nonsteroidal anti-inflammatory drugs: Medication to control pain and to reduce inflammation and swelling; also known as NSAIDs.

nosocomial (**nos**-oh-**KOH**-mee-al): A hospital-acquired infection that was not present on admission but appears 72 hours or more after hospitalization.

nuclear medicine: A diagnostic technique that focuses on physiologic processes to determine how well body organs or systems are functioning; also known as radionuclide imaging.

nuclear scan: The use of radionucleide tracers to gather information about the structure and function of organs or systems that cannot be seen on conventional x-rays; also known as a scintigram.

nulligravida (**null**-ih-**GRAV**-ih-dah): A woman who has never been pregnant.

nullipara (nuh-**LIP**-ah-rah): A woman who has never borne a viable child.

nyctalopia (**nick**-tah-**LOH**-pee-ah): A condition in which the individual has difficulty seeing at night; also known as night blindness.

nystagmus (nis-**TAG**-mus): Involuntary, constant, rhythmic movement of the eyeball.

O

obesity (oh-**BEE**-sih-tee): An excessive accumulation of fat in the body.

obsessions: Persistent ideas, thoughts, or images that cause the individual anxiety or distress.

obsessive-compulsive disorder: A pattern of specific behaviors such as repeated handwashing that are caused by obsessions and compulsions.

obstetrician (**ob**-steh-**TRISH**-un): A specialist in providing medical care to women during pregnancy, childbirth, and immediately thereafter.

occlusion (ah-**KLOO**-zhun): Blockage in a canal, vessel, or passageway in the body; coming together.

oligomenorrhea (ol-ih-goh-**men**-oh-**REE**-ah): Markedly reduced menstrual flow and abnormally infrequent menstruation.

oligospermia (**ol**-ih-goh-**SPER**-mee-ah): An abnormally low number of sperm in the ejaculate; also known as a low sperm count.

oliguria (ol-ih-**GOO**-ree-ah): Scanty urination.

oncologist (ong-**KOL**-oh-jist): A specialist in diagnosing and treating malignant disorders such as tumors and cancer.

oncology (ong-**KOL**-oh-jee): The study of the prevention, causes, and treatment of tumors and cancer.

onychectomy (**on**-ih-**KECK**-toh-mee): Surgical removal of a finger or toenail.

onychia (oh-**NICK**-ee-ah): Inflammation of the matrix of the nail; also known as onychitis.

onychitis (on-ih-**KYE**-tis): See onychia.

onychocryptosis (**on**-ih-koh-krip-**TOH**-sis): Ingrown toenail.

onychoma (on-ih-**KOH**-mah): A tumor arising from the nail bed.

onychomalacia (**on**-ih-koh-mah-**LAY**-shee-ah): Abnormal softening of the nails.

onychomycosis (**on**-ih-koh-my-**KOH**-sis): Any fungus infection of the nail.

onychophagia (**on**-ih-koh-**FAY**-jee-ah): Nail biting or eating.

oophorectomy (oh-ahf-oh-**RECK**-toh-mee): Surgical removal of one or both ovaries; also known as an ovariectomy.

oophoritis (oh-ahf-oh-**RYE**-tis): Inflammation of an ovary.

oophoropexy (oh-**AHF**-oh-roh-**peck**-see): Surgical fixation of a displaced ovary.

oophoroplasty (oh-**AHF**-oh-roh-**plas**-tee): Surgical repair of an ovary.

ophthalmologist (ahf-thal-**MOL**-oh-jist): A specialist in diagnosing and treating diseases and disorders of the eye.

ophthalmology (ahf-thal-**MOL**-oh-jee): Study of the eye.

ophthalmoscope (ahf-**THAL**-moh-skope): An instrument used to examine the interior of the eye.

optometrist (op-**TOM**-eh-trist): A specialist in measuring the accuracy of vision to determine if corrective lenses or eyeglasses are needed.

oral rehydration therapy: Treatment in which a solution of electrolytes is administered orally to counteract dehydration that may accompany severe diarrhea.

orbitotomy (or-bih-**TOT**-oh-mee): A surgical incision into the orbit for biopsy, abscess drainage, and removal of a tumor mass or foreign object.

orchidectomy (or-kih-**DECK**-toh-mee): Surgical removal of one or both testicles; also known as an orchiectomy or testectomy.

orchiectomy (or-kee-**ECK**-toh-mee): See orchidectomy.

orchitis (or-**KYE**-tis): Inflammation of one or both testicles; also known as testitis.

organic (or-**GAN**-ick): A disorder in which there are pathologic physical changes that explain the symptoms being experienced by the patient.

orthodontist (or-thoh-**DON**-tist): A dental specialist in the prevention or correction of abnormalities in the positioning of the teeth and related facial structures.

orthopedic surgeon: A specialist in diagnosing and treating diseases and disorders involving the bones, joints, and muscles; also known as an orthopedist.

orthopedist (or-thoh-**PEE**-dist): See orthopedic surgeon.

ostealgia (oss-tee-**AL**-jee-ah): Pain linked to an abnormal condition within a bone.

ostectomy (oss-**TECK**-toh-mee): Surgical removal of bone.

osteitis (oss-tee-**EYE**-tis): Inflammation of bone.

osteitis deformans (oss-tee-**EYE**-tis dee-**FOR**-manz): A disease of unknown cause characterized by extensive bone destruction followed by abnormal bone repair; also known as Paget's disease.

osteoarthritis (oss-tee-oh-ar-**THRIGH**-tis): Form of arthritis commonly associated with aging; also known as wear-and-tear arthritis.

osteoarthropathy (oss-tee-oh-ar-**THROP**-ah-thee): Any disease involving the bones and joints.

osteochondroma (oss-tee-oh-kon-**DROH**-mah): Benign bone tumors that occur as growths on the surface of a bone that protrude as hard lumps covered with a cap of cartilage.

osteoclasis (oss-tee-**OCK**-lah-sis): Surgical fracture of a bone to correct a deformity.

osteomalacia (oss-tee-oh-mah-**LAY**-shee-ah): Abnormal softening of bones due to disease.

osteomyelitis (oss-tee-oh-**my**-eh-**LYE**-tis): Inflammation of the bone and bone marrow.

osteonecrosis (oss-tee-oh-neh-**KROH**-sis): Death of bone tissue caused by an insufficient blood supply, infection, malignancy, or trauma.

osteopathic physician (oss-tee-oh-**PATH**-ick): A specialist in treating health problems by manipulation (changing the positions of the bones); may also use traditional forms of medical treatment.

osteoplasty (**OSS**-tee-oh-**plas**-tee): Surgical repair of bones.

osteoporosis (oss-tee-oh-poh-**ROH**-sis): Loss of bone density and an increase in bone porosity frequently associated with aging.

osteorrhaphy (oss-tee-**OR**-ah-fee): Suturing or wiring together of bones.

osteosarcoma (oss-tee-oh-sar-**KOH**-mah): A malignant tumor usually involving the upper shaft of long bones, the pelvis, or knee.

osteosclerosis (oss-tee-oh-skleh-**ROH**-sis): Abnormal hardening of bone.

osteotomy (oss-tee-**OT**-oh-mee): Surgical incision or sectioning of a bone.

ostomy (**OSS**-toh-mee): Surgical procedure to create an artificial opening between an organ and the body surface.

otalgia (oh-**TAL**-gee-ah): Pain in the ear.

otitis (oh-**TYE**-tis): Inflammation of the ear

otitis externa: Inflammation of the outer ear.

otitis media, acute (oh-**TYE**-tis **MEE**-dee-ah): Inflammation of the middle ear usually associated with an upper respiratory infection that is most commonly seen in young children.

otitis media, purulent (**PYOU**-roo-lent): A buildup of pus within the middle ear.

otitis media, serous: A fluid buildup in the middle ear that may follow acute otitis media or be caused by obstruction of the eustachian tube.

otolaryngologist (oh-toh-**lar**-in-**GOL**-oh-jist): A specialist in diagnosing and treating diseases and disorders of the ears, nose, and throat; also known as an otorhinolaryngologist.

otomycosis (oh-toh-my-**KOH**-sis): A fungal infection of the external auditory canal.

otoplasty (**OH**-toh-**plas**-tee): Surgical repair of the pinna of the outer ear.

otopyorrhea (oh-toh-**pye**-oh-**REE**-ah): The flow of pus from the ear.

otorhinolaryngologist (oh-toh-**rye**-noh-**lar**-in-**GOL**-oh-jist): A specialist in diagnosing and treating diseases and disorders of the ears, nose, and throat; also known as an otolaryngologist.

otorhinolaryngology (oh-toh-**rye**-noh-**lar**-in-**GOL**-oh-jee): Study of the ears, nose, and throat.

otorrhagia (oh-toh-**RAY**-jee-ah): Bleeding from the ear.

otosclerosis (oh-toh-skleh-**ROH**-sis): Ankylosis of the bones of the middle ear resulting in a conductive hearing loss.

otoscope (**OH**-toh-skope): An instrument used to visually examine the external ear canal and tympanic membrane.

ovariectomy (**oh**-vay-ree-**ECK**-toh-me): Surgical removal of one or both ovaries; also known as an oophorectomy.

ovariorrhexis (oh-**vay**-ree-oh-**RECK**-sis): Rupture of an ovary.

P

pacemaker: An electronic device to regulate the heartbeat to treat bradycardia or atrial fibrillation.

Paget's disease (**PAJ**-its): Disease of unknown cause characterized by extensive bone destruction followed by abnormal bone repair; also known as osteitis deformans.

palatoplasty (**PAL**-ah-toh-**plas**-tee): Surgical repair of a cleft palate.

palliative (**PAL**-ee-**ay**-tiv *or* **PAL**-ee-ah-tiv): A substance that eases the pain or severity of a disease but does not cure it.

palpation (pal-**PAY**-shun): An examination technique in which the examiner's hands are used to feel the texture, size, consistency, and location of certain body parts.

palpitation (**pal**-pih-**TAY**-shun): A pounding or racing heart.

pancreatalgia (**pan**-kree-ah-**TAL**-jee-ah): Pain in the pancreas.

pancreatectomy (**pan**-kree-ah-**TECK**-toh-mee): Surgical removal of the pancreas.

pancreatitis (**pan**-kree-ah-**TYE**-tis): Inflammation of the pancreas.

pancreatotomy (**pan**-kree-ah-**TOT**-oh-mee): Surgical incision into the pancreas.

pandemic (pan-**DEM**-ick): A disease outbreak occurring over a large geographic area, possibly worldwide.

panic attack: A mental state that includes intense feelings of apprehension, fearfulness, terror, and impending doom plus physical symptoms that include shortness of breath and heart palpitations.

Papanicolaou test (**pap**-ah-nick-oh-**LAY**-ooh): An exfoliative test for the detection and diagnosis of conditions of the cervix and surrounding tissues; also known as a Pap smear.

papilledema (**pap**-ill-eh-**DEE**-mah): Swelling and inflammation of the optic nerve at the point of entrance through the optic disk; also known as choked disk.

papilloma (**pap**-ih-**LOH**-mah): A benign epithelial tumor that projects from the surrounding surface.

papule (**PAP**-youl): A small, solid, raised skin lesion that is *less than* 0.5 cm in diameter; also known as a pimple.

paralysis (pah-**RAL**-ih-sis): Loss of sensation and voluntary muscle movements through disease or injury to its nerve supply.

paraplegia (**par**-ah-**PLEE**-jee-ah): Paralysis of both legs and the lower part of the body.

parasite (**PAR**-ah-sight): A plant or animal that lives on or within another living organism at the expense of that organism.

paraspadias (**par**-ah-**SPAY**-dee-as): A congenital male abnormality in which the urethral opening is on one side of the penis.

parathyroidectomy (**par**-ah-**thigh**-roi-**DECK**-toh-mee): Surgical removal of one or more of the parathyroid glands.

paresthesia (**par**-es-**THEE**-zee-ah): An abnormal sensation, such as burning, tingling, or numbness, for no apparent reason.

Parkinson's disease: A chronic slowly progressive, degenerative, central nervous system disorder characterized by fine muscle tremors, a masklike facial expression, and a shuffling gait.

paronychia (**par**-oh-**NICK**-ee-ah): An acute or chronic infection of the skin fold at the margin of a nail.

paroxysm (**PAR**-ock-sizm): A sudden convulsion, seizure, or spasm.

paroxysmal (**par**-ock-**SIZ**-mal): Sudden or spasmlike.

paroxysmal tachycardia: A fast heartbeat of sudden onset.

parturition (**par**-tyou-**RISH**-un): The act of giving birth to an offspring; also known as labor and childbirth.

pathogen (**PATH**-oh-jen): A microorganism that causes a disease.

pathologist (pah-**THOL**-oh-jist): A specialist in the laboratory analysis of tissue samples to confirm or establish a diagnosis.

pathology (pah-**THOL**-oh-jee): A condition caused by disease; the study of structural and functional changes caused by disease.

pattern baldness, female: A condition in which the hair thins in the front and on the sides, and sometimes on the crown.

pattern baldness, male: A condition in which the hairline recedes from the front to the back until only a horseshoe shaped area of hair remains in the back and temples.

patulous eustachian tube (**PAT**-you-lus): Distention of the eustachian tube.

pediatrician (**pee**-dee-ah-**TRISH**-un): A specialist in diagnosing, treating, and preventing disorders and diseases of children.

pediculosis (**pee**-dick-you-**LOH**-sis): An infestation with lice.

pediculosis capitis: An infestation with head lice.

pediculosis corporis: An infestation with body lice.

pediculosis pubis: An infestation with lice in the pubic hair and pubic region.

pelvic inflammatory disease: Any inflammation of the female reproductive organs not associated with surgery or pregnancy; also known as PID.

pelvimetry (pel-**VIM**-eh-tree): The measurement of the dimensions of the pelvis to determine its capacity to allow passage of the fetus through the birth canal.

peptic ulcer: A lesion of the mucous membranes of the digestive system caused by the bacterium *Helicobacter pylori.*

percussion (per-**KUSH**-un): A diagnostic procedure to determine the density of a body area by the sound produced by tapping the surface with the finger or instrument.

percutaneous (**per**-kyou-**TAY**-nee-us): A procedure performed through the skin.

percutaneous transluminal coronary angioplasty (**AN**-jee-oh-**plas**-tee): A procedure in which a small balloon on the end of a catheter is used to open a partially blocked coronary artery; also known as balloon angioplasty.

perfusion (per-**FYOU**-zuhn): The flow of blood through the vessels of an organ.

pericardiectomy (pehr-ih-**kar**-dee-**ECK**-toh-mee): Surgical removal of a portion of the tissue surrounding the heart.

pericardiocentesis (pehr-ih-**kar**-dee-oh-sen-**TEE**-sis): Drawing fluid from the pericardial sac.

pericardiorrhaphy (pehr-ih-**kar**-dee-**OR**-ah-fee): To suture the tissue surrounding the heart.

pericarditis (pehr-ih-kar-**DYE**-tis): Inflammation of the pericardium.

perinatal (pehr-ih-**NAY**-tal): Time and events just before, during, and just after birth.

periodontal disease: Inflammation of the tissues that surround and support the teeth; also known as periodontitis.

periodontist (pehr-ee-oh-**DON**-tist): A dental specialist in the prevention and treatment of disorders of the tissues surrounding the teeth.

periodontitis (pehr-ee-oh-don-**TYE**-tis): Inflammation of the tissues that surround and support the teeth; also known as periodontal disease.

periosteotomy (peer-ee-**oss**-tee-**OT**-oh-mee): Surgical incision through the periosteum.

periostitis (pehr-ee-oss-**TYE**-tis): Inflammation of the periosteum.

peripheral neuritis (new-**RYE**-tis): A painful condition of the nerves of the hands and feet due to peripheral nerve damage; also known as peripheral neuropathy.

peripheral neuropathy (new-**ROP**-ah-thee): See peripheral neuritis.

peritoneal dialysis (pehr-ih-toh-**NEE**-al dye-**AL**-ih-sis): Removal of waste products through fluid exchange in the peritoneal cavity.

personality disorder: An enduring pattern of inner experience and behavior that deviates markedly from the expectations of the individual's culture.

pertussis (per-**TUS**-is): A contagious bacterial infection of the upper respiratory tract that is characterized by a paroxysmal cough; also known as whooping cough.

petechiae (pee-**TEE**-kee-ee): Small pinpoint hemorrhages; smaller versions of bruises.

phacoemulsification (fay-koh-ee-**mul**-sih-fih-**KAY**-shun or fack-koh-ee-**mul**-sih-fih-**KAY**-shun): The use of ultrasonic vibration to shatter and break up a cataract making it easier to remove.

pharmacist: A specialist who is licensed in formulating and dispensing medications.

pharmacology: The study of the nature, uses, and effects of drugs for medical purposes.

pharyngitis (far-in-**JIGH**-tis): Inflammation of the pharynx; also known as a sore throat.

pharyngolaryngitis (fah-**ring**-goh-**lar**-in-**JIGH**-tis): Inflammation of both the pharynx and the larynx.

pharyngoplasty (fah-**RING**-goh-**plas**-tee): Surgical repair of the pharynx.

pharyngorrhagia (far-ing-goh-**RAY**-jee-ah): Bleeding from the pharynx.

pharyngorrhea (far-ing-goh-**REE**-ah): An abnormal discharge from the pharynx.

pharyngostomy (far-ing-**GOSS**-toh-mee): Surgical creation of an artifical opening into the pharynx.

pharyngotomy (far-ing-**GOT**-oh-mee): A surgical incision of the pharynx.

phenobarbital (fee-noh-**BAR**-bih-tal): A barbiturate used as a sedative and as an anticonvulsant.

phenylketonuria (fen-il-**kee**-toh-**NEW**-ree-ah): A genetic disorder in which an essential digestive enzyme is missing.

pheochromocytoma (fee-oh-**kroh**-moh-sigh-**TOH**-mah): A benign tumor of the adrenal medulla that causes the gland to produce excess epinephrine.

phimosis (figh-**MOH**-sis): A narrowing of the opening of the foreskin so it cannot be retracted to expose the glans penis.

phlebitis (fleh-**BYE**-tis): Inflammation of a vein or veins.

phlebography (fleh-**BOG**-rah-fee): A radiograph study of the veins with the use of a contrast medium.

phleborrhexis (fleb-oh-**RECK**-sis): Rupture of a vein.

phlebostenosis (fleb-oh-steh-**NOH**-sis): Abnormal narrowing of the lumen of a vein.

phlebotomist (fleh-**BOT**-oh-mist): An individual trained and skilled in phlebotomy.

phlebotomy (fleh-**BOT**-oh-mee): The puncture of a vein for the purpose of drawing blood; also known as venipuncture.

phlegm (**FLEM**): Thick mucus secreted by the tissues lining the respiratory passages.

phobia (**FOH**-bee-ah): A persistent irrational fear of a specific thing or situation. This fear is strong enough to cause avoidance of that thing or situation.

photorefractive keratectomy (ker-ah-**TECK**-toh-mee): Laser treatment to correct refraction disorders by reshaping of the top layer of the cornea.

pica (**PYE**-kah): An eating disorder in which there is persistent eating of nonnutritional substances such as clay.

pinealectomy (pin-ee-al-**ECK**-toh-mee): Surgical removal of the pineal gland.

pinealoma (pin-ee-ah-**LOH**-mah): Tumor of the pineal gland.

pinealopathy (pin-ee-ah-**LOP**-ah-thee): Any disorder of the pineal gland.

pituitarism (pih-**TOO**-ih-tar-izm): Any disorder of pituitary function.

placebo (plah-**SEE**-boh): A substance containing no active ingredients that is given for its suggestive effects.

placenta previa (plah-**SEN**-tah **PREE**-vee-ah): Abnormal implantation of the placenta in the lower portion of the uterus.

plaque (**PLACK**): A solid raised area of skin that is different from the area around it and *greater than* 0.5 cm in diameter.

plasmapheresis (plaz-mah-feh-**REE**-sis): A procedure in which the plasma is removed from donated blood and the red blood cells are returned to the donor.

platelet count: A laboratory test that measures the number of platelets in a specified amount of blood.

pleuralgia (ploor-**AL**-jee-ah): Pain in the pleura or in the side.

pleurectomy (ploor-**ECK**-toh-mee): Surgical removal of part of the pleura.

pleurisy (**PLOOR**-ih-see): Inflammation of the visceral and parietal pleura in the thoracic cavity.

pneumoconiosis (**new**-moh-**koh**-nee-**OH**-sis): An abnormal condition caused by dust in the lungs that usually develops after years of environmental or occupational contact.

Pneumocystis carinii **pneumonia** (**new**-moh-**SIS**-tis kah-**RYE**-nee-eye new-**MOH**-nee-ah): A form of pneumonia caused by an infection with the parasite *Pneumocystis carinii*.

pneumonectomy (**new**-moh-**NECK**-toh-mee): Surgical removal of all or part of a lung.

pneumonia (new-**MOH**-nee-ah): Inflammation of the lungs in which the air sacs fill with pus and other liquid.

pneumonitis (**new**-moh-**NIGH**-tis): Inflammation of the lungs.

pneumorrhagia (**new**-moh-**RAY**-jee-ah): Bleeding from the lungs.

pneumothorax (**new**-moh-**THOR**-racks): An accumulation of air or gas in the pleural space causing the lung to collapse.

podiatrist (poh-**DYE**-ah-trist): A specialist in diagnosing, treating and correcting disorders of the foot.

poliomyelitis (**poh**-lee-oh-**my**-eh-**LYE**-tis): A viral infection of the gray matter of the spinal cord that may result in paralysis.

polyarteritis (**pol**-ee-ar-teh-**RYE**-tis): Inflammation involving several arteries.

polyarthritis (**pol**-ee-ar-**THRIGH**-tis): Inflammation of more than one joint.

polycystic ovary syndrome: Enlargement of the ovaries caused by the presence of many cysts.

polydipsia (**pol**-ee-**DIP**-see-ah): Excessive thirst.

polymenorrhea (**pol**-ee-**men**-oh-**REE**-ah): Abnormally frequent menstruation.

polymyalgia (**pol**-ee-my-**AL**-jee-ah): Pain in several muscle groups.

polymyositis (**pol**-ee-**my**-oh-**SIGH**-tis): A chronic, progressive disease affecting the skeletal muscles that is characterized by muscle weakness and atrophy.

polyneuritis (**pol**-ee-new-**RYE**-tis): Inflammation affecting many nerves.

polyp (**POL**-ip): A general term describing a mushroom-like growth from the surface of a mucous membrane.

polyuria (**pol**-ee-**YOU**-ree-ah): Excessive urination.

port-wine stain: A large reddish purple discoloration of the face or neck that is present at birth and will not resolve without treatment; also known as a birthmark.

positioning: In radiography, the body placement and the part of the body closest to the film.

positron emission tomography: The combination of tomography with radionuclide tracers to produce enhanced images of selected body organs or areas; also known as PET.

postnatal (pohst-**NAY**-tal): Time and events after birth.

postpolio syndrome: Recurrence later in life of some polio symptoms in individuals who have had poliomyelitis and have recovered from it.

posttraumatic stress disorder: The development of symptoms such as sleep disorders and anxiety after a psychologically traumatic event such as witnessing a shooting, surviving a natural disaster, or being held as a hostage.

potentiation (poh-**ten**-shee-**AY**-shun): An interaction that occurs when the effect of one drug is increased by another drug; also known as synergism.

preeclampsia (**pree**-ee-**KLAMP**-see-ah): A complication of pregnancy characterized by hypertension, edema, and proteinuria; also known as toxemia of pregnancy.

premenstrual syndrome: Symptoms occurring within the 2-week period before menstruation; also known as PMS.

prenatal (pre-**NAY**-tal): The time and events before birth.

presbycusis (**pres**-beh-**KOO**-sis): A progressive hearing loss occurring in old age.

presbyopia (**pres**-bee-**OH**-pee-ah): Changes in the eyes that occur with aging.

prescription: An order for medication, therapy, or a therapeutic device given by an authorized person to a person properly authorized to dispense or perform the order.

primigravida (**prye**-mih-**GRAV**-ih-dah): A woman during her first pregnancy.

primipara (prye-**MIP**-ah-rah): A woman who has borne one child.

proctalgia (prock-**TAL**-jee-ah): Pain in and around the anus and rectum.

proctectomy (prock-**TECK**-toh-mee): Surgical removal of the rectum.

proctologist (prock-**TOL**-oh-jist): A specialist in disorders of the colon, rectum, and anus.

proctopexy (**PROCK**-toh-**peck**-see): Surgical fixation of the rectum to an adjacent tissue or organ.

proctoplasty (**PROCK**-toh-**plas**-tee): Surgical repair of the rectum.

proctoscopy: Visual examination of the rectum and anus.

profile: Laboratory tests frequently performed as a group on automated multichannel laboratory testing equipment.

projection: In radiography, the path that the x-ray beam follows through the body from entrance to exit.

prolactinoma (proh-**lack**-tih-**NOH**-mah): A benign tumor of the pituitary gland that causes it to produce too much prolactin; also known as a prolactin-producing adenoma.

prolapse (proh-**LAPS**): Downward placement.

prolapse of uterus: Falling or sinking down of the uterus until it protrudes through the vaginal opening.

prone: Lying on the belly with the *face down*.

prostatectomy (pros-tah-**TECK**-toh-mee): Surgical removal of all or part of the prostate gland.

prostatectomy, radical: Surgical removal of the entire prostate gland, the seminal vesicles, and some surrounding tissue.

prostatectomy, transurethral: Removal of all or part of the prostate through the urethra; also known as transurethral resection of the prostate.

prostate-specific antigen: A blood test to screen for prostate cancer; also known as PSA.

prostatitis (pros-tah-**TYE**-tis): Inflammation of the prostate gland.

prostatomegaly (pros-tah-toh-**MEG**-ah-lee): Abnormal enlargement of the prostate gland that may be benign or malignant.

prostatorrhea (pros-tah-toh-**REE**-ah): An abnormal flow of prostatic fluid discharged through the urethra.

prostrate (**PROS**-trayt): To collapse or to be overcome with exhaustion.

proteinuria (proh-tee-in-**YOU**-ree-ah): An abnormally high level of serum protein in the urine.

prothrombin time (proh-**THROM**-bin): A laboratory test to diagnose conditions associated with abnormal bleeding and to monitor anticoagulant therapy.

pruritus (proo-**RYE**-tus): Itching.

pruritus vulvae (proo-**RYE**-tus **VUL**-vee): A condition of severe itching of the external female genitalia.

pseudophakia (soo-doh-**FAY**-kee-ah): An eye in which the natural lens is replaced with an intraocular lens.

psoriasis (soh-**RYE**-uh-sis): A chronic autoimmune disorder of the skin characterized by red papules covered with silvery scales that occur predominantly on the elbows, knees, scalp, back, and buttocks.

psychiatrist (sigh-**KYE**-ah-trist): A physician who specializes in diagnosing and treating chemical dependencies, emotional problems, and mental illness.

psychologist (sigh-**KOL**-oh-jist): A specialist, other than a physician, in evaluating and treating emotional problems.

psychotic disorder (sigh-**KOT**-ick): The derangement of personality, loss of contact with reality, and deterioration of normal social functioning.

psychotropic drugs (sigh-koh-**TROP**-pick): Drugs that are capable of affecting the mind, emotions, and behavior.

puerperium (pyou-er-**PEE**-ree-um): The period of 3 to 6 weeks after childbirth until the uterus returns to its normal size.

pulmonary edema (eh-**DEE**-mah): An accumulation of fluid in lung tissues.

pulmonary fibrosis: The formation of scar tissue that replaces the pulmonary alveolar walls.

pulmonary function tests: A group of tests that measure the capacity of the lungs to hold air, their ability to move air in and out, and their ability exchange oxygen and carbon dioxide.

pulmonologist (pull-mah-**NOL**-oh-jist): A specialist in diagnosing and treating diseases and disorders of the lungs and associated tissues.

puncture wound: A deep hole made by a sharp object such as a nail.

purpura (**PUR**-pew-rah): A condition characterized by hemorrhage into the skin that causes spontaneous bruising.

purulent (**PYOU**-roo-lent): Producing or containing pus.

pustule (**PUS**-tyoul): A small, circumscribed elevation of the skin containing pus.

putrefaction (pyou-treh-**FACK**-shun): Decay that produces foul-smelling odors.

pyelitis (pye-eh-**LYE**-tis): Inflammation of the renal pelvis.

pyelonephritis (pye-eh-loh-neh-**FRY**-tis): Inflammation of the renal pelvis and of the kidney.

pyeloplasty (**PYE**-eh-loh-**plas**-tee): Surgical repair of the renal pelvis.

pyelotomy (pye-eh-**LOT**-oh-mee): A surgical incision into the renal pelvis.

pyemia (pye-**EE**-mee-ah): Presence of pus-forming organisms in the blood.

pyoderma (pye-oh-**DER**-mah): Any pus-forming skin disease.

pyometritis (pye-oh-meh-**TRY**-tis): A pus-containing inflammation of the uterus.

pyosalpinx (pye-oh-**SAL**-pinks): An accumulation of pus in the fallopian tube.

pyothorax (pye-oh-**THOH**-racks): An accumulation of pus in the pleural cavity; also known as empyema.

pyromania (pye-roh-**MAY**-nee-ah): A personality disorder characterized by a recurrent failure to resist impulses to set fires.

pyrosis (pye-**ROH**-sis): Regurgitation of stomach acid upward into the esophagus; also known as heartburn.

pyuria (pye-**YOU**-ree-ah): The presence of pus in the urine.

Q

quadriplegia (kwad-rih-**PLEE**-jee-ah): Paralysis of all four extremities.

R

rabies (**RAY**-beez): An acute viral infection that may be transmitted to humans by the blood, tissue, or saliva of an infected animal.

radial keratotomy (ker-ah-**TOT**-oh-mee): Surgery used to correct myopia by making partial incisions in the cornea causing it to flatten.

radiation therapy: Cancer treatment with the use of x-radiation.

radiculitis (rah-**dick**-you-**LYE**-tis): Inflammation of the root of a spinal nerve; also known as a pinched nerve.

radioassay: A laboratory technique in which a radioactively labeled substance is mixed with a blood specimen; also known as radioimmunoassay.

radiographs, bitewing: Intraoral radiographs that show the crowns of teeth in both arches.

radiographs, periapical: Intraoral radiographs that show the entire tooth and some surrounding tissue.

radiography: The use of x-rays to expose a film that shows the body in profile.

radiography, extraoral: In dentistry, radiographic projections in which the film is placed outside of the mouth.

radiography, intraoral: In dentistry, radiographic projections in which the film is placed within the mouth.

radioimmunoassay (**ray**-dee-oh-**im**-you-noh-**ASS**-ay): A laboratory technique in which a radioactively labeled substance is mixed with a blood specimen; also known as radioassay.

radiologist (ray-dee-**OL**-oh-jist): A specialist in diagnosing and treating diseases and disorders with x-rays and other forms of radiant energy.

radiology (ray-dee-**OL**-oh-jee): The use radiant energy and radioactive substances in medicine for diagnosis and treatment.

radionuclide imaging (ray-dee-oh-**NEW**-klyd): A diagnostic technique that focuses on physiologic processes to determine how well body organs or systems are functioning; also known as nuclear medicine.

rale (RAHL): An abnormal rattle or crackle-like respiratory sound heard while breathing in.

Raynaud's phenomenon (ray-**NOHZ**): Intermittent attacks of pallor (paleness), cyanosis (blue color), and redness of the fingers and toes.

recumbent (ree-**KUM**-bent): Any position in which the patient is lying down.

red blood cell count: A laboratory test to determine the number of erythrocytes in the blood.

reflux (**REE**-flucks): A backward or return flow.

refraction: An examination procedure to determine the ability of the lens of the eye to bend light rays so they focus on the retina.

refractive disorder: A condition in which the lens and cornea do not bend light so that it focuses properly on the retina.

regimen (**REJ**-ih-men): Directions or rules.

regurgitation (ree-gur-jih-**TAY**-shun): The return of swallowed food into the mouth.

renal colic (**REE**-nal **KOLL**-ick): Acute pain in the kidney area caused by blockage during the passage of a kidney stone.

renal failure: Inability of the kidney or kidneys to perform their functions; also known as kidney failure.

renal failure, acute: Sudden onset of renal failure that is characterized by uremia.

renal failure, chronic: A progressive disease that may be caused by a variety of conditions.

restenosis: The condition in which an artery that has been opened by angioplasty becomes blocked again.

retinal tear: The retina develops a hole as it is pulled away from its normal position.

retinitis (ret-ih-**NIGH**-tis): Inflammation of the retina.

retinoblastoma (ret-ih-noh-blas-**TOH**-mah): A malignant tumor of childhood arising from cells of the retina of the eye.

retinopathy (ret-ih-**NOP**-ah-thee): Any disease of the retina.

retinopathy, diabetic: A complication of diabetics causing damage to the retina of the eye.

retinopexy (**RET**-ih-noh-**peck**-see): Laser treatment to reattach a detached retina.

retroflexion (ret-roh-**FLECK**-shun): Abnormal tipping with the body of the uterus bent forming an angle with the cervix.

retroversion (ret-roh-**VER**-zhun): Abnormal tipping of the entire uterus backward, with the cervix pointing forward.

rheumatologist (roo-mah-**TOL**-oh-jist): A specialist in the diagnosis and treatment of rheumatic diseases characterized by inflammation in the connective tissues.

rhinitis (rye-**NIGH**-tis): Inflammation of the nose.

rhinophyma (rye-noh-**FIGH**-muh): Hyperplasia of the nose; also known as bulbous nose.

rhinoplasty (**RYE**-noh-**plas**-tee): Plastic surgery to change the shape or size of the nose.

rhinorrhea (rye-noh-**REE**-ah): An excessive flow of mucus from the nose; also known as a runny nose.

rhonchus (**RONG**-kus): An added sound with a musical pitch occurring during inspiration or expiration that results from a partially obstructed airway; also known as wheezing.

rhytidectomy (rit-ih-**DECK**-toh-mee): Surgical removal of excess skin to eliminate wrinkles; also known as a face-lift.

rickets (**RICK**-ets): Bone disorder caused by calcium and vitamin D deficiencies in early childhood.

rickettsia (rih-**KET**-see-ah): Small bacterium that lives in lice, fleas, ticks and mites.

rosacea (roh-**ZAY**-shee-ah): A chronic condition of unknown cause that produces redness, tiny pimples, and broken blood vessels.

rotator cuff tendinitis (ten-dih-**NIGH**-tis): Inflammation of the tendons of the rotator cuff.

rubella (roo-**BELL**-ah): A viral infection characterized by fever and a diffuse, fine, red rash; also known as German measles or 3-day measles.

S

salmonella (sal-moh-**NEL**-ah): An intestinal infection caused by nontyphoidal *Salmonella*.

salpingectomy (sal-pin-**JECK**-toh-mee): Surgical removal of a fallopian tube or tubes.

salpingitis (**sal**-pin-**JIGH**-tis): Inflammation of a fallopian tube; inflammation of the eustachian tube.

sarcoma (sar-**KOH**-mah): A malignant tumor that arises from connective tissue.

scabies (**SKAY**-beez): A skin infection caused by an infestation with the itch mite.

scale: A flaking or dry patch made up of excess dead epidermal cells.

schizophrenia (**skit**-soh-**FREE**-nee-ah): A psychotic disorder that is characterized by delusions, hallucinations, disorganized speech that is often incoherent, and disruptive or catatonic behavior.

sciatica (sigh-**AT**-ih-kah) Inflammation of the sciatic nerve that results in pain along the course of the nerve through the thigh and leg.

scintigram (**SIN**-tih-gram): The use of radionucleide tracers to gather information about the structure and function of organs or systems that cannot be seen on conventional x-rays; also known as a nuclear scan.

scleritis (skleh-**RYE**-tis): Inflammation of the sclera of the eye.

scleroderma (**sklehr**-oh-**DER**-mah *or* **skleer**-oh-**DER**-mah): An autoimmune disorder that causes abnormal tissue thickening usually starting on the hands, feet, or face.

sclerotherapy (**sklehr**-oh-**THER**-ah-pee): Injection of a sclerosing solution to treat spider veins.

scoliosis (**skoh**-lee-**OH**-sis): Abnormal lateral curvature of the spine.

scotoma (skoh-**TOH**-mah): Abnormal area of absent or depressed vision surrounded by an area of normal vision.

scratch test: A diagnostic test to identify commonly troublesome allergens such as tree pollen and ragweed.

sebaceous cyst (seh-**BAY**-shus): A cyst of a sebaceous gland, containing yellow, fatty material.

seborrhea (**seb**-oh-**REE**-ah): Any of several common skin conditions in which there is an overproduction of sebum.

seborrheic dermatitis (**seb**-oh-**REE**-ick **der**-mah-**TYE**-tis): An inflammation of the upper layers of the skin, caused by seborrhea.

seborrheic keratosis (**seb**-oh-**REE**-ick **kerr**-ah-**TOH**-sis): A benign flesh-colored, brown or black skin tumor.

sedative: Medication that depresses the central nervous system and produces calm and diminished responsiveness without producing sleep.

sedimentation rate: A laboratory test based on the rate at which the red blood cells separate from plasma and settle to the bottom of the container; also known as erythrocyte sedimentation rate.

seizure (**SEE**-zhur): A sudden, violent, involuntary contraction of a group of muscles caused by a disturbance in brain function; also known as a convulsion.

seizure, generalized tonic-clonic: A loss of consciousness and tonic convulsions followed by clonic convulsions; also known as a generalized seizure. See also convulsion, tonic and convulsion, clonic.

seizure, localized: A state that begins with specific motor, sensory, or psychomotor phenomena without loss of consciousness; also known as a partial seizure.

septicemia (sep-tih-**SEE**-mee-ah): The presence of pathogenic microorganisms or their toxins in the blood; also known as blood poisoning.

septoplasty (**SEP**-toh-**plas**-tee): Surgical reconstruction of the nasal septum.

serum bilirubin test: A laboratory test to measure how well red blood cells are being broken down by the liver.

serum enzyme tests: Laboratory tests to measure the blood enzymes.

sexually transmitted diseases: Diseases transmitted through sexual intercourse or other genital contact; also known as venereal diseases.

shin splint: Pain caused by the muscle tearing away from the tibia.

sigmoidectomy (**sig**-moi-**DECK**-toh-mee): Surgical removal of all or part of the sigmoid colon.

sigmoiditis (**sig**-moi-**DYE**-tis): Inflammation of the sigmoid colon.

sigmoidoscopy (**sig**-moi-**DOS**-koh-pee): Visual examination of the interior of the entire rectum, sigmoid colon, and possibly a portion of the descending colon.

silicosis (**sill**-ih-**KOH**-sis): A form of pneumoconiosis caused by silica dust or glass in the lungs; also known as grinder's disease.

Sims' position: Lying on the left side with the right knee and thigh drawn up with the left arm placed along the back.

single photon emission computed tomography: A nuclear imaging technique in which pictures are taken by one to three gamma cameras after a radionuclide tracer has been injected into the blood.

singultus (sing-**GUL**-tus): Myoclonus of the diaphragm that causes the characteristic hiccup sound with each spasm; also known as hiccups.

sinusitis (**sigh**-nuh-**SIGH**-tis): Inflammation of the sinuses.

sinusotomy (**sigh**-nuhs-**OT**-oh-mee): A surgical incision into a sinus.

skin tags: Small flesh-colored or light brown growths that hang from the body by fine stalks.

sleep apnea syndromes: A group of potentially deadly disorders in which breathing repeatedly stops during sleep for long enough periods to cause a measurable decrease in blood oxygen levels.

smoker's respiratory syndrome: A group of symptoms seen in smokers that include a cough, wheezing, vocal hoarseness, pharyngitis, difficult breathing, and susceptibility to respiratory infections.

somatoform (soh-**MAT**-oh-**form**): The presence of physical symptoms that suggest general medical conditions but are not explained by the patient's actual medical condition.

somnambulism (som-**NAM**-byou-lizm): The condition of walking without awakening; also known as sleepwalking.

somnolence (**SOM**-noh-lens): A condition of unnatural sleepiness or semiconsciousness approaching coma; however, a somnolent person can usually be aroused by verbal stimuli.

spasm: A sudden, violent, involuntary contraction of a muscle or a group of muscles; also known as a cramp.

spasmodic torticollis (spaz-**MOD**-ick **tor**-tih-**KOL**-is): A stiff neck due to spasmodic contraction of the neck muscles that pull the head toward the affected side; also known as wryneck.

speculum (**SPECK**-you-lum): An instrument used to enlarge the opening of any canal or cavity to make it possible to inspect its interior.

sperm analysis: A diagnostic test of freshly ejaculated sperm to determine the count, shape, size, and motility.

sphincterotomy (**sfink**-ter-**OT**-oh-mee): An incision into or division of a sphincter muscle.

sphygmomanometer (**sfig**-moh-mah-**NOM**-eh-ter): An instrument used to measure blood pressure.

spina bifida (**SPY**-nah **BIF**-ih-dah): A congenital defect in which the spinal canal fails to close around the spinal cord.

spirochetes (**SPY**-roh-keets): Spiral-shaped bacteria that have flexible walls and are capable of movement.

spirometry (spy-**ROM**-eh-tree): A testing method to record the volume of air inhaled or exhaled and the length of time each breath takes.

splenectomy (splee-**NECK**-toh-mee): Surgical removal of the spleen.

splenitis (splee-**NIGH**-tis): Inflammation of the spleen.

splenomegaly (**splee**-noh-**MEG**-ah-lee): Abnormal enlargement of the spleen.

splenorrhagia (**splee**-noh-**RAY**-jee-ah): Bleeding from the spleen.

splenorrhaphy (splee-**NOR**-ah-fee): To suture the spleen.

spondylitis (**spon**-dih-**LYE**-tis): Inflammation of the vertebrae.

spondylolisthesis (**spon**-dih-loh-liss-**THEE**-sis): Forward movement of the body of one of the lower lumbar vertebra on the vertebra below it or on the sacrum.

spondylosis (**spon**-dih-**LOH**-sis): Any degenerative condition of the vertebrae.

sprain: Injury to a joint such as an ankle, knee, or wrist involving stretched or torn ligaments.

sputum (**SPYOU**-tum): Phlegm that is ejected through the mouth.

staging: The process of classifying tumors with respect to how far the disease has progressed.

stapedectomy (**stay**-peh-**DECK**-toh-mee): Surgical removal of the stapes, which is a bone of the middle ear.

staphylococci (**staf**-ih-loh-**KOCK**-sigh): Bacteria that form irregular groups or clusters.

statins: Medication administered to reduce LDL cholesterol or other lipids in the blood; also known as cholesterol-lowering drugs.

steroids (**STEHR**-oidz): Naturally occurring hormones that help control metabolism, inflammation, immune functions, salt and water balance, development of sexual characteristics, and the ability to withstand illness and injury; artificially produced hormones used as medications to duplicate the action of naturally occurring steroids.

steroids, anabolic: Artificially produced hormones that are chemically related to the male sex hormone testosterone and have been used illegally by athletes to increase strength and muscle mass.

stethoscope (**STETH**-oh-skope): An instrument used to listen to sounds within the body and during the measurement of blood pressure.

stillbirth: A fetus that died before or during delivery.

stoma (**STOH**-mah): An opening on a body surface that can occur naturally or may be created surgically.

strabismus (strah-**BIZ**-mus): A disorder in which the eyes cannot be directed in a parallel manner toward the same object.

strain: Injury to the body of the muscle or attachment of the tendon.

streptococci (**strep**-toh-**KOCK**-sigh): Bacteria that form a chain.

stricture: An abnormal band of tissue narrowing a body passage.

stridor (**STRYE**-dor): An abnormal, high-pitched, harsh or crowing sound heard during inspiration that results from a partial blockage of the pharynx, larynx, and trachea.

stroke: Damage to the brain that occurs when the blood flow to the brain is disrupted because a blood vessel supplying it is either blocked or has ruptured.

stroke, hemorrhagic (**hem**-oh-**RAJ**-ick): Damage to brain tissue caused by the rupture of leaking of a blood vessel within brain; also known as a bleed.

stroke, ischemic: Damage to the brain caused by narrowing or blockage of the carotid artery and the resulting decreased flow of blood to the brain; also known as a cerebrovascular accident.

stupor (**STOO**-per): A state of impaired consciousness marked by a lack of responsiveness to environmental stimuli.

subluxation (**sub**-luck-**SAY**-shun): Partial displacement of a bone from its joint.

sudden infant death syndrome: The unexplainable death of an apparently healthy infant that typically occurs while the infant is sleeping; also known as SIDS or crib death.

supine (**SUE**-pine): Lying on the back with the *face up*; also known as the horizontal recumbent position.

suppuration (**sup**-you-**RAY**-shun): Formation or discharge of pus.

suturing (**SOO**-chur-ing): Closing a wound or incision by stitching or a similar means.

syncope (**SIN**-koh-pee): The brief loss of consciousness caused by brief lack of oxygen in the brain; also known as fainting.

synechia (sigh-NECK-ee-ah): An adhesion that binds the iris to any adjacent structure.

synergism (SIN-er-jizm): An interaction that occurs when the effect of one drug is increased by another drug; also known as potentiation.

synovectomy (sin-oh-VECK-toh-mee): Surgical removal of a synovial membrane from a joint.

synovitis (sin-oh-VYE-tiss): Inflammation of the synovial membrane that results in swelling and pain.

syphilis (SIF-ih-lis): A highly contagious sexually transmitted disease caused by the spirochete *Treponema pallidum*.

T

tachycardia (**tack**-ee-KAR-dee-ah): An abnormally fast heartbeat.

tachypnea (**tack**-ihp-NEE-ah): An abnormally rapid rate of respiration usually of more than 20 breaths per minute.

talipes (**TAL**-ih-peez): Congenital deformity in which the foot may be turned outward or inward; also known as a clubfoot.

tardive dyskinesia (**TAHR**-div **dis**-kih-NEE-zee-ah): Late appearance of dyskinesia as a side effect of long-term treatment with certain antipsychotic drugs.

tarsectomy (tahr-SECK-toh-mee): Surgical removal of a segment of the tarsal plate of the upper or lower eyelid.

tarsorrhaphy (tahr-SOR-ah-fee): Partially or completely suturing together the upper and lower eyelids to provide protection to the eye when the lids are paralyzed and unable to close normally.

Tay-Sachs disease: A hereditary disease marked by progressive physical degeneration, mental retardation, and early death.

teletherapy (tel-eh-THER-ah-pee): Radiation therapy administered at a distance from the body.

temporomandibular disorders (**tem**-poh-roh-man-DIB-you-lar): A group of complex symptoms related to the malfunctioning of the temporomandibular joint; also known as myofascial pain dysfunction.

tenalgia (ten-AL-jee-ah): Pain in a tendon; also known as tenodynia.

tendinitis (**ten**-dih-NIGH-tis): Inflammation of the tendons caused by excessive or unusual use of the joint; is also known as tendonitis.

tendonitis (ten-doh-NIGH-it is): See tendinitis.

tendoplasty: Surgical repair of a tendon; also known as tenoplasty.

tendotomy: Surgical division of a tendon for relief of a deformity; also known as tenotomy.

tenectomy (teh-NECK-toh-mee): Surgical removal of a lesion from a tendon or tendon sheath.

tenodesis (ten-ODD-eh-sis): To suture the end of a tendon to bone.

tenodynia (**ten**-oh-DIN-ee-ah): Pain in a tendon; also known as tenalgia.

tenolysis (ten-OL-ih-sis): To free a tendon from adhesions.

tenonectomy (**ten**-oh-NECK-toh-mee): Surgical removal of part of a tendon for the purpose of shortening it.

tenoplasty (**TEN**-oh-**plas**-tee): Surgical repair of a tendon; also known as tendoplasty.

tenorrhaphy (ten-OR-ah-fee): Suturing of a divided tendon.

tenotomy (teh-NOT-oh-mee): Surgical division of a tendon for relief of a deformity; also known as tendotomy.

testectomy: Surgical removal of one or both testicles; also known as an orchiectomy.

testicular self-examination: An important self-help step in early detection of testicular cancer.

testitis (test-TYE-tis): Inflammation of one or both testicles; also known as orchitis.

tetanus (TET-ah-nus): An acute and potentially fatal bacterial infection of the central nervous system caused by the tetanus bacillus.

tetany (TET-ah-nee): An abnormal condition characterized by periodic painful muscle spasms and tremors.

thalamotomy (**thal**-ah-MOT-oh-mee): A surgical incision into the thalamus to quiet the tremors of Parkinson's disease, to treat some psychotic disorders, or to stop intractable pain.

thalassemia (thal-ah-SEE-mee-ah): A group of genetic disorders characterized by short-lived red blood cells that lack the normal ability to produce hemoglobin; also known as Cooley's anemia.

thoracentesis (**thoh**-rah-sen-TEE-sis): Puncture of the chest wall with a needle to obtain fluid from the pleural cavity for diagnostic purposes, to drain pleural effusions, or to reexpand a collapsed lung.

thoracostomy (**thoh**-rah-KOS-toh-mee): Surgical creation of an opening into the chest.

thoracotomy (**thoh**-rah-KOT-toh-mee): A surgical incision into the wall of the chest.

thrombocytopenia (**throm**-boh-**sigh**-toh-PEE-nee-ah): An abnormal decrease in the number of platelets; also known as thrombopenia.

thrombolytic (**throm**-boh-LIT-ick): Medication administered to slow blood clotting and to prevent new clots from forming; also known as an anticoagulant.

thrombopenia: An abnormal decrease in the number of platelets; also known as thrombocytopenia.

thrombosis (throm-BOH-sis): An abnormal condition in which a thrombus develops within a blood vessel.

thrombotic occlusion (throm-BOT-ick ah-KLOO-zhun): Blocking of an artery by a clot.

thrombus (THROM-bus): A blood clot attached to the interior wall of a vein or artery.

thymectomy (thigh-MECK-toh-mee): Surgical removal of the thymus gland.

thymitis (thigh-MY-tis): Inflammation of the thymus gland.

thymoma (thigh-MOH-mah): A benign tumor originating in the thymus.

thymopathy (thigh-MOP-ah-thee): Any disease of the thymus gland.

thyroidectomy, chemical: The administration of radioactive iodine to suppress the function of the thyroid; also known as radioactive iodine therapy.

thyroiditis (thigh-roi-**DYE**-tis): Inflammation of the thyroid gland.

thyroidotomy (thigh-roi-**DOT**-oh-mee): Surgical incision into the thyroid gland.

thyroid-stimulating hormone assay: A laboratory test that measures circulating blood levels of thyroid-stimulating hormone.

thyromegaly (**thigh**-roh-**MEG**-ah-lee): An abnormal enlargement of the thyroid gland that produces a swelling in the front part of the neck; also known as goiter.

thyrotoxicosis (**thy**-roh-**tock**-sih-**KOH**-sis): A life-threatening condition resulting from the presence of excessive quantities of the thyroid hormones; also known as thyroid storm.

tic douloureux (**TICK** doo-loo-**ROO**): Inflammation of the trigeminal nerve that is characterized by sudden, intense, sharp pain on one side of the face; also known as trigeminal neuralgia.

tinea (**TIN**-ee-ah): A fungus skin disease affecting different areas of the body; also known as ringworm.

tinea capitis: A fungal infection found on the scalps of children;

tinea cruris: A fungal infection of the genital area; also known as jock itch.

tinea pedis: A fungal infection found between the toes and on the feet; also known as athlete's foot.

tinnitus (tih-**NIGH**-tus): A ringing, buzzing, or roaring sound in the ears.

tissue plasminogen activator (**TISH**-you plaz-**MIN**-oh-jen **ACK**-tih-**vay**-tor): A clot dissolving enzyme used for the immediate treatment of heart attack victims.

tonometry (toh-**NOM**-eh-tree): A test that measures intraocular pressure (IOP).

tonsillectomy (**ton**-sih-**LECK**-toh-mee): Surgical removal of the tonsils.

tonsillitis (**ton**-sih-**LYE**-tis): Inflammation of the tonsils.

total hemoglobin: A laboratory test that measures the amount of hemoglobin found in whole blood.

toxemia of pregnancy: A complication of pregnancy characterized by hypertension, edema, and proteinuria; also known as preeclampsia.

tracheitis (**tray**-kee-**EYE**-tis): Inflammation of the trachea.

tracheobronchoscopy (**tray**-kee-oh-brong-**KOS**-koh-pee): Inspection of both the trachea and bronchi through a bronchoscope.

tracheoplasty (**TRAY**-kee-oh-**plas**-tee): Surgical repair of the trachea.

tracheorrhagia (**tray**-kee-oh-**RAY**-jee-ah): Bleeding from the trachea.

tracheorrhaphy (**tray**-kee-**OR**-ah-fee): Suturing of the trachea.

tracheostenosis (**tray**-kee-oh-steh-**NOH**-sis): Abnormal narrowing of the lumen of the trachea.

tracheostomy (**tray**-kee-**OS**-toh-mee): Creating an opening into the trachea and inserting a tube to facilitate the passage of air or the removal of secretions.

tracheotomy (**tray**-kee-**OT**-oh-mee): An emergency procedure in which an incision is made into the trachea to gain access to the airway below a blockage.

tranquilizers: Medication administered to suppress anxiety and relax muscles; also known as antianxiety drugs.

transcutaneous electronic nerve stimulation: A method of pain control by the application of electronic impulses to the nerve endings through the skin.

transesophageal echocardiography (**trans**-eh-**sof**-ah-**JEE**-al **eck**-oh-**kar**-dee-**OG**-rah-fee): An ultrasonic procedure that images the heart from inside the esophagus.

transient ischemic attack (iss-**KEE**-mick): The temporary interruption in the blood supply to the brain that may be a warning of an impending stroke.

transmyocardial revascularization: A surgical procedure using a laser performed to provide more blood to the oxygen-deprived heart muscle; also known as transmyocardial laser revascularization.

transurethral resection of the prostate: Surgical removal of all or part of the prostate gland through the urethra; also known as a prostatectomy.

trauma (**TRAW**-mah): Wound or injury.

Trendelenburg position: Lying on the back with the knees bent and the legs elevated slightly higher than the head.

triage (tree-**AHZH**): Medical screening of patients to determine their relative priority of need and the proper place of treatment.

trichomonas (**trick**-oh-**MOH**-nas): A vaginal inflammation caused by the protozoan parasite *Trichomonas vaginalis*.

tricuspid stenosis: Abnormal narrowing of the opening of the tricuspid valve.

trigeminal neuralgia: Inflammation of the trigeminal nerve that is characterized by sudden, intense, sharp pain on one side of the face; also known as tic douloureux.

triglycerides (try-**GLIS**-er-eyeds): Combinations of fatty acids attached to glycerol that are also found normally in the blood in limited quantities.

tubal ligation: A surgical procedure performed for purpose of female sterilization.

tuberculin skin testing: A screening test to detect tuberculosis.

tuberculosis (too-**ber**-kew-**LOH**-sis): An infectious disease caused by *Mycobacterium tuberculosis* that usually attacks the lungs.

twins, fraternal: Two embryos resulting from the fertilization of separate ova by separate sperm cells.

twins, identical: Two embryos resulting from the fertilization of a single egg cell by a single sperm that has separated into two separate parts.

tympanectomy (**tim**-pah-**NECK**-toh-me): Surgical removal of all or part of the tympanic membrane; also known as a myringectomy.

tympanocentesis (**tim**-pah-noh-sen-**TEE**-sis): Surgical puncture of the tympanic membrane to remove fluid from the middle ear.

tympanometry (**tim**-pah-**NOM**-eh-tree): An indirect measurement of acoustical energy absorbed or reflected by the middle ear.

tympanoplasty (**tim**-pah-noh-**PLAS**-tee): Surgical correction of a damaged middle ear.

tympanostomy tubes (**tim**-pan-**OSS**-toh-mee): Tiny ventilating tubes placed through the eardrum to provide ongoing drainage for fluids and to relieve pressure that can build up after ear infections.

typhoid fever: An intestinal infection caused by *Salmonella typhi*; also known as enteric fever.

U

ulcer (**UL**-ser): An open sore or erosion of the skin or mucous membrane resulting in tissue loss and usually with inflammation.

ulcer, decubitus: An ulcerated area caused by prolonged pressure that cuts off circulation to a body part; also known as a pressure ulcer or bedsore.

ultrasonography (**ul**-trah-son-**OG**-rah-fee): The imaging of deep body structures by recording the echoes of pulses of sound waves above the range of human hearing; also known as diagnostic ultrasound.

uremia (you-**REE**-mee-ah): A toxic condition caused by excessive amount of urea and other waste products in the bloodstream; also known as uremic poisoning.

ureterectasis (you-**ree**-ter-**ECK**-tah-sis): Distention of a ureter.

ureterectomy (**you**-ree-ter-**ECK**-toh-mee): Surgical removal of a ureter.

ureterolith (you-**REE**-ter-oh-**lith**): Presence of stones in a ureter.

ureterolysis (you-**ree**-ter-**OL**-ih-sis): Procedure to separate adhesions around a ureter.

ureteroplasty (you-**REE**-ter-oh-**plas**-tee): Surgical repair of a ureter.

ureterorrhagia (you-**ree**-ter-oh-**RAY**-jee-ah): Bleeding from the ureter.

ureterorrhaphy (**you**-ree-ter-**OR**-ah-fee): To suture a ureter.

ureterostenosis (you-**ree**-ter-oh-steh-**NOH**-sis): A stricture of the ureter.

urethralgia (**you**-ree-**THRAL**-jee-ah): Pain in the urethra.

urethritis (**you**-reh-**THRIGH**-tis): Inflammation of the urethra.

urethrocele (you-**REE**-throh-seel): Hernia in the urethral wall.

urethropexy (you-**REE**-throh-**peck**-see): Surgical fixation of the urethra usually for the correction of urinary stress incontinence.

urethroplasty (you-**REE**-throh-**plas**-tee): Surgical repair of the urethra.

urethrorrhagia (you-**ree**-throh-**RAY**-jee-ah): Bleeding from the urethra.

urethrorrhea (you-**ree**-throh-**REE**-ah): An abnormal discharge from the urethra.

urethrostenosis (you-**ree**-throh-steh-**NOH**-sis): A stricture of the urethra.

urethrostomy (you-reh-**THROS**-toh-mee): Surgical creation of a permanent opening between the urethra and the skin.

urethrotomy (**you**-reh-**THROT**-oh-mee): A surgical incision into the urethra for relief of a stricture.

urinalysis (**you**-rih-**NAL**-ih-sis): Laboratory examination of the physical and chemical properties of urine to determine the presence of abnormal elements.

urography, excretory: A radiographic examination that traces the action of the kidney as it processes and excretes dye injected into the bloodstream.

urography, retrograde: A radiographic examination of the urinary system taken after dye has been placed in the urethra through a sterile catheter and caused to flow upward through the urinary tract.

urologist (you-**ROL**-oh-jist): A specialist in diagnosing and treating diseases and disorders of the urinary system of females and the genitourinary system of males.

urology (you-**ROL**-oh-jee): The study of the urinary system.

urticaria (**ur**-tih-**KAR**-ree-ah): A skin condition characterized by localized areas of swelling accompanied by itching that is associated with an allergic reaction; also known as hives.

uveitis (you-vee-**EYE**-tis): Inflammation anywhere in the uveal tract.

V

vaginal candidiasis (**kan**-dih-**DYE**-ah-sis): A vaginal yeast infection caused by *Candida albicans*.

vaginitis (**vaj**-ih-**NIGH**-tis): Inflammation of the lining of the vagina; also known as colpitis.

vaginocele (**VAJ**-ih-noh-seel): Hernia protruding into the vagina; prolapse or falling down of the vagina.

vaginodynia (vaj-ih-noh-**DIN**-ee-ah): Pain in the vagina.

vaginoplasty (vah-**JIGH**-noh-**plas**-tee): Surgical repair of the vagina.

vaginosis, bacterial: A sexually transmitted bacterial infection of the vagina.

valvoplasty (**VAL**-voh-**plas**-tee): Surgical repair or replacement of a heart valve; also known as valvuloplasty.

valvulitis (val-view-**LYE**-tis): Inflammation of a heart valve.

valvuloplasty (**VAL**-view-loh-plas-tee). Surgical repair or replacement of a heart valve; also known as valvoplasty.

varicocele (**VAR**-ih-koh-**seel**): A varicose vein of the testicles that may cause male infertility.

varicocelectomy (**var**-ih-koh-sih-**LECK**-toh-mee): Surgical removal of a portion of an enlarged vein to relieve a varicocele.

varicose veins (**VAR**-ih-kohs **VAYNS**): Abnormally swollen veins.

vasculitis (**vas**-kyou-**LYE**-tis): Inflammation of a blood or lymph vessel; also known as angiitis.

vasectomy (vah-**SECK**-toh-mee): A male sterilization procedure in which a portion of the vas deferens is surgically removed.

vasoconstrictor (**vas**-oh-kon-**STRICK**-tor): Medication that constricts (narrows) the blood vessels.

vasodilator (**vas**-oh-dye-**LAYT**-or): Medication that dilates (expands) the blood vessels.

vasovasostomy (**vas**-oh-vah-**ZOS**-toh-mee *or* **vay**-zoh-vay-**ZOS**-toh-mee): A procedure to restore fertility to a vasectomized male.

venereal diseases (veh-**NEER**-ee-ahl): Diseases transmitted through sexual intercourse or other genital contact; also known as sexually transmitted diseases.

venipuncture (**VEN**-ih-**punk**-tyour): The puncture of a vein for the purpose of drawing blood; also known as phlebotomy.

verrucae (veh-**ROO**-see): Skin lesions caused by the human papilloma virus; also known as warts.

vertigo (**VER**-tih-goh): A sense of whirling, dizziness, and the loss of balance.

vesicle (**VES**-ih-kul): A circumscribed elevation of skin containing fluid that is *less than* 0.5 cm in diameter; also known as a blister.

vesicovaginal fissure (ves-ih-koh-**VAG**-ih-nahl): An abnormal opening between the bladder and vagina.

viral (**VYE**-ral): Pertaining to a virus.

virile (**VIR**-ill): Possessing masculine traits.

viruses (**VYE**-rus-ez): Very small infectious agents that live only by invading cells.

visual acuity: The ability to distinguish object details and shape at a distance.

visual acuity measurement (ah-**KYOU**-ih-tee): An evaluation of the eye's ability to distinguish object details and shape.

visual field test: A diagnostic test to determine losses in peripheral vision.

vitiligo (vit-ih-**LYE**-goh): A condition in which a loss of melanocytes results in whitish areas of skin bordered by normally pigmented areas.

volvulus (**VOL**-view-lus): Twisting of the intestine on itself that causes an obstruction.

vulvitis (vul-**VYE**-tis): Inflammation of the vulva.

vulvodynia (vul-voh-**DIN**-ee-ah): A nonspecific syndrome of unknown cause characterized by chronic burning, pain during sexual intercourse, itching, or stinging irritation of the vulva.

vulvovaginitis (vul-voh-**vaj**-ih-**NIGH**-tis): Inflammation of the vulva and the vagina.

W

Western blot test: A blood test to confirm the diagnosis of HIV positive.

wheal (**WHEEL**): A smooth, *slightly elevated*, swollen area that is redder or paler than the surrounding skin that is usually accompanied by itching.

white blood cell differential: A laboratory test to determine what percentage of the total white blood cell count is composed of each of the five types of leukocytes.

white blood count: A laboratory test to determine the number of leukocytes in the blood.

X

xeroderma (zee-roh-**DER**-mah): Excessively dry skin.

xerophthalmia (**zeer**-ahf-**THAL**-mee-ah): Drying of eye surfaces characterized by the loss of luster of the conjunctiva and cornea.

Index

Page numbers in **boldface** indicate tables.

surgery on, 61
types of, 47
Juvenile
diabetes, 283
rheumatoid arthritis, 56

K
Kaposi's sarcoma, 133
Keloid, 262
Keratitis, 237
Keratoplasty, 240
Keratosis, 262
Ketones, 328
Ketonuria, 328
Keyhole bypass, 112
Kidneys, **186**
diseases, diabetes and, 284
failure, 190
pathology of, 191
stones, removal of, 195
treatment of, 195–196
urinary system and, 188–189
Kinesiology, 75
Kleptomania, 221
Knee–chest position, 326
Knees, 54
ligaments of, **48**
replacement of, 61
Koilonychia, 258
Koplik's spots, 130
KS, 133
KUB, 193
Kyphosis, 57

L
Labia, 166
majora, 300
minora, 300
Labor, 310
Labor and delivery, 310
Laboratory tests, **321**, 327–329
Labyrinth, 242
Labyrinthectomy, 244
Labyrinthitis, 243
Labyrinthotomy, 244
Laceration, 12, 260, 313
Lacrimal
apparatus, **230**, 233–234
bones, 51
canaliculi, 234
duct, 234
fluid, 233–234
glands, 233–234
sac, 234
Lacrimation, 234
Lactation, 311
Lacteals, 123
Lactiferous
duct, 300
glands, 300
Lactogenic hormone, **277**, 279
Lamina, 52
Laminectomy, 62
Laparoscopic
adrenalectomy, 282

cholecystectomy, 179
Laparoscopy, 25
Lap choley, 179
Large intestine, 172
digestive system and, **164**, 169–170
Laryngectomy, 155
Laryngitis, 151
Laryngopharynx, 146
Laryngoplasty, 155
Laryngoplegia, 151
Laryngoscope, 154
Laryngoscopy, 154
Laryngospasm, 151
Larynx, **142**, 146
pathology of, 151
Laser, 265
iridotomy, 241
trabeculoplasty, 241
Last menstrual period, 310
Lateral, **23**
epicondylitis, 84
projection, 332
Laxatives, 177
LDL, 108
LE, **129**, 261
Left, lung, 147
Left hemisphere, 210
Legal blindness, 240
Legs, 53–54
lower, 54
Leiomyoma, 304
Lens, **230**, 235
Lensectomy, 240
Lesion, 12, 258
Lesions
fluid-filled, 259, **260**
surface, 258–259
through the skin, 260
Lethargy, 216
Leukemia, 109
Leukocytes, **4**, 104
Leukopenia, 109
Leukorrhea, 304
Levator, 76
Level of consciousness, 221
LH, **277**, 279
Lice, 262
Lid lift, 266
Ligaments, 43, 47
Ligation, 12
Lipectomy, 266
Lipedema, 261
Lipid
panel, 328
tests, 328
Lipocytes, 256
Lipoma, 262
Lipoproteins, 108
blood levels, **109**
Liposuction, 266
Lips, 166
Liquid connective tissue, 28
Lithotomy, **8**, 196
position, 326–327

NOTES

NOTES

NOTES

NOTES

Flash Cards

Carefully remove the flash card pages from the book and cut them apart to create 160 flash cards.

There are three types of cards: **prefixes** (such as a- and hyper-), **suffixes** (such as -graphy and -rrhagia), and **word roots / combining forms** (such as gastr/o and arthr/o). For the prefixes and suffixes, the type of word part is listed on the front on each card. The definition is on the back.

The word root cards are arranged by body system. This allows you to sort out the cards you want to study based on where you are in the book. Use the "general" cards as they apply throughout your course.

Use the flash cards to memorize word parts, to test yourself, and as a periodic review.

By putting cards together, you can create terms just as you have done in the challenge word building exercises.

Word Part Games

These are games you can play with one or more partners to help you learn word parts using your flash cards.

The Review Game

Word Parts Up. Shuffle the deck of flash cards. Put the deck, *word parts up*, in the center of the desk. Take turns choosing a card from anywhere in the deck and giving the definition of the word part shown. If you get it right, you get to keep it. If you miss, it goes into the discard pile. When the draw pile is gone, whoever has the largest pile wins.

Definitions Up. Shuffle the deck of flash cards and place them with the *definition side up*. Play the review game the same way.

The Create-a-Word Game

Shuffle the deck and deal each person 14 cards, *word parts up*. Place the remaining draw pile in the center of the desk, *word parts down*.

Each player should try to create as many legitimate medical words as possible using the cards they've been dealt. Then take turns discarding one card (word part up, in the discard pile) and taking one. When it is your turn to discard a card, you may choose either the card the previous player has discarded, or a "mystery card" from the draw pile. Continue working on words until all the cards in the draw pile have been taken.

To score, each player must define every word created correctly. If the definition is correct, the player receives one point for each card used. If it is incorrect, two points are deducted for each card in that word. Cards left unused each count as one point off. Whoever has the highest number of points wins. *Note:* use your medical dictionary if there is any doubt that a word is legitimate!

prefix

A-, AN-

prefix

END-, ENDO-

prefix

ANTE-

prefix

HEMI-

prefix

ANTI-

prefix

HYPER-

prefix

BRADY-

prefix

HYPO-

prefix

DYS-

prefix

INTER-

within, in, inside

without, away from, negative, not

half

before, toward

excessive, increased

against, counter

deficient, decreased

slow

between, among

bad, difficult, painful

prefix

INTRA-

prefix

NEO-

prefix

PER-

prefix

PERI-

prefix

POLY-

prefix

POST-

prefix

PRE-

prefix

SUB-

prefix

SUPER-, SUPRA-

prefix

TACHY-

after	within, inside
before	new, strange
below	excessive, through
above, excessive	surrounding, around
fast, rapid	many

suffix

suffix

-AC-AL

-CYTE

suffix

suffix

-ALGIA

-DESIS

suffix

suffix

-ARY

-ECTOMY

suffix

suffix

-CELE

-ECTASIS

suffix

suffix

-CENTESIS

-EMIA

cell

pertaining to, relating to

surgical fixation of bone or joint,
to bind, tie together

pain, suffering

surgical removal

pertaining to

stretching, enlargement

hernia, tumor, swelling

blood, blood condition

surgical puncture to remove fluid

suffix

-ESTHESIA

suffix

-ITIS

suffix

-GRAM, -GRAPH

suffix

-LYSIS

suffix

-GRAPHY

suffix

-MALACIA

suffix

-IA

suffix

-MEGALY

suffix

-IC

suffix

-NECROSIS

inflammation	sensation, feeling
breakdown, separation, setting free, destruction, loosening	record
abnormal softening	process of recording
enlargement	state or condition
tissue death	pertaining to

suffix

-OLOGIST

suffix

-OTOMY

suffix

-OLOGY

suffix

-PATHY

suffix

-OMA

suffix

-PAUSE

suffix

-OSIS

suffix

-PEXY

suffix

-OSTOMY

suffix

-PLASTY

surgical incision

specialist

disease, suffering, feeling, emotion

the science or study of

stopping

tumor

surgical fixation, to put in place

abnormal condition

surgical repair

surgical creation of an opening

suffix

-PLEGIA

suffix

-PNEA

suffix

-PTOSIS

suffix

-RRHAGIA, -RRHAGE

suffix

-RRHAPHY

suffix

-RRHEA

suffix

-RRHEXIS

suffix

-SCLEROSIS

suffix

-SCOPE

suffix

-SCOPY

abnormal flow or discharge	paralysis
rupture	breathing
abnormal hardening	prolapse, drooping forward
instrument for visual examination	bleeding, abnormal excessive fluid discharge
to see, visual examination	to suture

-STENOSIS

ARTER/O, ARTERI/O

-TRIPSY

ATHER/O

-URIA

CARD/O, CARDI/O

ANGI/O

HEM/O, HEMAT/O

AORT/O

PHLEB/O

artery

abnormal narrowing

plaque, fatty substance

to crush

heart

urination, urine

blood, pertaining to the blood

pertaining to blood or lymph vessels

vein

aorta

Cardiovascular System	Digestive System
THROMB/O	**COL/O, COLON/O**
Cardiovascular System	Digestive System
VEN/O	**DUODEN/I, DUODEN/O**
Diagnostic Procedures	Digestive System
ECH/O	**ENTER/O**
Diagnostic Procedures	Digestive System
RADI/O	**ESOPHAG/O**
Digestive System	Digestive System
CHOLECYST/O	**GASTR/O**

colon, large intestine	clot
duodenum	vein
small intestine	sound
esophagus	radiation, x-rays
stomach	gallbladder

Digestive System

HEPAT/O

Endocrine System

THYR/O, THYROID/O

Digestive System

SIGMOID/O

General

ADIP/O

Endocrine System

ADREN/O, ADRENAL/O

General

ALBIN/O

Endocrine System
Reproductive Systems

GONAD/O

General

CEPHAL/O

Endocrine System
Digestive System

PANCREAT/O

General

CERVIC/O

shield, thyroid gland

liver

fat

sigmoid colon

white

adrenal glands

head

sex gland

neck, cervix (neck of uterus)

pancreas

CORON/O

LAPAR/O

CYAN/O

LEUK/O

CYT/O

LIP/O

ERYTHR/O

MELAN/O

HIST/O

MYC/O

abdomen, abdominal wall

coronary, crown

white

blue

fat, lipid

cell

black, dark

red

fungus

tissue

General

PATH/O

Immune System

ONC/O

General

PY/O

Integumentary System

CUTANE/O

General

PYR/O

Integumentary System

DERM/O, DERMAT/O

General

SARC/O

Integumentary System

HIDR/O

Immune System

CARCIN/O

Integumentary System

SEB/O

tumor

disease, suffering, feeling, emotion

skin

pus

skin

fever, fire

sweat

flesh (connective tissue)

sebum

cancerous

Integumentary System	Muscular System
UNGU/O	**MY/O**

Integumentary System	Muscular System
XER/O	**TEN/O, TEND/O, TENDIN/O**

Lymphatic System	Nervous System
ADEN/O	**ENCEPHAL/O**

Lymphatic System	Nervous System
SPLEN/O	**MENING/O**

Muscular System	Nervous System
FASCI/O	**NEUR/I, NEUR/O**

muscle

nail

tendon, stretch out, extend, strain

dry

brain

gland

membranes, meninges

spleen

nerve, nerve tissue

fascia, fibrous band

COLP/O

OOPHOR/O, OVARI/O

HYSTER/O

ORCH/O, ORCHI/O, ORCHID/O

MEN/O

SALPING/O

METR/O, METRI/O

UTER/O

OO/O, OV/I, OV/O

VAGIN/O

ovary

vagina

testicles, testis, testes

uterus

uterine (fallopian) tube,
auditory (eustachian) tube

menstruation, menses

uterus

uterus

vagina

egg

Respiratory System

Respiratory System

BRONCH/O, BRONCHI/O

PULM/O, PULMON/O

Respiratory System

Respiratory System

LARYNG/O

TRACHE/O

Respiratory System

Skeletal System

PHARYNG/O

ANKLY/O

Respiratory System

Skeletal System

PLEUR/O

ARTHR/O

Respiratory System

Skeletal System

PNEUM/O, PNEUMON/O

CHONDR/O

lung

bronchial tube, bronchus

trachea, windpipe

larynx, voice box

crooked, bent, stiff

throat, pharynx

joint

pleura, side of the body

cartilage

lung, air

Skeletal System

COST/O

Skeletal System
Respiratory System

THORAC/O

Skeletal System

CRANI/O

Special Senses
Integumentary System

KERAT/O

Skeletal System
Nervous System

MYEL/O

Special Senses

MYRING/O

Skeletal System

OSS/E, OSS/I, OST/O, OSTE/O

Special Senses

OPTIC/O, OPT/O

Skeletal System

SPONDYL/O

Special Senses

OT/O

chest

rib

horny, hard, cornea

skull

tympanic membrane, eardrum

spinal cord, bone marrow

eye, vision

bone

ear, hearing

vertebrae, vertebral column, back bone

Special Senses	Urinary System
RETIN/O	**NEPHR/O**
Special Senses Integumentary System	Urinary System
SCLER/O	**PYEL/O**
Special Senses	Urinary System
TYMPAN/O	**REN/O**
Urinary System	Urinary System
CYST/O	**URETER/O**
Urinary System Digestive System	Urinary System
LITH/O	**URETHR/O**

kidney

retina

renal pelvis, bowl of kidney

sclera, white of eye, hard

kidney

tympanic membrane, eardrum

ureter

urinary bladder, cyst, sac of fluid

urethra

stone, calculus